Colin Griffith MCH, RSHom is a highly respected and effective practitioner. He studied at the College of Homoeopathy and, instead of writing a thesis, he set up a supervised drop-in clinic which continued for eleven years and became a teaching clinic where students under his supervision set up their own tables. He has always preferred to work in multi-disciplinary practice where other complementary therapies are offered: cranial osteopathy, reflexology, counselling etc. He is a founder member of the Guild of Homoeopaths; he lectures regularly at the Centre for Homoeopathic Education, Regent's College, London and has lectured in America, Canada, Japan and Greece.

To my mother, who cared passionately about homoeopathy
and always wanted to know more

THE COMPANION TO
HOMEOPATHY

THE PRACTITIONER'S GUIDE

COLIN GRIFFITH

WATKINS PUBLISHING

LONDON

Distributed in the USA and Canada by
Sterling Publishing Co., Inc.
387 Park Avenue South, New York, NY 10016-8810

First published in the UK and USA in 2005 by
Watkins Publishing, Sixth Floor, Castle House,
75–76 Wells Street, London W1T 3QH

This edition published in paperback in 2010

1 3 5 7 9 10 8 6 4 2

Designed and typeset by Jerry Goldie and Westkey

Printed and bound in China by Imago

Library of Congress Cataloging-in-Publication Data Available

ISBN: 978-1-906787-72-1

www.watkinspublishing.co.uk

For information about custom editions, special sales, premium
and corporate purchases, please contact Sterling Special Sales
Department at 800-805-5489 or specialsales@sterlingpub.com

CONTENTS

PART 3 THE HIERARCHY OF THE MIASMS

ACKNOWLEDGEMENTS

For some seven years my wife, Sofi, has endured the writing of this book. She has had to put up with the moods, the late meals, the postponed shopping trips, the forgotten chores and a host of other things that have gone on in the house – or not. She has had to read passages late at night because I wanted a trustworthy critique NOW! Though her patience has worn thin on occasion, her loving support and enthusiasm have been unstinting from the first. I could not have contemplated writing a book on homoeopathy without her.

Nor could I have written anything without my four children – Richard, Nicholas, Bella and Rafa – who were not much help in a practical sense, but who make Sofi's and my life so worthwhile. They have grown up with homoeopathy not only in the house but also as a means of remaining well and happy. I have watched as homoeopathic remedies have healed their troubles, great and small, and have brought out in them facets of their character that are imbued with a strength that, had we remained in ignorance of the gift of homoeopathy, might not have come to light. All four children, so different from each other, have afforded me more lessons in life than it seems I can ever have taught them.

My heartfelt thanks are due to Janice Micallef, our family homoeopath, who has inspired so much love, trust and faith in her patients. Heaven knows where we'd be without her and only she knows how many remedies she gave me just to get me through all these pages; though the research in books and on the internet was fascinating, collating the cases and then writing them up often made me feel that I was reliving each one. (When you reach the section on the miasms you will see why!) Janice was careful to follow my progress throughout. Just as people start scratching when someone mentions the words 'nit' or 'flea' so students of homoeopathy temporarily take on the characteristics of what they study.

I have to thank Janice too, for giving me what insight I have into Karma and its significance. By her patient exposition of what she was given to see of the progress of three generations of my family, I came to understand that medicine and health remain limited concepts if no account is taken of the past and the future

It was Janice, too, who set up the meditation group which eventually formed the basis of the Guild of Homoeopaths. I must thank all my friends in this group – Martin Miles, Terry Howard, Jill Wright, Sylvia Treacher, Diane Pitman, Maureen Rose, Jill Ward and the late but much loved Fred Harker – who were such a fantastic support network. For over ten years this group met regularly to practise meditation and to experience new remedies, many of which have become invaluable in clinic. The Guild of Homoeopaths, a brainchild of my mother's as much as of the group's, was founded in 1996. It was formed to disseminate the practical knowledge not just of using new remedies but also of a wide range of prescribing techniques and styles: it became akin to a homoeopathic *atelier*, an artist's workshop for homoeopaths. Had I not been involved in the Guild there would have been little inspiration to write this book.

Thanks are due to my colleagues, the craniosacral osteopaths who have taught me so much more about healing and the functioning of the human body than I ever learnt at college or would have picked up through practical experience on my own: Mary Patton, Maria Fenocchi, Lizzie Spring, Phillip Williamson, Ivo van Gils and Jean Draisey have all given me so much of their valuable time in explaining their view of just how the body works as an integrated whole. We might learn about holism during our training but it is not until we witness, 'hands on', just how perfectly and harmoniously it functions that we realise the power of the body's will to self-heal.

From my student days, I am indebted to Kate Diamantopolou for kick-starting me into practice. An extraordinarily skilled practitioner with a no-nonsense manner, she was the woman who first made clear to me the vital importance of considering miasmatic history from the beginning of every case. No less should I acknowledge Robert Davidson whose particular and provocative talent for drawing out the hidden intuition in any half-willing novice built my self-confidence and provided exactly what was needed to cope on a daily basis with the exigencies of a full diary.

For enthusing me about the whole subject of dentistry in homoeopathy I am very grateful to my colleague Kyriakos Hajikakou whose diligence in his own enquiries into the subject has been so enlightening.

What would any homoeopaths do without having reference to the prescribing giants of the past who left us such a rich legacy of literature? No student of homoeopathy has done his homework unless he has read all (well, nearly all) that Samuel Hahnemann wrote or that James Tyler Kent wrote. The dictionary of Dr James Clarke and the little volumes of practical experience written by James Compton Burnett are books that should be among the first to be rescued from a burning building. Dr Dorothy Shepherd's accounts of her work in practice are concise masterpieces of simplicity that both fascinate and entertain. Were all these people with us today I should sit happily at their feet, listening – or rather observing – as they would not have had time to talk.

Two people from the world of books must be mentioned; without their invaluable support and help this book would never have made it into print at all. Fiona Spencer-Thomas, both literary agent and qualified homoeo-path, has proven herself to be something of a crusader for homoeopathy. Her unstinting enthusiasm has kept me buoyed up throughout the publish-ing process and I cannot imagine anyone else being able to convince me that I should write another book! Victoria Eldon must also know how grateful I am as she was the first to read a draft copy of my early efforts; her scribblings in the margin and crossings-out on the page taught me in double quick time to concentrate on essentials.

Finally, I have to acknowledge the contribution made by my patients. I have learnt from every one of them. The basis of a secure practice of homoeopathy is the exchange of energy between patient and practitioner. While there are those who do not want medicine to be on this level, my patients for the most part have worked hard at creating their own progress. They show me even more about the tools of my trade, the remedies, about prescribing strategies, and the creative side of my work. A profound 'thank you' to them all.

PREFACE

Some time ago now, while I was a first-year student of the College of Homoeopathy, my neighbour, Mrs D, came up the field in distress to ask for help with her geriatric tomcat. This brute was no favourite of ours as it had a long history of rape and pillage; those days were clearly over now and it was in need of all the help it could get. Mrs D explained that for some while the cat had been sneezing violently and was breathing with increasing difficulty. She had consulted the vet who had diagnosed cancer of the throat and had given a damning prognosis. He had advised that with such a large growth on the wall of the pharynx, the animal had only days to live and that it would be kinder to put it out of its misery. He had offered to come back on the following day when she had had time to decide what she wanted to do. Mrs D went on to comment on how thin the cat now was and, though she did not like to speak ill of the dying, how bad tempered it was. Was there anything I could do? I had no idea but said that I would do some searching in my books to see what might turn up.

I looked up the 'throat' chapter in the homoeopathic repertory, the book of symptoms, and found the rubric: 'cancerous'. Listed were just three remedies, none of which I knew anything about. Nevertheless, I looked them up in the *Materia Medica*, the descriptive book of medicines, and found that only one covered the symptoms suffered by the cat. The remedy was *Carbo Animalis* (which is made from the charred remains of burnt oxhide). Mrs D gave her cat a daily dose of the remedy in a very low potency (the 6th) for several weeks. Such was the efficacy of this remedy that the cat died of old age some two years later.

This story illustrates the point that one does not need faith in either the remedy or the practitioner to benefit from homoeopathy. A blank pill – a placebo – would have done the cat no good whatever. Animals and small children are amongst the most successfully treated patients of homoeopathy – largely because their energy is so relatively unpolluted – and neither has ever heard of the placebo effect.

Faith does help, of course, but belief in anything that takes time and effort to understand is often born of experience – this is certainly true in the field of alternative treatment. To experience the elimination either of troubling symptoms in oneself or in one's child, as a result of taking homoeopathic medicine is to become a believer in the healing potential of the intrinsic energy – *atomic energy* – of minerals, plants and even animal products; a healing power that has been harnessed in what may seem arcane ways but, as we shall discover, by a quite simple process of refining raw materials to the point where the crudity of chemistry is left behind. (Simple though this process may be, it requires a full explanation and a leap of imagination on your part to grasp the full implications.)

Sometimes it takes time for faith to take root. I had been an unquestioning patient of homoeopathy for twenty years before I became interested in studying it as a profession. I had just accepted that 'the little white pills' were doing me good. They had helped me to deal with insomnia and irritable bowel and to overcome my teenage neuroses. I had no clear idea that homoeopathic remedies were responsible for easing my low self-esteem and poor confidence. Then, at a career crisis point and through a series of serendipitous events, I took up the whole subject. Since then it has become a lifetime study.

As I began to find out about the apparent mysteries of homoeopathy and alternative medical thinking, my initial intuitive inspiration began to need some back-up. My intellect, having been on a sabbatical in my previous occupation as a teacher of English as a foreign language, became engaged; I began to question everything that I was learning – I wanted to know how it all worked; how the homoeopathic clock ticked. This was faith tempered by enquiry. Those first student weeks of enthralling discovery – during which I had so innocently prescribed for a cat with terminal cancer – gave way to many months of struggling to understand what on earth I was doing. Only later did it become clear that college was a place where the blind led the blind. Hundreds of hours of frustration in searching for whys and wherefores were aggravated by conflicting and contradictory answers from the teachers. The reference books fed my fascination; treating patients at the college clinic provided a fund of anecdotes to stock my conversation for years to come; I was ready to take up the cudgels and defend homoeopathy to the death…yet so much of it made confusion, not sense.

I used to wonder whether not being a scientist handicapped my vision and progress – but then none of the teachers were noted for being particularly analytical and their knowledge was almost exclusively experiential. It was uncomfortable for me that, though some (if not many) of the great books on homoeopathy had been written by doctors (originally trained in conventional medicine), current practice was now mainly in the hands of 'lay practitioners' – people hardly qualified to question the precepts of scientific thought despite their brave efforts to define what appears to be indefinable. Yet their everyday practice was a continual process that bore witness to homoeopathy at work. Even now, after years in my own practice, I still find it little short of amazing that homoeopathy initiates the healing ·process – and in such profound and yet diverse ways.

But there was the other side of the coin: it used to worry me that science – usually in the guise of medical journalism – wanted either to *explain* homoeopathy so that it could be 'packaged' and pigeon-holed or to condemn it altogether. That homoeopathy might after all be found to be less worthy of our consideration than conventional medicine was a threatening thought. (I felt I had a personal stake in this as orthodox medicine had failed me when I most needed therapeutic help in my teens.) I wanted homoeopathy to be accepted generally and shown to be capable of offering proof of healing even if in quite unorthodox ways.

Allopathy[1], another term for conventional orthodox medicine, seems superficially not to have to prove itself: of its nature it is generally approved of and accepted. By dint of its sheer professionalism, its unrivalled knowledge of physiology and pathology, its long experience of prodigious feats of surgical skill and the vast cornucopia of chemical drugs, it has an almost unchallenged history of apparent success. Allopathic medical practice is part of the status quo of everyday faith. Paradoxically, it is a far younger system of medicine than most.

Though allopathy has its historical roots in herbalism, it is the biochemist's laboratory that is its crucible. Medieval rhizomists were collectors of roots and plants, some of which still form the basis of our modern drugs – think of digitalis. Today, plants are still eagerly examined for their medicinal properties though it is the biochemist who artificially synthesises the end product. The vast commercial production of drugs, the enormous battery of diagnostic equipment and the mushrooming understanding of the body's biochemistry and genetic make-up have all kept pace with the speed of technological development. We stand in awe of technology and the expertise that creates it. It is this that is mainly responsible for our unquestioning acceptance of allopathy's pre-eminence in the field of medicine. Yet what we think of as orthodox medicine arose chiefly as a result of the Industrial Revolution. The pharmaceutical industry, worth billions of dollars per annum and mass-producing staggering quantities of chemicals, would, on the face of it, seem to suit our exceptionally materialistic age. There is now, though, a crisis of faith in the conventional wisdom of allopathy that needs to be addressed. Disillusioned and frustrated patients are looking for alternatives to invasive surgery or synthetic drug treatments and forcing the orthodox medical profession to take account of systems of holistic therapy that are hard to countenance in a laboratory.

The difficulty that scientists have is the acceptance of anything that would undermine the supreme authority of its present practice. Some alternative practices, such as osteopathy or chiropractic, can be readily accommodated as they do not disturb the horizons of acceptable scientific thought. Reflexology and aromatherapy do not impinge on orthodoxy sufficiently to make waves but this is more to do with the fact that neither of them makes spectacular claims and they are content with a supporting role. Acupuncture, which can claim roots going deep into pre-Christian history, has too long and trusted a history of success to be dismissed even though its very oriental philosophical approach would superficially appear to be alien to western culture and to be dependent for proof only on clinical evidence. All these therapies have an obviously practical application; they are all 'hands on' treatments – unlike homoeopathy.

Of the major alternative therapies only homoeopathy, in spite of some very serious-minded enquiry, and some 200 years' worth of literature and practice, has been forced to remain 'below stairs'. For those who have dismissed homoeopathy as a placebo, a 'faith' medicine that may not do any particular good but that does not do any harm, it has been safely left to eccentrics. As patients begin to broaden their perspectives in search of ways of treating illnesses for which conventional medicine has only palliative or no answers, this Cinderella is seen by some to be stirring the pot.

Homoeopathy seems to have reached a tricky moment in its history: the point of either mass discovery or of being proved to be not much more than a dotty aberration. There are simply not enough qualified practitioners in full-time practice to cope with mass discovery despite the encouraging numbers of graduates emerging from the dozen or more professional colleges in Britain. Further dismissal would not greatly affect those who have experienced the benefits but might well keep Cinderella amongst the shadows and ashes for another generation or more – at a time when she needs to be above stairs and at the ball.

Why is it that homoeopathy has been so neglected by the establishment? Why have science commentators so frequently sought to put it down? Why has it got the reputation of being so difficult to come to terms with? What has prevented the weight of respected opinion (some of it royal) from establishing homoeopathy beyond reasonable doubt as a powerful healing system – one to match the great eastern philosophies of medicine and even to be a first choice for creating vital health?

The answers to these questions lie in the philosophy of healing that underpins the whole structure of the system. Every medical system has a philosophy even if the patient is unaware of it. The principles of homoeopathy cause controversy only because they turn orthodoxy on its head. To accept homoeopathy we have to unlearn what we have previously taken for granted – just as our forebears found that they had to change their minds about living, first on a flat earth and then on a planet that was not the centre of the universe.

One of the problems we come across in our search for evidence of homoeopathy's effectiveness is that we believe that scientists are the best people to explain our world to us. For the most part this is true but there are no scientists of undisputed authority who are steeped sufficiently in homoeopathic tradition to guide us to any new understanding; they are too firmly entrenched in a rational and materialist view of the world and busy with all the technology that seems so successfully to prove their point. That leaves us with the explanations of the homoeopaths of the last two centuries, many of whom were scientists in the true sense of the word: seekers of knowledge. Most of their writings are, by nature, *evolutionary*. Even though they were guided by the few immutable basic principles of homoeopathy, its practice is so flexible that it appears to change from generation to generation; different commentators set down their thoughts in print only to have them superseded then qualified by the next wave of authors. Worse still, more recent books, articles and conference papers show that there is constant debate and conflict between homoeopaths as to what they should be thinking and doing. Furthermore, authors writing for the general public have sought to explain homoeopathy in simple terms – for example giving an infinitesimally small dose of something to cure what a larger dose of the same would cause – which is confusing and inaccurate. It is no wonder that such inconsistency should have bred scepticism. Yet 200 years of evidence show how well documented, practical and inexpensive a system homoeopathy is and how the basic core of principles remains unchallenged and unchanged.

Scientists hold a unique position of academic authority that would allow them to demonstrate officially just how phenomenal this natural healing system is as a curative and preventative method of medicine. We have come to trust scientists to illuminate our understanding; their sure grip on the ball and sceptre of knowledge has given them credence and obliges us to listen. Their position has been achieved through inspired guesswork and imaginative experimentation – not to say bumbling about in the dark! Scientists are explorers by nature, driven by a need to discover that is every bit as imperative as that felt by Columbus or Livingstone. Medical technology – beginning with the microscope: one of the spectacular early fruits of their discoveries – has become one of the main factors that shapes medical exploration even though the technical approach tends to obscure the human element. Chemistry, too, although it can effect powerful change on a sick body, tends to obscure all but the pathology of a patient.

The pioneers of homoeopathy were also driven by the imperative force of inspiration. The difference between them and their allopathic colleagues was that the homoeopaths' discoveries were all based on the *observation* of particular and peculiar reactions of *individual* patients. This did not lead on to any results that could be packaged and marketed; textbooks on homoeopathy tended to emphasise the differences and individuality of sick people rather than the identifying common factors that described each ailment which could then be treated with a stock procedure. Nor was there any commercial reward to speak of if you were experimenting with homoeopathy. Meanwhile allopaths, basing their thinking on a very material, biochemical view, were making discoveries that demanded plenty of appliances and technological activity that have, over the last two centuries, provided a thoroughly sound commercial base to fund further research and development. The focus of allopathy is the treatment; at its core is the process of applying patients to therapeutic procedures. The focus of homoeopathy is the individual patient; at its core is the moulding of homoeopathic thinking towards the patients' own self-healing process – a process that takes time and effort to grasp and to which the first part of this book is devoted.

Homoeopathy has no need whatever of modern technology either to prove itself or for its general application in everyday practice. No expensive equipment is required[2]. Scientists who would be so well placed in the public mind's eye to undertake research into the principles of homoeopathy are at a disadvantage: there is almost no commercial incentive to do so; in fact, the opposite is true. The medicines used in homoeopathy are so comparatively inexpensive that it is highly unlikely that any pharmaceutical company would ever fund the work. Furthermore, in seeking to understand it themselves, rationalist scientists would be faced with the fact that there is a viable system of medicine that contradicts fundamental beliefs in what disease is and the way that medicine should be practised in order to combat it. To the trained rationalist mind homoeopathy is both too simple and without a sound basis of logic; it can appear to be homespun and unprofessional.

For scientists logic and reason are paramount. Despite the lip service paid to empiricism, modern orthodox medicine is rationalistic and its basis is formed of theories about disease rather than people. If experiments do not justify the theories then their awkward findings are all too often relegated to dusty archives. Homoeopathy is genuinely empirical: there are very few incontrovertible principles as its foundation and almost every likely rule is qualified by the many exceptions to it. The very ground on which homoeopathy stands allows for flexibility and variation as diverse as the patients who seek its healing effects.

The few incontrovertible homoeopathic principles are immutable laws of Nature rather than the intellect; they can be explained simply enough even though they may take a bit of swallowing. The forces of Nature that make homoeopathy possible are electrodynamic and, like magnetism, are seemingly easy to prove by demonstration but very hard to prove through repeatable experimentation. Scientists have, historically, either fought shy of or ferociously attacked any such demonstrations because of the intrinsic impossibility of replicating the tests exactly. Within their own terms of reference they are right, of course. It is not the doctors who are wrong about the research; it is the methodology of the research itself that needs to be adapted. Homoeopathy is simply not susceptible to the usual double-blind trials that so convincingly provide orthodoxy with its statistics and data.

Scientists have yet to understand the absolutely fundamental truth that homoeopathy is the art of healing the *individual* by means of selecting a remedy based on the patient's peculiar and characteristic symptom picture – and not according to the name of the diagnosed disease. As every patient is as different in their disease as they are in facial features or in personality traits, it is impossible to create experiments to test homoeopathy by means of conventional laboratory procedures. The best that can be hoped for in such circumstances is to find *similarities* of results and then to offer *expectations* rather than exactitude. Though no two people are the same it is always possible to see similarities between them; 'expectations' are not as limited as the word might imply. The edifice of homoeopathy is built on the comparison of similarities between people expressing their individual symptom pictures and the effects of homoeopathically prepared medicines on those healthy and willing to test them. It will be seen to be a scientific process even if an unconventional one.

This book is an attempt to set down on paper the explanations I am asked to give so often in clinic. It contains my own particular and hard-won understanding of the vagaries of this vast and mercurial subject – though I am well aware of the continued need to study it in ever greater depth. Much of what is written here will be subjective opinion and I do not expect all readers to accept blindly what is, after all, another person's experience. I was not trained as a scientist so do not look for quantifiable or statistical data[3]. Such things have little place in a homoeopath's surgery. This is not a textbook or a first-aid book; it is intended as a companion to such books, one that will suggest answers to many of the awkward questions that arise in considering alternative and complementary medicine. It is important to explain, in as far as it is possible, why and how natural medicines and people interact in the way they do. It is my hope that this book will motivate you to embrace homoeopathy with some basic knowledge as well as intuitive trust.

Being ambitious for the future of homoeopathy I want to initiate your own further investigation into the process of personal development that begins with healing, to help you to foster the notion that chronic illness is the body's attempt at creating in symptoms a metaphor for a general condition of imbalance and negative energy. This is to begin seeing healing and medicine in three dimensions: discovering the history of a chronic condition, describing its present manifestation and understanding its purpose.

This book will help all those who intuitively feel the need to seek alternative and practical self-help medicine and who want to understand that the reasoning behind the practice of homoeopathy is neither whimsical nor eccentric but purposeful and full of common sense.

Introduction

I can think of many times in my life when this book would have been helpful to me: as a home prescriber puzzled by the mixed results I got from my 36 remedy kit; as a patient puzzled by not getting help for a serious complaint from four different homoeopaths – then cure from the fifth; as a student puzzled by the different viewpoints of different homoeopathy 'schools'; and then as a practitioner learning to communicate with my own patients about what I do.

Imagine being able to sit down with an experienced homoeopath for a deliciously long dialogue. Imagine being able to ask him any and every question under the sun about homoeopathy, about how and why it works from every angle you can think of. You have just imagined this book! *The Companion to Homoeopathy* isn't a textbook: it is an 'insider's view of homoeopathy'. It is a book for every person who wants to understand more about the whole homoeopathic process by engaging in a series of in-depth discussions.

This book is jam-packed with fascinating metaphors and thought-provoking analogies that dust off the theories and begin to paint them into life. Hundreds of cases complete the process of describing a three-dimensional process of healing.

Patients will find this book riveting: they will be astonished at the depth of thinking and intricate analyses that go into the selection of their little white pills.

Students will enjoy this book enormously. It will complement their classroom education through cases that breathe life into the philosophy. This book does not simply present a practitioner's best cases. A myriad of issues surrounding case analysis, methodology and case management are discussed, including the author's blunders.

Virtually every homoeopathic stone is here, conscientiously turned. How nice then that this book is written in a refreshingly conversational tone that makes it easy to access. This 'companion' is ultimately about the humanity of homoeopathy. It unravels the tangle of suffering encountered by patients and describes a process of healing that is unique to homoeopathy. Practitioners, students and patients alike cannot fail to be humbled and impressed by the workings of the Vital Force as Colin Griffith describes this healing journey from the inside out.

Miranda Castro, November 2004
www.mirandacastro.com

PART I

THE CINDERELLA OF MEDICINE

CHAPTER 1

TAKING HEALTH INTO YOUR OWN HANDS

The essential difference of approach between conventional and homoeopathic thinking

The normal thing to do, if you are feeling unwell, is to tell your doctor of the symptom that is interfering with your well-being. He will listen carefully in order to select a treatment that is appropriate to effect the removal of the problem – as if it were an obstacle, or an inconvenient nuisance. He will either write out a prescription for a drug that you will take to the chemist or, if the problem is considered serious, will refer you to a consultant who, in turn, will decide whether chemotherapy (drug-based therapy) or surgery is appropriate. The philosophy underlying this procedure is called *suppression*.

The beauty of this system is its comparative simplicity. The patient is required only to answer questions, to undergo an examination or tests and to follow instructions. The responsibility for the condition that is being treated no longer belongs to the patient. The practitioner has assumed responsibility for the outright cure. In order to achieve success the physician sets out to eradicate the offending symptom. Antibiotics kill off bugs and cooties; anti-inflammatory drugs reduce swellings; analgesics kill pain; and so on. The purpose of all drugs and surgery is the restoration of the body's normal function by means of a chemical agent or the knife which are employed in order to reduce and to remove the symptom. The symptom is viewed as the disease.

At a very basic level this is akin to taking your car to the garage to find out why it takes so long to start it in the morning – the mechanic replaces the spark plugs or the fan belt and all is well. In allopathic medicine the diagnosis of conditions is refined to an extraordinary degree and technology has provided so many additions to the physician's tool kit that we are left in awe of the whole system – yet it remains a very mechanical and materially-based therapy. Even if the physician recognises an emotional or traumatic element to the condition under examination, the therapeutic response will be, many times out of ten, to subscribe a drug of some description.

The basic premise of homoeopathy is that the symptom, unless it is the result of an accident, is a *representation* of the disease and not the disease itself. To remove the symptom simply takes away a window onto the nature of the illness. Symptoms are manifested by the *whole* body. Put another way, if a body is displaying symptoms of disease or illness, it is the body *as a whole* that is not well, and these symptoms are there to help us to read the map of the disease state.

The Romans, it is said, towards the end of their empire, would execute any messenger of bad news. The consequence was that they never saw the true nature of the enemy at the gate. Symptoms are messengers of an underlying state that affects the whole body; the local part announces the distress of the whole. The homoeopath, in examining the patient, asks exhaustive questions about every aspect of a symptom: size, colour, shape, type of pain, times of day it occurs, what makes it feel easier or worse and how long it has been there. In addition, he asks questions about changes of temperature, appetite and mood. The practitioner is building up a unique picture of not only the offending symptom but also of the whole body. The characteristics will lead to the selection of a remedy, not to suppress the symptom but to encourage the body to alter its energy so that it heals itself by a process of elimination and adaptation – an *evolutionary* process.

A patient that chooses to start such a positive evolutionary process is choosing to develop and grow and is always, even if he or she is unaware of it, actively participating in the healing process. In allopathy there is very little room for 'patient power' and many patients feel simply swept along on a tide of professional expertise. Let's compare the following examples.

The allopathic approach

A man of forty complains of recurrent 'migraine' headaches. The doctor asks how long he has suffered from them and what he has done so far to help himself. (He might reply that he has been taking paracetamol or Nurofen.) The doctor then asks whether the headaches are bilious or stress-related; whether they affect the vision or body temperature, or if they might be attributable to any head injury. The patient then has his blood pressure checked and some dietary changes might be suggested. The resulting prescription takes account of all these factors though if there are no complications such as high blood pressure, then the selected treatment is not likely to be much different from the paracetamol that the patient has been taking since the headaches began. If blood pressure were a factor then tests would follow and the drug treatment would be more radical as it would be supposed that the cause of the headaches was a disorder of the circulatory system, possibly complicated by any digestive problems. The tests would mean hospital appointments and the treatment would involve drugs, possibly for life. The end result might well be a reduction or elimination of the headaches but would the patient have been 'cured'?

The homoeopathic approach

A man of forty complains of recurrent 'migraine' headaches. The practitioner spends some time on the headache *symptoms* – they might be like this: the pain comes on each day at the same time, just as he is leaving work at 5 p.m. It centres on the forehead and it feels as if the temples are being pressed together; there is some throbbing felt there too. He feels a bit light-headed and irritable. All he wants to do is to get home and eat his tea as this clears the giddiness and the mood. After eating, it takes a while for the head pain to ease but it has usually gone by later in the evening though he is very tired and good for nothing other than sitting in front of the TV, where he sometimes falls asleep.

The homoeopath then needs to know of the rest of the circumstances: the headaches began some months before, soon after the patient was given a promotion. The new responsibilities demand more time and organisational skill than he was used to, and although he knows that challenge is good for him he feels that he might not succeed to his manager's satisfaction. In addition, now that there is more money available, his wife wants to look for a private school for their young son, which worries him, as money is still tight.

Headaches in the forehead usually suggest that the liver is involved in the illness; so the homoeopath then asks about digestion. Yes, the patient does get indigestion and feels bloated and heavy after meals; yes, he does have flatulence which can at times be quite embarrassing; yes, he has always had a slight tendency to this but it has all been much worse since the headaches began.

By this process the homoeopath gathers information about the headaches themselves, about the causative factors and about how the whole economy of the body is affected. The resulting three-dimensional 'picture' is illustrative of the patient's general state and tells the practitioner that the patient needs just one or two doses of a particular remedy: *Lycopodium* – which is made from a particular variety of moss. The result of such a prescription, from experience, is that the patient's headaches would clear up, the digestive symptoms would ease considerably to the extent that the patient is no longer aware of them and would be far better able to deal with pressures at work. If the patient's blood pressure had been high then this would come down to a normal level. As a result the patient would probably make some very effective decisions regarding money and schooling for his son as well.

The point of this illustration is that the homoeopath goes to the heart of the patient's condition by finding out the whole story. In this case the patient is suffering from a crisis of confidence, which became established as the result of what might be seen as excellent circumstances – a job promotion. The headaches developed out of the stress of having increased responsibilities and greater demands on his time. The homoeopath takes account of the whole picture because he knows that he can find a remedy that will cover not just the distressing symptoms and their effects on the rest of the body but also the original reason for their being there in the first place. (Even when such a potentially serious problem as high blood pressure occurs, remedies will act curatively.)

Lycopodium is known to be one of the most important remedies to deal with conditions that arise from a lack of self-confidence which can affect the body by producing sluggish liver function and disordered digestion, combined with flatulence and hypoglycaemia – low blood sugar. It is also used for dealing with problems that arise between 4 and 8 o'clock a.m. and p.m.[1] That the patient's headaches (which, incidentally, are not in this case migraines – a common misnomer) happen to be the presenting complaint is only incidental to the whole; they were what disturbed the patient's equilibrium enough to want to seek treatment – he could have lived with the flatulence, perhaps.

Take a further and similar example: a man of forty complains of 'migraine' headaches. This patient has pains in the back of the head that are accompanied by dizziness and nausea and come on whenever he feels stressed. He works in uncongenial circumstances and under considerable pressure. He constantly has to meet deadlines and yet is expected by his company to spend extra time wining and dining clients. The patient is very sensitive and his temper is very 'close to the edge'; a medical practitioner of any persuasion would recommend dietary changes here. Surely the real 'cure' is for the man to change his circumstances, to leave his job. Yet the patient is too full of anxiety about the future and his career to risk such a drastic prescription.

The homoeopath would give *Nux Vomica* to this patient because the causation, circumstances and symptom picture all match what we know from experience will be treated and cured by it. The result will not just be the elimination of the headaches; there is a considerable possibility that the medicine will also afford the patient the energy and clarity of thought to find a way of changing his circumstances. The result? He will no longer get into the sort of situation which would bring on the symptoms of irritability from stress and overindulgence that tax his general physical and emotional sensitivity to the limit. (Tales about *Nux Vomica* and its effects include one of a man who hated his job and his wife. He was given the remedy based on its characteristic symptoms; whereupon he went home and told his wife that he wanted a divorce, went to work the next day, walloped his boss on the jaw and handed in his notice. He reported feeling considerably better.)

7

Both these case illustrations have satisfactory outcomes in that the patients shed their illness and alter their perspectives.

Under allopathic care only the symptom is treated, often leaving the patient in the same position as he was before or worse, perhaps, as the drug so often suppresses not only the symptom but also the patient's general energy. Take the drug away and the symptom will often return. Under homoeopathic treatment the prescription is based on everything pertaining to the problem. The effects of the prescribed remedy, working as it does only on the electrical energy of the body (i.e. the central nervous system), bring about creative changes in the whole system so that not only does the presenting symptom disappear but the patient can also shift perspectives and make choices to feel more in charge of his or her being. Though it is the homoeopath's work to be responsible for selecting the prescription, it is the patient himself (mostly unwittingly) who is taking responsibility for his own well-being once he has embarked on treatment. The changes created within restore him to health, yet the remedial agent that brought this about, being of an electrodynamic yet virtually imperceptible force, can only instigate any such changes because they potentially exist in the body already.

To put it another way: an allopathic drug imposes an external chemical force on the system which creates artificial changes intended to obliterate the symptom; while a homoeopathic remedy (being of an electrodynamic nature) sparks off a series of events within the body system that relieves the body of a disease energy that usually affects not only the physical body but also the mind and emotions as well. It makes no difference, as you will come to see, whether that disease energy is psychosomatic or of bacterial or viral origin. The body has a programme for well-being and will always return to health if given the right stimuli for setting the healing process in operation. This point cannot be stressed enough: however sick or damaged the body might be or become, it always retains the memory of its 'wellness' and, given the appropriate stimuli, will always endeavour to return to that state.

All this begs a few questions. Is homoeopathy a cure-all? Are all drugs and surgery bad? (Of course not, is the answer to both questions!) Is there ever a meeting place for the two systems? Can we use the two therapies side by side? (Of course, is the answer to both questions!) Surely homoeopaths cannot take so simplistic a view of health as to believe that illness is all in the mind? (Certainly not!) Isn't it rather far-fetched to describe medicine as electrodynamic – so called 'energy' medicine? (Yes, so it needs extensive clarification.) What does self-healing really mean?

CHAPTER 2

SELF-HEALING

One of the difficulties in understanding the human self-healing mechanism is that it seems to be different things to different disciplines. For example, in Chinese medicine the health of the whole (body, mind and spirit) is dependant on the balance between yin and yang (polar but complementary opposites of the whole, or any part of the whole, and its function as growth and development occur) and the integrity of Qi, (chi), often loosely translated as vital energy. To this must be added the concepts of Earth, Air, Fire and Dampness (Water) and their balance and interaction within the body.

In Ayurvedic medicine (practised on the Indian subcontinent) there is a similar focus on the balance of the constitution as influenced by, among other things, Earth, Air, Fire, Water and Ether, there being three basic types of constitution for these to play on: vata, pitta and kapha. Although one type may be more strongly represented than the others, each of us is an integrated mixture of vata (dry, cold, light, changeable, subtle, hard and rough), pitta (hot, fluid, sharp, soft, interactive) and kapha (chill, wet, heavy, slow, dull, smooth, impenetrable). These may seem strange philosophical ideas to our western minds but they come from disciplines that have withstood the test of thousands of years of practice.

While the philosophic principles of homoeopathy do not take account of the 'elements' as eastern medicine does (or, indeed, as early European medicine used to) many homoeopaths are familiar with such concepts. Most schools of alternative practice accept that it is essential to see the body in terms of the elemental forces of nature and therefore the study of oriental medical philosophy is included to a greater or lesser extent in their curricula. Nevertheless, in homoeopathy our concept of self-healing is based not on apparently abstract notions of the balance of elemental energies but on a patient's subjective description of his ills and an objective observation of his condition. The 'picture' that is built up includes not just the distressing symptoms of the moment but also the history of the ailment, the history of the patient's general health and the description of what is 'normal' for the patient when they feel well. (This may not necessarily be good health but what the patient views as his/her own norm.)

What is being studied here is the way energy is expressed by the whole: spirit, emotion and physical body. (In simple, acute pathology, spirit and emotion may not form part of the equation. In chronic illness they always do.) Homoeopathy is the study of the changes instigated and wrought on the whole (or part of) the body by the electrodynamic energy that courses through it – not so very far from the oriental philosophy of healing.

Allopathy, by contrast, remains firmly grounded in the material world. Here it is biochemistry (the constant reactive interplay between chemicals necessary for the vital functioning of the body) and the immune system (the body's SAS) that maintain health. The term 'immune system' is used to describe the lymphatic system – the waste-disposal unit of the body – and all immune responses. It drives the deployment of leucocytes and lymphocytes through the body, to seek out and destroy invading organisms and ensure our safety from attack.

This is a materialist's view of the way we deal with disease but, though extremely limited in its scope, it is none the less valid as far as it goes. It also has the merit of being very easy to comprehend. Unfortunately, if this approach to healing is used exclusively, it becomes very hard to imagine how the body copes when the self-healing system breaks down. Allopaths have to resort to using methods of treatment from outside the body's resources – foreign bodies. Allopathic philosophy does not yet extend to allowing for, let alone encompassing, the idea that there is a critical faculty within us (one that is programmed deliberately to work in harmony with the central nervous system and the endocrine glands and biochemistry) that seeks to maintain equilibrium: a status quo of optimum health. Allopathy does accept that we have a self-healing faculty that can cope with acute conditions: we can mend a broken bone (once it is set); we can heal a cut; we can get over a cold – all by ourselves and without

11

intervention – yet such self-healing is seen as part of the body's chemistry set. There is no allopathic confidence that the body could have a far broader and deeper reaching faculty that is inherent and intelligent[1] and capable of healing on the profoundest level of our existence. This really would be just too close for comfort to accepting 'the ghost in the machine', a 'higher self', or the spiritual dimension.

We *are* born with a self-regulating system; one that is indeed based extensively on chemical interaction. When well, we know when we are hungry or thirsty, in need of sleep, uncomfortable or in danger; we have a heart that beats perpetually and unattended; we have a waste-disposal unit with a variety of outlets; we have a 'body clock' that keeps everything ticking over automatically according to a diurnal rhythm – and a monthly and annual rhythm as well. We also have the 'Home Guard', the immune system which is, when working well, ruthlessly efficient. Is this assemblage of parts simply the result of chemicals reacting intimately to provide such a resilient yet fluid structure? Is this the whole story? Must we accept culturally alien medical philosophy if it is not? We need to look a little more closely at the way the body reacts when the balance is tipped.

If you cut yourself badly enough to need a sticky plaster you will probably curse because of the pain and worry in case of infection. You might hold the cut under the cold tap to staunch the bleeding and get out the antiseptic cream and plaster. Stop – the self-healing process is being compromised! Allowing a wound to bleed a little (common sense dictating how much) encourages leucocytes (white blood cells) to reach the site and deal quickly with any staphylococcal bacteria that might make a home in the wound. (Staphylococcus is mostly responsible for wounds becoming infected.) By using antiseptic cream you kill off some of the white blood cells as well as the staphylococci. If you are too hasty with the cream and plaster you may well, from a strictly microbiological view, be trapping some of the microbes within. As well as that, the delicate tissue fibres that start to grow towards each other over the wound to form new skin are 'burnt' and clumped by the cream; so as they grow they are more likely to form heavier scar tissue. By covering the wound with a waterproof plaster or a tight bandage you are preventing the air from circulating around the area. (The air is not laden with toxic and malevolent microbes just waiting for a chance to breed – to believe this is to forget that staphylococcus is normally an indolent tenant of the skin anyway.)

Even the deepest cut will heal itself despite our anxieties. The healing does involve chemistry: for one thing, vitamin K is necessary to cause clotting. Then there is all that phagocytosis – leucocytes feasting on foreign bodies; white blood cells ingesting foreign bacteria. The body 'knows' what to do but we have almost forgotten how to trust it. Allopathy has taught us so much about the chemistry of the body that we expect chemistry to put things right when they go wrong. Antiseptics do kill germs but take no account of what the body's own chemistry does when there are no antiseptics available. But what initiates the body's own chemistry?

Physics vs. chemistry and the role of the Vital Force

Chemistry comes to life only when some force of energy puts two or more chemicals together to create reaction. For the body's chemistry to work there has to be a dynamic force within, creating the environment for any chemical changes to happen. We know what the *instrument* of this force is: the central nervous system. This all-pervading, tree-like network of nerves, is dependant on water and chemicals held within the body for its full functioning. It provides the pathways for all messages to be received and delivered – including information about trivial cuts at the extremities. Nothing, in a healthy person, escapes the nervous system's attention. It is programmed for survival and it is alive with electrical impulses. It is the engine of self-healing. The intrinsic critical faculty that drives it and that links body, mind and spirit is known in homoeopathy as the Vital Force.

To reduce this to its essentials: healing occurs at that moment when the physics of the nervous system sparks chemistry into action – and that is where science has left it, for the moment. Yet this is where all ancient forms of healing begin.

The Vital Force cannot be described directly as it has no *material* presence. It cannot be identified by any specific location in the same way that the heart or liver can be. It remains unseen and can be described only by its effects on the whole. (In this it has something in common with magnetism.) It can be witnessed in the way it organises the system for survival and

13

quality of life and by the signals of distress that it creates when the whole is unwell. It is as nebulous as instinct. It can be left to its own devices to deal with minor acute problems such as cuts or bruises. We become aware of it only when the general balance it creates is upset – for it is responsible for creating all the persistent physical, mental or emotional symptoms that threaten to become chronic.

The Vital Force is not seen as spiritual energy in the sense of 'soul' but it is seen to act as both link and chain between the physical body and the subtle bodies of mind, emotions and spirit. The electrical impulses created by the central nervous system and the way they play on the endocrine system (made up of the organs that produce all the vital hormones) are the mode of expression of the Vital Force. They have the ability to create changes in the physical body, the emotions and the spirit. The Vital Force works on the spirit as well as on the mind that reflects it and on the physical body that houses them both. As such, the concept of the Vital Force is not so very far from the esoteric philosophies held by other, more ancient cultures. It equates to the Chinese concept of Qi.

A straightforward cut, even if it is a deep one, is hardly likely to persuade anyone that there is a Vital Force even though such a simple acute situation has often been the occasion for homoeopathy to be first witnessed as a viable alternative therapy. (Anyone who has seen a septic wound heal under the influence of *Hypericum* or *Calendula* will testify to the swift curative response these remedies trigger within the body.) Some further illustrations might help to focus attention on this self-healing aspect and show how practical and well organised the body is, thanks to its self-regulatory programme.

Drainage and discharge: the release of waste as a positive step towards cure

Inflammation of the middle ear (otitis media) spells fear for many mothers. Allopathically speaking, it can be a viral or bacterial infection causing fever, partial deafness, pain and swelling of the eardrum. However, the original onset can be triggered by events such as: teething, by catching a chill or after a bout of furious anger. Whatever the initial reason for it, the body will create a fever to speed the process of reaction and ensure the arrival of leucocytes in the Eustachian tube behind the drum to deal with the bacterial infection that results. As they set to work on the bacteria, pus is formed. The drum bulges, causing excruciating pain, until – if it is not prevented by a hasty dose of antibiotics – it bursts. This releases all the foul debris that has been lying behind the drum. When the discharge finishes, the drum heals and hearing is fully restored. Sometimes the pus will not need to be eliminated in such a dramatic way: if the patient develops a cold then the muck to be eliminated will run down the Eustachian tube into the back of the throat and join the rest of the mucus that is being coughed and sneezed out. This is how an otherwise healthy body would work if left to fend for itself.

Many a parent can testify to the fact that their child's high temperature reduced as soon as the eardrum burst. (Though this description is not meant to advocate leaving a patient to cope with intense pain without appropriate homoeopathic treatment.) As soon as the body is aware that the *vent* it chose for the elimination of all the toxic debris has worked thoroughly then the blood circulation is returned to normal. What is more, the body of a healthy person 'knows' when to start the process of healing the drum (once the discharge is over) and this can happen without causing scar tissue (which would impair the quality of hearing).

Contrary to popular belief, it is perfectly possible to deal with such an unpleasant ordeal *without* drug intervention; there is no need to suffer anything worse than possible fever and initial pain – which announce the problem – and a resultant discharge from the ear. With no chemical drug treatment, the fever can subside when the leucocytes have completed their job and the discharge is underway. This is most satisfactorily achieved with indicated remedies.

Unfortunately but not unreasonably, this condition is so painful and distressing that it is seldom allowed to run its course without intervention. Antibiotics do relieve the situation very efficiently in most cases but they also prevent the body *completing the natural process of discharging waste*. The suppression has interrupted a process set up by the body, designed not only to heal but also to teach the body how to react in future. The drum never releases the rubbish through the vent that was chosen and the consequence is that the patient is likely to suffer another bout which will in turn be suppressed again and again.

The point here is that the body sets up a pattern of self-healing and one that is efficient even if, when left to its own devices, it is painful. It even has a measure of aftercare in the form of earwax which is produced to protect the middle ear for a while after the event. The body may seem to be responding on a chemical level to the presence of multiplying organisms but even after their demise the self-healing continues – on tissue regeneration and protection. The response has been initiated and organised totally by the body's integrating energy. (Homoeopathy is able to assist the self-healing mechanism with otitis media. There are several remedies that might be called for – *Chamomilla*, *Silica* and *Pulsatilla* are the most common – and when indicated and given as soon as the symptoms can be 'read', they not only speed the process but also help the body to do it *without pain*.)

This system of drainage is evident at all times in any pathology that is properly managed; here are some examples:

- Headaches can be relieved by nosebleeds, by passing a motion, by passing quantities of water or by releasing emotions that underlie the physical problem.
- A sore throat can be relieved when the tonsils finish exuding matter.
- Bronchitis can be healed when the lungs are encouraged to discharge lots of phlegm.
- Food poisoning is cured when the body throws out the problem by vomiting and diarrhoea.
- A fever will resolve if a profuse sweat or copious urination is initiated.
- Most asthma/eczema sufferers would tell you that they can breathe better if their eczema flares up and exudes matter; the skin acting as a discharge point rather than the lungs.

Discharges can be thoroughly messy and obnoxious but they are *always* to our advantage unless, it should be added, they are continuously profuse and weaken the system. Suppression is very bad news because it prevents the completion of drainage and is therefore one of the reasons for a compromised Vital Force.

Functions of the Vital Force

The self-healing mechanism is not only geared for 'cure'. It is also geared to find alternative means of expression, damage limitation and survival. Think of the teacher who develops a streaming cold as soon as the stress of the end of term exams is over and the holidays begin. The timing may be awkward but it is a way of releasing pent up negativity. If a chronically nervy person suffers from frequent bouts of diarrhoea before any event where he is called on to perform, he is only expressing through his bowels how he feels in his mind. A student who develops glandular fever may really be expressing exam stress – as a way of opting out or because the stress is too much. A person who has recurrent tooth abscesses may actually be suffering from suppressed boils or a suppressed breast abscess – that may have developed years before. A child suffering from eczema on the hands may develop it in the creases of the elbows or the armpits instead if steroid creams are used to put a stop to the expression of the eczema on the original site. It is not chemistry but the Vital Force that chooses the most ecologically economical and least damaging option of how and where a person's physical symptoms should represent the distress of the whole being and it does it in striking, diverse ways – often creating symptomatic metaphors for the underlying negative state.

More often than not, the Vital Force chooses a symptomatic response that elegantly illustrates the underlying problem. Take the case of the wife whose mother-in-law came to stay. The younger woman found her guest overbearing and insufferably condescending. She developed severe toothache from clenching her jaws and grinding her teeth at night. She felt unable to say what she really wanted to say in case she offended her husband: she had 'to bite it back'. (The remedy that relieved these symptoms entirely was *Staphysagria* – the common delphinium – that has the dubious reputation of being the 'mother-in-law's remedy'.)

Another example is shown in the case of the child who was always slapped on the legs and told not to cry whenever she became upset. She

17

learnt not to cry but was brought for treatment by her grandmother when she became unable to stop wetting herself or her bed. She was well in other respects. *Pulsatilla*, a remedy that is often given for children who are tearful and dependant, cured the symptom of frequent urination as well as helping her to be less dependant – which meant in turn that her mother's low level of tolerance was not sparked by her child's whining. It is not uncommon for water, stopped from one source, to leak away from another.

Sometimes, however, the Vital Force is obliged to demonstrate the body's distress rather more dramatically. Migraine headaches are a case in point. So often, migraines are a sign of what might be termed malignant stress. The patient is often experiencing external pressure from uncongenial circumstances as well as internal trouble from an overloaded liver – the organ most inclined to carry suppressed anger – or even a suppressed sex drive.

Another example of deeper pathology eloquently expressing whole body distress is in the case of stomach or duodenal ulcers. They often occur in people who are unable to express their dissatisfaction with their creative professional lives. Unable to find a means of adapting and changing their circumstances they produce a pathology that seems, with its accompanying irritable temper, to beg the question: *"What's eating you?"*

Haemorrhoids or piles can show up the effects of suppressed or unexpressed emotions too. Piles are varicose veins, blood vessels whose walls have become incompetent and enlarged from laxity of the tissue and from pressure on the venous system (the veins that carry used blood back to the liver and lungs). In almost all cases there is a certain amount of 'toxic overload' in that organ, in addition to any stress factors occurring in the life of the patient. (Though it *can* be an entirely physical problem, as in the case of piles during pregnancy.) More often than not the root cause is both dietary and emotional. It may seem odd or extreme to think that the liver is an organ that might suffer from the patient's emotional state. However, it is very well known in alternative medical thinking that the liver responds negatively to negative emotions and most noticeably to anger – especially if it is repressed. The liver is vital not only to most chemical functions of the whole system; it is also the organ that 'stores' any toxic waste that cannot immediately be 'dumped' (via bowels or bladder). It can easily be seen that a compromised liver can lead to a state of general toxicity and unwellness.

Imagine a businessman on the morning rush hour train, having to stand all the way, trying to read through a report needed for the next meeting, having gobbled his breakfast after a short night that followed a late but heavy meal. His liver is upset because he has taken no account of his body clock that prefers not to have to deal with food after about 8 p.m.; because he did not have time to go to the lavatory satisfactorily before catching the train; because he was just too late on the platform to get that last seat in the compartment and it was his wife who had persuaded him not to pay the extra for first-class travel this year; because the report he has been reading has been prepared sloppily and he knows that there should be more data; because it is Wednesday and he will have to do all this again tomorrow and the next day. When he gets to work he has a chance to go to the lavatory but is depressed because there is blood in the pan again. He feels his body is letting him down. Actually it is doing him a favour: the bleeding pile is a release of pressure for the liver.

This is his body's expression of physical and emotional stress. Our commuter's body has chosen a very satisfactory point of discharge because it is safer for the system to have trouble in the anus than in the liver. That the Vital Force has chosen this place to express the body's problems seems fanciful until you see what happens if the haemorrhoids are suppressed by surgery or injection. Suppressed piles very often lead, in time, to a hiatus hernia. This is a condition of the cardiac sphincter, a ring of muscle (that resembles the anal sphincter), which acts as the entrance to the stomach and opens and then closes when we swallow food or drink. It can become incompetent and lax and let the stomach acids through, up into the oesophagus when we bend or lie down. There is distressing heartburn as the acid burns the delicate tissues of the gullet. Flatulence and chest pain can lead patients and doctors to misdiagnose this problem as the early signs of angina – which, indeed, it can eventually become if it is mistreated and suppressed.

If it is not hiatus hernia that results from the suppression of piles then it might be a peptic ulcer, some form of irritable bowel condition or high blood pressure – or a combination of these. If the site chosen by the Vital Force for the original expression of distress is taken away (through surgery or drugs) then the next disease 'event' will go deeper into the body. The body may be sick but it will still find ways of limiting the damage done to the whole by putting its symptomatic distress signals as near to the surface as possible. The Vital Force is intent on survival even when the whole is ailing.

The case of a severe mastitis with a threatening breast abscess offers a prime example of the Vital Force finding a means of diverting potentially serious pathology to a site that carries less risk. A woman had a very painful right breast; she also had a high fever and swollen glands. Treated with anti-biotics, which immediately reduced the fever, she developed a painful area on the breast that began to harden. On receiving indicated remedies the gathering abscess resolved but she developed a tooth abscess on the lower right jaw. She again took indicated remedies and the gum abscess swelled grotesquely and, for a while, painfully. It then burst and let out a mass of foul pus. The patient felt entirely relieved of all symptoms. The Vital Force had found a site closer to the surface (the gum) to discharge the toxic waste. Breast and gum were restored to normal.

If the Vital Force is compromised

If we look at the other end of the spectrum of disease where chronic ill health has compromised the Vital Force to the point where it cannot re-establish its original balance, we can find examples of the way the body organises itself to create a tolerable if often an uneasy status quo. Take gout, for instance. This is the bane of many an imbibing businessman. It is suf-fered mostly by middle-aged men, though by no means exclusively. There is a hereditary link as well. In allopathic terms gout is caused by high levels of uric acid in the blood. Where uric acid becomes concentrated in certain joints (the big toes are favourites), crystals form and cause acute pain and inflammation. However, underlying the problem is poor liver function. The liver has many functions; it is the chemical post office of the body. It organ-ises the storage and subsequent disposal of toxic waste either of the body's own making or of ingested materials such as drugs or poisons (including alcohol). An attack of gout occurs when the liver can no longer process any more than is absolutely essential. Too much red meat and soft French cheeses or overindulgence in wines can easily tip the balance. Rather than create immediate and serious liver damage, the body does something far more subtle. It sends the excess toxic waste in the form of uric acid to the furthest extremity of the body, to be stored as crystals in the convenient spaces between the bones of the toes, where it will do the least damage to the vital functioning of the liver and kidneys. To send such a sudden excess of toxic waste out through the kidneys might have caused damage to this delicate pair of organs. As and when the patient stops the intake of rich foods (especially those heavy in proteins), so the body is able to reduce the crystal formation in the joints and gradually release the waste safely through the bowels and urine.

The Vital Force works even in severe conditions

Crohn's disease is an extremely unpleasant condition in which the walls of the small intestine or, occasionally, the colon become chronically inflamed. There are phases of acute pain and debility and the passing of blood in the motions. Allopathy does not commit itself to a known cause for this condition, but the presence of infection, ulceration and oedema (swelling due to water retention) suggests that the usual treatment should include steroids (to reduce swelling) and antibiotics (to kill off any associated bacteria). Success under drug therapy is variable and most sufferers continue to have recurrent bouts of symptoms. The inflammation of the intestinal wall can be so severe that it creates a complete blockage allowing nothing to pass through.

If this situation were left unattended, there would be serious danger of autointoxication from the build-up of faecal matter at a site where ulceration of tissue allows infection into open blood vessels. The body's response is to do something practical, inexpensive and simple: it forms a fistula. A fistula is a hole made in the healthy part of the loop of the bowel wall, just before the inflamed area, which extends through to an adjacent loop, which is just *beyond* the diseased part. This isolates the inflammation thus giving the area a chance to 'rest' (during which time a certain amount of local healing takes place) and provides an alternative outlet for the faeces. This means that digestion can continue relatively unimpeded. This process does not happen just once. When the inflammation settles down the fistula closes up

21

and the usual passage is restored. However, stressful situations tend to aggravate the patient into suffering another bout so the whole process starts again.

This remarkable feat of engineering, performed as a survival technique by a partially crippled self-healing system, cannot be described simply as chemistry. The cell structure of *healthy* soft tissue has been reorganised to create a vent or drain for potentially dangerous toxic waste. The response occurs in a place where the cells that make up the local tissue are not affected by inflammation and disease so would not normally be expected to change their function and organisation so drastically. Furthermore, if this reaction was solely chemically inspired then one would expect to find a textbook description of the disease. (The action of chemicals being fixed and invariable according to their relationships.) Indeed, medical books attempt such a description but ruefully note that surgery to remove the offending section of bowel is unsatisfactory as the problem develops in another part soon after. Though all Crohn's patients suffer similar pathology, the symptoms by which it is identified can actually differ widely. It does not always happen in the same location. The quality of pain can vary enormously; some feel burning, others have cutting or stabbing and yet others may have dull aching. Many suffer anaemia and while some develop anorexia there are those who may gain excessive weight from water retention.

Although rationalist theories of invasive bacteria are suggested as the likely cause (Mycobacterium Paratuberculosis being the most obvious candidate), what is universal is that all such patients have a history of some form of stress that pre-dates the onset of symptoms. Even scientists now recognise that stress causes chemical changes in the body – but chemicals cannot 'feel' nor dictate where symptoms should act as metaphors; they can only react with each other when an energy puts them together.

Stress and its energy

Stress factors can vary widely between grief, anxiety, unexpressed anger, hatred, fear, depression or guilt. Stress in these guises creates perverse forms of mental and emotional *energy* which, often unable to find adequate expression on an emotional level, then proceeds to disturb the economy of the physical body, which is then disposed to suffer disease.

If it is accepted that such energy belongs to the science of physics and that chemical activity is the material result of energies that threaten the normal harmony of the body then, in disease reactions, we are witnessing an end product of an event that took place *before* the disease was manifest. *The physics of the cause creates the chemistry of the disease.*

Suppression of the symptom rather than the cause leaves the rogue energy that initiated the problem free to do it all over again. In other words, suppression takes no account of the history of the condition. Treating the negative chemical changes of the body with chemistry encourages the suppression of symptoms – and the causes are left untouched. Treating the causes which inspire those chemical changes with matching 'energy medicine' encourages physical processes of elimination and less susceptibility to the stress factor.

Each patient needs a specific and characteristic *energy medicine* to relieve him or her of their symptom picture but no-one gets better unless the causative energy factor is taken into account in the selection of that remedy. All of which indicates that *the physics of the self-healing process inspires the chemistry of symptom relief.*

Unless the spirit, mind and emotions (so often involved in the causation of disease) are treated in a patient, the body will either not respond to treatment or will react only partially, only to succumb once again. From this it is clear why steroids and antibiotics create only a temporary relief and why surgery, on its own, is no permanent answer. Though drugs and the knife may be needed they should always be viewed as palliative and not curative. They do their best work when they afford the patient time to gather together the resources of the Vital Force necessary for recuperation.

How the self-healing system might be damaged

So, if there is such a thing as a Vital Force, why does it fall short of its task and allow the body to suffer? Could it be that all disease is essentially psychosomatic? What is it that happens in order for a psychical disturbance to have such a damaging effect on the physical body? If the psyche or the physical body are maimed, does this permanently compromise the so-called Vital Force?

First of all, emotions such as grief and anger are not the only things to affect the psyche – the mental 'body'. Shock in the form of fright or bad news, general anaesthesia and surgery, an accident and even overwhelming joy can all disturb the system sufficiently for it to go into a long term or chronic crisis. The imprint of the shock or the trauma is such that it is stamped on the system, compromising its ability to re-establish its former balance. The Vital Force itself is maimed; the shock is enough to keep it 'stuck' in a habit of reaction. We need an example to illustrate how this might occur.

A man of sixty-four came for treatment. He explained that he felt a fraud, as he did not have much wrong with him. However, he said that he felt tired most of the time and his limbs ached. He complained of poor sleep and how he could never feel comfortable when he sat or lay down. He had a fear: he was afraid that arthritis would set in. Though he was fairly uncommunicative, unused as he was to talking about himself, he did say that he was *"more ill-tempered than not most of the time"* and that this had caused his wife to send him along for treatment. He was then asked if he had ever received any medical advice for this condition. *"Good Heavens, no! What on earth for? What do I need a doctor for?"* he replied with a scowl.

The rest of the interview was taken up by taking details of his present and past circumstances to find out if there were any predisposing factors that might reveal why he should feel as he did. He was asked how long he had felt like this. *"I'm not sure but my wife seems to think it's been years but it's now getting worse."*

People who clearly have something wrong with them but say that they do not need any treatment, medical or otherwise, often need the remedy *Arnica*. Though a few other medicines also cover this odd state, *Arnica* is usually confirmed when the patient complains of aching, bruisy limbs and restlessness in bed – and even more especially where there is moroseness as well. He was given *Arnica* and asked to return for a follow-up appointment in six weeks. When he came back he appeared quite a different person. His expression was lighter; his complexion was not so grey; he had sparkle. He could hardly wait to speak of his reaction to the remedy.

"What was in that medicine!? Within three days of taking it a massive bruise came out on my chest and then on my abdomen. It seemed to work its way down my whole body, here on the left side and then onto my leg as well. There was no pain, just a deep-purple bruising. It was there for a week and then it was gone! But the amazing thing was that as it went down my torso all the aches and pains I've had for years started to go. My wrists aren't painful and they don't click any more. My knees are fine and I can run up and down stairs now. It's fantastic. I'm sleeping and I'm rested when I get up – and now my wife can sleep because I'm not tossing and turning all night. So what happened? To get a bruise like that I'm sure I'd have noticed doing something to myself – and then it wasn't painful, that was the extraordinary bit."

He was asked if he had ever in his life been involved in a car accident. He thought a while and then remembered that he had indeed been in an accident and that he had been hurt on the left side of his body. As he thought back about the incident he recalled the fact that no bruising had ever come out despite the severity of the pains and that it had puzzled the doctors who had kept him in hospital for a short period of observation. As he seemed to improve he was allowed home. *"But that was forty years ago!"*

He needed no further treatment and has remained well to this day. It was as if his body had been unable to express the physical accident in an immediately acute form – i.e. bruising. There *should* have been bruising. It is natural for the body to bruise after physical trauma but this man had not produced any reaction even though he had been so severely traumatised. *Arnica* is the prime remedy for bruising – both physically and emotionally – and has earned an unassailable reputation for this (even to the point where nurses have been known to supply hospital patients in their care with it). That extensive bruising on the area of a body severely injured even so long ago should come out, suggests that the body is capable of holding the memory of unexpressed trauma deep within. Had this man been given *Arnica* at the scene of the accident or soon afterwards, he would not have suffered the symptoms he came to have treated forty years later. Instead, the effect of the accident, which *should* have resulted in bruising, was held deep within the system, to be inappropriately expressed over the following years as aching, restlessness and moroseness – all of which was a chronic and latent expression of what should have been experienced acutely, immediately after the accident[2].

In other words, it is as if the self-healing mechanism or the Vital Force itself was handicapped by the initial shock and rendered incapable of dealing satisfactorily with the physical symptoms (even if he was able to continue a comparatively normal life otherwise). This case can be taken to illustrate the immutable fact that *homoeopathy does not treat chronic disease; it treats the handicapped self-healing process.*

The natural corollary of this is that once the integrity of the self-healing mechanism is restored it can then set about repairing the body and dealing with the disease state.

A homoeopath is always searching for how and why a patient's Vital Force or self-healing mechanism might be compromised. Though the essential details of any chronic condition suffered (i.e. the symptoms) are important – because they are the whole body's physical expression of the disease – they are seldom sufficient on their own (except in the case of mechanical injury) to determine the full story. There is always a context for the illness, which includes the patient's general susceptibilities as well as actual causation. We need another example to illustrate this point.

A man with the early signs of either Crohn's or ulcerative colitis came for treatment. (The doctors were uncertain of a clear diagnosis.) He described his condition in this way: *"From time to time I get this terrible pain in my insides. It feels as if someone is cutting me open. It always makes me exhausted and I feel so sick as well. The pain lasts for about an hour or so and then I have to go to the loo."*

He went on to add that when he got the pain he had to stop what he was doing and bend over double while pressing his clenched fists into his belly. At the same time he would break out in a cold sweat and would tremble. If his wife were to attempt to help him at such a moment then he would be furiously angry and tell her to leave him alone – this was a noteworthy symptom as he was, by nature, a very mild and even slightly effeminate man who was very much in need of support. (He brought his rather forbidding wife to the consultation with him and would frequently look towards her when answering.) It transpired that he had had this condition ever since he had been humiliated by some of his pupils who had substituted waste paper for his lecture notes in his briefcase. Until the moment he came for homoeopathic treatment he had been trying various different nostrums and potions from the chemist – antacids chiefly. He had been to his doctor who had prescribed painkillers and bowel binders.

These had had no effect at all, he said. He felt intimidated by his doctor who had told him that if his prescription did not help he would refer him to a specialist who would undertake tests, which would include taking a barium meal. The patient had come to homoeopathy not because he knew it would work but because he was afraid of hospitals and blood tests and wanted to rid himself of the symptoms as fast as possible in order to avoid the trauma and ignominy of investigation.

Though the pathology was potentially serious – he already felt that the symptoms were more frequent and severe than they had been at the start – the symptom picture was crystal clear. He was given *Colocynth* in a high potency and within two days he had no further symptoms whatsoever. Why? Because the remedy *Colocynth* addresses all the bowel and general symptoms as they were suffered by this man *after being humiliated* (the negative energy of humiliation being central to this medicine). It was the humiliation that had struck this man's self-healing mechanism. His body expressed his feelings in this way because he was unable to do anything, or to say what he felt about his pupils and, being unable to find words or actions to meet the situation, his body became stuck in the pattern of symptomatic pain. After taking the remedy he said he was able to 'switch off' from thinking over and over about the incident; as it was now past history he could 'let it go'.

In a case like this, allopathy puts the cart before the horse by treating the physical symptoms – and treating them with chemicals. When these do not work it is necessary to investigate the physical body with blood tests and X-rays. Even if the patient had been particularly prescient and had told the doctor that his problem was entirely due to a particular psychological stress, it would probably still have led to a chemical solution in the form of an antidepressant. One of allopathy's handicaps is that it has divided itself between pathology (of the physical body) and psychiatry (of the mind).

Treating the Whole

Though allopaths know perfectly well that psychiatrically unstable patients also suffer psychosomatic *physical* conditions they do not know how to treat the patient as a whole. This is because drugs and surgery only treat symptoms manifesting in a part of the Whole. Yet, many generations ago, Plato stated:

The cure of the part should not be attempted without the treatment of the whole. No attempt should be made to cure the body without the soul. If the head and body are to be made healthy you must begin by curing the mind; for this is the greatest error of our day in the treatment of the human body, that the physicians first separate the soul from the body.

The word 'soul', in our age, has heavy connotations but it should not detract from the thrust of Plato's words. It might be summarised as: you cannot treat and cure the body without taking the emotions, the mind and the spirit into consideration.

The first step to understanding susceptibility to illness

I hear you object: "That's all very well when it comes to psychosomatic conditions but what about bacterial and viral infections? These are not to do with spirit, mind or emotions. These are outside agents of disease."

Indeed they can be viewed this way but the body must be *susceptible* to the disease condition associated with the bug for it to produce its characteristic symptoms. A healthy body is no fit place for a bacterium or a virus to flourish. If fifteen children attend a birthday party held in a hot village hall and one sneezing individual is brewing a cold or 'flu or chickenpox, not *all* will develop the disease. Even if we subscribe wholeheartedly to the orthodox view of aggressive and invasive bugs it still has to be accepted that bugs rely on chance to find a system weakened by injury, previous illness, emotional trauma or age to find a suitable breeding ground. Without such predisposition bugs could not take hold any more than a tree seed will germinate if it falls on uncongenial soil.

You must have encountered a multitude of types of cold virus in your time and never shown the slightest symptom, not even a sniffle. Your immune system worked for you in each case and you were never aware of it. Yet it is equally true that people develop colds after an emotional upset, after a fall, after getting wet, after heavy exercise and then getting chilled – without encountering anyone else's infection! Children develop tonsillitis, not due to being brought low by the *streptococcal* bacteria but because their self-healing mechanism is weakened or deployed elsewhere, making them susceptible to the invasion. Times of teething or growth spurts are common for this; poor nutrition due to eating too many sweets and too much junk food is another pre-disposing cause. There is also the heredity factor to consider: it is common enough that one or other parent suffered the same problem when they were at the same age. In other words, where the Vital Force or self-healing mechanism is either temporarily weakened or otherwise engaged, the body becomes susceptible to the ravages of infectious diseases. It is not the other way round. *A vitally healthy organism does not become sick for no internal reason!* It certainly does not have to be a psychological reason; as we can see, it might also be due to physical trauma, lack of foresight for our physical welfare or a hereditary disposition.

Should drugs be the first resort?

Once susceptible to a bug or a cootie, why should we not use a drug to deal with it especially if the self-healing mechanism has been struggling? Antibiotics have a secure reputation for dealing with these infections so why should they be abandoned when they work so quickly? Steroids often come to the rescue in controlling severe breathing troubles and inflammatory conditions so should they, too, be left on the shelf? Can alternative means be as effective and speedy?

There are several reasons why, in short-term acute ailments, we should avoid the chemical drug solution *if we possibly can*. First of all, the self-healing mechanism is usually destabilised only temporarily (though this is not so for patients with underlying chronic illness). Once the system is aware of imbalance – from whatever source – it creates a set of symptoms in reaction. *It is not the disease agent that causes the symptoms; it is the body's reaction to a negative stimulus that creates symptoms.*

If, say, antibiotics are used to squash symptoms then the body has been stopped from doing what it does naturally – creating symptoms. Like any organism that is told that it is getting it wrong in spite of doing only what comes naturally to it, it becomes confused.

The point and thrust of all such reactions (either in short or long term illness) is *elimination through discharge*. Antibiotics stop discharges, dead! We have come to see discharges as inconvenient and disgusting and we look forward to having them stopped, yet the body really wants to get rid of waste products, often faster than the bowels or bladder could do it on their own.

So why are antibiotics so effective? Because they do kill off the bugs and this in turn means that the body no longer has to show a symptom reaction. However, this leaves the body with two problems: (i) the body's immune system has been bypassed and made redundant; (ii) nothing has been done about the original susceptibility to the disease.

Initially it might not matter that the immune system has been bypassed but if this happens too often then the body is rendered ineffective without the support of the chemical agent. The body becomes used to needing the drug and so 'believes in' its own incompetence. Here we find all those patients who resort to drugs at the first sign of symptoms. Patients with eczema, asthma, hay fever, bronchitis, cystitis, ulcers, or gout, all resort too soon to drugs they have become familiar with; they are stuck with a habit. It is none too rare these days to come across quite young patients who are on long-term antibiotics – 'just in case'. This is appalling but all too easily defensible using the rational philosophy of allopathy. No account is taken of susceptibility as a background cause for the recurrent problem because *Allopathy has no method of treating patients for their characteristic tendency to suffer particular conditions.* Treatment therefore remains the same for all: steroids for skin and lung problems; antibiotics for infections; anti-inflammatories for inflammation and so on.

Yet, suppose that someone developed a simple cold after a fit of anger, or hearing some really bad news – do not for a moment doubt that this can happen – and then the cold is neglected and the symptoms progress to a threatening bout of bronchitis. Inevitably, this would be dealt with by antibiotics, because the focus of attention has shifted away from the emotional distress and onto the opportunistic bug that is busy colonising the lung tissue. The original cause of *being susceptible* to fostering the virus is forgotten even though it was the degree of negative emotion that caused the patient to feel low enough about himself for his body to allow the cold to initiate a worse crisis. The antibiotics may kill off the opportunistic bug but the patient now has to deal with a suppressed immune system as well as the original emotion that brought on the whole episode. In homoeopathy, the treatment would have dealt with both the physical symptoms *and the psychological ones* – in one go. Thus the cold would not have developed to bronchitis. This is possible because homoeopathic remedies are not restricted to influencing the self-healing of physical symptoms but also the restoration of balance in the mental and emotional sphere as well – a distinct advantage over straightforward chemistry.

A positive view of infection

Surely, though, a common cold could not be regarded as a physical outlet for a set of feelings? Here is an example:

> A patient starts snuffling and sneezing and gagging on thick mucus in the throat pit; there is a cough which soon develops but is worse in the morning on waking up and then later in the evening. The nose feels blocked up but nothing comes out when it is blown. In spite of a dry throat and a claggy tongue the patient has little sense of thirst and even remarks on this and wonders if it is a potential problem. In addition there is a noticeable rise in body heat though, when the temperature is taken, there is no fever. Feeling so warm becomes irksome and the patient needs to be either in a room with the window open or outside in the fresh air. Being cooped up indoors makes her feel light-headed and air-hungry. Furthermore the patient admits to feeling very weepy and downhearted.
>
> *"The whole thing started after my cat died."* If this person were given *Pulsatilla* then the cold would clear up and the emotional symptoms would be eased with it. The real problem was not the cold; those symptoms were merely an *expression of reaction* while the immune system and the emotions were below par – a situation caused by, in this event, bereavement. *Pulsatilla* is a remedy that is often needed for such a situation and it is justly well known as a remedy for tearful grief – however apparently minor the cause.
>
> Had the initiating cause been not the death of a pet but, say, the loss of employment, then the story might have been different. The likely emotional symptoms of anger, disappointment and anxiety might then have been accompanied by a different physical symptom picture: runny nose with profuse sneezing and a sore top lip from having to use a hanky frequently; a hot head with a chilly body and a dry mouth and throat which call for sips of ice-cold water. Such a situation would demand

Arsenicum Album to deal with it. The result in both cases is the relief of the physical symptoms as well as the emotional ones. The bug is ousted, the immune system is restored and the susceptibility is eradicated. In effect, the *character* of the instigating 'trigger' as well as the patients' reactions, when individually assessed, announces exactly what needs to be done.

If antibiotics were used then only the bugs and, sometimes, the mucus would go, leaving in the first case the dry throat and temperature variation, light-headedness and weepiness or, in the second, the anxiety, restlessness and disappointment. Both patients would continue to feel distressed and would spend far longer recuperating.

For those who resort to antibiotics infrequently none of this may seem relevant but increasingly and especially among the younger generations, there is a markedly poor response to them combined with, paradoxically, an increased use of them. It is also well known that bugs are keeping pace with the development of new antibiotics. They simply mutate to render the drugs ineffective – but we should not be surprised by evolution, as this is what nature does best. The bugs want to survive and their simple life styles are geared to adapting to their environment.

Fortunately, though, our response to infection remains similar to the way it has always been: we still produce characteristic symptom pictures that can be matched by homoeopathic remedies.

Side effects and why they occur

There is a further reason for avoiding drugs: the side effects. Much of the bulk of the *British National Formulary* (BNF) – the allopathic doctor's *Materia Medica*, the descriptive book of drugs – consists of listed side effects and cautions on the use of drugs. If patients took the trouble to find out what is written about some of the drugs that are prescribed to them it is doubtful that they would take the prescription to the chemist, let alone swallow the pills.

Chemical actions have immediate and demonstrable results so it is easy to understand how we have come to rely on drugs. They work! But the laws of physics state that every action has a reaction. For every action of a force there must be a result. Chemicals are material substances; when they are applied medicinally it is the *primary* action of suppression that is required. What we see *first* is the reduction and elimination of a disease agent (such as bacteria) or the reduction of a swelling, so we initially believe that the drug is working positively. *Yet we have to remember that the symptoms being suppressed are creations of the body and not of the disease.*

Once the chemicals have completed their allotted task of suppression then the body reacts (the secondary action) to the fact that a foreign agent has been introduced into the system. If the chemical agent is relatively harmless then the reaction will be mild, even unnoticeable. If the chemical agent is toxic then the reaction will be proportionately severe. The awakened self-healing mechanism does not discriminate between a toxic chemical agent and a disease agent and will react in the most appropriate way to eliminate either one for its own safety. Hence the healthy person will have a short bout of diarrhoea after a course of antibiotics; the bowels are eliminating the toxic agent as swiftly and as conveniently as possible. The diarrhoea, therefore, is a direct (though secondary) result of a drug's action.

Everyone is aware, though, that nothing is as simple as that. If the patient's general system has been weakened by the condition as well as by the introduction of a drug to treat it, then the self-healing mechanism can react by becoming stuck in the mode of elimination so, for example, a state of chronic diarrhoea is set up. (Though, confusingly, in some cases the opposite happens and long-term constipation is the net result of the drugs.)

Frequent and recurrent use of a drug will always result in a progressively weakened response from the body. One of the fears most commonly expressed by severe asthma sufferers is that their drugs will become increasingly less effective. They base this fear on their experience with antibiotics. The same is often true for those who use steroids. Their dependency is not supported by confidence. This negative state of dependency often overrides the fact that many people on drugs (especially long-term) suffer accompanying symptoms – side effects. Their relief at losing the main symptoms of the condition often outweighs the inconvenience of sundry others. While the body's natural symptoms are being suppressed, others are cropping up as a result of the self-healing mechanism's attempt to rid itself of a foreign agent.

Look in the *BNF* and you will read that antibiotics can cause skin rashes, diarrhoea or constipation, hormonal changes and depression. Steroids can cause rashes, oedema, acne, adrenal insufficiency and atrophy (causing debility), peptic ulceration (stomach ulcers), inflammation of the joints and a host of other symptoms. We call them side effects but they are more properly the body's response to an outside, artificial and invasive chemical agent. The problem is that these drugs are always given in overdoses. They have to be given in this way in order to work because the body would otherwise eliminate them as a foreign body before they had achieved what they had been administered to do. Chemical drugs have to be given in doses large enough to overcome the body's natural reaction to the introduction of material that is alien to it. (Remember the instruction that you must finish the whole course of antibiotics? Now you know why.)

Getting the body to heal from the inside

Now look at the whole picture from the other way round. Suppose, as alternative practitioners believe, that symptoms are the body's *reaction* to a primary force – be it an epidemic (as in 'flu or cholera) or a psychological stress (as in grief or anger) or a mechanical trauma (as following injury). The cure should be found in administering something that stimulates the self-healing mechanism into appropriate *eliminative* action.

In healthy people it may not be necessary to prescribe anything as the healthy body often finds ways of stabilising: the fever will run its course, the bruise will fade, the distress will ease with time. In those whose Vital Force (and therefore the self-healing department) is either already compromised or severely handicapped by the *cause* of the present condition or by a pre-existing problem, the illness can take on a potentially chronic and threatening aspect. These are the patients in need of help from beyond the body's resources.

If an illness that is not spontaneously improving is the manifestation of a handicapped self-healing mechanism (that is producing symptoms in response to a force stronger than itself) *then the balance will remain in favour of the disease state*. Where drugs are administered long term (as in asthma, rheumatism, heart disease and so on) they can maintain an uneasy status quo but the body is, nevertheless, to some degree not its own master. It is forced to support a drug-governed regime as well as the suppressed cause of the original problem. *Drugs, given in large enough doses, are stronger than the Vital Force and quell symptoms created by it.*

In alternative medicine generally, the whole thrust of administering healing agents – whether herbs or acupuncture needles or homoeopathic pills – is towards promoting and stimulating the self-healing mechanism. If the Vital Force, under stress, has begun its work by producing certain symptoms of disease but has then got stuck and become incompetent to continue dealing with the illness, then the cure has to be in giving the system a boost that would *encourage the self-healing mechanism to finish the job that had been started.*

If a fever is the body's reaction to an epidemic cold or 'flu but the Vital Force cannot complete the process, thus leaving the patient in the same state for too long, then the cure will be found in something that will stimulate the body *to continue and finish the fever.* If a patient is too weak from unresolved pleurisy and pneumonia, then the cure will be found in a therapy that encourages elimination of waste (mucus), restoration of balanced body fluids and repair to any damaged tissue (i.e. in the lungs). (If you can believe that lacerated surface skin can be self-healed then you should have no doubt that internal tissue damage can be equally successfully repaired. It just usually takes longer because the damage takes place in situations where the self-healing mechanism is likely to be more handicapped.)

Cases to illustrate the need to stimulate the Vital Force

A five-year-old girl developed a fever after lunch. By 3 o'clock the temperature was 104°F and the child's face was bright red, the carotid arteries (in the throat) were pulsating, the pupils were dilated and delirium was setting in. The mother administered Calpol and put cool flannels over the forehead. By 5 o'clock the child was raving and seeing visions of monsters on her bedroom walls. Further doses of Calpol did nothing and the mother called the doctor and the homoeopath. The doctor, when he came 1½ hours later looked for telltale signs of a body rash and asked if the child had been screaming in pain or arching her back. (He was checking for meningitis.) Before he arrived the mother had already given a *Belladonna* to the girl on the advice of the homoeopath and the fever was somewhat reduced and she was calmer in herself. She had even fallen asleep for 20 minutes. The doctor checked the little girl's throat and found that she had very inflamed tonsils so he prescribed antibiotics and told the mother to call him if there were any adverse developments. The antibiotics were left on one side. The child was given one more dose of *Belladonna* that night when the fever began to climb again and by morning she had recovered, except that she now had a cold and was streaming with mucus from her nose. The child was kept home from school and within two days the last symptoms of the cold were gone.

Without explaining for the moment about the way a remedy works, suffice it to say that *Belladonna* was the energy medicine that was needed to trigger the self-healing mechanism into *completing the action of the fever* and creating a drain for the tonsils, pregnant with bug-heavy mucus. *Belladonna* (deadly nightshade) is famous for its affinity for fevered organisms. In recognising the specific characteristics of the *Belladonna* fever – it starts at 3 p.m., affects the head but leaves the extremities cold, pulsating arteries, delirium with visions of monsters, etc. – the homoeopath was able to select it as the remedy for this fever. No other fever remedy would have worked.

A more serious case will illustrate the depth to which the remedies are asked to go:

A man phoned from hospital to say that he had been suffering from what had been tentatively labelled myocarditis (inflammation of the tissue of the heart). He had severe stitching pains on both sides of the chest and was having difficulty breathing. He had a deep cough with rattling in the lungs but was unable to bring up any mucus. The doctors had done all sorts of tests and were puzzled and unsure of their diagnosis but had found that there was a shadow on the left lung and oedema of both lower lobes of the lungs. They had given him antibiotics and had drained the lungs of excessive fluid. He was very weak and unable to move without pain. What is more he was in deep depression and his girlfriend reported that he kept saying he was "worthless and good for nothing". He felt and said that he was sure that he would die. The homoeopath directed the girlfriend to give him *Aurum* (gold) in homoeopathic potency.

Within 24 hours all the depression had lifted. He was able to breathe more easily and he could walk about the ward. He still had the deep cough, although he was now bringing up quantities of thick, foul, green and yellow mucus. The man reported that he had urinated profusely after the remedy and had felt much better for that. What is more, he claimed he now felt much more at peace with himself than he did before he became ill; he felt able to tackle his work, which had been causing him great difficulties before. He did need other remedies to finish off the remaining symptoms of his chest but these were resolved within ten days. (It was absolutely appropriate that this patient was in hospital; he needed constant nursing. The problem was that the doctors were unable to treat the fundamental despair and feelings of worthlessness – feelings that were stronger than the state of infection.)

A homoeopath would interpret this as being an example of how the patient's self-healing mechanism had become incompetent through getting bogged down in emotional difficulties over his work and his perception of his own self-worth. *Aurum* is well proven in homoeopathy as a medicine that will encourage the Vital Force to redress imbalances brought on by low self-esteem and profound depression. Look how this man got better: he urinated his problem away! His body found the appropriate channel of elimination for excess water in the system. Once the bladder and kidneys were functioning as eliminative organs, the lungs stopped being water-logged and were able to get on with their job of gathering up infective mucus and ejecting it by coughing. His temporarily handicapped self-healing system was kick-started into action by gold – and nothing else would have done. It had to be gold because only gold has an affinity with such a bleak and depressive outlook in combination with pathology that affects the heart. (As it turned out he had had endocarditis with pleurisy and pneumonia but these labels hold little significance when what is really wanted is the *description* of symptoms that will individualise the required remedy.)

The right tools for the job

There is of course no irrefutable scientific proof that such a thing as the Vital Force exists, but there is absolute proof that there is a self-healing mechanism. There is a discriminating faculty within us that determines in what way a symptom picture should portray the cause of distress. What science refuses to see is that this mechanism can do more than simple repair jobs; that it is, in fact, capable of dealing even with major, life-threatening pathology *as long as it is given the correct stimuli when it appears to falter*.

The history of epidemic diseases and the way mankind has been ravaged by them goes a long way to explain why we should doubt our ability to get better without applying powerful agents (such as chemotherapy and surgery) to disease processes. So too does the study of some incurable chronic conditions for which no-one has found satisfactory 'cures'. Allopaths refer to 'spontaneous remission' in inexplicably cured cases of incurable diseases.

Since time immemorial, medicine men and their increasingly allopathic descendants have been applying herbs, minerals and the knife to both our everyday ills and serious pathology. It is not unreasonable to ask why this should not continue. The answer is that modern medicine has the technology and expertise – produced with the best of intentions – to develop ever more aggressively powerful means of suppression that are capable of compromising or even destroying the body's self-healing mechanism. Though allopathy is loosely based historically on herbal medicine, long gone are the days of an intimate and exacting knowledge of the natural use of medicinal plants. When scientists diligently search the jungle canopies for new cures and ask indigenous healers about their use, they make the fatal error of enquiring about diseases rather than people. The chemistry of the plants becomes the focus of attention and not what changes they can inspire in the life force of patients. Drugs are synthetically produced and thus the original natural resources are taken out of their natural context. The Vital Force of a sick body is not being matched by an equal force of nature when treated with steroids or antibiotics, beta-blockers or antidepressants; it is being faced with the stronger force of synthesised chemistry.

While Chinese herbal medicine, a holistic system that uses herbs as the medicinal basis for healing chemistry, is fully capable of restoring balance to the body's whole economy through treating a complaint of one part or organ and taking into account its relation to the rest, allopathic drugs could never be used in the same way. It is impossible to imagine an allopathic drug being used to restore order to a diseased body in any way other than simply as a suppresser of local symptoms. Indeed, most remove symptoms from one part while creating others elsewhere.

It is only in our modern times that the concept of a self-healing mechanism or the Vital Force has been so largely forgotten. Alternative practitioners remain content to believe in it – and without exhaustive laboratory based tests to prove it. It is enough to witness its actions through the positive influence of the tools of their particular therapeutic trades. They do have to make assumptions to explain the therapeutic actions of remedies – just as is suggested by the above *Aurum* case – yet those assumptions are based not just on the improvement in health of this or that patient but also on what we know of our means of effecting cure. Remedies used by homoeopaths; needles and meridians (energy channels) in the body used by acupuncturists, herbs by herbalists and so on, provide each practitioner with clinical observation and experience; so-called *empirical* medicine. Each knows from experience what the remedial agents of their profession are capable of.

Alternative practice in general is irrefutably experiential. Homoeopathy, not being exclusively chemically orientated, will not render its mysteries up to scientists who refuse to see that healing occurs only when physics takes charge of chemistry; when body energies are galvanised to create a new distribution of chemical reactions. Unfortunately, alternative practitioners have often laid themselves open to reasonable criticism by indulging in 'New Age speak' which has been making do for any explanation that would be acceptable to a trained scientist. Homoeopaths have not completely shed the 'caftan, pot and Jesus sandals' image of the 1960s so when we read of 'cosmic connections' between medicine and man, a chorus of sceptical objection is only to be expected. This is sad because it can discourage serious consideration of the whole concept of alternative therapy – not because there are no cosmic connections but because scientists find it impossible to quantify such things in terms of medical 'evidence'.

Homoeopathy, acupuncture and the other alternative medicines work without the necessity of believing in cosmic forces; such things are irrelevant to the experience of the healing process itself. Tiny babies and animals have no inkling of the finer points of philosophy but they do become well on homoeopathic medicine. Yet it is true that almost all homoeopaths do believe in the connection between the Vital Force and the energies of the cosmos even if they cannot find adequate words to express it. They see humanity as a refined expression of the same energies that made the planet Earth. They see man's self-healing mechanism as part of his Vital Force and see the link with Earth and her own healing force of nature; none of which need impinge on our acceptance of what one famous nineteenth century homoeopath called 'the testimony of the clinic'.

Observation of individual patients is time-consuming and gathering statistics on homoeopathy in the quantities that science would require would be astronomically expensive. In the face of ever-increasing technological advances and expanding knowledge of chemistry and genetics, there is very little incentive for science to bother itself about alternative views on any putative self-healing mechanism. If anything needs to be tested there are laboratories especially equipped and stocked with animals similar enough to us in terms of biological and genetic make-up to provide the necessary information. Yet laboratory protocols miss out on vital steps to true knowledge.

It is vital to understand not just the concept of a self-healing system, whatever name might be given to it, but also its *endless range of individuality*. Homoeopathy is meaningless without the aspect of individualisation – the very quality of life that is missing in the laboratory. While the biochemist's life work is dedicated to searching for the norm and the average, homoeopathy is the art of selecting a uniquely identifiable energy from nature's resources (a remedy) in order to stimulate a compromised or crippled self-healing mechanism. To understand how the process works it is necessary to know about the nature of the medicines, the nature of disease and the way these two forces interact.

CHAPTER 3

A DOSE OF YOUR OWN MEDICINE

'Like with like' and 'When a little equals more'

Homoeopathy suffers badly from explanations composed of neat and memorable catchphrases such as 'like cures like'. Here is a typical example taken from a national daily paper:

> ...the basic principle is treating like with like, meaning that a minute dose of a drug will cure symptoms which the drug would cause when given in a larger dose. For example, Belladonna (deadly nightshade) causes high temperature when given in large doses to a healthy person. Homoeopaths use it in tiny doses to treat some fevers.

And another:

> A substance that would cause the symptoms in a healthy person that are manifest in the patient to be treated, is diluted to a point where there is no measurable material substance and the result is given to cure the sickness.

It really is not surprising that homoeopathy is not taken seriously. There is no effort to explain the concept of 'like cures like' and there is no mileage whatever in trying to explain how a *dilution* of a substance can cure what a concentrated dose of it is capable of causing. Nor is there any guide as to what on earth is meant by 'tiny doses', a term that becomes especially confusing when the phrase is qualified by stating that the doses become more powerful the more they are diluted.

To find comprehensible descriptions of the principles of homoeopathy you need to go to textbooks that are written, all too often, in an impenetrable and didactic style mostly dating back to the 1800s. (There are exceptions such as George Vithoulkas's *Medicine of the New Man*, published by Thorsons). You really should not be asked to believe that a simple *dilution* of a substance would cure what a large dose will cause. You do not have to accept that a 'tiny dose' of anything will remove a disease caused by a 'larger dose' of the same thing. It is frankly absurd once it is then realised that the 'tiny dose' is one that has been diluted beyond the point of molecular reality. You need not wrestle with the concept that as a substance becomes more and more *diluted* it becomes more powerful. Homoeopaths who persist in giving out this explanation are making a rod for their own backs. The truth is both simpler and more complex than that and it takes a while to explain.

Poisons that demonstrate that 'like cures like'

We cannot move past the concept of 'like cures like' without thoroughly understanding what it means. The most usual way of beginning the explanation is to discuss one of the poisonous remedies – such as *Belladonna* or *China Officinalis* (the source of quinine). It is easy to comprehend that a dose of deadly nightshade would cause anyone to have symptoms. The same is true for *Arsenic*, *Mercury*, *Bromium*, *Stramonium* (a hallucinogen) or the venom of the bushmaster snake, *Lachesis* – to list but a very few of the sometimes deadly poisons used by homoeopaths. Each one of these substances is more or less toxic and would cause unique and very characteristic symptoms in anyone who took a material dose.

So to say that a patient might be suffering from a disease that looks like a case of poisoning by one of these substances is not too far fetched. Let's take an example:

> The patient is restless and anxious; suffers nausea and diarrhoea; has a dry mouth and throat, with dry cracked lips; is thirsty but only for small amounts of cold water; has burning in the abdomen which feels better when well wrapped up; is very chilly and shivery yet cannot bear too much heat around the head and is petulant and demanding. This description would have been very familiar to Agatha Christie as the symptom picture is that of arsenic poisoning. It also bears strong similarities to the characteristics of gastro-enteritis. Because of this

symptomatic match a homoeopath knows that the patient will respond to
the remedy made from this poison. Naturally the actual chemical poison
is not administered; only pharmacists and those with a licence are
permitted to handle such toxins. (We will come to how the remedy is
rendered not only harmless but also curative in due course.)

Anyone who has a condition with symptoms that have similar characteristics to the effects of the poisoning would be relieved of their illness by
taking *Arsenicum Album* in homeopathic potency. This is true not only for
gastro-enteritis; it is true for any disease state that is marked by these characteristics even if only part of the whole arsenic poisoning picture is
present. *Arsenicum* is one of the most usual remedies for the common cold:
blocked up nose with profuse, runny mucus which causes burning soreness
of the top lip; dryness of the mouth and throat with parched lips and the
need for sips of water; restlessness and irritability; chilliness with shivering
but a need to have fresh air circulating around the head. *Arsenicum* has an
assured place in any homeopathic first-aid kit: it deals with food poisoning,
coughs, croup, bronchitis, hay fever, fever, sore throats and asthma attacks.
It is also an important remedy for chronic heart, lung and stomach conditions as well as mental and emotional problems, all of which bear the
signature of the poison: restlessness, anxiety, chilliness, a demanding temperament and an underlying fear of their illness even to the point of a
profound fear of dying.

What is true of *Arsenic* is true of other substances. Here is another
example:

sore throat with dark red, almost purple discoloration of the mucous
membranes of the pharynx; swallowing is excruciatingly painful; the neck
looks and feels swollen, is discoloured a darkish red and any pressure
around the throat is unendurable. On examination it is very hard for the
patient to open the mouth or to protrude the tongue; when the tongue
does venture out it is trembling and pointed; the sore, constricted pains
start on the left side of the throat and move across to the right. The mood
of the patient is extremely unpleasant – he makes vicious remarks that are
intended to hurt. Depending on the severity of the symptoms the patient
would be diagnosed as suffering from tonsillitis, a viral infection of the
throat, or quinsy – but such a picture is similar in every respect to that of

someone who has been bitten by (and about to die from) the bushmaster or Surukuku snake from South America, which homoeopathy knows as *Lachesis*. A few doses of the remedy prepared from the snake's venom would cure outright a bad sore throat such as this. However, *Lachesis* is no less valuable a remedy than *Arsenicum*. It is used in many different types of pathology from boils and abscesses, piles, menstrual conditions such as fibroids, headaches, fever, high blood pressure, heart complaints and thrombosis. Wherever it is indicated there will always be those peculiar and characteristic symptoms of the snake: congestion of parts with stagnating blood, dark red or purplish discoloration of the skin and membrane surfaces, the intolerance to pressure, the shifting of symptoms from the left to the right side of the body and the typical sharp or even spiteful temperament. In psychosis, the *Lachesis* condition is evident from the similarity to the snake itself: wary and suspicious with a venomous tongue, restless and uneasy, timid at times but ready to go on the attack and with an inability to tolerate pressure from stressful situations.

Non-poisonous substances that show that 'like cures like'

These descriptions are easy on the intellect because we all understand the concept of poisoning by a chemical agent. The effects of non-poisonous substances are equally interesting however. Suppose we consider a substance that seems relatively harmless and has no record of poisoning at all. Camomile, for example, far from being a poison, is used as a soothing herbal tea. Once prepared into a homoeopathic remedy it will cure a patient (most often a baby or toddler) of any extreme pain that is accompanied by spiteful, irritable, unreasonable and demanding behaviour. The patient asks for things and when presented with them refuses them or throws them away; he may shout or scream in agony; a child may demand to be picked up and carried about – to be still would bring on the screaming again. The cause of the pain might be a toothache or teething; it might be an earache or a stomach cramp; it might be period pains. All these conditions will respond to the remedy made from camomile: *Chamomilla*. How do we know all this? Where does this come from? This does not seem to be 'like cures like' at all. Camomile is supposed to encourage sleep in those who enjoy it as a digestive drink!

Samuel Hahnemann: the first to notice a profound paradox

We need to step back a moment to see from a different perspective. Samuel Hahnemann (1755-1849) would not have been able to build the edifice of homoeopathy based on the herbal properties of camomile. His first inklings about what he came to call homoeopathy were connected with a plant that, though not a poison in the same class as arsenic, certainly had side effects when ingested. He was intrigued by a treatise that he found, written by a Glaswegian doctor on the herbal drug cinchona (which we know as quinine or, in homoeopathy today, as *China Officinalis*) which was made from the bark of a tree native to Peru, and which was making that country a fat profit as a cure-all for any type of malarial fever, by being exported to Europe. The paper described the effects of the drug on the body and these corresponded closely to the symptom picture of malaria (a condition he knew well as he was a medically trained chemist). At that time malaria was a major scourge of the armies tramping round the boggy battlefields of Austro-Hungary.

What intrigued Hahnemann was that cinchona bark had a reputation for *curing* malaria. He did not understand why the *cure* should also produce the *symptoms*. Being insatiably curious he set to work on *himself*, taking doses of the substance and then noting down the effects. He promptly produced the characteristic sweating, shivering, thirst, fever and weakness that belong uniquely to cinchona.

Being a true scientist he was intent on reproducing the results of the experiment – so he began experimenting on family, friends and colleagues by giving them doses of cinchona and observing the outcome. He found that they too produced similar symptoms – though he was far too keen an observer not to notice that each guinea pig had his own variations on the principle 'theme' of the drug.

Like a ferret after a rabbit, Hahnemann went on to study other substances that might demonstrate a similar pattern. He quickly noted the connection between the poisoning picture of deadly nightshade and scarlet fever. Mercury was already well known as a medicine for syphilis so he was furnished with information on the consequences of poisoning by this liquid metal and saw how, in some sufferers, the disease and the poisoning had similarities.

Imitating nature to find a cure

Hahnemann began to formulate the idea that *true cure was effected by imitating nature*; that patients suffering from a disease with a certain characteristic symptom picture would be cured of that disease if they were administered a substance that symptomatically imitated that disease. The *artificial disease* of the poisoning – that is the disease state produced by being given doses of poison – he began to believe, would act curatively on the patient with a pattern of symptoms similar to that brought on by a real disease agent. Once the patient had recovered from the side effects of the poisoning it would be seen that the disease symptoms had also gone.

The problem was that the cure was so terrible that many patients suffered horribly due to vicious side effects. (Which is what happened to patients who used mercury to cure syphilis.) The effects of the poisoning removed the symptoms of the disease though they all but destroyed the patient in the process; this was true of most of the metals and poisons that were in use at the time.

Hahnemann began to apply his new-found knowledge to his treatment of patients. In his effort to reduce the appalling side effects of these poisons Hahnemann began to dilute them. At first, in preparing dilutions of one drop of the tincture (in the case of plants) to ninety-nine of pure alcohol (which he regarded as inert and thus incapable of influencing the nature of the substance to be used), he was using material doses. This means that there was still raw plant material in the medicine; there were molecules of chemical substance that had the potential to influence the physical body. He called this first step the first potency. Not satisfied with this, due to the persisting (albeit milder) side effects, he diluted the tincture further and at the same solution of one drop to ninety-nine; which creates 100 drops that in Latin translate to a 'c' potency. (The successive potencies became known by their number: second, third, fourth, and so on.) His intention was to reduce the intensity of the side effects – which were referred to as 'aggravations'. Because the aggravations continued to be noted he persisted with the process of dilution, believing that he was seeking the minimum amount of the *material substance* that would effect the swiftest and gentlest cure.

He had, as yet, no clear concept of the Vital Force of the body, let alone of the intrinsic electrodynamic energies held within the atomic structure of the medicines he was experimenting with. He was no more of a biochemist than any of his contemporaries and had no means by which to measure his experiments except the clinical observation of results.

Hahnemann's inspired guess: 'Less can be turned into more'

With each process of dilution he 'succussed' the mixture – that is he repeatedly banged the phial of liquid on a firm surface (a leather bible) thus jarring the contents. Hahnemann noted that the further he got from the material, undiluted dose, the swifter and gentler was the cure. He was also aware that the further he got from the material dose, the more harmless any poison became; hence he was able to use lethal substances with less and less danger of causing harm. Being a marvellously gifted polymath he was quite aware that by the time he had reached the sixth dilution he was dealing with something *beyond the confines of Chemistry*. (Hahnemann eventually took remedies up to the 30th potency.) He knew that it could not be *only* the effects of dilution that brought about the more effective and gentler cure. He reasoned that there was some, as yet unexplained, natural force *within the body of the patient* that responded to some sort of *stimulus* inherent, after *succussion*, in the apparently diluted solution. This was the Vital Force responding to the dynamically transformed medicinal agent. His critics had a field day; they treated him with derision – much as they do today. Yet Hahnemann's basic premise has been expanded and developed beyond anything that contemporary science is able to measure: his modest scale of potencies up to the 30th now stretches to astronomical limits. Available to any working homoeopath are remedies in the 100c, 200c, 1M (the equivalent of one thousand c), 10M, 50M and CM (hundred thousand c). Although these numbers indicate the degree to which the medicines have been diluted, they can only make any sense to us if we see them as describing the depth of healing effect that a remedy's atomic energy would have on a patient's Vital Force.

It was Hahnemann's realisation that, while there was a Vital Force within each of us – a marshalling of the resources of body, mind and spirit – there was also a correspondingly potent force within the succussed liquid of any medicinal substance that he chose to test – whether poisonous or not! Genius though he undoubtedly was, he could not have explained the 'Why?' and 'How?' – any more than we can today. Hahnemann had to content himself with speculating that the Vital Force amounted to some form of electromagnetic energy – an idea that we have held onto since. He also realised that succussion (and trituration – a system of grinding the substance with milk sugar – in the case of insoluble minerals such as gold and silver) was in some way vital to the whole process and was the key to unlocking whatever unidentifiable energy he had been tentatively using to heal patients; patients who were increasingly demanding his attention. He knew nothing of quantum physics but he was bang on the mark. The electromagnetic forces within the atoms that make up every molecule of any substance were unknown to him but he would not have been surprised by their discovery. His intuition, one hundred and fifty years ahead of his time, served him well.

'Proving' medicines

Having stumbled on the curious and revolutionary notion that the toxic effects of certain substances mimicked and yet would also cure specific sets of disease symptoms and that this was not an anomaly shared by only a few of the known poisons, it did not take much more than his intuition to take the next step. This was to see what other substances, once processed through succussion and dilution, would do. He began to give prepared, 'potentised' medicines to 'provers' – healthy people who had no illness.

His intention was to see whether and how these healthy people would react to the medicines. He had already discovered that he and his provers could replicate, startlingly precisely, artificial malaria symptoms by taking the *material* dose of cinchona; and that this same plant in *potentised* dilution would cure the actual disease gently and efficiently. (Hahnemann gained a substantial reputation for being able to cure malaria among a particular army of soldiers – to the eternal gratitude of their commanding officer.) Having seen how patients got better having taken the potentised remedies (i.e. <u>succussed</u> *dilutions*) he had so far studied, he saw the importance of testing such preparations on the same premise as that which had governed cinchona.

The provers, following strict guidelines, registered any symptoms that arose as a result of taking repeated doses of whichever potentised medicine was to be proved. The details of each prover's experience of each remedy were collated and the symptoms that were common to all the provers quickly established in what disease states that remedy would be of curative value. It was the core symptoms that described the individuality of the medicine and that would, by and large, be present in any case that indicated its use. Provings also showed that while each medicine almost always had a hard core of universally produced characteristic symptoms, there were also other symptoms that were produced by a substantial number of provers (but not all) and there were a few symptoms that were evident in only one or two provers. This suggested that provings were subject to the individual susceptibilities and sensitivities of the provers; it was shown that some people were more sensitive to some remedies than others and produced more and abstruse symptoms.

Individual sensitivity is equally apparent in the differing responses of patients to the conventional chemotherapy of today. There is absolutely no guarantee that every patient given a particular drug will react in the same way. Some will produce no side effects while others might react horribly. Yet there is no system within orthodox medicine by which individual patients can be tested for side effects *before* they take their drugs. Though clinical trials on people do take place (often on medical students), these furnish us only with a list of *potential* side effects and do not tell us what type of person is likely to produce them. If you were prescribed a drug for, say, high levels of cholesterol, there would be no guide to tell you that you were particularly at risk of any adverse reactions (such as raised blood pressure – a common enough reaction!) A list of potential side effects is included in the *British National Formulary* (*BNF*) but if you were to ask your doctor whether you personally were safe from any unpleasant symptoms as a result of taking his prescription he would be quite unable to say 'Yes' with any certainty.

The system of proving remedies on healthy people has enabled us to build up a vast store of knowledge about many hundreds of substances. Hahnemann was an inveterate experimenter and his experiments were conducted under conditions that would have satisfied the scrutiny of any sceptical scientist of his day – had they troubled to investigate what he was doing. His evidence is still in print today. He proved over a hundred sub-stances and he used them to heal all those who sought his help in spite of the bad press he received. He handed down his knowledge, skill and meth-ods to pupils who continued his work. Over the following two centuries the *Materia Medica*, the book of descriptions of the established homoeopathic medicines, begun by Hahnemann and added to ever since by his disciples, has swelled enormously and includes remedies to raise the eyebrow of many a scientist – such as camomile or dog's milk (*Lac Caninum*), nitro-glycerine (*Glonoin*) or scorpion!

Each substance proved has its own characteristic symptom picture

Hahnemann discovered that harmless substances were, when potentised in the method he precisely laid down, as capable of becoming curative agents as poisonous ones. Each medicine that he produced and every one that has since been proved demonstrates a unique symptomatology – each of them has a distinct symptom picture, their own signature if you like, that is instantly recognisable. This reflects the fact that the *movement and relation-ship* of electrons and protons and whatever else may be within the atoms that are bound together by electrodynamic force to make up the molecules of any given substance are unique to itself. In other words, the electrical vi-brations of the building blocks of each substance are what distinguish it from any other. These movements can be different in terms of speed as well as intensity and so it is that we find that remedies have the reputation for be-ing either fast or slow, of having a short or long duration of efficacy. It is also why some remedies are said to suit tall, thin, 'sparky' people and others may suit short, fat, pale people; why some remedies are known for healing, say, inflammatory processes and others for healing blood poisoning.

Putting Hahnemann's discovery to the test

Orthodox medical science complains that there is no proof that any of Hahnemann's findings are true, and yet not one scientist, critical of the principles of homoeopathy, has yet set up a proving of a remedy using

Hahnemann's guidelines with the express intention of proving Hahnemann wrong. Why not? Hahnemann was absolutely clear in his description of the procedures for proving medicines. It would be perfectly straightforward to follow his 'recipe'. A selection of somewhere between twenty and forty volunteers would be needed. A proportion of them would be 'controls' and would take only placebo pills. The remainder would take a remedy in a selected potency (say the 30th) at the rate of two or three doses per day. The provers would be asked to continue taking the remedy either for a prescribed period of time (perhaps a week or a month) or until the symptoms produced were so uncomfortable as to cause distress to the individual. If *just one* prover were to produce one symptom (mental, emotional or physical) as a direct result of taking the potentised remedy – and then lose that symptom as soon as the remedy was stopped – then homoeopathy would have demonstrated its potential. (It should be noted that most provers need to take the remedy that they are testing for quite some time for *physical* symptoms to become manifest – which would provide the most convincing result. Homoeopathy still remains one of the safest systems of medicine ever devised and anxious mothers of recalcitrant children who swallow the little white pills as sweets need have no fear.)

A summary of the basic principles of 'like cures like'

To summarise:

i) All substances have an atomic structure which is possessed of physical energy created by the movement of its constituent parts – which add up to what we might loosely (and very unscientifically) call 'vibrations'.

ii) The characteristic energy patterns of each substance are identifiable by their specific effects on the body, mind and emotions of a healthy subject who takes the homoeopathically potentised preparation.

iii) Energy occurring in natural substances produces symptoms of a disease state peculiar to itself when taken by a healthy person. This is an artificially induced disease state that is temporary.

iv) When the prover stops taking the remedy his Vital Force will re-establish its normal equilibrium – though sometimes the effects on a sensitive subject are so profound that the symptoms need to be eased by the administration of another and antidotal remedy.

v) A remedy, capable of causing an artificial disease state in a healthy person, when given to a sick person who is suffering from a condition with the same or similar symptoms as the artificial disease, will provoke the Vital Force into re-establishing a balance as close as possible to health.

vi) The artificial disease, being superimposed on the sickness, stimulates the self-healing mechanism to respond to it and in the process removes both. This is 'like cures like'.

There is something much closer to home that demonstrates 'like cures like' as well.

An old wives' principle

Anyone who has a hangover knows about the 'hair of the dog' – i.e. taking another drink as a cure. In earlier generations, before the advent of the ubiquitous Calpol, mothers knew that wrapping a feverish patient in a blanket in a hot room would often cure a fever. Old soldiers will tell tales of camp or desert fevers cured by wrapping the patient up and sitting them in a tin hut to sweat it out. These are all examples of mimicking the disease in order to cure it.

Here is a curiosity from a casebook:

> A patient complained of a severe pain in the big toe, which he said was caused by stubbing it on a door frame. He suspected that the bone was cracked and as it was not healing even after two months he felt that homoeopathy might help. (He had had no other treatment.) He was prescribed various remedies over the next several weeks but there was no improvement in spite of the affinity of the remedies chosen for damaged bone. (These were *Ruta* – common rue – and *Symphytum* – comfrey.) However, when he returned for the next appointment he said that the toe

was completely better and he went on to explain what had happened. He recounted how the original injury had been caused by stubbing his toe on the door frame of the French window when he lashed out with his foot at a neighbour's marauding tomcat. The toe got better only after another visit from the same cat and following the same infuriated reaction from the patient. He was unimpressed by the failure of the remedies but he was struck by the truth that 'like cures like'.

Not all fevers are susceptible to being sweated out just as not all hangovers are responsive to taking another drink. It is the concept of 'likes' that needs to be established. 'Feed a cold and starve a fever' was a favourite maxim of the nursery yet not all colds respond well to this treatment. In some cases this should be altered to '*If* you feed a cold then you *will have* to starve a fever.' A patient suffering from a feverish cold that would respond well to *Phosphorus* would probably feel very hungry and do better if he ate; one enduring the cold symptoms that correspond to *Pulsatilla* would probably show no appetite at all and would suffer more if persuaded to eat anything.

'Like cures like' even when it's different

Here is a case that compares the different medicinal approaches of allopathy and homoeopathy:

Melinda, a girl of seven, was brought for treatment. She did not look at all unwell but the mother explained that she had undergone a change of personality. She was unable to be exact as to when the change had come about but she knew her daughter had 'not been right' for at least three years. The girl, she said, was always angry and would fly into a rage at the slightest provocation. She would go red in the face, shout, scream, throw things and bite anyone who came anywhere near her. She would also spit at people who tried to reason with her. When she was not being angry she was delightful. At night she suffered terrible nightmares and she would, at times, appear almost delirious with them. The mother explained that her daughter was quite clever and "*until all this started she was so docile – my little angel!*"

Melinda sat silently through her mother's description and showed no emotion on her face at all. When asked if she agreed with what her mother had said she nodded her head exaggeratedly. Further questions elicited the information that whereas the girl had always been prone to feeling the cold, she now always felt hot.

Enquiring about the child's history brought out a significant clue about the personality change. Some three years before she had had a very high fever – 104°F – that had continued for so long that the doctor had been called to the house. He had prescribed antibiotics, which had had no effect. Eventually she was sent to hospital where she was packed in ice to reduce the fever artificially. After a while the fever reduced and the child was permitted home. The mother was intrigued by the thought that the behavioural changes might have begun soon after the suppression of the fever – by such radical means – but asked how her present condition could be treated so that she could *"have my little girl back"*.

The girl was given *Belladonna* 10M – a very deep-acting potency). Two months later the mother reported that the girl had completely recovered – and had done so within three days of beginning the remedy. She was no longer angry; she was no longer so hot; she no longer had nightmares. Since then she has remained well.

The doctor was not wrong to send Melinda to hospital. According to allopathy he was not wrong to prescribe the antibiotics. There could be no criticism of his caring attitude or that of the nurses who looked after her once she was in the ward. It was the procedure of suppression that was wrong. Ice does not *cure* fever! So immense was the effect of the shock to her system of packing her in ice that her body, driven to reduce the fever, had to put the fever into some other form. In other words, the fever was transformed into a more generalised, chronic state of unnatural permanent body heat and into behavioural disorders probably brought about by the excessive heat in the head. What had been a straightforward though very unpleasant fever had become something far more sinister – a personality disorder that, had it not been treated successfully, would undoubtedly have handicapped the child's whole life, as well as disturbed the family dynamics permanently.

How can we be so certain that it was the suppression of the fever that caused the personality change? How can we be sure that it was not some coincidence that brought on the disagreeable behaviour pattern at approximately the time of her experience in hospital? The answer is absolutely direct: because the remedy that *would* have treated her original fever and the one that *did* treat the personality change successfully were one and the same: *Belladonna* – a medicine that covers both brain fever and raging delirium.

Medicines have personalities

How is it that a fever remedy can treat psychological disorders? If *Belladonna* does treat these two seemingly quite separate types of disorder then do other remedies have equally wide horizons? In allopathy drugs are viewed as being therapeutic for specific disorders: antibiotics are for infections, steroids are for bad asthma attacks, *Digitalis* and its derivatives are for heart conditions and so on. In homoeopathy medicines are not seen specifically in this therapeutic light. Though homoeopaths talk loosely of fever remedies, ulcer remedies or gout remedies, they are actually speaking about medicines that have an affinity for patients with these conditions. In general, most homoeopathic medicines have far wider applications than therapeutic limitations would imply. The medicinal energy of *Lachesis* might be indicated in tonsillitis, inflammation of the gall bladder or a breast abscess; *Lycopodium* might be indicated in appendicitis, eczema or pneumonia of the right lung. The heart of understanding the relationship between patients and homoeopathic medicines is that remedies have affinities for people who produce symptoms that are similar to the symptomatic effects they have on healthy people; the artificial disease state that provers produce: comparing 'like with like'. What is more, each remedy has its own characteristic affinities for areas of the body (left or right; chest or heart; circulation or glands) which are intrinsically part of the personality of the medicine. *Belladonna* favours the right side in earache and sore throat while *Pulsatilla* favours the left; *Mercurius Solubulis* (mercury) is a right-sided medicine in throat, gland and lung conditions but *Lachesis* is principally left-sided but with the habit of shifting to the right. Furthermore, remedies induce psychological states in their provers; people who have mental and emotional symptoms that accompany their physical symptoms are not manifesting anything separate from their disease state. On the contrary, they are showing the wholeness of their condition. It is by knowing the physical affinities as well as the psychological profiles of the homoeopathic medicines we are able to prescribe on the whole person.

The answer to the question as to whether a remedy like *Belladonna* can treat two apparently different disorders lies in studying the *Materia Medica* which is based on provings of the remedies and clinical evidence of healing gleaned from two centuries of practice. You have only to look in the homoeopathic *Materia Medica* to read what symptoms are listed there, to find out what a particular remedy will cure because only symptoms either manifested by the provers or that have been cured through the administration of the medicine will appear in the descriptions. Each remedy is set out in a specific manner.

There is first the generalised description of each of the disease states that are covered, followed by: what parts of the system are affected chiefly; what character of symptoms – such as quality of pains (whether sharp, dull, hot, neuralgic, throbbing etc.) or quality of discharges (whether thin and watery or thick and purulent etc.). Such information is known as the 'generals' as it covers that which affects the whole system. For example, *Belladonna* is described in the following manner:

Chief action is on the brain and nerve centres causing changes to the special senses which include twitching, convulsions, pains, excitement even to fury. Blood circulation is also altered and blood vessels become dilated, full and congested with pulsation. There are surges of blood into the head leaving the extremities with reduced circulation. The effects are sudden and violent. The chief characteristics are heat, redness and throbbing with dryness of the skin and mucous membranes. Pains felt anywhere in the system can be sharp, cutting, spasmodic or fleeting. Pains can be accompanied by a sense of local constriction or more generalised jerking or twitching. There is great sensitivity to light or noise both of which can induce spasms of other symptoms. Causation can include ill effects of hair cutting or washing the hair; air sickness; eating bad meats (esp. sausages); sunstroke; becoming chilled after being overheated. Acts as a prophylactic in scarlet fever. Very common in childhood diseases esp. for fevers; tonsillitis; teething. Also resolves boils and carbuncles with characteristic symptoms as well as insect stings, infected animal bites; also exophthalmic goitre; thyroid toxaemia, hydrophobia. Symptoms are often on the right side of the body.

This is very specific information and is very wide ranging. It shows that *Belladonna* not only acts on the physical body as a whole but also on individual parts and organs as well as on the sensorium (the central nervous system) and the mind and emotions (notice the word 'fury').

The next part of the written description is about what causes aggravations and amelioration. This is what makes the patient feel better or worse while they have the general symptoms.

> *Worse for: the sun; becoming overheated; draughts esp. to the head; light; noise; being touched. Suppressed sweating. Any pressure; letting the affected part hang down; lying down. 3 p.m. Looking at running water or shining objects. Vaccination.*

> *Better for: resting; leaning head against something hard; bending head or body backwards; light covering.*

The next section described is labelled 'Mind'. This covers all the effects of the medicine on the psyche and in *Belladonna* they are rich indeed.

> *Excited, nervous and ferocious. Quarrelsome with biting, spitting, striking and tearing. Cries out in fury or in delirium or fear of imaginary things. In nightmares or feverish delirium sees monsters, wild or black dogs or other outlandish things. Desire to escape or run away and hide. Very restless. Talks fast in excitement. Tends to dance, sing and whistle then becomes taciturn with a tendency to weep followed by fury. Easily startled or frightened by the approach of others esp. strangers. An angel when well but a fiend when sick. All mental symptoms accompanied by excessive body heat and redness (though can become pale during a fever). Has its greatest influence on those with strong intellect and plethoric constitutions so often needed by children.*

The rest of the description of the remedy is composed of sections for each part of the system affected by or with an affinity for the medicine. These include head, eyes, ears, nose, face, mouth, throat, stomach, abdomen, bladder, male and female generative organs; respiration (chest and lungs), heart, neck, shoulders and back, extremities, skin, sleep and fever. It would be tedious to read through all this information unless one had a particular purpose in doing so. Suffice to say that the information is exhaustive and covers all that we know about the symptomatology of the remedy.

It would be naïve to imagine that a single patient could possibly suffer all the symptoms described in any one remedy; it is clearly impossible, and knowledge of many of the remedies reveals that they have contradictory states as well. (*Sulphur*, for example, can be either very hot or sometimes freezing cold.)

The *Materia Medica* is a listed description of all the *possible* effects that have been produced by a large number of provers and patients. Not everyone reacts in the same way to a particular stimulus. Where one prover of, say, *Calcarea Carbonicum* (calcium carbonate) may suffer a loss of appetite, another would develop a craving for pasta and yet another would crave indigestible things such as chalk or uncooked potato. However, all the major remedies that we use all the time (some 150–200 of them) have very characteristic portraits that are unmistakable. We can almost always tell when a patient needs *Pulsatilla* (the pasque flower) because the core symptoms of dependency, a tendency to weep, a sense of slight (or considerable) claustrophobia, a marked lack of thirst and need for air, are present in the condition, whether it be a fever or a cold or a stomach upset. We can tell when *Lycopodium* is needed because the core symptoms: flatulence, bloating, a drop in energy, or aggravation of the symptoms between 4 and 8 p.m., are so often present in whatever illness has been diagnosed and often in a person who maintains a front of self-confidence but who is really only truly secure when bolstered by close family and friends.

Diagnosis by symptom picture and not by labels

Because it is not the disease that is important but the way the Vital Force reacts to (or in) a disease state, homoeopaths do not usually concern themselves with disease labels, though they can be a useful pointer as to which direction the body might be taking. If the practitioner knows that the patient is suffering from multiple sclerosis (MS) then he knows that he is likely to be dealing with a different and probably narrower range of remedies than if it were thyrotoxicosis (a suffering thyroid gland). Yet several remedies listed in the treatment of MS also appear in the literature as being of value in healing the thyroid: *Natrum Muriaticum* (rock salt), *Lycopodium* (club moss) and *Phosphorus* for example.

There may be no difference in remedy choice for the patient suffering from gall stone colic and one suffering from haemorrhoids; or one with gastro-enteritis and another with a peptic ulcer. *Nux Vomica* has a well-established record in instigating the cure of both piles and liver problems; *Arsenic* has an equally distinguished career in dealing with ulcers, asthma *and* diarrhoea and vomiting. The homoeopath is always looking for the telltale *signature* of a remedy within the symptom picture that will lead to the selection of what is referred to as the 'indicated remedy'. The signature is always made up of keynote symptoms: *Belladonna* is always 'red, hot and throbbing'; *China* is always oversensitive and delicate, bloated, thirsty and much worse for having lost too much body fluid; *Apis* (bee sting) is always fidgety, irritable and dozy by turns and suffers stinging pains and puffiness of affected parts.

Some of these marking or keynote symptoms are quite abstruse and some are glaringly obvious. Some are psychological and some are exclusively physical. Much of a student homoeopath's time is spent studying these medicines and learning their sometimes very subtle differences. This is the stage at which the student starts to describe a person as being a '*Belladonna* patient' or an '*Arsenicum* patient' or a '*Lycopodium* type' or a 'typical *Sulphur*' which can seem rather patronising. It is also when students begin describing some medicines as 'constitutional remedies' and others as 'acutes'. In other words a process of compartmentalising goes on. This has led to a certain amount of 'homoeopath-speak' that can be confusing and contradictory.

Suffice to say that some remedies are used more commonly than others. These medicines are the ones that seem to be more useful because they cover so many of the different but typically common ills that the Vital Force needs help to resolve.

Remedies such as *Arsenicum*, *Calcarea Carbonicum*, *Sulphur*, *Silica*, *Phosphorus*, *Thuja* (one of the *cupressus* trees) and *Lycopodium* are known as '*polychrests*' because they are used in so many different types of disorder. Others such as *Menyanthes* (buck bean), *Spartium Scoparium* (common broom), *Oxytropis* (locoweed) and the like are often unused from one year's end to the next because the kind of mental and physical reactions inspired by disorders treated by these medicines are less common, or because these medicines have not yet had a thorough proving and are therefore incomplete pictures. They are, however, just as vital because if any one of these so-called minor remedies is indicated by the patient's symptom picture then nothing else will do. We can illustrate this point:

> A woman of fifty came for treatment. She said that she had been going through the menopause for the last few months and that she felt that she had been doing rather well. She had been to her doctor for a routine check-up as she was going to Australia for a long stay with her daughter and "*wanted to be sure that all was as it should be*". The doctor had found that her blood pressure was high. He was concerned that the long flight to the Antipodes would cause her physical distress so he prescribed for her. "*I didn't fancy the idea of beta-blockers or anything like that,*" she said, "*so I thought I'd try out something herbal or alternative.*"
>
> The patient seemed fit and well in every respect. She did not appear to have any physical disorder in the respiratory or digestive system; she did not have any stress apart from the fact that her daughter lived so far away: "*but then I'm doing something about that, aren't I?*" She said herself that she felt that her condition was to do with the menopause as she did feel hot at night and this was a new symptom even if it did not distress her. She knew that she was "*supposed to feel hot at this time of life.*"
>
> For people who are constitutionally well with only a raised body heat and no other abnormal signs *Sulphur* is probably the most indicated remedy. She was given a dose of *Sulphur* 100 and asked to return in a fortnight to have her blood pressure checked. This she did and said that she felt well and that her energy certainly had had a boost. "*I felt better in myself.*" Yet her blood pressure was still too high which surprised her. She was then prescribed *Spartium Scoparium* 1x in drops. (This potency is made by succussing one drop of the mother tincture – the original plant material steeped in ethanol – in only nine drops of pure alcohol rather than one in ninety-nine. So in this prescription there was very definitely still some of the material substance of the remedy present making it a herbal medicine in part, as well.) She was asked to take one drop per day.
>
> When she returned she explained that she had only ever taken one drop because she had felt the effects of the remedy at once. It had made her feel hot all over and then weak. She fell into a deep sleep and woke in the morning slightly disorientated but feeling better. She did not care for the experience so she went back to her doctor and asked him to check her blood pressure thinking that she would probably have to take the drug he had offered her before. She was delighted to find that her blood pressure was normal. The doctor had quite rightly asked her to return in

two weeks to see if there would be any further variation. (It is common enough for blood pressure to fluctuate quite widely and such cases should be monitored regularly to find out if there is a pattern.)

She kept her appointments with the homoeopath in the following months before going to Australia but she needed no further treatment as the blood pressure remained steady and at a healthy level. *Sulphur*, one of the most universally used remedies in the entire homoeopathic canon, had to bow to the single drop dose of tincture made from the common broom plant. (Patients with high blood pressure should note that *Spartium* is a mild poison and should only be prescribed by a professional practitioner.)

Making the most of our plant life

Many of the plants used in homoeopathy are also familiar to chemists. *Belladonna* and *Digitalis* (foxglove) are, perhaps, the most famous. There is a swell of interest in the yew tree, *Taxus Baccata*, as it is reckoned to be the most promising potential cure for some kinds of cancer. The forests of Brazil and Malaysia are the source of many exciting plants that may yield their extraordinary healing properties to diligent scientists and their menageries of rabbits, mice and monkeys. The idea for the use of such plants often stems from the local folklore. Many plants have been used as cures for hundreds of generations.

Is Hahnemannian potentisation the only difference between homoeopathy and allopathic use of such natural medicines? No, it is not. Biochemists study plants at the microscopic level. Each plant is made up of not just one substance but of many and sometimes of hundreds. In the laboratory the plant is analysed for all its chemical constituents. Through tests on slides, dishes and animals, the potentially useful chemicals are isolated and, if proved to be suitable for further testing as drugs, they are synthesised. There is often no necessity to use the original plant, as the chemical composition is reproducible *artificially*.

Two differences in the homoeopathic approach stand out like beacons. The first is that no homoeopathic remedy is ever tested on anything other than humans. The second is that homoeopathy is interested in what healing powers the *whole* plant has. The plant is as it is because of the interrelation and interaction of its constituent parts. Natives of the areas from which plants are taken know what the plants will do to heal – and they have never had the benefit of a test tube in their lives. When a homoeopathic pharmacist makes a remedy from a plant he uses either the *whole* plant: root, stem, leaf and, when appropriate, flower as well, or a sample of it that contains the full complement of its constituent chemicals.

Ancient Roman women knew well that deadly nightshade would enhance their beauty by dilating their pupils to increase their allure; hence the name *Bella Donna*, 'beautiful woman'. Biochemists extract atropine from the plant – used by eye specialists to dilate the pupils artificially – yet the rest of the plant's composition is ignored. Taken as a whole plant and subjected to the process of potentisation in the homoeopathic pharmacies, *Belladonna* is the most common childhood fever remedy and proves itself as such on an everyday basis. In addition, as we have noted, *Belladonna* will cause a patient to have a self-healing reaction that will deal with any condition that has at its core great internal heat with pulsation and redness – even if there is bacterial or viral involvement. This response might cover not only fevers but also boils, bites and behaviour patterns as we have witnessed in Melinda's case.

Herbs, homoeopathy and modern medicine

It is worth underlining the difference that exists between what modern science and alternative practitioners make of natural remedies. Chemists search for chemicals that will cause *specific* and often *local* functional reactions in patients and that will most speedily remove symptoms. These chemicals, being so often inspired by nature in the form of plants, are synthesised to mimic the active ingredients found in plants: synthesised drugs are chemical substitutes for the original raw material. (It is far more cost effective to manufacture drugs in a laboratory than to maintain farms for the propagation of herbal remedies. Synthesised chemicals are also far more stable and reliable than anything grown under conditions that might vary due to weather, pollution or soil quality.) The patient, reacting to the chemical, makes no general effort to get better; his physical body, unable to create its own curative process, allows the drug to work on his sick tissues.

Herbal medicines, on the other hand, when chosen for their affinity to the individual expressing his or her peculiar condition, though still very much material chemistry, are capable of encouraging not just the elimination of symptoms but also the instigation of cleansing discharges. Discharges are simply not within a chemist's sights. Indeed, drugs are most commonly prescribed by allopathic doctors with the express intention of *stopping* discharges. We have created a situation in which we have a natural and abundant resource which we have put to polar opposite uses in the vain hope of achieving the same end.

Plants have been the main medicine chest for thousands of years and it is only with the advent of modern allopathy that we have lost the lore and ancient traditions of healers. This has only taken a few hundred years. Herbalists carry on a practice that carries a history that far outstretches any other art of healing. Modern homoeopathy is an extension of herbalism; broader in its scope only because of the accidental discovery of the electro-dynamic properties inherent in the atomic structure of the biochemistry of any substance and the depth to which a potentised remedy can provoke the Vital Force to dig into the body's healing resources.

Modern drugs have been around for a relatively short time – less than one hundred years in most cases. All the nostrums of the immediately preceding age (which at the time was viewed as a renaissance of medical thinking) have been abandoned. Mercury, lead and leeches have all been found to be ineffective in the cure of chronic health problems (though leeches are making a discreet return). They were all once seen as part of the vanguard against the ravages of disease.

There has always been a desperate race to find ever more effective combatant drugs to deal with the increasing number of threatening ills. The drive to discover new antibiotics to replace those that are no longer as effective is accelerating. The desperate search for vaccines to deal with the ever-increasing population of mutant and malignant viruses goes on apace, but never fast enough. The race to find cures for heart disease and cancer has been soaking up billions of dollars for years; some of the results of research have been striking and of value, but very little advance has been made in halting the advance of these disease conditions. It is only the promise of genetic engineering that has been taking the heat out of the panic. (As we shall see in Part III, genetic medicine will face different but equally frustrating brick walls.)

The truth is inescapable: chemists can never rest because the demand on them to produce ever more curative (suppressive) drugs is fuelled by the swollen and swelling population of sick people – and this at a time of unparalleled understanding about hygiene and nutrition and universal free treatment. Yet the term 'curative drug' is used by scientists to mean medicines that treat *parts* of the body, not the whole. This is to deny that disease serious enough to require treatment from outside the body's own resources has *history. No chronic symptom exists in isolation and without cause or context.*

Putting homoeopathy into a contemporary perspective

There is no doubt that people are becoming less and less constitutionally well and more and more susceptible to illness, and this process has partly followed the increasing reliance on chemotherapy and other suppressive methods of treatment (to which we will return later). Apologists for orthodoxy sometimes cite the vast increase in the population of geriatrics as a statistic to prove that our general health is better because we are now living longer. Yet the *quality* of life of those people is not put in with the same data: many older people do little more than survive, living on drug regimes that lengthen life but do little more. Though patients' heart, liver, lung or kidney tissues might continue to function, their general state of well-being and the life-enhancing quality of positive energy is normally compromised. (The exception to this rule is the patient who is able to maintain his or her sense of creative purpose.)

Doctors' and consultants' surgeries are quite likely to be filled with people under thirty with an astounding variety of severe complaints, while children need medical attention far more regularly than they ever did in the past except when there were epidemics of acute diseases. The staggering increase in patients with respiratory complaints who require long-term medication is a case in point.

This is a very depressing picture and is obviously not attributable solely to incautious or excessive drug administration. There are other factors, separate from medical philosophy, that have contributed. Universal pollution from a host of different sources is but one factor; another is the absurd speed at which we are all expected to live. Compounding this is the extraordinary level of stress heaped on us in our formative years at school while trying to cope with academic and peer pressure, then exaggerated by television's rapacious invasion of our homes.

To keep things in perspective it also has to be said that, in spite of all the opprobrium that is heaped on drug therapy by alternative medical thinkers, there is a vital place for allopathic drugs in the treatment of chronically ill patients. Sadly, there are many so-called classical homoeopaths who cannot countenance this and refuse to treat patients if they are taking any drugs for existing conditions – but this is to deny them access to an alternative source of treatment that really can become *complementary*. (As we shall see, there is no earthly reason why those on long-term chemotherapy should not also derive safe benefit from any of the alternative practices.)

The comment that, "There is a vital place for drugs in the treatment of chronically ill patients" is, on the face of it, extremely impertinent: but an understanding of homoeopathic medicines and the reasons for prescribing them reveals that orthodox drugs *should* be entirely redundant in a vast majority of cases. That they are not is a sad reflection not only on the history of homoeopathy, its practice and its relation to the commercialisation of companies producing drugs but also on the desire to remove symptoms at all costs as quickly as possible, and on the fact that there are those who have a hidden agenda in remaining symptom-bound. Patients are most likely to consult the physician who promises to remove symptoms as quickly as possible, or who will prescribe drugs or treatment that will ensure the relief of pain and discomfort without the necessary effort of dealing with the history of the problem.

It is partly the philosophy of the 'quick fix' that has provided the market for the staggering success of allopathy. The 'quick fix' market is generated by patients (albeit ignorant of alternative thinking) while drugs companies follow the laws of competitive commerce. Big business follows only where inspirational ideas have demonstrated the possibility of a substantial financial return. Homoeopathy is neither fundamentally a big earner nor is it a quick fix. It is a system of medicine in which the patient has to do all the work while the practitioner remains no more than a catalyst.

In homoeopathy there are already known remedies that would cover all the 'labelled' contemporary disease conditions of humanity. That is not to state that homoeopaths can cure them but it is most definitely to say that there are remedies that have the *potential* to cause sufferers of almost all known maladies *to heal themselves* through their self-healing force. This is not splitting hairs. It is a way of saying that practitioners of homoeopathy can be as fallible as those in any other discipline. They may not perceive how to use the remedies to effect the cure required, or that the patient has either no wish to get better or has an investment in remaining unwell. In such circumstances allopathic drugs become not only useful but vital. (There are situations too in which, in spite of the most assiduous efforts of both patient and practitioner, the energy of the *disease* – some cancers and certain heart conditions are typical examples – is greater than the combined efforts of the patient's self-healing mechanism and the indicated remedies. A discussion of this belongs properly in Part III.)

A cornucopia of medicines

In Dr Clarke's *Dictionary of Materia Medica* there are well over a thousand remedies listed, most of which have a comprehensive description (though he does include a good few that have never received a proper proving but lay claim to inclusion because of success in individual cases). This is the stuff of thousands of hours of careful and painstaking research that has involved many hundreds of dedicated practitioners and their faithful patients. This work continues today. There are already many more remedies than Dr Clarke knew about when he published his dictionary in 1901. No-one would be surprised to find in it many of the plants and minerals and metals that are common to everyday language: *Allium Cepa* (the onion), *Thuja Occidentalis* (common enough in the suburban garden where it is often clipped into a hedge to line the drive); *Urtica Urens* (the stinging nettle); the ubiquitous *Sulphur*, *Calcium* (in its various different chemical guises), *Silica*; *Ferrum* (iron), *Argentum Metallicum* (silver) and *Aurum* (gold). Then there are the animal remedies such as the various kinds of snake venom and spider poisons: *Naja* (cobra), *Crotalus Horridus* (rattlesnake); *Tarentula Cubensis* (Cuban tarantula), *Theridion* (orange spider). There are also remedies made from other animal products like *Ambra Grisea* (from the secretion of the sperm whale), *Mephitis* (from a skunk), *Moschus* (from the musk deer). There are acids: *Sulphuric, Hydrocyanic, Prussic, Nitric* and *Carbolic*. Medicines have been made from radioactive material as well: *Radium Bromide, Uranium Nitricum, Strontium Carbonate* and even *X-ray*. There are some remedies that cause revulsion because they have been made only by killing the creature that provides the unique cure: *Apis* (the bee) and *Scorpion*, a recent addition, come to mind.

Hahnemann, not being content to find remedies in obvious places and realising that diseases were also part of the natural world, made remedies from disease material. He made and proved a remedy from the fluid within the vesicle made by a scabies mite on the surface skin. This remedy became known as *Psorinum*. This extraordinary, seemingly repulsive remedy was followed in the next generation of homoeopaths by *Syphilinum* (made from syphilis), *Medorrhinum* (made from gonorrhoeal pus) and *Tuberculinum* (of which there are various examples but all made from tuberculous material). They are known as 'nosodes'.

Remedies start out as ideas in the mind of a practitioner who believes that a particular substance or energy source would, perhaps, make a useful addition to the *Materia Medica*. The sample material or energy is then taken to the homoeopathic pharmacy where it is potentised in exactly the way laid down by Samuel Hahnemann, two centuries ago. (In the case of remedies where there is no material dose – *Luna* (moonlight), for example – a different process is needed. A phial of ethanol – pure alcohol – is placed in the light of the moon for up to three weeks and the resulting liquid is then potentised as any other medicine would be. Risible? Perhaps, but only until the curative effects are witnessed. Then such things become serious and quite wonderful.)

In search of the role of disease

This is all very well but none of it has explained so far how remedies work on the body or how the relationship between the physical, emotional and spiritual aspects of the whole are integrated. It is not enough to say that homoeopathic medicines work on the central nervous system or that they stimulate the body's self-healing mechanism. There is more to understand if we are fully to see the importance of the homoeopathic alternative philosophy of medicine. We need to see homoeopathy in action within the context of the patient which means that we must also look at the role of disease. This is not a subject to which many people are attracted. It is, nevertheless, fascinating because humanity and disease have a curious and paradoxical symbiotic relationship. The host on which disease plays its tunes is the body – the *whole* body – and there is a purpose in its doing so.

CHAPTER 4

THE HIERARCHY OF
THE BODY

The whole or the part?

One of the clichés of alternative therapy is that it is the *whole* body that is treated and not the part. What does this mean? Isn't a cold just a cold in the head? Isn't a boil just an eruption on the skin? Is asthma more than a lung condition? Can eczema be anything more than the sloughing off of flakes of skin? Surely, if someone is suffering from heart disease then it has nothing to do with arthritis in the little finger?

'Holism' derives from the Greek and means the tendency in nature to produce wholes out of ordered groups of units. The body begins as a single cell containing the duality of male and female traits and is just such an ordered grouping which creates a whole. Inherent in that grouping is an integrated system of parts functioning in a way that is completely interdependent. The system is hierarchical in the sense that some parts are more vital, delicate and vulnerable than others are and require greater degrees of protection. Some parts are designated specifically to protect and others to support; like any well-designed city with a rubbish-collection system and a comprehensive self-defence strategy, the body knows how to clean itself up as well as how and when to defend itself. Furthermore, it operates a self-regulating repair programme that is part of a continual self-renewal process.

The first lines of defence are the skin and the central nervous system. The skin is waterproof and yet breathes; it also copes with the cold (by shivering and raising body hair) and the heat (by releasing sweat) as well as with rashes and eruptions that result from acute childhood diseases or an overloaded liver. The skin deals with allergic reactions to insect bites and stings and reactions to plants (through rashes and histamine release); through touch it is integrated into the nervous system. The five senses provide us with an early warning system in emergency situations.

The second line of defence and the main *internal* system of management is the lymphatic system. This operates via a network of tubes and glands throughout the body that collects waste products and carts them off to be excreted. The tonsils, which are throat glands, are the usual sites for early trouble in children. The tonsils are very close to the largest orifice in the body and therefore close to a very useful drainage point. Tonsils that swell and produce pus are painful and look threatening but the mucus from the throat and muck from the crypts in the tonsils need to be eliminated as fast as possible. If such rubbish were sent through the usual channels to be excreted in urine and faeces then the process would take much longer to resolve and would be expensive in energy – and even possibly threatening to the kidneys. Some patients produce swollen glands in other parts of the body – favourite places are the mesenteric glands of the abdomen and the inguinal glands of the groin and it takes longer to get better than if they had had the problem in the throat because these glands are deeper in the system and not so close to a drainage point.

The lungs also play a vital role in keeping the body clean. They produce mucus from the membranes. This is sent upwards and therefore outwards by tiny hairs (cilia) that wave the fluid towards the throat, carrying with it any unwanted material. The lungs can easily become trouble spots because of their structure of sponge-like tissue threaded through with greater and smaller air tubes (bronchus and bronchioles). At the end of these tubes are the waiting 'terminals' of the blood vessels (alveoli), which is where the exchange of gases takes place (where blood picks up fresh air and carbon dioxide is excreted). As this part of the system is a 'cul de sac' it is important that there should be as little debris as possible. It is easy to understand why mucus and pus in the lungs can be more threatening than mucus and pus in the throat.

The alimentary canal is basically a tube from mouth to anus. From the gullet to the stomach is a straight drop. If anything nasty is deposited in the stomach then the reflex action of vomiting will eject it smartly. However, if there is a problem brewing in the intestines it may well take rather longer to resolve as the drainage point might be anything up to thirty-two feet away and certainly not as the crow flies.

By the same token it is easier for the body to deal with a bladder condition than with a kidney problem. The kidneys are extraordinarily delicate constructions of tiny tubules that filter all the exiting fluid in the body. They cannot afford to fail for they ensure that vital minerals remain within the body. The bladder on the other hand is a bag with a drain; it acts as a reservoir with an overspill.

Some parts are designed to put up with illness better than others

Some parts of the body are better designed to put up with illness than others. This may appear to be a very simplistic view, but consider that: it is safer for the body to have disease of the skin than it is to have disease of the throat glands; it is safer to have an illness of the throat glands than it is of the lungs; it is safer to have trouble in the lungs than in the heart; it is safer to have a condition of the stomach than of the liver or pancreas; it is safer to have a problem with the bladder than in the kidneys. The body always has greater success in healing itself if there is a convenient point of drainage. The skin and the orifices are drains and should be respected as such.

Skin: the first line of defence

We should look at the skin first. Medicated shampoos are specifically formulated to eradicate dandruff yet those who use them know not what they do. The speedy overproduction of skin cells that leads to the itching and flaking of the scalp is actually a form of discharge. The body is attempting to throw off something that is unwanted by the system. While many people are strong enough constitutionally not to notice side effects from the chemicals that suppress the dandruff, there are some who suffer in other ways as a result of using the shampoos.

A boy of ten who had had yellow, flaky dandruff that had been suppressed for some years with shampoos and chemicals like coal tar, suffered from excessively loose motions and headaches once the scalp was under control. When he stopped using the proprietary applications the bowel and head symptoms disappeared and the yellow dandruff reappeared. He also became more cheerful and more energetic. His mother was not happy: the boy came from a family of psoriasis sufferers and she was afraid that her son would go on to develop the problem. This troubled her more than the fact that he seemed to have a perpetual cold in the nose from which he poured profuse yellow mucus. He was given several doses of *Kali Sulphuricum* (potassium sulphate), which is well known for the yellowness of its discharges, and the nose and scalp troubles both cleared up.

Sweaty feet, a condition of the lymph system as much as of the skin, is another common problem which people try and suppress ruthlessly even though it is often difficult to achieve and it quickly returns. It is particularly common for patients who have forgotten that they used to have sweaty feet and who are now seeking alternative treatment for swollen lymph glands – either in the groin or in the armpits – to experience the return of the sweating. They may not care for this reversal of fortune as they had hoped that the foot symptoms were history. Yet when asked if they feel generally better in themselves the reply is invariably positive. There are even recorded cases of mammary tumours arising as a result of suppressing perspiration of the feet. Fortunately there is a remedy that covers this symptom: *Silica*. Cases that have been treated with *Silica* have been resolved by first restoring the foot sweats which have in turn responded favourably to the same medicine. Sweat, prevented from occurring at its natural point of discharge, has had to seek another, less appropriate route; the lymph system, attempting to do the right thing by putting its waste products through the pores of the skin, becomes confused and the discharge, sent into reverse, blocks up the glands. The only true cure has to be a return to the original function of the skin.

What about eczema? A common story in alternative practice is that of the child who had eczema suppressed by cortisone creams and who now suffers from chronic throat and chest infections. The acute infections have invariably been suppressed by antibiotics which in turn has led to a diagnosis of asthma, for which steroid inhalers and bronchodilators are the stock allopathic answer. A wise homoeopath will always advise the patient or the parents of such a patient that the chest troubles will undoubtedly clear up given time, but at the expense of the skin condition returning. This is often a daunting and heart-rending process because the skin, being a drainage system, will become involved in the expulsion of the suppressive treatments that went before. The drugs that were used to stop the eczema, chest infections and the asthma need to be removed from the body.

In such a patient the elimination system of bowels and urine excretion has not been able to keep pace with the suppression, leaving the liver to store what it cannot deliver. The application of indicated natural remedies instantly encourages the removal of the drugs through the fastest routes. The net result of prescribing homoeopathic remedies in these cases is initially for the bowels to evacuate very loose motions and for the discharge through the returning eczema lesions of clear or pus-filled serum. Many parents find this as hard to bear as the patient (and not simply for obvious cosmetic reasons) but the return of the skin condition is absolutely essential in order to relieve the internal organs of the onus of bearing the disease. It is safer to scratch than to cough. It is easier to treat eczema than asthma. A child relieved of asthma at the expense of the old skin problem will be a healthier individual, despite temporarily *looking* to the contrary.

Further into the system

Tonsillitis is another common topic among practitioners. The majority of children suffer throat infections (for reasons that will become apparent later on) and as these are so often accompanied by fevers the usual treatment is with antibiotics. Children who have persistent bouts of tonsillitis and who are treated allopathically, frequently go on to suffer otitis media – 'middle ear'. Ear trouble is viewed by parents and practitioners as more threatening than tonsillitis because perforated eardrums are both excruciatingly painful and a potential threat to hearing. In tonsillitis pus gathers in the tonsil glands; there is frequently an accompanying fever that is the body's way of promoting the whole process to be performed at speed. If this process is suppressed then the body must find another outlet for the pus. The nearest outlet to the throat is the Eustachian tube, a channel that leads from the back of the throat up into the back of the ear. This is unfortunate because the channel is blocked by the eardrum. In otitis media the pus collects behind the drum and causes local inflammation and swelling even to the point of causing the drum to burst. It is usually safer to have tonsillitis than a perforated eardrum. If a patient has not eventually developed trouble in the ears then he has probably advanced to lung problems.

Asthmatic patients find out about steroids the hard way. In this disease the lungs fill with phlegm of a wide variety of descriptions and become both obstructed by drying mucus and constricted by muscular contraction. This dual affliction causes enormous pressure on the chest. Steroids suppress inflammation and adrenaline-inspired spasm in the muscles of the walls of the air passages (which causes the constriction). All asthmatic patients know that the drugs do not cure the problem but hold it at bay and afford the blessed relief of snatching another full breath. Yet how many of these people eventually go on to suffer heart troubles? The answer is: a depressingly substantial number. The heart, being in the middle of the chest, is geographically in prime position to take aggravation resulting from suppressed lung conditions. If the heart is not the site of future disease then the kidneys could be – not least because the adrenal glands, which sit on top of the kidneys and have a very close relationship with them, are suppressed by the use of steroids.

Therefore, it will be no surprise to learn that a suppressed bladder condition can easily reflect negatively on the kidneys – or on the uterus. (Men do not have the luxury of this extra drainage point though repeated bladder or urethral infections can lead to prostate conditions.)

The healthier the constitution, *the closer to the surface any evidence of disease will be*. Comparatively healthy children begin their biography of disease by producing skin conditions and disorders of the lymph and liver. They may produce acute rashes either as reactions to allergens or as the result of childhood ailments. They might produce eczema but this more complex disease has to do with hereditary factors. Whatever the skin condition and its cause, the internal state of the body may remain well with all the functioning organs continuing to perform their allotted tasks perfectly. Lymph glands may swell from time to time but this natural reaction is a demonstration of internal activity in the waste disposal unit and will be followed by some form of discharge – either through bowels, bladder, skin or sinuses.

The liver is a 'boiler' and is the origin of any fever which it stokes in order to 'burn off' a disease. Again, the result of this is often a discharge. How many children with a fever then either vomit or have diarrhoea or sweat profusely or wet the bed?

The less interference there is in the body's functions the healthier it remains. The more suppression or downright abuse it suffers, the more disease ventures inward. ('Abuse' covers anything from alcohol and smoking to aggressive parenting and emotional trauma – anything that disturbs the equilibrium of the body's harmony.) The more the body is left to its own devices to slough off disease, the more disease becomes externalised. The childhood diseases are a perfect example of this. Chickenpox is a disease apparently of the skin yet once the pocks have arrived on the skin the patient has reached the end stage. The first stages of the disease are often mistaken for a cold or a threatening chest infection. As these symptoms ease off, so the spots come out. The same is true of measles and rubella. Even mumps can often finish up with a skin rash after the swollen glands have gone down.

Patients who suffer from skin complaints that alternate with internal problems such as eczema and asthma experience greater vitality and lifting of spirits when the lung trouble is relieved even though the skin symptoms aggravate. (The main problem here is that the infuriating itching and the distress felt over the cosmetic appearance lead to the further suppression of the eczema which brings back the difficult breathing.)

The physical effects of emotions

Emotions also need full consideration. Lack of emotional expression is an ample reason for the physical body to become involved.

> Consider a child aged five, whose parents divorce under a cloud of acrimony and recrimination. No one has told her that she is not involved in the dispute and that it is not her fault. All she knows is that Mummy and Daddy have been rowing but *"it will all be OK because nothing is really going to happen"*. Then it does happen and she is the subject of a custody battle. People keep telling her not to cry because everything will be settled soon and she has to be a big, grown-up girl. So she does what she is told

and produces raging eczema instead. This raises the stakes in this tragic game. She becomes the focus of medical attention and is given creams to plaster all over her body. Soon she develops restricted breathing and a persistent cough, for which she is given inhalers and is labelled an asthmatic. Her personality, which was sunny and open before the parents' rowing started, is now depressed and closed.

The cure lies in the natural expression of her emotions – tears of rage and grief. These are externalised emotions. Emotions should be seen as a form of discharge too so they need to be included in the hierarchy of the body. Other examples might serve to illustrate this.

The child whose pet rabbit died suddenly and unexpectedly developed frequent and distressing urination and enuresis (bedwetting); she had not grieved properly for her 'friend' and the crying she had been suppressing was expressed through another water system of the body. She was given a high potency dose of *Natrum Muriaticum* (rock salt), amongst the symptoms of which is 'unable to cry'. The bladder problem stopped and she spoke for the first time to her parents about her unhappiness and of how she had suspected her younger brother of having 'done something' to the rabbit.

A little boy of three who had been sent to playgroup developed a persistent dry, hacking cough; he was clingy and weepy and, every time his mother left the room, he howled in deep distress. The mother was very caring but, having two other very demanding children who spent their entire time bickering and at each other's throats, she had not realised that the youngest might be coughing from emotional distress. After he had said one day that he was afraid that Mummy would not be there any more, he was given *Pulsatilla* (one of the most naturally weepy and clingy remedy states) and then *Thuja* (a remedy that is often needed to cover states of concern and anxiety about personal security) and the cough resolved within a week – (*"Don't want Mummy gone"* were his actual words and they might be interpreted as an expression of his fear of her death, a surprisingly common fear among children – and one that frequently needs *Thuja*.)

A business woman who suffered blinding, bilious migraines knew that she worked too hard and too long hours but confessed that she could not stop – she needed the money and had had her father's work ethic instilled in her at any early age. She had a list of remedies a yard long that had been given to her over a few years but, although her general constitutional health improved, it was not until she was ready to examine and resolve her difficult relationship with her father that the migraines began to ease off. To get to this point she needed *Ilex Aquifolium* (a form of holly), a remedy noted for its affinity for people who have been unable to resolve their relationship with their father. (Her long-dead father had had migraines all his life too.)

A woman who had been raped some 15 years previously and felt too ashamed to speak of it suffered from severe uterine symptoms and infertility. Down-to-earth and practical, bouncy and confident, she nevertheless suffered from terrible menstrual cramps which were due to a twisted pelvis. In spite of excellent osteopathic treatment for this, the problem kept recurring until she was ready to look at the trauma of the rape. Once she had been given appropriate remedies (*Staphysagria,* the delphinium and, later, *Xanthoxyllum,* the prickly ash) and was able to express her anguish and humiliation over this incident, she began a steady improvement. She went on to produce two healthy children.

All of these instances serve to illustrate that the body 'discharges' its emotional pathology – and if it is unable to do so then the physical body will often assume the role of memory bank and cause physiological changes (for example, the twisted pelvis and spasmodic pains) that are held until a healing process is initiated. It also illustrates that, even in the face of severe, physical symptoms, unless a particular vital organ is dangerously weakened, it is often the mental and emotional symptoms that lead us to the core of a problem.

The hierarchy: past, present and future

So, to sum up: a *healthy* body has a hierarchy. The skin is affected first, only to be followed by internal organs if the skin is unable to deal completely with the problems. The internal organs usually go into distress only as a consequence of either emotional or drug-induced suppression. The big problem is that most of us do not have robustly healthy constitutions and so each story becomes more complex and more interesting. We erroneously congratulate ourselves for living in an age where the average life span extends into the seventies, forgetting that it is not length of life that is important but the quality of life. Cavemen, whose constitutions were prodigiously tough, died at very young ages, not from cancer, heart disease or Alzheimer's but from fire, flood and wars. Mammoth and sabre-toothed tiger hunts and flash epidemics of acute diseases wiped out the unfit and left the rest with a better immunity. Later we will see how the earliest diseases that affected man and mammal were of the skin and not of the internal organs.

Now that we have come so far down the road of suppression and technology we can make most skin diseases tolerable and survive their consequences for longer – for undoubtedly the advance of chemotherapy has enabled us to support the internal consequences of our external suppression even though there is an increasing awareness of the risks of going down this road.

We are left with the question: "Is it worth it?" A chorus of yeses is inevitable from those with the conventional, materialist view of medicine; but the whole picture must be examined. What happens when the inward progress of disease runs out of places to go? We are staring terminal illness in the face even if we can stave it off for years. Any illness that is not resolved completely is a handicap to the continued perfect functioning of the body. What is more, any serious condition that is suppressed is registered somewhere in the DNA and can be passed on to any children. (The hereditary aspect of disease is so important that it requires a whole section of this book to itself.)

A doctor reading this section on the hierarchy of the body might be justified in dismissing the idea as he would be used to patients arriving at his surgery complaining of a stomach ulcer or of high blood pressure who have never had a skin disease in their lives. If the skin and lymph systems really are the healthy person's symptom producers why should it be that so many people do not suffer from their chronic symptoms in either department? Do they become ill so quickly that the usual system is completely by-passed?

The skin and lymphatics are most readily used as chronic symptom producers when we are children, barring any profound suppression. We have, as children, the centrifugal energy to push our problems onto the surface in a way that becomes more difficult after puberty and certainly more so in our middle years. By the time we are adults it is harder for the physical body to register illness that has its origins in suppressed or unresolved emotions as symptoms on the surface; our symptom metaphors have to be expressed by internal functions and organs that best illustrate our distress.

CHAPTER 5

THE HIERARCHY OF DISEASE

Compartmentalising the bits of the body

Our view of disease is very limited; it is one-dimensional and mostly confined to what we fear. Allopathy and journalism have contributed greatly to both our superficial knowledge and to our misapprehension of what disease is. Science has devoted much patient study and research into individual diseases and their functional disturbances of the body. There are labels for almost every imaginable condition and it is common for patients to feel better once they know the name of the condition they are suffering from. The knowledge allows them to feel confident that their problems have been witnessed before and that doctors will therefore know what to do for them. Nor do they have to worry about the other conditions that might have been wrong with them – they can concentrate on the one named thing. Patients focus their attention on the symptoms that they suffer from and the parts of the body that are producing them. If they can relate their symptoms to the doctor, then the doctor can remove them. That is the theory. Once treatment begins both doctor and patient continue to watch the part or parts that are distressed. If the original problem is resolved but another springs up to create a new priority then the second condition is regarded very often as a separate issue – particularly if a gap of time elapses before the second condition arises – more than likely in a different part of the body.

Allopathy separates health problems to such an extent that the whole system of orthodox medicine is carved up into specialist fields. If your doctor cannot deal with the condition presented to him he will refer you to a consultant. He is being entirely practical and realistic because he knows that a specialist is more likely to know what specific thing needs to be done according to allopathic thinking.

The great disadvantage of this system is that while the part may be attended to, the whole is not. A cardiologist knows all that might be needed to know of the heart; the oncologist is conversant with the details of cancer; a urologist is familiar with all things pertaining to the bladder and kidneys. Each of these experts also has a deep understanding of the workings of the whole body but, because the focus of their efforts is on the parts of the patient that they specialise in, they are chiefly interested in achieving successful cure of those and those alone. A patient who is receiving treatment from a urologist but who then begins to suffer migraine headaches will be sent to a different specialist. A dermatologist who is treating someone for psoriasis will send his patient back to his or her general practitioner if there is occurrence of asthma.

This fragmentation has led to a loss of understanding that disease, in whatever form it takes in each person, affects – indeed, is created by – the whole body. Any system of medicine that compartmentalises the body is working at the level of a garage repair shop. Disease and humanity are far more sophisticated than that. We should, for the sake of clarity, look more closely at the hierarchy of disease by separating out all the strands that go to make up the formidable rope which is so intimately bound to us.

Acute conditions

Disease can be subdivided into two main categories: acute and chronic. Acute diseases are those from which we either recover or die within a specified time. The body produces them in specific ways that are definable and characteristic and often very easily identifiable. Most of these conditions are either bacterial or viral. They include all the childhood diseases: chickenpox, measles, mumps, whooping cough, scarlet fever and German measles. As we shall see later, these diseases have a special place in our health history and have a strong link to our disease-ridden heredity. Epidemic diseases such as typhoid, cholera and yellow fever belong in this group too though they are often regarded as 'tropical' – erroneously in the case of the first two as it is not so very long since both cholera and typhoid existed in western Europe. Tetanus, polio and hepatitis ('A', 'B' and 'C') are also on the list though tetanus, being a condition caused by the release of a neurotoxin, is unique in its natural history and is not in any way infectious.

Then there are all the varieties of colds and influenzas, the number of which is legion. Even when well we can become as predisposed to their unwelcome appearance through lowered immunity as we are to any other viral or bacterial infection. The immune system becomes depressed for a variety of reasons, some of which have already been suggested: getting wet or chilled, accidents, emotional difficulties and so on. *When we are vulnerable we become a suitable temporary host for a bug to occupy while it develops and reproduces. The disease is the body's negative reaction to accident, chill or grief; the bug's presence is the result and not, as we shall see, the cause.*

These common and not so common bugs and cooties are to be regarded as life forces of nature as much as we are or trees or sheep are. They have a life plan and span that are clearly defined – though in the case of 'flu and cold viruses modern methods of suppressive treatment may lead these to vary due to mutation. *Infectious and epidemic diseases have purpose and intention: survival and reproduction. The important thing is that the survival of these diseases depends entirely upon us and on our continued expression of them.* We happen to be their vehicle of expression. We should not lament this too quickly.

Our relationship with acute diseases is symbiotic; we gain something from them[1]. When we have a dose of 'flu or a cold we sneeze as part of the infectious agent's reproductive cycle. In the process we produce lots of phlegm to clear the system of unwanted toxins – of which there is often a build-up, in spite of the efficiency of the waste-disposal unit, especially if we have not been maintaining a purely natural lifestyle. When we have chickenpox we cough, sneeze and scratch but we also strengthen our immune system – and, as aware parents will notice, children make concurrent developmental leaps in growth and learning ability. The same is true when suffering from measles, scarlet fever and mumps. It is significant that the most infectious stage of these diseases is *before* the appearance of any skin or glandular symptoms.

Strange as it may seem, humanity has a purpose in promoting epidemics of these acute diseases, as they are so much part of our hereditary history – see Part III. (It is also interesting to note that they cannot be 'cured' in the conventional sense – there are no drugs for them; the patient can only be *nursed* while the body finds its own way back to health.)

In gastro-enteritis the diarrhoea and vomiting that occur clear out not only the invading and multiplying bacteria but also any preponderance of unwanted bowel flora that might have been accumulating in the intestines and that could have caused the temporarily lowered immunity. (Healthy bowels are inhabited by friendly bacteria, which are vital to aid the process of digestion. However, sometimes one or other of them gets out of hand and multiplies out of its normal proportion to the others. This excess of one type causes an imbalance.) In spite of the extreme discomfort of vomiting and passing liquid stools, the healthy body very quickly restores itself to a normal state.

The net result of suffering an acute disease is heightened immunity; a healthy person who has a cold at least once or perhaps twice a year will be none the worse for it and will be free of such viral infections for long stretches of time. Someone with a strong constitution who has just had gastro-enteritis will be unlikely to have it again within the next few years. It may seem a cliché to say that having the childhood illnesses builds up immunity but the truth of this is too easily forgotten or dismissed in our age of media scaremongering and mass vaccination.

The key to freedom from acute infection is a healthy immune system. We know that a balanced diet of quality food, plenty of physical activity and awareness of hygiene are contributing factors as well. Nevertheless even the fittest amongst us succumbs to illness from time to time and having disease actually helps prevent further, more frequent and more serious bouts. So it is homoeopathic prophylaxis to have the odd cold or 'flu.

Unfortunately there are some acute disease conditions that are so virulent that at first it appears imperative for there to be some form of intervention through suppressive means. Impetigo presents an obvious example. This is a skin disease for which the staphylococcus bacterium seems to be responsible. The symptoms are itching and red or dark red, sometimes scabby or crusty lesions, often on the face, that spread like fury. Once the disease is established it needs to be dealt with promptly because of its speed of progress and the high degree of contagion. Antibiotic creams are the stock allopathic answer and usually they do the job successfully. However there are homoeopathic remedies that are more satisfactory. The trouble with using them is that they do not always work in quite the way that is expected of a curative agent. As in the case of any other acute disease, the patient has become susceptible to impetigo not just because of proximity to another sufferer. There is always another predisposing factor that antibiotic creams would be wholly inadequate to cover; it might be emotional or hereditarily constitutional. In using an appropriate homoeopathic remedy to clear up the skin problem, the emotional distress that had been successfully covered up will now be appropriately discharged – usually in the form of an emotional release such as tears or anger or both. (Sometimes, as the eruptions fade, a cold develops and with it the patient becomes aware of understanding more about some problem that had been causing distress.) If the underlying cause was constitutional – as is so often the case in children – then the patient will appear to be healthier and more energetic than he or she was before falling foul of staphylococcus. (Indeed, children who overcome impetigo through natural means often show obvious developmental progress: they have a growth spurt or their vocabulary suddenly broadens. This is equally true of all the childhood illnesses as was noted above.)

To illustrate this apparently bizarre concept, meet the woman who developed impetigo on her face and breasts.

The woman was extremely worried as she was breastfeeding her daughter and feared that the infection would spread. The symptoms of impetigo are often subtly different from one patient to another and where they differ they call for a different remedy. This woman needed *Graphites* (pencil lead) in potency. Within a few days the lesions on her breasts were worse but those on her face had all but gone; only a stain was left where the open sores had been. By this time she was frantic about the possibility of her daughter catching the disease and expressed herself angrily, saying that the impetigo was no better. She was then asked if anything untoward had been going on in the house before she developed the problem. It transpired that her husband had recently given up his job and had decided to become a gardening handyman. He had done this without consulting her. As she began to speak about this she started to weep, pulled out her hanky and twisted it about her fingers nervously. She went on to say how angry she was that her husband could be so selfish when she had had to give up her very responsible and well-paid job to have the baby. Now she felt trapped and isolated while her husband was able to be out and about. Then she apologised for letting off steam: *"It's not something I usually do at all."*

She was given *Sepia*, a remedy that is often indicated in women whose wrath is invoked by their husbands' uncaring attitude. Within two more days the impetigo was gone completely. The baby never developed any sign of the condition.

What of the woman who fell hopelessly in love with her local but married vicar? She was friendly with him and his wife and sometimes went round for tea. She had a history of unfortunate relationships partly because she had a penchant for married men. She developed facial impetigo which disfigured the left side of her face. It was violently itchy and looked revolting. She was very distressed by it but was given *Antimonium Crudum*, which not only addresses skin conditions that are itchy and tend to be pustular but also the psychological state of being hopelessly and romantically lovesick. Though she endured the skin condition for some six weeks – a wholly unacceptable length of time in allopathic terms – she was not only relieved eventually of the impetigo but also the emotional attachment. This might seem an almost comical history until one realises just how pathetically affected was the woman. Had she used creams to suppress the skin complaint she might have been badly scarred, not by the impetigo but emotionally by unrequited feelings that would not have come so readily to the surface.

The constitutional effects of healing impetigo by homoeopathy are illustrated by two of the children in a family of four.

Only the two middle siblings developed the symptoms. The lesions broke out around their mouths and were furiously itchy and very crusty. Within a week both had 'beards' of dried orange pus. The little girl had never had particularly robust health and frequently succumbed to colds; her hair was lank and did not grow; her moods were unpredictable and she was often weepy. Her brother was healthier but inclined to be thin and pale and had a poor appetite. They remained off school for five weeks due to the impetigo. Nevertheless, with the administration of *Sulphur* they both cleared their condition without any antibiotics and the net result was an improvement in their constitutional health. The girl's hair began to grow, she put on weight, her moods improved and she felt the need to create 'scenes' less often. Her brother's appetite improved dramatically and he became far more outgoing.

A disease that can progress at terrifying speed and can have fatal consequences, is meningitis. Meningitis is feared by all, to the extent that doctors and homoeopaths alike are consulted for advice on almost any type of severe, unexplained fever with headache – and not unreasonably as many children produce fevers with headaches and rashes that could so easily be the early signs. Meningitis tends to strike at those whose immune systems have been compromised in some way, where there is a predisposition for an acute fever state.

Meningitis is usually associated with either bacteria or viruses. Viral meningitis is the more usual problem today. It can seem to come out of the blue or be regarded as having a link with an acute infection such as measles or mumps. If any such infection has lowered the system sufficiently then it is possible for the delicate coverings of the brain (the meninges) to be affected, producing the characteristic symptoms of violent headache and head rolling or back arching along with the frantically high fever. Yet look again at our friend *Belladonna*: it covers the throbbing headache with pulsating carotid artery; the red face with cold extremities; the dilated pupils and photophobia; the arching back; the delirium and screaming. Though it is not by any means the only remedy homoeopaths might be called on to use in meningitis, *Belladonna* is probably the most usual one. This is not to say that patients with meningitis can dispense with hospital care. What is meant here is that it is both possible and desirable to treat the disease homoeopathically. Antibiotics and drips are vital when nothing else is available – which is ninety-nine per cent of the time; yet if there were enough homoeopaths with the confidence to deal with meningitis then many patients would be able to get better by non-chemical means.

Quality of life after suppression

Does it matter very much *how* one gets better from such a dangerous disease? Yes, it does. The after-effects of meningitis can be very unpleasant. There are often severe headaches, visual impairment, lassitude, lowered immunity and susceptibility to a host of minor but pestilential conditions such as *candida albicans* or herpes simplex. There can also be disturbance of the psyche: patients can become very irritable, even irascible. They may be

85

safe from the disease itself, the bug having been killed off, but their quality of life can be impaired.

We can cite the case of the twenty-one-year-old man who was taken to hospital completely incapacitated with severe headache and high fever. He was kept in overnight for observation. This was, it was explained to the parents, because the doctors were not certain if it was viral or bacterial meningitis. The parents remained by his bed but called the homoeopath. The most striking symptom was that every noise or movement seemed to be a torture to him. He was restless but felt worse for moving or even whispering his answers. He also complained of feeling giddy whenever the door opened or closed or if anyone spoke above a whisper. He said he could feel noise go right through him.

There is only one remedy that can cover this degree of sensitivity: *Theridion*, a remedy made from the orange spider. He was given a dose of the 200th potency. Within twenty seconds he was burning with high fever. His face was bright red and he became slightly delirious. He was given a *Belladonna* 1M . Within fifteen minutes he had quietened down and had become sleepy. He asked for the urine bottle and passed nearly half a litre of dark, vinegar-coloured urine which, when it had stood a while, had a thick sediment at the bottom. After he had slept for about half an hour the fever showed signs of returning. This was not surprising as it was by now 3 o'clock in the afternoon – *Belladonna*'s bad time of day. He had a second dose of the 1M. By the next morning he was well enough to leave hospital. The *Theridion* had been needed as the condition was having an effect deep within the central nervous system, causing all the symptoms of extreme sensitivity. Once the remedy had stimulated the self-healing mechanism the frank fever came out and was distinctly observable and recognisably obvious as a *Belladonna* state. Simply by letting the body express its symptom picture it became possible to avoid any drug intervention.

This is in marked contrast to the girl of fifteen who was given a measles and rubella vaccine, went on to develop measles and then suffered meningitis within the space of four weeks. She was treated with drug therapy and subsequently went on to develop all the desperate symptoms of myalgic encephalomyelitis (ME).

To study colds and meningitis is to study the extremes of the range of acute diseases. Between them there is a host of well-known and not so well-known conditions that can equally well be treated alternatively.

When is an acute disease not acute?

There is a more difficult type of acute situation: the acute flare-up of a chronic condition. These are acute episodes that stem from the patient's general state of chronic unwellness. A typical example is bronchitis in a chronic asthmatic. Gout, haemorrhoids, migraine, menstrual cramps and recurrent boils are just a few examples among many. The underlying state of illness is ever-present in these patients and can be very mild (even to the point of being apparently negligible) or extremely severe.

Whatever the condition of the constitution, the flare-up still comes into the general category of 'acute' due to the fact that it is a crisis that is marked by beginning with worsening symptoms and a more or less predictable end. However, in these diseases the crises are most often determined by drugs as the patients have by then learnt not to trust their bodies at all and seek the suppressive route unhesitatingly. Though homoeopathic prescribing for these acute crises is trickier than for ordinary acutes, it is nonetheless both feasible and possible.

In straightforward acute cases, such as in accidents, minor fevers and mild infections, it is possible for the patient to take charge of his own pre-scribing. In the case of acute crises, however, this is seldom advisable, no matter how competent and conversant he or she may be with remedies and the reasons for their administration. The reason for this is that, until the patient is familiar with the way his or her body might react to the chosen remedy, a professional assessment is needed to gauge the quality of the body's response. A seasoned practitioner needs to oversee these episodes, at least until the patient has experienced several bouts and has learnt to 'listen to his body'.

Take as an example, Nigel, an asthma patient who succumbs to bouts of wheezing and coughing every time he gets a cold – which is frequently as his immunity is severely depressed through the constant use of steroids. In the past he always used antibiotics; so common was this that he had a regu-lar prescription for them at his local surgery.

Since Nigel was introduced to homoeopathy he has begun to learn about the remedies for acute asthma attacks. His usual symptom picture is quite specific: he wakes up in the small hours coughing and wheezing and feeling he cannot get enough breath because he cannot expand his chest walls; he has to breathe from his abdomen. His chest is full of rattling phlegm, his cough sounds like that of an old smoker and he is unable to clear his airways. To breathe at all he has to sit bolt upright in bed. His wife watches him helplessly as he turns bluer and bluer. For this acute condition he was given *Antimonium Tartaricum* 30 to take as he needed, up to every fifteen minutes. He quickly discovered that this remedy worked faster for him than the antibiotics or the steroid inhalers.

Nigel has other occasions when his asthmatic breathing gets the better of him and when *Antimonium Tartaricum* is of no service at all. If he overdoes any physical exertion and especially if he climbs any hill or goes upstairs too quickly, or too often, then he finds that he becomes short of breath and very anxious and restless; he gets a parched mouth and feels chilly and clammy. He also feels faintly nauseous. He soon discovered that *Arsenicum Album* would relieve not only his distressed breathing but also the palpitations that accompany the other symptoms. Nigel feels that he will never be one hundred per cent clear of his asthma but he is 'thrilled' to have found natural alternatives to the inhalers. *"I feel I'm in charge of my own body!"*

Gout is one of the most excruciatingly painful conditions to suffer. Overindulgence in good food and wines is a common trigger for an attack so it could be said with ample justification that patients tend to bring it on themselves. One such patient, though, has learnt to accommodate his gout very well. He has discovered that *Sulphur* 200 will completely clear him of any pain. Taking it upon himself to experiment, he decided to take a prophylactic dose before going off on a drinking binge. He found that it worked so well that he was able to take a glass of port to finish off his gourmet meals. It happens that *Sulphur* is homoeopathic to his particular condition (i.e. the remedy is similar in its effects to the gout that he suffers) and by taking it before he overdoses on liver-bashing meals he, so to speak, inoculates himself against the worst excesses. Others have found the same applies to other remedies which are specifically homoeopathic to their own symptom pictures.

The purpose of a sub-acute condition

What is the significance of these sub-acute episodes? The answer is clear: each acute attack is the body's attempt to clear out the worst of the excess of problems within. Just as volcanoes are a safety valve for the earth's boiling mass within, so these sub-acute flare-ups temper the underlying distress of the suffering body. Unfortunately, such attempts are often thoroughly unsuccessful in terms of finding satisfactory resolutions to underlying long-term problems. The flare-up is recognised all too often only as an acute state that needs to be eradicated as quickly as possible. Gout seems to be simply an episode of diabolical pain; pneumonia is apparently a bacterial or viral invasion; gastric pains from a peptic ulcer are superficially just that.

Yet each symptom picture tells a story to those who can read it. Each symptom picture carries a purpose. The main objective of any acute crisis is discharge – recurrent boils gather toxic waste from the body's core and discharge it on the surface; diarrhoea and vomiting are the body's way of discharging bacteria from the alimentary canal; sputum relieves the lungs and bronchus of toxic waste and so on. The less successful the body is at creating such a discharge, the more severe is the acute crisis and the less likely the body is to create any real relief for the chronic condition underlying it.

The action of the body's healing energy system is *centrifugal* in its effect and because alternative therapies enhance this it stands to reason that using remedies to promote discharge is far more practical and makes more common sense than using suppressive drugs. Hence the homoeopathic remedies that deal with gout will promote the secretion of sweat and urine to help wash out the system. Remedies called for in a bout of pneumonia promote excessive sweating and the expulsion of phlegm from the lungs. Remedies indicated to assist the healing of ulceration of the stomach lining would promote the secretion and subsequent expulsion of mucus in and from the stomach as well as repairing damaged tissue. Remedies needed to relieve the swelling and inflammation in rheumatoid arthritis promote speedier evacuation of bowels and bladder. None of these events can happen without stimulating rather than suppressing.

It is because the body finds it very hard to resolve these flare-ups using only its own resources that outside (allopathic) help seems so imperative – and it is imperative where there are no alternatives. It is in severely chronic cases that can become acute emergencies that drugs come into their own and play a vital part in relieving great distress and saving lives. The great successes that they have had have blinded us to the down side of immediate suppression. We become tempted to rely on suppression all the time, not realising *that every flare-up artificially removed weakens the integrity of the whole*; thus a gout patient put on Alopurinol will have fewer, if any, attacks of pain in his left big toe but he will eventually be talking to his doctor about the beta-blockers he needs for high blood pressure and angina. To understand why the inappropriate but sometimes, paradoxically, necessary allopathic treatment of acute and sub-acute conditions should eventually affect the body adversely, it is necessary to look closely at the nature of chronic disease.

Chronic disease

Chronic diseases are usually comparatively slow to progress and are less easily defined initially than any acute condition. These are conditions for which the body has only a partial or no answer, and is therefore incapable of self-healing without either a radical change of lifestyle or some form of outside intervention – even if that is as apparently slight as dietary advice. Such diseases seldom have a well-defined beginning and often have to be traced back through a range of minor problems that pre-date the existing illness but that have contributed to it – usually through their neglect or suppression. It is also true that minor problems that gradually accrue over years have a decided tendency to become more troublesome or more serious as time goes on. Almost always to be found beneath the surface of distressing symptoms that illustrate an advancing chronic state is a history, either short but intense, or long and detailed, of emotional crisis. It is unquestionable that there are no long-term chronic conditions that exist without a rich seam of psychosomatic causation to mine.

A stomach ulcer is a chronic illness and may have taken several months or even years to advance to a stage where the patient feels uncomfortable enough to consult a doctor. The preceding history of this condition could well be indigestion with bloating and flatulence combined with an intolerance of rich food. If the patient ignores the symptoms and puts up with the discomfort but continues to indulge in heavy and spicy foods, relying on proprietary antacids, then the net result will be a chronic gastric and hepatic disorder. The tougher the constitution, the longer the body will put up with the abuse. Stopping the antacids and denying himself the rich food might well improve the patient's now-established chronic state but such measures are unlikely to complete a cure except in one with a very good constitution who has been able to deal with any outstanding emotional issues.

The stomach ulcer is usually the result of a more advanced pathology than indigestion resulting from indiscretion. It affects the system on a deep level so the patient would need correspondingly deep homoeopathic treatment or a radical change in regime. This is before we mention the frustration and resentment that often underlie this problem. We can ask almost all ulcer patients the question "What's eating you?" Though orthodox science would like the responsibility for internal ulceration of mucous surfaces to be laid at the door of *Helicobacter Pylori*, an opportunistic bug that is so often present in such cases, the truth is that the underlying cause is to be found within the psyche that has been unable to express its negativity purposefully.

All of us have a minor chronic condition that more or less frequently disturbs the even flow of our chosen lifestyles. It may be no more than dandruff or peeling skin on the soles; it might be no more troublesome than a small pile that bleeds occasionally; it could be no more threatening than a nervous tic at the corner of one eye. Such things are easily ignored. Nevertheless, we are each predisposed to the gradual onset of more and more serious health problems as we age and we tend, in this, to follow hereditary patterns. These are not always easily recognised though it is common knowledge that patients with particular conditions such as eczema and asthma, heart disease and arthritis often have forebears with the same troubles.

The process of history behind chronic disease

The ageing process shares similarities with what geology has to tell of the earth's history. We build up different strata, layers of health history. When a patient speaks of the arthritis in his hands he is talking only of the surface symptoms. He does not think to mention all the life events that went to make up his present complaint. It would seem ridiculous to mention how sad he felt twenty years ago when his best friend died and that he was devastated when his dog was put down but that he did not cry or tell anyone of his emotional pain. How would a woman suffering from pre-menstrual tension and severe menstrual cramps know that the fall she had on her coccyx at the age of sixteen and the history of having taken the contraceptive pill for six months contributed significantly to her condition? Would the angina patient speak much more than cursorily to the heart specialist about her chronic asthma and its treatment or would she be listening to long-term strategies for dealing with the heart? Would it ever be mentioned that she developed the first symptoms of asthma when her parents showed their disapproval of her choice of future husband and of angina after choking on a ginger biscuit?

The point here is that chronic disease, even if it can be given some complicated label, never results from just one thing. It is the result of a series of events in life. These events can be and often are of a traumatic and emotional nature. We are so good at putting off what we have no time or inclination to sort out that unresolved problems become buried and forgotten and we therefore have little realisation of just how much they contribute to our increasingly poor health. Physical trauma plays a part too. Though the body can compensate well for pain sustained through injury, it always leaves an indelible imprint on future chronic conditions unless well treated straightaway. Many a patient has complained that he or she has never felt well since a fall or a whiplash. If the injury is forgotten, the chronic complaint (say, migraines or vertigo) does not get better until the history of the injury itself (even though apparently long since gone) is treated – often by using cranial osteopathy, shiatsu, acupuncture or homoeopathy itself.

Some infectious or acute diseases have chronic, long-term implications: malaria and polio are two obvious examples. Hepatitis too, can cause chronic indisposition by damaging the liver; whooping cough can do the same to the lungs through excessive coughing; rheumatic fever can affect the valves of the heart. Other childhood complaints such as otitis media or tonsillitis, especially when suppressed with drugs, can cause damage to the ears, lungs and immune system as a whole, thus setting up chronic problems.

The three dimensions of our medical histories

To the homoeopath, every patient is like a jigsaw. To take the case of anyone suffering from a chronic condition is to gather pieces of information about the condition, about its history, about the person's lifestyle, emotional state and about significant past events; about the family history of disease and anything else that is an influence on his or her life. Homoeopaths see people in layers; one is put in mind of a cut-away diagram of a mountain in a geography book. Treating chronic conditions is akin to medical archaeology. In considering the individual history of each patient it is always essential to take into account three things:

1. The patient's present symptom picture – because that is the present manifestation of their history.
2. The patient's emotional and health biography – because today's complaint is the net result of this history.
3. The patient's heredity – because this is where the pre-conditions for all subsequent complaints are laid down.

These factors make up *three-dimensional medicine*. The terrain of the present complaint is combined with the context of the patient's biographical details and the soil of heredity in which the whole is rooted. This can be taken one step further by restating the obvious: that this happens within the integrated whole of our physical, emotional and spiritual bodies. Nature views the soul as the most significant factor in the hierarchy, and the emotional body as more significant than the physical. In the same way that the body will attempt to keep its disease states as near as possible to the surface or to drainage points so that vital organs will be able to function as well as possible, so damaging emotional trauma that is too terrible to sustain without adequate expression will be transmuted to the physical body. If the soul body is traumatised (which often occurs in the form of suppressed creative aspiration) then the psyche will express such distress until the emotional body is unable to sustain it further; depending on hereditary disposition, the patient will either manifest psychosis or physical disease: heart disease or cancer are the most usual long-term outcomes.

It takes enormous amounts of emotional and physical energy to sustain grief, fright, fear, hate, humiliation, unrequited love and the rest of the range of feelings to which we are subject and that we so frequently suppress. We could not keep up our purposeful lives for long if we did not find a way of securing these loose cannonballs. Ideally we need to find an appropriate way of expressing negative emotions so that they are discharged. Unfortunately this is frequently impossible and for a tidal wave of reasons.

Unexpressed emotions are an investment in illness

Tears are often an inadequate way of expressing sadness once we are beyond our childhood years. Many people are taught from an early age that angry tirades are unacceptable; tantrums are squashed all too often without a search for their root cause (although they can be a symptom of disease). Children are told not to be so silly about their fearfulness; they are told to pipe down, shut up, stop snivelling, and to wipe their eyes in case someone sees. Little incidents like this are part of the emotional conditioning because it makes things easier for parents. How often does a husband or wife or parent shame or quite carelessly embarrass someone into silence? What do we do with the unspoken emotions – frustration, humiliation or rage? Parental, educational and social pressures maintain the process of suppression of ready self-expression. In order to safeguard the integrity of the mind and emotions, *the body will assume responsibility*. This is what makes chronic disease more than a set of physical symptoms.

Anyone who has been diagnosed as having cancer and who has gone on to achieve a genuine cure knows how much they have had to change not simply their daily regime of exercise and diet but also their attitude to life and relationships. Not only the physical body but also the emotional and spiritual bodies have to be nurtured. Curative treatment of chronic complaints has to cover all three dimensions. This is why asthma does not get better on drugs; asthma is an emotional condition – the patient is emotionally stifled. (This refers to true asthma, not the bronchospasm that so many children suffer from these days. It looks like it, but is a result of repeatedly suppressed ear, throat and chest infections in those who have been vaccine damaged.) This is why rheumatism does not get better on steroids and anti-inflammatories. Rheumatism owes much of its force to buried resentment, anger and a history of friction within relationships. This is why gallstones do not get better permanently but keep recurring; gallstones are the result of bitter anger that has been suppressed. This is why ulcerative colitis is not curable with sulphur drugs; ulcerative colitis is the result of unforgiving anger in a fearful patient. Hypothyroidism (underactive thyroid) is not cured by taking thyroxin; it is held in balance by it and often with difficulty. Hypothyroidism is an emotional disease that has its roots in the feeling of 'When is it going to be my turn?' The list is as long as the list of named (and unnamed) chronic conditions.

> Because allopathy uses only chemical agents and surgery to treat physical pathology, 'cure' is inevitably limited. Doctors and consultants are at a distinct disadvantage in dealing with chronic illness. Most of them would not think of referring their patients to psychiatrists unless there were a specific and potentially diagnosable psychiatric condition – one that could be given a convenient label. Some, however, will refer their patients on to counsellors or psychotherapists. There can be no question that there are many patients who do well by taking this route of orthodox treatment plus non-interventionist counselling. They do better still if common-sense dietary and exercise advice is also available.

Many patients become adventurous and then go in for esoteric therapy; they take up yoga and meditation in the knowledge that relaxing the three bodies is an essential part of healing. Though the role of the drugs or surgery is obviously important to the resolution of the physical aspect of the disease, it is the patient's determination to attend to their negative reactions to stress and emotional trauma that actually affords the cure. Drugs and surgery give a temporary space for the patient to set about healing everything else, which includes the predisposing factor of emotional imbalance. There is absolutely no true and lasting cure of any chronic disease without the resolution of the history of emotional disturbance. Only the patient can heal this, no-one else can.

Many patients of deep pathology achieve a temporary respite in their illnesses only for a return of symptoms to draw them into another round of suffering. These are the patients who have not been able or have not sought to discharge, through emotional expression, all their past grief. Take, for example, the story of Rosalind.

> Rosalind astonished her doctors by recovering from cancer of the pancreas. She had had an earlier operation to remove a breast lump. Some two years later they found that some of the lymph glands in her armpit were affected so they removed those and gave her radiotherapy treatment. Throughout this time Rosalind had homoeopathic remedies and nutritional therapy; she also practised yoga and transcendental meditation. For a while it seemed as if she had recovered but when she developed some worrying digestive symptoms more tests were done. The pancreas was now affected.
>
> Rosalind determined that she was going to do all she could to improve her health. She continued her homoeopathic treatment and went on a special diet. During her appointments with the homoeopath she went into her life story of passions and grief – which was considerable, involving as it did sexual and physical abuse. Within six months the doctors could find no evidence of cancer.

Some months later however, there was a sudden and marked turn for the worse. Within a space of just three months Rosalind lost weight and became dramatically weaker. She was hospitalised and treated for the last stages of liver cancer. No-one involved could understand how such a delightful, gifted and positive person could have taken such a dramatic turn for the worse. Then, just a few days before the end, Rosalind asked to see her sister, someone with whom she had had no words whatever for nearly thirty years. These two women met at last and openly forgave each other for the grief of their confused and tragic relationship and all the wasted years of no communication.

Rosalind's daughter related how her mother had said to her that she felt 'really better' once she had spoken to her sister. The quality of her final hours was infinitely enhanced by being able to resolve the bitterness and hatred that had lain buried in her heart for so long. The few minutes of resolution became a lifetime achievement.

The reality and value of the hierarchical model

How can we confirm that there is this hierarchical system? There are no orthodox textbooks that even hint at such a thing. There are few alternative medicine books that state it unequivocally. The answer must be in the study of case histories of those who have achieved cure. Anything else remains just theory. Before looking at some illustrative case histories it is worth summarising the hierarchy of the body and the hierarchy of disease.

i) Acutes are clearly defined conditions that have a specific cause and progress. They range from the negligible to the fatal. They may or may not involve fever but they usually involve discharges from one or more orifices or the skin.

ii) Chronic diseases are of slower onset involving a variety of predisposing factors (which usually include a hereditary aspect) for which the body has no intrinsic cure beyond the patient's own recognition that there is a need for radical change – which, if instituted, can bring about a reversal of the disease unless damage to internal organs is so severe as to be irreversible.

iii) Sub-acutes are flare-ups of acute conditions arising in patients that have a more or less chronic problem which requires some form of immediate release due to a toxic build-up (either biochemical or emotional) within the system. (It should also be added that there are many cases where the flare-up is triggered by the patient's emotional dependency and is nothing short of manipulation of those caring for them – a distressing form of emotional blackmail.)

iv) The three bodies that form our integral 'whole' – body, emotions and spirit – are subject to a natural law of priority in which the spirit has the highest priority followed by the emotions and then the physical body.

v) The physical body in turn prioritises its constituent parts according to what it can afford to allow to suffer pain or disease. (Epidemic diseases such as malaria or whooping cough are not subject to any prioritising as they affect specific organs – but even here there may be hereditarily hierarchical reasons for their existence as we shall come to see.)

vi) Disease, suppressed or neglected, strikes inwards. The more it is suppressed in whatever form it manifests *the more it will be obliged to change its location, its intensity and its description.* While isolated incidents of suppression can be supported with few or no harmful effects, frequent or long-term suppression becomes the principle agent of the worsening disease state.

We can add to this summary a fuller answer to the question of why disease might appear in an internal part or organ without any prior skin or immune system problem. The Vital Force will often make use of a part or organ for its symptoms that will demonstrate *illustratively* the cause of the problem: a bladder infection with frequent urging to urinate in one who is grief-struck but unable to cry; asthmatic breathing in one who has been stifled for much of his or her life; irritable bowel syndrome in one who is perpetually anxious but who has to suppress the outward signs of it. It is rare indeed for a disease state not to match and illustrate its causation. There is also the other reason for disease first manifesting in inner parts: heredity. A patient may well present symptoms in an internal organ of an otherwise healthy body because the condition is mimicking one that has occurred in a previous generation.

As proof that these facts are so it is necessary to demonstrate the possibility of cure by natural means. Taking as the premise of cure the return of the body to a state of health where (i) the patient is no longer suffering any symptoms of the complaint treated and (ii) the patient is free of any predisposing factors that would encourage the return of the same symptoms, the cases in the following section show that healing not only comes from within and is therefore achieved by the patient (and not the practitioner) but also that healing is the very reverse of the disease process. Furthermore, the case studies demonstrate a notion that has been gaining ground for years even if painfully slowly; that there is a *positive* aspect to illness; that disease is actually an integral part of our potential development; that it might be considered part of an individual's Karma or 'life-lesson'. By going through a process of natural healing, the patient is ridding him or herself of that which is restricting personal evolution – some might take this as far as seeing this as *soul growth*.

CHAPTER 6

THE LAW OF CURE

Hering's Law

Constantine Hering, that gifted disciple of Samuel Hahnemann who did so much for the advance of homoeopathy, established the four points of the Law of Cure. They are useful as a guide to the way treatment is going, whether positively or negatively, in acute, sub-acute or chronic conditions. They also neatly encapsulate the process of healing that we have illustrated so far. Hering's four points describe the process of cure as a *reverse* of the way acute disease transmutes towards chronic illness:

1) Symptoms move from the top of the body downwards, towards the extremities.
2) Symptoms move from within to the surface of the body.
3) Symptoms move from more important organs to less important ones.
4) Symptoms reappear in the reverse order of their first appearance.

These four points are not incontrovertible. There are times when the healing body will do something to contradict the rule. An asthma patient whose breathing is improving at the expense of his skin may find that the skin eruption (eczema, say) is spreading *upwards* over the torso. This is because the lungs need to be healed completely and to do this the skin will show the *full* extent of the original disease and the natural reaction to the suppressive treatment that was instituted before the asthma took hold.

Sometimes an old symptom returns in an organ that is more delicate and vulnerable than the one for which treatment is presently being given. A bowel condition may be healing well when suddenly a kidney infection blows up – but this is possibly because there was a history of suppressed or neglected cystitis and kidney infection in the past, one that needs to be tackled as a 'return of an old symptom'. A patient will not conveniently repeat old symptom pictures in a neat reversal of chronology; the pattern will be more to do with whichever old condition the body views as a priority. Ultimately it is the body – or, more properly, the Vital Force – that is the arbiter of the process of 'cure'.

If the healing process is going according to the general ethos of the four points then the 'cure', as far as it is possible, will take place. If it is not then it is not the Vital Force that is in charge but the disease state – remembering, of course, that disease is a creation of the whole body. The 'Law of Disease' is the very opposite to the 'Law of Cure'. By looking into the way that homoeopaths think, we can see the Law of Cure in practice. To do that we need to go back and consult Samuel Hahnemann again before going on to illustrate the Law with cases.

The gentlest method of cure

When Samuel Hahnemann set out on his life of medical exploration he was armed with a formidable intellect, a zealous nature and a profound desire to be of service. He had no notion that there was a Law of Cure. Nevertheless, he wrote down, in a book that he called *The Organon*, his understanding of the processes of healing. This and a later publication: *The Chronic Diseases*, would lead Hering to make his list[1]. So possessed was Hahnemann of certainty that he was right in following his path away from suppressive medicine, that it is not surprising that he eventually clashed with so many of his contemporaries. Nevertheless, he was not so rigidly convinced that he could not subtly change his mind as experience showed him more: he wrote six versions of *The Organon* over the course of his long life. What he never changed his mind about was the idea that the process in search of a cure for every individual should be as gentle as possible: a contradiction in terms for the revolutionary times he lived in!

If Hahnemann were alive today he would have been incensed that conventional medicine still so often renders the patient passive and that the participation of the sick in their own healing process is still reduced to listening to advice and taking the pills. He would have recognised in patients the more or less mute acceptance that side effects are inevitable and shaken his head. How differently Samuel Hahnemann saw things! In *The Organon* he wrote:

> The highest ideal of therapy is to restore health rapidly, gently, permanently; to remove and destroy the whole disease in the shortest, surest, least harmful way, according to clearly comprehensible principles.

As described earlier, it was the very side effects of the drugs in use in medical practice at the time that caused Hahnemann to abandon conventional methods and to devote his life to experimenting with naturally occurring substances until he stumbled on the system of potentisation that he developed into homoeopathy as we know it today. Not for him the leech or the curette, the bleeding-cup or the ice bath.

In the third paragraph of *The Organon* he wrote the following:

> If the physician clearly perceives what has to be cured in disease, i.e. in each individual case of disease; if he clearly perceives what it is in medicines which heals, i.e. in each individual medicine; if he applies in accordance with well-defined principles what is curative in medicines to what he has clearly recognised to be pathological in the patient so that cure follows, i.e. if he knows in each particular case how to apply the remedy most appropriate by its character, prepare it exactly as required and give it in the right amount and repeat the dose exactly when required; if in each case he knows the obstacles to cure and how to remove them so that recovery is permanent, then he knows how to treat thoroughly and efficaciously and is a true physician.

The implications within this paragraph are enormous.

i) A patient is an individual and his or her disease is individual to him or her.

ii) Medicines should be curative and not suppressive and each one should be perceived to have qualities and characteristics that are definable and unique to itself.

iii) There is an affinity and relationship between a patient producing characteristic symptoms and a medicine that has been proved to produce (in a healthy person) the same symptoms that it will heal.

iv) Every patient suffering from a disease displays symptoms that will be healed in the gentlest manner only by the administration of the chosen indicated medicine in a dose appropriate to that individual.

v) There is clear recognition that there are potential reasons for a patient's lack of response to treatment and that these need to be taken into account before prescribing.

However caring an allopathic doctor may be it cannot be said that the patient is always and at all times viewed as an individual. He or she is a 'heart patient' or a 'cancer patient', has a stomach ulcer or multiple sclerosis. The patient is labelled by the condition that can be looked up in a textbook, where the suggested specific therapeutic course of treatment is described for *all* such cases. The patient is on the way to becoming a statistic.

Drugs are suppressive and not curative. In patients with healthy constitutions drugs can halt a symptom sufficiently for the patients' self-healing mechanism to reassert itself and thus take over the cure but it is *not* the drug that cures.

Allopathic drugs are recognised only as having an affinity for diseases and not for patients.

Individualising the patient

There is very little differentiation in allopathy between a short, balding, intemperate beer-swiller with a heart problem and a tall, quick-witted, warm-hearted priest with a heart problem. The same drug is likely to be prescribed to deal with a condition with the same label in individuals of totally different constitutions. While allopaths do as much to ensure the correct dosage as they can, they are dealing with drugs that have potentially harmful side effects. Every dose administered needs to be stronger than the Vital Force of the patient under treatment. If not, as has already been noted, the body would excrete the drug as an invading toxin. In other words, drugs *are always given in large doses*; too little will be worse than useless, an excessive amount might have damaging (and occasionally lethal) consequences, just right and the symptoms will be suppressed.

Furthermore, there is scant recognition in allopathy of the reasons why a patient should *not* get better. The suppressive treatment is designed to remove *only* the physical symptoms; where the suppressive treatment fails to achieve a 'cure', the recourse for the patient is to undergo tests or exploratory operations. By looking only at the disease the doctor or consultant is often unable to determine whether there are spiritual, mental, emotional, hereditary or, and this is very common, physical reasons for lack of progress towards cure. In psychiatric cases the same is essentially true. No allopathic drug has ever been produced that has the potential for treating the *underlying cause* of illness.

The most positive reports about practitioners are about those who know their patients as individuals, as part of a family and within the community; who know the characteristics and foibles of their patients; who are able to step outside the purely physical aspects of a condition they are treating. Their patients' histories are familiar to them. Such family doctors, who inspire so much trust, are increasingly in the minority and we are the poorer for it. These are individuals called into their profession by a healing mission and their chief assets are their patience and their ability to listen. Whatever the medical philosophy of the practitioner, the healing that needs to be performed begins with this *patience* – to observe in every detail – and the ability to *listen*. When these are combined with warmth and generosity of spirit then healing can often begin even before the prescription has been written out.

What a practitioner looks for as a guide

Patients produce symptoms that we can hear about and see; they can be both subjective – *"I feel sick and chilly"* – and objective – *"the patient was doubled up in pain and driving her fists into her belly"*. There are few illnesses that do not announce an internal disorder either subjectively or objectively; any one or all of the five senses ensure that we can relate or demonstrate our unwellness. No cure can be initiated until the *complete* symptom picture is taken into account – and it is best done when there is empathy between patient and practitioner.

To prescribe medication for a 'sore throat' or an 'ear infection' is to miss the individuality of the patient's condition; it is not enough to hear how the patient feels in himself and in the part affected. Observation of the general and then the particular and active listening as the patient describes how he or she feels, are vital to natural healing and are the prerequisites of any prescription – allopathic or alternative. By this process the patient becomes an active participant in the healing process and the practitioner becomes the 'listener'; passive until the moment of putting pill into packet. This may seem obvious but it is far from common practice.

In our attempts to control disease we all want there to be specific cures for our ills. It is comforting to think that there might be a well-known procedure for eradicating every condition. Allopathic scientists promote this attitude all the time by releasing to the press information on the latest research into newsworthy diseases, holding out promises of cures for potentially terminal illnesses. Having spent the best part of a century attempting to find solutions to cure anything from colds to cancer scientists are gradually abandoning research into chemotherapy and starting work on manipulating DNA, the very building blocks of life. From their indefatigable research they want to gather answers to be able to write the textbooks that will fix the solutions to the interminable problems of disease. The recipes for cure must be cast in stone and patented by commercial enterprises.

Individuals and the constant flux of nature

Nature never stands still. Disease is not immutable; it is infinitely plastic. People are not universally similar; they are infinitely varied. Cure, if there is truly such a thing, must take place within the individual and, as far as the world of science is concerned, with ten billion people on the planet that is a professional nightmare.

In alternative practice there is never – or *should* never! – be any attempt to 'fix' anything into any rigid form. The whole essence of observation and listening is to see how things differ from the accepted norm of the patient, not to see how similar he or she is to the description in the book of pathology. The only immutable laws are those of nature and they can be understood only by observing patients as they become sick and as they heal.

While disease and health are both subject to the laws of nature, the body – home to both – is intent on survival. In order to survive, nature has given us a straightforward survival plan; one which is observable in every particular if you look in the right place in the right way. *Healing can be witnessed.*

The nature of cure

What is 'cure'? The answer is obvious in the case of acute conditions. It is the relief and eradication of all acute symptoms of the disease, leaving the patient completely restored to former health. This is true also of those who have suffered from accidents and trauma.

When we look at sub-acute illnesses such as bronchitis or gout then the answer becomes less clear-cut. The underlying chronic condition remains after the symptoms of the flare-up have been dealt with. For example, antihistamines may relieve the body of all hay fever symptoms but the problem will come back next year because the allergic susceptibility has never been addressed. For chronic complaints there are no cures at all except through patients' own efforts at creating positive change in their lives – with whatever means they may use to achieve that, alternative or allopathic. We need to illustrate these points with cases so that the underlying pattern of healing is plainly seen.

Case 1
A young woman had suffered a severe surface burn on her right calf. About the size of a saucer, it was sustained as a result of standing too close to her boyfriend's motorbike exhaust. The area was deep pink and looked scorched. It wept a thin, clear fluid and she complained that it felt very sore. She had been putting lint plasters on it for the three weeks since she had been to the outpatients' department in the hospital. There had been no change to the lesion since then. She was very anxious about the wound and was worried that it would leave a scar, which would be cosmetically unpleasing. The remedy given for this was *Causticum* 30, one twice a day for five days. She was asked to report at the end of this time. She rang back one week later and said that the wound was much better and no longer hurt. When asked about her levels of anxiety she said that she had not thought about feeling anxious since shortly after her visit to the homoeopathic clinic. Over the week the wound had at first dried up

and then begun to itch. The surface skin began to peel away leaving fresh, healthy coloured skin on the surface.

A point to notice here is that the healing began with a relaxation of the mental attitude – *Causticum* is a remedy that covers anxiety. *Causticum* was also responsible for encouraging the wound to stop discharging lymph inappropriately. As the damaged surface began to itch and peel, so new skin was formed below the wound. When the patient next presented for treatment, for an unrelated problem, the skin on her leg showed not the slightest evidence that there had ever been a burn.

Case 2

A mother brought her eight-year-old daughter to the 'drop in' clinic. She was not sure whether the girl was suffering from measles or from mumps; both were going the rounds at the local school. There were no signs of the telltale Koplic spots in the mouth that would have confirmed measles but this was not taken as conclusive evidence. The girl looked cheerful but said that she had a headache in the back of her head. She also looked pale and lacking in energy. Her mother mentioned that she was extremely thirsty and, unusually for her, she wanted ice in her water. ("*I can't bear it when she crunches up the ice cubes!*") The girl's lips were unusually red and glistened with saliva. It was noticeable that she was dribbling from the corners of her mouth and it caused her to keep slurping. She agreed that she had been feeling first hot and then cold, especially at night and that this temperature variation had kept waking her up. She reported, too, that she sweated profusely at night. "*And her breath is awful!*" whispered her mother. Only *Mercury* has this symptom picture and it matters not at all that the condition might have been mumps or measles. She was given *Mercurius Solubulis* (*Merc. Sol.*) 30, one to be taken four times a day for three days. The mother returned the following week with her daughter who felt completely well except that she had a rash on her abdomen. After the remedy had been started it quickly became evident that the problem was with mumps. The parotid glands on both sides of her neck became swollen. "*There was no pain at all which I always thought there was supposed to be,*" said the mother. The temperature changes and sweating ceased within two days and the glands went down soon after. On the fourth day the rash on the abdomen appeared and was obviously fading now.

Notice how the body was attempting to eliminate by salivation and sweating profusely. Once the body began responding to the remedy the disease was announced clearly by the production of the characteristic swelling of the neck glands. As the condition became easier the child eliminated more satisfactorily through excessive urination. The final phase was the appearance of the rash on the skin of the abdomen; very typical in the case of any of the childhood diseases. It is noteworthy that all these symptoms were pain or discomfort-free as soon as she took the remedy. (The headache had disappeared by the morning after the first dose.)

Case 3

A man came for treatment for an abscess under the right nipple. He was embarrassed by it but so anxious to get better that he had decided to have it examined. The abscess looked swollen and was dark pink in the centre but with a mixture of bluish and greenish tinges around the edges. He complained that it was very painful with sharp stabs every so often. He was feeling extremely irritable. He kept frowning and, on being asked what he would prefer to be doing at this moment, he said that he wanted to be left alone to sit in front of the fire with a hot cup of tea. *"I wish the bloody thing would come to a head and burst!"* This symptom picture is typical of *Hepar Sulphuricum*, Hahnemann's compound of sulphur and oyster shell (calcium). It covers just this degree of irritability, the wish to be left alone, characteristic stabbing pains, boils and abscesses. The man was given *Hepar Sulph.* 30 to be taken three times a day for three days. He reported back that the abscess had simply faded away over the three days, that he was far more cheerful and had been since waking up after the first night of the remedy. A small head had appeared just beside the nipple which had some white pus in it but that was now gone and there was only a slight itching of the area. He was asked whether he had found that he had needed to pass more water than usual and he said *"No"* to this. *"However, I have been sweating like a pig and it doesn't smell very nice! Can you do anything for that?"* He was asked to allow the perspiration to continue as this was helping him eliminate the toxic waste. When next he came for a consultation, months later, he said he had no recollection of the smelly sweats. Once again, notice how the mood and general state of the patient improved while the body found a way to discharge the physical symptom. The body externalised the internal problem.

Case 4

A fifteen-year-old girl was brought to the 'drop-in' clinic. She was suffering from an unexplained rash. It was bright pink and slightly raised; it covered her torso and there were patches on her back. She felt that it was also beginning to creep up to her neck and her face, and it felt dry and irritated. There was no apparent explanation for the rash in spite of her and her parents' every effort to think of possible causes. She was asked how she felt 'in herself' and she replied that she *"felt a bit down"*. Her mother then chipped in that the girl had been very tearful. She had a demure expression and did not raise her head much or her voice above a whisper. With every question she was asked, she would look at her mother for reassurance. (Though her mother would say, *"Go on then, you've got a tongue in your head!"*) She was asked if she felt too warm to which the eventual answer was *"Yes, but I want to keep wrapped up."* As she sat there in the close atmosphere of the clinic she was fanning herself with a letter she was holding.

She was given *Pulsatilla* 1M in a single dose and asked to report back within three days if the rash had not gone. There was no news from her for three months when she returned with exactly the same problem. She said that the original rash had cleared up by the time she woke the next morning though she had noticed that it had travelled to her forearms overnight. By the end of the day it had also gone from there. When asked if her skin had peeled at all she looked surprised and said that the soles of her feet had only just stopped doing so. On this occasion the rash was not so strong but it had reached her neck and face quite quickly. She again had the rather contradictory temperature condition and her mood was the same as the first time. This time she was asked if anything had made her unhappy. She hesitatingly said that she was being teased at school by one or two other girls, one of whom was her best friend – *"or so I thought."* She was given *Pulsatilla* 10M with the same instruction to call back. This time she rang to say that the rash had gone but now it had gone down her legs as it disappeared from her torso. Her feet had not peeled as much but her fingertips were doing so now. She sounded much more confident and was clearly interested in what her body had done to heal itself. Asked about her friendships she replied, *"I don't have anything to do with that girl any more. I realise that she was just using me."*

The next few illustrative cases also demonstrate this externalising process; the body's centrifugal force.

Case 5

Two children from the same family had gone down with gastro-enteritis. The elder, a boy aged eight, felt sick but could not vomit; he kept passing very watery, foul-smelling diarrhoea; he was very anxious and restless. He was getting quite weak but refused anything to eat; his mother was worried because, although he said he was very thirsty, she had noticed that he only drank a little at a time and she was afraid that he would become dehydrated. His sister, aged five, behaved differently in that she kept being sick but had passed no motions for thirty-six hours, which was unusual for her. She also was restless and intermittently anxious especially just before she vomited. She refused all food but drank copiously of cold water, which she would bring up again within a few minutes. She kept complaining of pains in her abdomen that she described as "*hot*". Both children were given *Arsenicum Album* 30, one every two hours. The boy was sick within fifteen seconds of the first dose. Less than twenty minutes later he asked for food and soon after he had a piece of dry toast and half a bowl of porridge, he fell asleep and did not wake till the following morning. He needed no further doses.

His sister stopped vomiting altogether after the first dose but complained that her tummy hurt a bit more. She told her mother that it was "*growling*" and still hot. She asked to be taken up to bed where she lay quietly listening to a story (which she had not been able to do before). After about quarter of an hour she began stirring again but said that she did not feel sick at all. Very shortly after that she gave a baleful wailing whimper and rushed to the bathroom where she passed "*an enormous quantity*" of dark ("*almost black*") diarrhoea. Within a few minutes she was back in bed and fast asleep.

These two children demonstrate that two people, even though their symptom pictures differ in some respects, can call for the same medicine if the essential core of the condition is the same. Both children were restless and anxious in the manner that is peculiar to *Arsenic* but individually they produced different aspects of *Arsenic's* pathology. Because the disease affected them similarly *in general* (restless and anxious) then *Arsenic* was able to help both of them re-establish well-being even though *the particular* (vomiting or diarrhoea) were apparently different. (Actually, *Arsenic* is one of the most common diarrhoea and vomiting remedies.) The main physiological difference was that the boy had a focus of pathology in the stomach while the girl had a focus in the small intestine. In both cases the body discharged the problem appropriately and speedily.

Case 6

A boy aged fourteen was brought in to the clinic as an emergency. He had frightful pains across his abdomen that caused him to double up and ram his fists into his midriff. He was quite unable to stand up straight and could not walk. He was carried from the car. In addition he complained of severe aching in the kidney region which he felt was in some way connected with the other pains. He was crying out in pain and noticeably irritated by questions. Beads of sweat were standing out on his brow and he felt nauseous with the pain. He was given *Colocynth* 200 on the spot. Within thirty seconds he began to stand up straighter. He began to smile and had the expression of someone dazed, as if coming out of a dream state. He was asked how long ago he had passed water to which he replied that he had *"not been to the loo all day"*. His mother later reported that on arriving home he passed almost two pints of urine; that he no longer had pains in the abdomen or kidneys; that he now felt that he had an irritation in the bladder and the penis. He described it as a sensation as if there were more urine to come all the time. No further prescription was given but he was directed to drink more water. All symptoms were cleared by the following morning.

This case was potentially extremely serious as the kidneys were a focus of the condition. Had he been treated allopathically he would probably have been given antibiotics and a urine sample would have been taken. (It is perhaps unlikely that any bacteria would have been discovered as the urine that the boy passed after taking the remedy was absolutely clear in colour and consistency.) He would have been given a painkiller such as pethidine but this would not have dealt with the underlying problem. After he had recovered he agreed that he had been extremely angry shortly before the acute pain came on. He had felt humiliated and furious over an incident at school in which he had been passed over in a selection process for a responsible position. With the removal of his symptoms he also said that he was no longer worried about the school issue. Had antibiotics been used it is highly likely that the problem would have recurred.

Case 7

One more case demonstrates acute symptoms responding to acute prescribing:

A young woman came to the 'drop-in' clinic complaining of a sore throat. She had recently returned home from somewhere in Africa. She said that her throat felt very constricted and that it was very painful to swallow. The left side of her throat was worse but it now felt as if the right side was also becoming more painful. She was unable to protrude her tongue and she refused to open her mouth: *"No way! It's absolutely disgusting in there!"* She was asked how she felt in herself. Her reply was a gesture: she made her hand into a two-fingered claw, which she held up and, while going *"Siss, Siss!"* she imitated a snake biting. *"I feel so venomous,"* she added in a whisper. She was given *Lachesis* 30, from the venom of the bushmaster snake, and the report was that within twenty-four hours her throat symptoms had cleared and she was completely well twenty-four hours after that. She also said that she felt a great deal better than she had before the throat symptoms had begun. *"However, I've coughed up the most amazing amount of the most foul looking mucus. Was that part of the cure?"* The answer, naturally, was *"Yes"*.

The remedy here was not difficult to spot. She even illustrated the snake energy with her gesture. So it was not just the patient's throat that was affected by the condition but her whole being, including the psyche. (This patient had no prior knowledge whatever of homoeopathy; she had never had any alternative treatment before and had wanted to try out homoeopathy before going to the doctor.)

From these cases several points of importance can be observed. Firstly, symptoms heal from within towards the surface. The scorched skin of the first case healed when new skin developing from within was able to replace the damaged and sloughed off skin. Eruptions, just below the skin, as in Case 3, can either be eliminated by forming a head and discharging directly onto the surface, or through the body – absorbing the toxins into the lymph system and discharging by way of sweat, bowels or bladder. The exit points of the lymph system are the bladder and kidneys, the bowels, the skin and the mucous membranes. It is often difficult to tell which of these routes the body will choose for elimination but one or other of them must be employed for the satisfactory expulsion of waste. (It should not be forgotten that the uterus is also an organ of elimination.)

In Case 4, a second observable point is illustrated: that symptoms go from above towards the extremities. The girl's rash left her body only by degrees. It travelled away from the torso, first to the forearms and then, on the second occasion, to the legs. This phenomenon of a rash or eczema eruption travelling away from the centre towards the extremities and downwards, is so commonly seen in the progress towards cure that it almost goes without saying that if the skin symptoms do the opposite and travel upwards and towards the centre then the disease is not progressing towards cure.

In Case 6 the third point of importance is seen. Internal symptoms that affect the more important organs are relieved by throwing the burden of elimination onto less delicately balanced organs. Notice how the boy's kidneys were relieved through the elimination of urine from the bladder; he also had symptomatic sensations in the bladder and penis, where he had had none before, prior to his complete restoration to health.

These points are, in some form, observable in any case that is 'cured'. When a patient suffers a symptom that is striking inwards in spite of treatment then cure will not take place. If a more important organ is affected by symptoms after treatment has begun – say the heart suffers while the lungs are being treated – then cure will not take place. Except in very complex, chronic cases, the same is true if symptoms do not travel downwards or outwards; no cure will come about unless they do.

If we now take a look at a more complex batch of cases then certain other points of interest will emerge.

Case 8

Edward, a child aged four, was brought for treatment suffering from 'asthma'. The mother had just had the diagnosis from the doctor who had prescribed ventolin and steroid inhalers. These had not yet been used as the mother was doubtful about the implied seriousness of her son's condition. She explained that the boy had had a persistent cough for only six weeks. She had gone to the doctor so that he could listen to her son's chest and check his lungs. She had been surprised to hear that the problem was asthma. The coughing had begun after a cold; it sounded dry and wheezy at one time and then loose and rattly at others. He was unable to blow his nose so he tended to swallow any phlegm that was manufactured by the sinuses. He felt queasy as a result and sometimes he would retch and bring up quantities of creamy mucus. In the mornings he was wheezy but his breathing always sounded easier by lunchtime. The cough was always made easier when he was outside in the fresh air and worse if he was indoors watching the TV (the only activity that would keep him inside). Edward's mood was good most of the time though he was of a mild and rather yielding temperament anyway. The prescription was for *Pulsatilla* 1M, three doses at two-hour intervals. The result of this remedy was that the cough stopped by the next morning but was followed by a sore throat like the one he had had prior to the cough. He remembered it because he felt as if there were something sharp in his right ear whenever he swallowed. (This symptom would have been treated by *Hepar Sulphuricum* had the case been 'caught' earlier. It is common for acute symptom pictures to change quite quickly from one remedy state into another. It is through the body's habit of returning through past states in order to get back to original health that we see these 'missed' remedy pictures.) The throat symptoms did not last for more than the day and by evening his nose was streaming; first he poured green, then yellow and then clear mucus. This process took forty-eight hours. By the time his nose was clear he had no further symptoms at all.

Here we have not just the elimination process going on but also the return of the original problem of the sore throat that, having developed into a cough, never satisfactorily resolved. The body went back to reproduce the symptoms that had, so to speak, gone off at a tangent. Instead of the body dealing with the throat by elimination, somehow the disease energy had been diverted to the lungs – in fact, the mother had used a eucalyptus balm to ease congestion which could have been the factor that caused the switch from throat to lungs. This return to a previous and unresolved state en route to cure is very common and very important. You might also note how the green, infected mucus that first started to run from his nose after the remedy was given gradually became clearer. This demonstrates that 'infected' mucus – i.e. mucus that is full of bacteria – is part of the elimination process and not the disease process.

The following cases are further examples of healing reversing the history of a complaint:

Case 9

A boy aged three had developed symptoms of asthma. He had a history of eczema and ear infections. For these earlier problems he had been prescribed a lot of antibiotics. The mother was afraid that he responded less well to the antibiotics each time he was given them and now she was sure that he had adverse reactions in the bowels. He had steroid creams to put on the affected areas of his skin (the hands, backs of his knees and his ankles). Every time he developed cold symptoms he would start coughing and become wheezy. Both parents had noticed that their son's skin improved dramatically whenever his asthmatic symptoms worsened.

The child was always warm and would tolerate only the lightest covering, day or night. He always kicked his shoes off whenever he could. He was also a very sweaty person, most particularly on the head. He objected to washing, not least because contact with water aggravated his skin. He spent most of the night scratching and by morning the backs of his knees in particular would be blooded. However, the skin trouble was not the parents' main consideration; they wanted the asthma to be dealt with.

Before prescribing it was also learnt that the boy was very thirsty, always hungry, had perpetually loose bowel motions and never stopped talking. He was given *Sulphur* 6 to be taken twice daily. However, the parents were advised that the skin symptoms were likely to get worse. They did.

After several weeks the mother phoned to report that the eczema was appalling and that she did not know what she should do. She was on the point of going back to the doctor. Through questioning it transpired that he had had no difficulty with breathing at all. After the first few doses of *Sulphur* he had had one spectacular bout of diarrhoea *"that went everywhere"* and had smelled rank; he had then had *"a runny nose for a week at least"* and had then developed a pain in the right ear which came to nothing. The eczema was now very red, oozing a clear fluid and forming crusty scabs. Not only was it all over his hands but it had spread from the backs of the knees to the ankles and over the calves.

Apart from anything else, the mother was anxious in case the skin lesions became infected. In fact there was an infection of the right wrist as the area had become inflamed, very red and sore. For this local infection he was given *Belladonna* 30 which, after several doses, reduced the site of the inflammation to the state of the rest of the local skin. It was immediately after this that the right ear became acutely painful and seemed threatening. Along with the ear pain came extreme thirst for water, profuse salivation and foul breath. This called for *Mercury* 30 which swiftly soothed the ear but led to a throat infection. The right tonsil became inflamed and his temperature went up to 102°F. The mother was frankly alarmed by these developments especially as she now feared that the asthma would come back with the throat symptoms. She was remembering how his old pattern of symptoms worked.

Nevertheless, she agreed to give him a dose of *Belladonna* 200. This brought the fever down within hours and he slept deeply until the next morning. He was well for most of the day but began to spike a fever again at around 3 p.m. A further dose of the *Belladonna* 200 dispatched the temperature for good. The throat symptoms eased off considerably over the next day and were gone by the morning of the third day. (*"I can breathe again,"* said his mother.)

Over the next few months a similar pattern of events reoccurred twice, each time with less intensity. After each episode the eczema would worsen a little but then subside, until all that was left of the bloody, scabby, oozing eruptions was dry skin that was roughened like fine sandpaper. Except at the times of acute flare-ups of the ears and tonsils, *Sulphur* 6 was administered throughout at the rate of two per day. On two occasions other remedies, *Tuberculinum* and *Psorinum* (see Part III), were used to treat the underlying, hereditary disposition for producing eczema; they were needed intercurrently[2] with the *Sulphur* in order that it should complete as much of its action as possible. The eczema was cleared for the most part but the roughened skin suggested that further constitutional treatment would be necessary. Of the so-called asthma there was absolutely no further trace.

(Over the following two to three years the boy received regular prophylactic treatment; his roughened skin is now a thing of the past.)

So, what went on? *Sulphur* is a well-known remedy for the symptom picture displayed by this boy: warm-blooded, sweaty (on the head), thirsty; susceptible to eczema which bleeds and itches on becoming hot (especially in bed). It is also well known for the treatment of those whose conditions have been suppressed by drugs. In effect, it is an antidote to the effects of many allopathic drugs; it will allow the body to create reverse reactions to those set up by such medicines as antibiotics. The initial reaction to the *Sulphur* 6 was in the fastest eliminator of all: the bowel. After the explosive diarrhoea his motions returned to a normal consistency. Then the skin began to aggravate, which is very common with *Sulphur*. The oozing fluid was discharging as an expression of the suppressive steroid creams. They were being pushed out the way they had gone in.

It is also usual for the skin to harbour bacteria that can cause sepsis. *Belladonna* sorted this out as well as the fever with the throat infection; both had the same essential picture of redness, inflammation and heat. It was no surprise to find the ear and throat troubles resurfacing because these were old symptoms that had never been allowed to finish naturally; they had always been driven underground by antibiotics. They returned under the influence of the *Sulphur* in order for the body to have the opportunity of dealing with them naturally.

It is significant that the mother confirmed that both the ear and throat acutes manifested in exactly the way they had always done. This meant that whenever he had had an acute attack of ear pain he produced the same *Mercury* picture and whenever he had produced an acute attack of throat infection he would have the same *Belladonna* symptoms. There is only a theoretical explanation as to why the acute flare-ups recurred twice more but in less severe form: for the body to have suffered the acute flare-ups all in one go would have weighed heavily on the body's healing resources so it set about curing itself in stages. This is a frequently observable phenomenon most particularly amongst those patients who have had a considerable amount of suppressive treatment.

This case illustrates both the aggressive nature of suppression – the eczema suppressed becomes an onslaught on the ears and throat (lymphatics) and then, with further suppression, on the lungs (asthmatic breathing) – and the equally forceful but eliminative capacity of the body's healing process. The lungs were relieved at the expense of the skin and, temporarily, of the tonsils and ears (both orifices near the surface). The tonsils and ears provided acute relief for the whole system as well as being the sites of previous acute illness that had been treated suppressively. Casting off the disease took some time – to the distraction of the poor mother who had to witness the surfacing of the symptoms. Only a parent with a strong will and a determined sense of what is right in nature – or one who has done everything else and is desperate – will put her child through such apparent suffering. Chronic and suppressed disease does not always leave the body easily. Try as they might, homoeopaths cannot always ensure that healing is as gentle as it is thorough, as swift as it is permanent. There are so many reasons for 'cure' being a process beset with adversity and it is why it is necessary to devote a whole section of the book to them (see Part II).

A case and its analysis that demonstrates 'the Law Of Cure'

In another case to develop the theme of the Law of Cure the patient concerned is suffering from a long-term, chronic complaint. It is instructive to set out the case as you might see it in the homoeopath's casebook. In this way you will get some idea of how searching and thorough the homoeopath needs to be to become acquainted with a person's full history, in order to arrive at a strategy for treatment and then make a prescription.

The following symbols have been used:

$$< \ = \ \text{aggravates or worse for}$$
$$> \ = \ \text{ameliorates or better for}$$
$$+ \ = \ \text{likes}$$
$$++ \ = \ \text{craves}$$

J.N. (b. 1949) Woman of 45

Presenting complaint:
IBS (Irritable Bowel Syndrome). Began 4 years ago.

Pains:
"colicky"; < lower abdomen; < when bloated; < after bread or cabbage; > hot drinks; rest; > eating little but regularly.
"The pains tend to start here on the right side and then move across to the left-hand side. Sometimes they do the opposite but not very often."
Pains < ileocaecum. (The area of the appendix.)

Bloating:
< after eating esp. eating late in the evening.
< late afternoon (5 - 8 p.m.); > passing wind.

Stools:
Normal or slightly loose. Colonoscopy (investigation of the bowel) showed only slight inflammation of the walls of the sigmoid flexure (the lowest section of the large intestine, just before the rectum).
"*I get indigestion a lot. I feel full and nauseated which is worse if I have a large meal or after rich food. I get a sensation of a tight band round my midriff; that's there most of the time.*"
With indigestion (she) tends to feel uncomfortable unless she keeps moving about the house doing simple things. Feels < for sitting down.

Liver:
Pain in the right side – palpation indicates in right lobe. Pain extends through to back; into lower corner of scapula. Pain often wakes her at 4 - 5 a.m.
"*It feels as if the pain comes through from the front and into my back; it's like a deep stitch there.*"

Appetite:
Small; lost interest since onset of IBS when was given special diet.
Feels generally < eating onions, spices, fats. + rice which >.

Thirst:
+ weak tea. ++ hot water with lemon which > digestion.

Bowels:
"*My bowels always react to stress. If I'm upset about anything I'll get the pains.*"
Used to be constipated before the IBS.

Bladder:
Passes more water in the morning than in the afternoon yet drinks more in the p.m. Urine is normal except after an attack of pains; then it's "*orangey yellow*".

Menstruation:
Hysterectomy six years ago. Surgery recommended after profuse haemorrhaging each month. Uterus only removed.

"I'm still aware of my cycle though and the tummy pains are much worse at around that time – the middle of the month. I do get so uptight around then."

Sleep:
Needs at least eight hours but seldom gets that. Sleeps on right side till the liver becomes uncomfortable and then turns onto back and sleeps fitfully.

Environment:
+ Sun. < cold, damp. (Feels depressed.) Would hate to live anywhere far from the sea. Claustrophobic in crowds and in hot stuffy atmospheres. Feels the cold quickly but < for becoming overheated.

Temperament:
"People say that I'm a bit of a worrier. I'm always a bit nervous in case I've done anything amiss. I'm a timid sort of person really. I don't like confrontation. I'll do anything to avoid conflict. I think I had enough of that at home. I have an older brother – quite a bit older – and he was constantly at loggerheads with father. They had such rows. I think that's why I married my husband – he hardly says a word; it exasperates the children. Actually it has got to me recently. I find myself always bullying him – it's quite unlike me. I find it rather annoying when he makes comments on my condition – it's usually in front of other people and I do hate that. He does it because he's embarrassed for me; he tries to explain my diet because people get so upset when you don't eat what they provide. I don't like going out as much as I used to because of that."

"Yes, I do get despondent. It's been so long since I was well and sometimes I feel I'm going crazy which is so silly – I can't believe I'm saying all this! I sometimes think I'll never get well." Tends to be restless and yet lethargic. Feels she *"fritters away the time on trivial activity"*. Becomes tired easily esp. after talking for a long time. Has a fear of cancer.

Family history:
Mother: Died 5 years ago of bowel cancer. Had had 'shadows' on her lungs: probable TB (tuberculosis) in youth.
Father: Died in his 60s of heart attack.
Maternal Grandfather: Emphysema (d. 79)

Maternal Grandmother: High blood pressure; angina. Gall bladder removed.
Paternal Grandfather: Killed WW1.
Paternal Grandmother: Died in her 90s.
Paternal Aunt: Cancer of the pancreas (d. 55)

Personal history:
Frequent chest infections as a child. Stopped when family moved to the coast. Has always lived by the sea since.
Age 5: Fell off swing and landed on coccyx – can still remember the pain.
Age 9: Trauma: cousin died in a boating accident.
"She was a bit older than me but she was so good to me. I still think of her and the waste! I didn't cry at the time and I can remember wondering why I couldn't. I s'pose I just bottled it up. I tend to do that."
Age 12: Menses started. Took the pill for four years at twenty-two and felt unwell most of the time – headaches, nausea, weight gain. Stopped when she wanted to conceive.
Age 27: 1st child – forceps delivery; episiotomy. Haemorrhoids ever since.
Age 29: 2nd child.
Age 41: Hysterectomy: prolapse and haemorrhaging prior. Still has sensation of prolapse – operation made no change to sensation.
"Sometimes it feels in the front but it can also feel heavy and dragging in the back passage as if it's all connected to the bowel problem."
Age 42: Mother died. Was shocked.
"I had no idea she was so ill. She would never let on, of course. I knew something was wrong because she looked so drawn and we kept telling her that she should go to the doctor but she tutted in her way and told us to mind our own business. She hated anything to do with doctors – she was such a private person. But for all that she was so warm-hearted. She would do anything for you… for anyone! I miss her still – I even find myself talking to her as if she were in the room. I s'pose it's comforting to think her presence is still there. That's what I feel anyway – you'll probably think I'm very strange."
(Weeps now and apologises.)

Set out in this way it is quite easy to see the *three-dimensional nature* of the case. There is the present (IBS), the past (grief over her mother, her cousin; deep in the past, the family relationships when she was a child; the gynaecological history) and heredity: the family history of both cancer and TB, 'shadows' of which are counted as genetically-carried influences.

How she presently feels emotionally and the way that her symptoms influence her view of her own future are important to the prognosis (the opinion as to the probable result of treatment) which is for the practitioner to assess. He needs to evaluate the general picture to judge the following:

(i)   the degree of seriousness of the complaint;
(ii) the strategy of treatment (i.e. the method of applying the remedies, dietary advice etc.);
(iii) how well the patient will respond to treatment, and
(iv) how she will make positive use of whatever 'cure' takes place – though this last point is what the patient should experience.

One of the practitioner's rewards is to witness the creative use to which patients put their restored Vital Force.

There were two foci of treatment for J.N: the IBS and the unresolved grief. The patient had not asked for any help beyond treating the IBS so it was not appropriate to delve further than the patient had already revealed as to her emotional state. It was enough to acknowledge the strong element of grief. Because homoeopathy is so rich in its ability to heal psychological conditions, the homoeopath is often faced with the temptation to dig into the deepest emotional history too soon, hoping that a remedy will be revealed that will heal everything at once. Indeed there are remedies that have just this ability but they are usually more useful to patients who have not had many years of their complaint and have not had surgery. (Besides, patients do not take kindly to having their suppressed emotional histories exposed until there is a bond of trust between them and their practitioners.)

So, of the two foci, the remedial spotlight fell on the bowel condition. By setting up healing in the bowel and liver function the patient would become, both physically and mentally, more ready to allow her suppressed grief about her mother to be expressed – if she so wanted.

IBS is one of the most common digestive problems but it is a label that is very loosely applied to a host of illnesses, some of which are very mild and others which are pernicious. It is a label with little intrinsic meaning until the nature of the symptoms is investigated.

From the patient's story it was gathered that the condition began after the hysterectomy and her mother's death: a physical and an emotional causation. How could a hysterectomy be a trigger for a bowel problem? Operations on the viscera (soft tissue of the abdominal cavity) can lead to adhesions which are areas of scar tissue that pull on adjoining tissue thus causing 'drag' on nearby organs. (This is, for example, fairly common after appendectomies where the resulting scar tissue can cause trouble for the right ovary.) In this case the adhesions from the hysterectomy pulled on the lower bowel which is why the patient felt that the gynaecological symptoms and the IBS were connected. This fact would not be possible to treat allopathically except by further surgery to excise the scar tissue. Even then there would be no guarantee of success as some patients form scar tissue very readily and so the process might well begin all over again.

To arrive at a satisfactory prescription that would help the patient's body begin the healing process it was necessary to take the symptom picture of the IBS as she related it. The physical symptoms of bloating, wind, bowel pains (and their location and time aggravation) and the excretory process have to be considered together with the liver pains she described as well as her dietary preferences and aggravations. In addition, it is vital to consider as part of the condition, her *present* mental attitude (which is different from the suppressed grief). She said quite clearly that her behaviour towards her husband was not like herself; she also said that her digestion was influenced by stress and she used the word 'despondent' to describe how she felt about her condition generally. She also admitted to fear of cancer. The IBS, therefore, was interfering not just on a physical level but also on a mental, emotional and spiritual level – the spiritual aspect must be included because her *sense of purpose* in life had been affected; witness her words about frittering away the time. Few chronic cases of ill health are without a spiritual aspect – even if one has to hunt for them.

Seeing a case in this way is to take as much of the whole person that is in view as possible – no adult is so completely transparent that the whole is visible at once! Once as much of the whole as possible is in view then the remedy that displays similar characteristics to the patient's presenting condition should be apparent. In this case the remedy that covered all the significant characteristic symptoms was very obvious — not least because the case revealed a symptom that is unique to just one remedy. The pain at the lower corner of the right shoulder blade that felt as if it came through from the front of the body is a keynote of *Chelidonium*.

Chelidonium is the homoeopathic remedy made from the greater celandine, a plant usually regarded as a weed. It has bright orangey yellow flowers (a pointer towards its being a 'liver remedy' — i.e. one to treat conditions arising from unhealthy livers), irregular, slightly hairy leaves and is full of a violently acrid, orange-coloured poisonous juice. As a homoeopathically prepared energy it was given to the patient in the 30th potency once each day. She was asked to report on her progress in ten days — which she failed to do. Instead she waited until her next appointment which was six weeks after the first consultation. She explained that she had forgotten to phone in with an update as she was feeling so much more positive and had begun to "*get on with my life*". She had continued to take the remedy and wanted still to do so. She found that it gave her considerable relief from all her symptoms but that she was not yet confident of her ability to do without it. She also mentioned that her husband was pleased with her progress as she was no longer shouting at him as she had been. Nevertheless, she said that she was more aware now than ever of the feeling of prolapse, especially as it affected the bowel. She was conscious most of the time of the feeling of a drag in her lower abdomen and the pull it exerted on the rectal passage. In addition, she now complained of a low backache.

> "*It is exactly like the backache I used to get before I had my hysterectomy. At the same time, I have to say, my piles are playing me up. They do bleed quite a lot after I have been to the loo. Really, if there were something you could do for that I would be most grateful.*"

The IBS symptoms were indeed better but the patient was still expressing symptoms — this time old ones from her past history. Because the hysterectomy had removed the offending uterus the patient could no longer manifest symptoms there. The IBS, by her own admission, had always had a hormonal element in that it was always worse around the middle of her menstrual cycle (which was no longer there in the form of a menstrual discharge). Now it was as if her body was reproducing as closely as it was able the symptom picture of her pre-hysterectomy days. In addition to the low backache and the bleeding pile, there was also the increased sense of prolapse and, she admitted, *"a tremendous tiredness that comes over me in waves. I have to keep going; if I sit down I collapse!"* (She added that she did not wish to give the impression that her greater sense of well-being had gone; her sense of renewed purpose and enthusiasm was still very much evident.) She agreed that this was how she had felt all the time when her periods had been so troublesome. She was given *Sepia* 200 (to take one dose every two hours for three doses).

Sepia is one of the most commonly needed remedies for women who have such difficulties with their periods. This remedy is made from the ink of a squid. This sea creature releases its ink for two reasons: one is to protect itself from predators and the other is to confuse its own prey before it darts forward and strikes. The symptomatic parallel is that patients in need of *Sepia* often have, temporarily, a distinctly antisocial attitude. They do not want to expend any more energy than is absolutely necessary on dealing with other people – so they will create minor subterfuges to avoid contact – and also display a snappy temper. They say quite wounding things (especially to those closest to them) without compunction (though they often quickly regret this). In addition, it has been noted that the squid is basically constructed like a living bag which, once it has released its eggs into the ocean, becomes a spent force and sinks, flaccid, to the seabed where it dies. This incident of underwater drama has been likened to the flaccidity of the uterus after childbirth and years of menstruation. Homoeopathy is full of such parallels both imaginary and realistic, so readers need not be offended by the comparison with a flaccid bag! (*Lycopodium* is another example. This is the wolf's claw moss. It was once one of the largest plants on earth but, through evolution, has become one of the smallest. It is a very common remedy, particularly for boys and men who have problems with self-confidence.)

Sepia had a remarkable effect on the patient. The bleeding stopped and the pile contracted. The backache was relieved over the course of the following week. The quality of the patient's energy improved considerably and she no longer felt exhausted. (She confessed then that what had chiefly made her so tired was the thought of doing so much housework. She had now employed a cleaning lady to help her and felt much more positive about the home situation.) She also reported that the prolapse sensations had all but disappeared; occasionally she could feel a slight drag but that was only if she had been a little bit constipated (old symptom!) and had to strain.

However, when she came for her third appointment she was rather subdued and withdrawn; her complexion was grey. Significantly she held a lacy handkerchief, which she kept twisting round her fingers; she never used it, in spite of sniffing through the interview. She still wanted to keep taking the *Chelidonium* 30. *"If I don't take it for any reason, then after a while I get that pain back in my shoulder blade."*

The progress of the rest of the interview was much slower than the previous ones and the patient was reluctant to make any eye contact. She was asked how she felt emotionally but she evaded the question and began talking, not without acerbity, of her children. Without digging and probing into emotional issues it was not possible to clarify her state of mind but, based on how she had progressed in her physical well-being and how she had achieved this by retracing her medical footsteps, it was judged that she was near to expressing her grief for past and buried circumstances.

The most common (but by no means the only) remedy for deeply held grief, that follows well after the particular remedies that she had had so far, was *Natrum Muriaticum*, rock salt (sodium chloride). In order to confirm the need for this remedy at this point in her treatment some arbitrary and leading questions were asked: Did she find that she had been thirstier for water recently? Did she also find that she had been taking more salt than usual? Did she also, perhaps, feel that she was brewing a drippy cold and that her eyes were rather dry and sand-papery? *"Yes"* was the answer to all these questions and it confirmed the prescription, because these symptoms are common to those in need of the remedy. She was given *Natrum Muriaticum* (*Nat. Mur.* for short) 1M. She went home and wept for a week.

"I just couldn't stop. It was so awful. I had to stay in my room. I know I had to do it. I just kept thinking of my mother – all the time – all the things I never said to her; all the thoughts I had at the funeral came flooding back. And I found that I was so angry! They were bitter tears indeed. But, you know, it's odd: I've tried to hold on to her image but I find it's increasingly difficult. Her face used to be so clear in my mind but it's begun to fade. Is that wrong?"

After a little while longer she found that she could do without the *Chelidonium* on a daily basis. When she returned in three months for a check-up she was able to report that she only needed it when she was under stress at work. (She was a legal secretary and viewed by her employers as a general factotum.) She considered that she had undergone a transformation and was wholly satisfied with the 'cure'. She said that it was only now that she realised how fulfilling her life really was. Nevertheless, she would not care to be without the bottle of *Chelidonium*.

A look at the notes on *Chelidonium* in the 'Mind' section of the *Materia Medica* reveals that this remedy covers a state of anxiety in which one feels one has done something wrong; has a fear of going crazy; timidity. It also covers, paradoxically, feeling quarrelsome and irritable. Such contradictions are almost common enough amongst remedies to prove the rule and only reflect the contradictory nature of the human psyche. In this case the irritability and quarrelsome feelings were relieved but the slightly timid, cautious temperament remained as it had always been – she continued to give the impression of someone who lacked self-confidence even though she herself felt that this had improved.

She continued well until some months later when she felt that some of her bowel symptoms were returning. She still felt full of energy and motivation but she was beginning again to complain of the bloating and wind as well as some vague nausea. She had had a cold and a chesty cough shortly before and she felt that this had *"lowered my resistance"*. She also noted that the need for salt had come back *"with a vengeance!"* and she was extremely thirsty again. She was given a further dose of *Nat. Mur.* 1M but this time it did nothing for her.

Her symptoms continued for some three weeks before she phoned to say that nothing had changed. She was now rather anxious in case all the original treatment was coming to naught. It was at this point that a return to the notes of the first interview was needed. The family history showed that there were severe chronic diseases – cancer, emphysema and heart problems – amongst the close relatives. These are extremely relevant and no homoeopath would ignore them for it is here in the heredity that a major piece of the human health jigsaw is found. The implications are far greater than is at first apparent.

In this case, the family history shows there was a strain of TB running through it. The patient was given the remedy *Tuberculinum* 1M and within days she was feeling well again. Not only that, but her outlook on life was radically different. She was able to consider the rest of her life with a positive and creative urgency. She has been recently able to report that she has continued generally well to this day and if she has felt unwell at all it has been due to a bug in the office or an extra helping of roast potatoes at the weekend.

A question arises from this case about the sequence of remedies. If emotional suffering is so significant why was she not given the *Nat. Mur.* as the first prescription? The principle of treating thoroughly by means of the swiftest, gentlest means has to be qualified: what appears to be the swiftest way to the heart of a matter may not be the most effective or the gentlest. If this woman had been given *Nat. Mur.* first then it would have been quite likely that her IBS symptoms would have aggravated severely. Her liver, full of toxic waste, would therefore not have been able to function well as part of the eliminative process. By first treating her compromised liver and the symptoms that generally expressed her physiopathology it was possible to prepare her body for the day when she could discharge her emotions without physical pain being a complication. Being respectful of a person's sensitivities leads to far greater trust in the process.

The tubercular strain in her inheritance proved to be a block to the complete effectiveness of the three remedies that had apparently done so well on the physical and emotional levels. They were not sufficient to create a state of total and permanent well-being. Once the remedy made from the disease material of TB itself – horrific though this might sound – had been given, her healing system was able to establish more permanent equilibrium. This enormous subject of inherited strains of chronic disease is of paramount importance and is covered in Part III.

The 'black box'

Imagine that the body has a 'black box'; a flight recorder such as an aircraft has to record all that happens on a flight. This faculty would be ready to inform the body on a cellular level of all that had happened to it. It would record negative events in pregnancy, birth, childhood ailments, accidents, operations and emotional traumas. The purpose would be part of the body's continuing need for preparation and protection. The cells, in other words, would have their own learning curve and the experiences of the whole would be registered on this microbiological level. As a result of this the body would have the facility to call on its 'cell memory' in order that, at a propitious moment, negative experience could be reversed by the Vital Force, the body's organisation for well-being. We have this 'black box' faculty and it is always functioning and it is forever at the service of the Vital Force. Together these two will react to any natural healing agent positively. Together they will react negatively to any form of suppression – even where circumstance demands that suppression is temporarily the safest course of action. (Such suppression might be an appendectomy or the removal of a very diseased kidney; the use of antibiotics in galloping septicaemia where no other remedial treatment is available; having to talk to the police about a fatal accident and then being strong for the rest of the family instead of being allowed time to weep.)

Fantastical? Hardly when we consider that the freshly fertilised egg that becomes implanted on the wall of the uterus contains all the information necessary for the full maturation of a human being. Every one of the cells of our mature bodies contains the same information even if individual cells have different functions. For the body to be an integrated whole this has to be so. What is more, the microbiological wonder that this is does not start with the individual; it begins with the very information that we inherit from our forebears. We inherit a compendium of influences that have the profoundest consequences on health; the way we express disease individually is predetermined before we are born. This is why one child suffers earache when he teethes and another suffers colic and burning, acidic diarrhoea; why one youth has warts all over his hands and another has raging acne; why one geriatric suffers dementia and another angina. We inherit susceptibilities. We also inherit the influence of the quality of the Vital Force response to disease and trauma energy suffered by our forebears. One only has to hear, for the umpteenth time, a mother reporting on a sick child that the child reacts in exactly the same way as she used to, or acknowledge that many children react to trauma in the same way that one of their parents would have done at the same age.

Steps in the right direction: searching for hidden blocks to cure

Whatever is registered on this microbiological cellular library matters, whether it is part of the biography of the patient or of his or her forebears. The threads of human disease energy are rooted deeply in the past. One of our life's tasks is to attempt to heal these threads so that heredity becomes far less of a Pandora's box.

Before we look at the medical minefield of hereditary disease patterns we should take time to focus on all those other circumstances and conditions that prevent us from achieving a swift, gentle and comprehensive healing – some are to do with lifestyle while the key to others is held in the 'black box'. In homoeopathy we call them 'maintaining causes' and this term covers anything that prevents the chosen form of natural healing from working. They range from the mundane (e.g. antidoting remedies) to the extraordinary and unexpected (living over underground streams). At least one of them is highly controversial: artificial immunisation. All of them are potential blocks to cure.

PART II

MAINTAINING
CAUSES

INTRODUCTION

Why can't I get better?

One of the challenges to the homoeopath is to recognise all the possible reasons why the Vital Force should find itself incapable of throwing off disease. There are many factors that, until they are removed, will prevent the patient's full recovery.

Practitioners of any healing art are constantly faced with patients who do not get better. Every apparent failure seems to refute the thinking behind the last prescription. So often this leads the practitioner to let his focus slip away from the patient and the all-important hunt for the underlying reasons for the continued illness. Attention is turned instead to fruitless speculation about the inadequacies of either his or her analysis or, worse, the patient's part in the failure.

"Did you take the pills at the time specified?" "Are you sure you've been remembering to take the drops every night?" "Have you been drinking coffee since I saw you last?" Questions like this tend to put patients on the wrong foot. We are all ready, when interviewed by experts, to feel unnecessarily guilty in case we have sabotaged their efforts inadvertently. This is due partly to our readiness to abdicate responsibility for our own health to another who, by nature of his or her training, would claim to hold the key to the return to wellness. It is true that there are times when simple instructions are misunderstood or ignored and this can lead to lack of success, but in the practice of homoeopathy we should be ready to offer the benefit of the doubt. Patient error is not as common as the dozens of other, less immediately

obvious reasons, probably because patients are keen on exploring the possibilities of natural healing, are predisposed towards the peculiarities of the medicines and because they are paying.

Part II is an exploration of those different reasons why patients might not be getting better under homoeopathic (or, indeed, any other) treatment. It is a discussion of causes that spoil or pervert the course of treatment. They are known as 'maintaining causes' because, while they exist, they maintain the symptom picture that is being addressed and/or the state of general ill health despite all the willingness of the patient and expertise of the practitioner.

CHAPTER 7

THE PHYSICIAN'S POSITION

A patient's inability to get better may sometimes have more to do with the practitioner's lack of perception than with the patient. Although the patient, living with his or her problem(s) so intimately, might be puzzled by anyone's inability to see what needs to be healed, it is nevertheless frequently difficult to assess what is wrong and how best to create a strategy to deal with it. (This is especially true bearing in mind that the patient often erroneously considers that his symptoms need treating whereas in reality the symptoms are the surface manifestation and it is the underlying *causes* that should be treated.)

The task is easiest if practitioners are dealing simply with what is presented *now*, this moment – as happens with acute conditions. With acute disease one is basing treatment on consideration of two dimensions: the patient and the immediate symptom picture and, where there may not be a great deal of 'history' to the complaint, not much more than a singular event such as getting chilled or taking a tumble. However, in patients with a chronic condition there is always the complex history of how the patient arrived at their present state to take into consideration as well. To prescribe on the whole person, in three dimensions, as demonstrated in Part I, one needs to know not only about 'now' but also about 'before' and in quite some detail; often about aspects that may appear to have very little to do with the presenting complaint.

The classical view

You would think that 'classical' homoeopathy was the system that was handed down by its originators: Samuel Hahnemann and his pupils. This is to underestimate the effect of two hundred years' worth of playing 'Chinese whispers' with the philosophy of their vision. This was not helped by the fact that Hahnemann wrote the core textbook, the *Organon*, six times and would undoubtedly have gone on to write several more versions had he lived longer. Not only that but Hahnemann did not always practise precisely what he preached.

In so-called 'classical' homoeopathy, the ideal system of treating non-acute problems takes the description of the whole (including the 'before') and selects a remedy that most matches the state described by the symptoms (particularly emotional ones and the most peculiar physical ones); the indicated remedy mirrors the aggregate of general and particular symptoms more than any other. This includes all the mental and emotional symptoms that are either volunteered or elicited that might have a bearing on the case. Hence there are remedies that are listed, in the 'Mind' part of the book of symptoms, under 'Ailments from Grief' or 'Ailments from Bad News', 'Complaints from Fright' or 'Ailments after Mortification'. These each imply a historical event that has caused a symptom picture that has arisen in the past, that has developed and has now reached a pitch at which the patient is sufficiently discomfited to seek help – even though the symptoms that are causing the discomfiture may be only physical rather than obviously emotional, the latter having been closed off from consciousness some time before. (As indicated before, it is one of the physical body's functions to produce physical symptoms in order to relieve the overstressed mind and emotions which, without this safety valve, would otherwise be overwhelmed by the excessive burden of emotional pain.) So the contemporary classical ideal is to identify a single remedy that energetically represents the same thread of energy that is manifest as pathology in the patient and that runs through all three levels of body, mind and spirit.

This model – the one remedy that will lead the patient back to full health even after years of sustained symptoms – is gratifyingly simple. It is based on the assumption that every one of us has an energy 'theme' which is the underlying common denominator of any symptom and that the theme characterises the illness being treated. For example, someone who has gradually developed heart pains, palpitations and waking with a start, accompanied by a strong thirst and a craving for salty food, ever since their much loved grandmother died five years ago, would need *Natrum*

Muriaticum because it covers deep bereavement in addition to the presenting physical symptoms. A woman, widowed in her early forties, who becomes increasingly timid and easily frightened of life and who suffers from mental confusion and is developing an uncertain gait and a tremor in her hands would need *Conium Maculatum* (hemlock) as this remedy covers grief from the death of a husband that remains unexpressed.

This broad-canvas view of remedies relating to emotional origins of pathology can be witnessed in terms of constitution as well. A thin, pale and weedy nineteen-year-old youth of narrow outlook who has frequent colds, tends to be very chilly yet who prefers all his meals cold (sandwiches or salad) and whose hobby is to make plastic model aeroplanes, presents with recurrent whitlows on his fingers. Such a person requires *Silica* as this remedy covers not only the recurrent suppurative boils on the fingers but also the poor constitution with nutritional insufficiency, the peculiar chilliness with a desire for cold things to eat and drink and the wish to focus creative attention on small and undemanding activities.

Pursuing this ideal, the modern classical homoeopath would be expected to prescribe the single indicated remedy and wait – and wait for a lengthy period if need be. This is to allow time for the pent up negative energy within to express itself fully; firstly as physical discharge and then as emotional expression.

The basic assumption is that, despite the vicissitudes of everyday emotional life, the individual's core remains constant enough for an ideal curative response to the prescription of the remedy that most matches that core 'picture'. Someone who was born with a long and lanky body, who has always sweated a lot, gets especially hot in bed, who has always been very thirsty, has had a predilection for salty and spicy foods, who has been prone to skin conditions and to having long philosophical discussions that lull everyone else into a stupor, would inevitably be given *Sulphur*. If this picture were strongly presented, any homoeopath would be expected to give this remedy, almost completely confident of success – whatever the physical pathology that might accompany it.

If someone seeking treatment for severe constipation is also recorded as being very introverted, shrunk and emaciated; chronically shy and lacking in self-confidence, to the point of avoiding almost all social contact;

dull-witted to the extent that he can only do menial work for a living and with a tendency to catch colds easily, then he would be given *Baryta Carbonicum* (barium carbonate) as this remedy covers this constitutional state perfectly.

There are dozens of remedies that have archetypal pictures. Here are a few examples described briefly:

Antimonium Crudum (antimony): The patient is sentimental and given to weeping; he is prone to feeling lovesick, especially when it is full moon. He becomes a glutton, eating his food at speed and between meals. His digestion is easily upset (not surprisingly) and this makes him bad-tempered. He finds fault and moans about his fate yet he might be consulting the practitioner about his painful corns.

Argentum Nitricum (silver nitrate): The patient is nervous and anxious, cripplingly so. He cannot take an exam or make a speech without the most agonising worry. He paces the floor; he chain smokes; he forgets what he most needs to remember. This is the acute state he gets into when faced with an ordeal. Yet he has other anxieties. Most importantly, he suffers vertigo even from looking up at tall buildings; he might also complain that he becomes clumsy and unsteady on his legs. His digestion, too, can be easily upset and he might be consulting the practitioner about chronic diarrhoea with colic and embarrassing flatulence.

Platina (platinum): This is often viewed as a woman's remedy. She is proud and haughty and does not suffer fools gladly. She is highly strung and temperamental. She is the mistress of the 'put-down' remark and she can be extremely unkind. She is brusque and quarrelsome and makes her husband's life a misery with her jibes. Yet she has a high sex drive that causes her to make an idiot of herself when in lively company: she can sing and dance or tell silly stories which may make the rest of the group cringe in embarrassment. When she is alone she feels that she is truly alone in the world and that no one really cares; she feels abandoned. She presents a dichotomy of contemptuousness, arrogance and vitriol as opposed to weak, pathetic loneliness. The pathology that she brings for treatment is most likely either to be of nervous origin (such as tics or neuralgia) or to have a fundamentally hormonal basis; her menstrual cycle might well be causing her trouble.

Kali Carbonicum (potassium carbonate): This person is conscientious to a fault. He likes routine and principle; he runs his life by them. He has a sense of duty, even honour, and he has a stiff upper lip. He needs to be in control or he feels insecure. 'Rigid' is his middle name. He has a narrow view of the world and tends to cut out everything that is not immediately relevant to his existence. Hence he has a tendency to be more interested in his bank statement than in the arts section of the *Times*. He is likely to suffer from myalgia (muscle pains), a stiff back and constipation. More seriously he might have asthma or heart disease.

Rubus Quercus (oak): This is a person of considerable sticking power who nevertheless is prone to becoming world weary and exhausted but with no idea of when to stop. He is tough and reliable but has had a tendency to allow himself to be overloaded by other people's problems. Despite this dependability he is quite unable to make anything significant of his own life: the creative urge is thwarted or set aside in favour of others. The patient might well present a history of injuries and traumas with a consequent picture of muscle or skeletal problems.

These thumbnail sketches serve to show that remedies can illustrate constitutional states that might be thought to capture the essential nature of particular patients. From the beginning of their training homoeopaths are taught to see that the psyche is the most significant aspect of the patient and the aspect that requires the most attention, hotly followed by consideration of the general constitution. Thus it is that classically trained homoeopaths will often pay less attention to diagnosed diseases with their attendant physical symptoms and more to the underlying causes that lie in the distressed psyche and peculiarities of the general state. This would only seem to follow the precepts not only of Samuel Hahnemann but of Paracelsus, Galen (before he saw more advantage in siding with the allopaths of his day) and Plato.

Here is an example of a 'classical prescription':

Maisie, a woman of forty-eight, asked for help with her menopause. She had had a hysterectomy some five years before but was still suffering the same symptoms that she had before the operation. She had painful bloating and wind from which she could find no relief. She had distressing hot sweats which seemed to affect her throat and head. She had feelings of constriction in her throat and abdomen. She dreaded the nights as she could not stay asleep but would wake frequently feeling breathless and fearful after frightening dreams. She only felt better when *"my hormones switch off"*. She also felt that her marriage was suffering because she kept being so aggressive towards her husband. She knew that she was being paranoid but she could not get rid of the idea that her husband was seeing another woman.

"I know he's not really. He's just not like that. But I find myself checking his wallet and the phone bill. He says I do nag him. But, you know, this is how it was with my first husband. Looking back I realise that I must have driven him to distraction and that's why he went off with someone else – my best friend it was."

The patient was suffering symptoms that she had displayed in one form or another for over thirty years, ever since her periods had begun. The hysterectomy had done nothing to correct the problem. She still suffered from suspiciousness and an uncontrollable temper. She still experienced sensations of pressure and heat and had the feeling of being throttled and of being 'pregnant' with bloating. The mental, emotional and physical symptoms that had always bedevilled her cycle – and thus influenced her whole adult life – were all covered by the one remedy: *Lachesis*, the venom of the bushmaster snake. She was given *Lachesis* 200. She spent the weekend going through thirty years of symptoms.

In turn she passed quantities of urine that smelt of ammonia; she had copious diarrhoea (something that used to happen immediately prior to the menstrual bleed); she developed a high fever with drenching sweats (*"it was like a hot flush to end all hot flushes!"*); she had a series of abdominal cramps that felt as if she were having labour contractions – which came on when she began to weep hysterically towards the Sunday evening. (She had failed to mention that she had had an abortion in her twenties – the memories of which came flooding back.)

By the middle of the week she said that she had not felt so well in many years. She was *"a new woman"* and felt positive for the first time she could remember. Her husband reported that he could see the change in her colouring and her energy but that he would wait a while before commenting on her moods. What is of further interest in this case is that the patient had had very little orthodox medical suppression beyond the removal of her uterus. She had never taken the contraceptive pill. She had never trusted painkillers so had avoided them. She had refused HRT outright. Her Vital Force had been left intact to express itself as it had always known how. It is not everyone who has the constitution to react to remedies so swiftly and thoroughly.

Broadening the horizon

In modern homoeopathic repertories of symptoms there are rubrics in which to look up remedies that resolve the ill effects of environmental changes, old injuries, past diseases, excessive quantities of common but harmful foodstuffs, poisonous substances and a mass of other influences. Any or all of these influences may be at work much of the time, adding layers of diverse energies that complicate symptom pictures. Though constitutionally healthy, patients may continue to represent these influences in the form of symptoms that do belong to their 'single' remedy constitutional state; alas, not everyone is able to maintain such a continuum.

We are seldom a simple expression of one energy state but a layered and woven tapestry of hereditary, parental and environmental influences, toxicity (we live in a world of pollution, we are vaccinated and we eat contaminated food), past illnesses, accidents, unresolved grief (we vastly overestimate our capacity to support negative emotional experience) and of offence taken – appropriately or otherwise. Those involved with the western development of eastern philosophy would add Karma to this list – which understands each one of us to have life lessons to work through, the blueprint of which we are born with.

When this depth of history (and prehistory) is to be considered along with the present pathology (which can be critical) it is clear that part of the practitioner's acquired skill is to judge nicely just *which* historical aspect may be the origin of the presenting complaint. In a case of multi-layered complexity that will take several months or even years to treat, it is also important to see the priority of events that has led the patient to their present parlous state. *For the treatment of chronic conditions is nothing less than the unfolding and resolution of past history through the present expression of physical and emotional and spiritual states.* Our very tissues have a memory of what occurs to the body throughout life. We carry our histories with us.

The system of treatment that faces the force of such complex structures of negative energy needs to be flexible and susceptible to being employed strategically. This means that it is naïve to expect one remedy (however vast the number and variety of symptoms it might cover) to restore back to a perfect balance of health those with a long, complex, confused history of physical and emotional trauma. It also means that practitioners have to acquaint themselves with more than just the 'classical' principle which for some, it must be said, remains an intellectual ideal. Every student homoeopath's learning about the treatment of chronic pathology begins with the identification of the single most indicated remedy, drawing on the symptom picture of the patient and chosen as a result of analysing and distilling to what has come to be termed (for good or ill) an 'essence': then giving that remedy in the minimum dose to effect the speediest but most gentle cure.

It is worth noting that contemporary classical practitioners credit Hahnemann and his philosophical descendants with promulgating the notion of the single constitutional remedy. However, few of these alternative pioneers would have taken kindly to being restricted in their prescribing to such a narrow philosophy and certainly did not consistently practise according to this principle. The current practice of 'essence' prescribing, i.e. of prescribing a single constitutional remedy to cover all ills in a patient (that is nevertheless based chiefly on the psychological profile of the patient), is a phenomenon of the late 20th century. It is a philosophy that has evolved not least through the work of the celebrated Greek homoeopath, George Vithoulkas, whose life's work has been the interpretation of Hahnemann's *Organon* and the expansion of the psychological profiles of all the major and many of the minor remedies. His career has been of immense value but one that has been subjected to misrepresentation and misinterpretation by many erroneously seeking to simplify homoeopathy to what they consider a fundamentally immutable philosophy of healing that is really little short of prescribing by numbers.

The different means to the same end

This brings up the issue of the different styles of homoeopathy that are practised in Britain, Europe and elsewhere. Methodology in homoeopathy is a minefield. There are many different approaches that nevertheless are variations on the original theme. At first, to most students, the differences seem to be thoroughly bewildering.

It is perhaps surprising that any system of medicine should be susceptible to different approaches especially when the basic principles of the healing art are so fundamentally simple. Yet it would seem there are different and equally satisfactory methods of arriving at a prescription that will trigger the patient's Vital Force to curative activity – even, on occasion, allopathic ones. However, as any equestrian knows, there are horses for courses; not everyone will do well with any or all of the methods. Some practitioners will only feel comfortable with one particular style. Others feel hampered by the straightjacket of having to stick to the classical line. The issue of individuality in alternative practice starts with the exchange of energy between the patient and the practitioner. It is not uncommon for patients to find that they do not establish a rapport with their first choice of practitioner and they have to go in search of one with whom they do feel comfortable; this may have as much to do with the style of practice as with personality.

Students of homoeopathy study different methodologies unless they are fed on a diet of strict classicism. They learn how to diversify. They learn how different patients need different approaches; how one patient will do well on a single remedy with a long period of action; how and why another will require a low potency of a remedy given daily over many months; how yet another will need careful and frequent monitoring with a relay of complementary remedies. They go on to find out about prescribing remedies in liquid form or how some practitioners habitually give remedies in ascending potencies (e.g. *Sulphur* 6, 30, 200, 1M, 10M given over a period of several weeks in stages) and others do the opposite. They learn about those who prescribe rote 'recipes' of strategically organised remedies that are designed to programme the patient through detoxification on each of the body levels. They find out that in France and Germany homoeopaths practise polypharmacy (the admixture of many remedies, the combination of which is designed to cover all symptoms), anathema to classicists but too successful in its own terms to be dismissed easily.

Unfortunately, with such a diversity of methodologies – and there are more than are suggested here – homoeopathy becomes a disputatious subject and its practitioners are inclined to join one school of philosophical thought or another. This leads to philosophical convictions. Convictions inevitably lead to fixed ideas that ultimately mean stultification. The opposite can happen too. Homoeopaths can also be susceptible to the siren call of eclecticism. Practitioners who try out every new homoeopathic theory on their patients tend to end up in ungrounded confusion. Practitioners from either end of this greasy pole may serve a caucus of their patients extremely well – those who respond to the particular style and personality of the individual – but there will be many who fall outside the limitations.

The successful practitioner treads a cautious but inquiring path of balance, gaining experience by discovering what works best for the patients who come to him or her and by being open to all the exceptions to any given rule. It is the exceptions that not only prove the rule but also teach the most, both about personal limitations and the breadth of potential for healing, even in the most rare of circumstances. The experienced practitioner who is open to new ideas, who is prepared to be wrong and who is content to learn from his patients is a confident practitioner. Without this flexibility patients are not being well served. Different methods of approach do not arise simply on a whim because someone has become bored and taken time out to invent a new way of presenting remedies. Methods arise out of the necessity to diversify. Practitioners would not promote their pet theories for long if there were no clinical evidence to support their propositions. It is for the rest to hear what is said and take from it what they need and put it into practice. Didactic academics would do well to remember that theory, however steeped in historical precedent, should bow to clinical results.

Every generation of homoeopaths needs to develop its own tide of energy; every individual homoeopath needs to develop his or her own particular style which works best for him or her. Homoeopathy is not only a science but it is a craft and an art too. However, those who slavishly follow a narrow method to the exclusion of all else will be successful with only a correspondingly narrow cross section of patients. Strictly classical homoeopaths run this risk just as much as those who practise nothing but polypharmacy.

The first maintaining cause to consider might well be the practitioner's limitations. The inclusive study of methodology in homoeopathy allows practitioners breadth. It gives them a greater range of operation. *Being able to tailor the practice to the patient* rather than the other way round enables the practitioner to adapt responsively and responsibly to whatever may be presented. Where homoeopathy fails most frequently is when prejudice, lack of insight and lack of knowledge of the infinite flexibility of the system prevails.

A good example of this can be found in some countries where the use of disease nosodes such as *Syphilinum*, *Medorrhinum*, *Tuberculinum*, *Psorinum* and *Carcinosin*, are eschewed either because practitioners are not taught the methodologies of their use or because they are unavailable in the pharmacies due to what amounts to a medical embargo. Though practitioners may all have been taught about the individual 'pictures' of the nosodes from the various provings, caveats on their employment inhibit some practitioners from using them. For some the disease nosodes are potentially hazardous and this prejudice is handed down to the next generation of homoeopaths. If these practitioners were to discover just how liberal many British homoeopaths were in prescribing nosodes, they would be surprised.

In England there is a perfectly valid school of thought that promotes such frequent use of indicated nosodes either as *support*[1] or to underpin remedies in cases that are deeply affected by a hereditary thread of a chronic disease pattern. Practitioners brought up in a different tradition may be left in a quandary as to what to do when patients become 'stuck', having hit a hereditary block to cure, and are ideally in need of one or other of the nosodes to shift them forward. Misplaced concern about these particular remedies removes a key tool in their 'kit'.[2]

Do allopathic doctors make good homoeopaths?

Despite the fact that most of the very greatest homoeopaths of the past have qualified as allopathic doctors, many who take up homoeopathy tend to suffer from the limitations of inadequate training in alternative thinking that fails to shift their rationalist perspective of disease. With few notable exceptions, doctors tend to remain wedded to their earliest mindset. They think *therapeutically* which means that they think in terms of ridding the body of symptoms and not in terms of what positive aspects might be inherent in the patient's purpose for falling into illness, nor of the underlying cause. If they do look beyond the symptom picture it is often to hunt for the trigger that set off the present symptoms. This approach is appropriate in dealing with acute conditions but only incidental when looking into chronic pathology.

This inability to see beyond the symptoms means that allopathic doctors do not form strategies for healing. They do not look to the individual's creative purpose in getting well. So the removal of symptoms, the central focus in the conventional, rationalist approach, remains an end in itself. Though homoeopathic remedies may be used and are therefore unlikely to suppress any symptoms, they do not know which direction to take to maintain health after the presenting symptoms (so often only the tip of an iceberg) are expunged. The common result is a relapse or the emergence of a new set of symptoms as a manifestation of the untouched underlying distress felt in the psyche.

Doctors in Britain who study homoeopathy are generally taught through the study of the *Materia Medica*. Their study of the *philosophy* of healing is distinctly rudimentary though it is based on Hahnemann's teachings. They get half the picture. Nor are they discouraged from resorting to allopathic drugs to overcome difficult sub-acute episodes. In fact, it is common practice for a doctor–homoeopath to advocate the use of drugs and homoeopathic remedies at the same time[3]. This is most common in severe skin complaints when a prescription will be issued for steroid creams as well as the chosen remedy. This means that as fast as the body receives the stimulus to create an eliminative process, the body's chosen method of elimination is stymied! This is self-defeating and absurd bad practice. Yet it is done for the best if most misguided of reasons: the practitioner wishes to minimise the distress of the patient without realising that an aggravation (a discharge through the skin) needs to occur before true healing will take place[4].

It is interesting to note that even Marjorie Blackie, homoeopathic physician to royalty and doyenne of the London Homoeopathic hospital in the middle of the last century, on occasion saw no difficulty in using antibiotics to deal with acute infections. Yet this practice is to overlook the body's need to go through an acute disease in order to teach itself how to cope with fever and infection. When self-healing in such a situation becomes difficult or impossible, the administration of a homoeopathic remedy sets the body's healing process back on track. (Though, once again, it must be noted that there *are* occasions when one's best efforts are defeated for reasons best known to Nature and then antibiotics become lifesavers.)

Are homoeopaths adequately trained?

It is only right to be even-handed in criticism. Where homoeopathic training often falls short in the colleges of homoeopathy is in the very area in which allopathic doctors should be respected. The study of anatomy, physiology and pathology is, for the most part, inadequate. A new graduate of homoeopathy might be expected to be as knowledgeable as a newly qualified nurse would be. The difference, though, between a nurse and a graduate of homoeopathy is that the latter would have only 'book knowledge' and not have had the distinct advantage of hands-on experience in a hospital ward.

On the face of it this should not make much difference to a practising homoeopath; the study of homoeopathy is not about the diagnosis of specific diseases or being versed in reading charts or checking electronic monitors. Nor is it about taking urine and blood samples to look for the incidentals of pathology. It is more about identifying in Nature what is most similar in energy to the symptomatology of the individual patient.

This is the theory, and reality does prove the theory to be true – most of the time. It also demonstrates that homoeopaths become far more effective and professional if they have a very thorough grounding in the regular scientific aspects of healing the body. To know, for example, how the great psoas muscles that cross the abdomen are attached into the groin below and up into the diaphragm above is to understand how leg injuries can disturb digestion. To know that a blocked ethmoid sinus (above the bridge of the nose) can cause pituitary malfunction and therefore hormone insufficiency, is to see that someone with chronic sinus problems might well begin to present a picture of, say, underactive thyroid; this becomes of primary importance when one knows that ethmoid congestion can be the result of a fall on the coccyx!

Theoretically such information is of very little value to fulfilling the criteria of a homoeopathic prescription. One might expect to consider the symptoms of the digestive problems or the hypothyroidism and prescribe on the *general* effects that these conditions would have on the patients, but this is not really enough. All too often the indicated remedies chosen in such circumstances either fail to act or they begin changes that the body simply cannot sustain. Treating conditions complicated by physical trauma and/or functional congestion often requires combining a therapeutic approach (prescribing an organ support remedy for the part that is sluggish or blocked) with the indicated remedy (the so-called whole-body *similimum*), as well as the ability to refer patients to other complementary therapies (such as osteopathy) that can facilitate the deeper and more lasting results of the remedies.

For example: a little boy of twenty months was brought with perpetual congestion of the left ear and nasal sinuses as well as conjunctivitis of the left eye. All his general symptoms as well as those of the eye and ear indicated *Pulsatilla* as the remedy. (He was weepy and clingy, pale and whiney. He had yellow pus oozing from the affected eye and he moaned from time to time that his left ear caused him pain – a classic example of *Pulsatilla*.) A dose of *Pulsatilla* did help for a while but the symptoms returned. A dose of *Tuberculinum* (as there was a history in the family of TB on the mother's side) also relieved the problem for a little while. An examination of the child's cranium revealed that it was misshapen and asymmetrical; that the left side was considerably more compressed downwards than was the right side. This had come about through a traumatic birth after a long labour. The net result was that the drainage of the left sinuses was blocked and the space deep within the head – which houses the pituitary gland – was also compressed. When tissues containing mucous membranes are pulled out of shape they tend to step up their secretions. If the pituitary gland is compromised then the system becomes sluggish and the immune system can become vulnerable. A thorough knowledge of the mechanics of the cranium reveals that the sphenoid bone can become stuck and immobile through damage to the cranium. This is a wing shaped and mobile bone required to rock back and forth to act as a pump to cerebrospinal fluid washing past the pituitary gland as it secretes hormones to be sent out to the rest of the body. *Pulsatilla* would not be able to reverse this problem; nor would *Tuberculinum*. It is unlikely that most students of homoeopathy are taught about the mechanics of the sphenoid even if they are expected to know about the pituitary gland. Yet as this case shows it is important as such information can provide an answer to an otherwise insoluble problem[5].

These observations about allopathic doctors and graduate homoeopaths are broad generalisations. They are offered in order to point out that areas of ignorance and prejudice in any practice can compromise the effectiveness of treatment.

Flexible prescribing

We should illustrate some of the points made so far for the sake of clarity.

> A patient with gall bladder pains had severe pain intermittently in the right side of her abdomen below her ribs and felt as if she would explode with flatulence. What was worse, she explained, was a nagging, drilling pain in her back at the level of her shoulder blade. Her emotional state was tearful and dejected and she said she was lonely as her husband was away and it was the anniversary of her mother's death.
>
> She was asked if she had a fever with any of the symptoms. "No", was the reply but on occasion she felt faint, dizzy and in need of fresh air. She added, when asked about it, that she was not thirsty and had hardly drunk anything all day. A homoeopath straight out of college would be forgiven for assessing everything on the mental/emotional attitude – for this is what he would have been taught to do. This at first glance would indicate *Pulsatilla* – tearful, lonely, in need of company and support – and this would be neatly confirmed by the general physical symptoms of dizziness, faintness and air hunger as well as lack of thirst. It is only the *particular* physical symptoms of the gall bladder that might suggest something else would be needed.

The remedy that is indicated by the gall bladder trouble is *Chelidonium*, which features the remarkable pain in the bottom corner of the right shoulder blade, particularly manifest with cholecystitis (inflammation of the gall bladder). The woman had been given *Pulsatilla* on its own in the previous year when she had first come with the complaint. Though she had felt much stronger generally in herself, the gall bladder pain had not improved, in fact it had got considerably worse and caused nausea and vomiting – the result being that she spent an anxious night in hospital. When, on the present occasion, she was given *Chelidonium* 30 to take twice daily after the initial dose of *Pulsatilla* 200, she began to feel well. All the gall bladder symptoms eased away. Not only was her general state being considered (*Puls.*) but also the much more delicate condition of the gall bladder which on the previous occasion had been unable to cope with 'keeping up' with the improvement of the rest of the body.

This prescription runs counter to the classical ideal of 'one remedy at a time'. The first prescription of *Pulsatilla* on its own, which would fit within the classical model, proved to be less than adequate. What was needed here, beyond a broad knowledge of the relationship of remedies, was the recognition that the condition of the gall bladder was far weaker and more volatile than the rest of the body. The necessity of addressing the needs of the suffering organ – whose symptoms did not match *Pulsatilla* – as well as the Whole was amply illustrated by the night in hospital.

Any homoeopath deciding to treat only the gall bladder with just the *Chelidonium* would run the risk of missing the whole picture. The painful symptoms might well go away and thus make the patient feel temporarily much better and more energetic. However, unless the *Pulsatilla* followed soon to take care of the Whole then the patient would soon relapse into the old pattern of physical symptoms. (To assuage any sense of guilt that one is not towing the 'classical' line it helps to know that *Chelidonium* is a remedy entirely complementary to *Pulsatilla*.)

It is not uncommon to meet patients in a similar predicament where there is advanced organ pathology showing an independent energy pattern from the Whole. Anyone unsympathetic to or not realising the potential of simultaneously prescribing complementary remedies where they are indicated would have difficulty in sustaining the continued therapy of complex chronic pathology.

In a nutshell, the depth and clarity of the practitioner's perception of what it is to be healed combined with the knowledge of how to match it with a strategy of remedial action is of primary importance. Without this comprehensive view, treatment can become bogged down or grind to a halt.

As we shall see a little later, this means that homoeopaths cannot afford to stop learning.

Here is another example of a case where it was necessary to look beyond the obvious and to see that no one remedy would be able to achieve lasting results:

> Joyce, a woman in her early forties, complained of *"pain in the tummy"*. She said that she had not felt well since she had had an operation to remove her gall bladder by keyhole surgery. Her pains were located directly below the scar of the operation. There were very few other symptoms. She simply kept repeating that she did not feel well.
>
> *"I don't know what it is. I just don't feel right in myself. I can't put my finger on it but I'm just not 100 per cent."*
>
> She sat on the very edge of her seat twisting her fingers round and round. She admitted that she had lost her appetite and that she was not thirsty. She was always in floods of tears and she was cross that her husband was forever out of the house *"doing his own thing"*.

At this point it is reasonable to assume that Joyce was still in a certain amount of shock from the operation. She was also upset about her domestic situation that had probably been heightened by her recent ordeal. We might also take into consideration that her physical body had not recovered from the operation itself. Many patients who 'go under the knife' suffer the persistent sensation that they can feel the slice of the surgeon's incision. Had this been the focus of the case then Joyce would have needed *Staphysagria* (delphinium) which covers this peculiar symptom. We might also take into account the underlying cause of the gall bladder problem: resentment and bitter anger. These were undeniably there as Joyce had spoken several times before about her emotional state but now their point of expression, the gall bladder, had been removed. (In a classical assessment these emotions should have formed the target of remedial response.) Finally we could suspect that beneath the incision scar tissue had begun to form thus gathering and puckering surrounding tissue, pulling the area out of shape. (Not so usual after keyhole surgery but still a possibility.)

Joyce finally gave a clue regarding the true focus of her condition in an off-the-cuff remark made towards the end of the interview. *"I just wonder if this pain is cancer or something."* She spoke with a scared look and pinched tone in her voice.

She was given a single dose of *Carcinosin* 200[6] and within twelve hours her pain had gone and her whole demeanour was radically different. Over the phone she reported that she felt *"ever so much better"* and that she couldn't imagine how silly she had been to be so depressed about everything. *"I'm absolutely fine! I've just turned out the dining room and that always makes me feel better."*

At her next appointment she did not even recall feeling so scared about cancer; nevertheless, she was feeling tearful and moody. She still was not eating properly, tending to browse on chocolate and biscuits. Her complexion was bad. She was not drinking nearly enough fluids and she was getting hot flushes. Every time she had a flush she felt very angry and snapped at whoever came near. She had her period at that moment and she felt that she was losing more menstrual blood than usual. She was tired, achy and *"really peed off"*.

Joyce was presenting two pictures at once: (a) her underlying state of tearfulness, changeable moods, feeling down and lonely and (b) the temporary symptoms of her period: irritable, weak from blood loss, fed up and intolerant. The former is answered by *Pulsatilla* and the latter by *Sepia*. She was given *Sepia* 200 to be taken immediately and *Pulsatilla* 10M to take in three days' time. She rang six weeks later and asked the receptionist to cancel the next appointment she had in the following week and to make another in three months; she said that she felt very well. When she did return she explained that she had started divorce proceedings against her husband, that she had found a new man in her life and that she was really happy. The only problem now was that she had very uncomfortable corns and could they be treated, please.

Physician! Heal thyself

It is said that practitioners get the patients they deserve. In other words, patients often turn up with complaints that teach practitioners what they need to know – about their craft or about themselves. This may be in the form of their worst fears. Newly qualified homoeopaths are often faced with patients who are suffering from the complaint that they most fear having to treat. (This is frequently a skin condition that they are afraid will go badly 'wrong' as a result of remedies they might prescribe.) Or it could be in the form of digging up feelings from the practitioner's own past that lie unresolved. (An example might be that of a case of traumatised emotions resulting from a messy divorce being treated by a practitioner who had suffered badly in a similar situation.) In either case the healer's judgement can be compromised.

It is not uncommon for practitioners to find themselves asking leading questions that stem from their own experience rather than that of the patient. Inevitably the resulting prescription can be as much or more to do with the homoeopath. Though the experience of meeting and interacting with patients with a similar negative context can be healing for the practitioner it still behoves him or her to be conscious of the importance of professional impartiality. It's too easy for empathy to become sympathy; this is when patients can get confused signals and the practitioner can lose his way. Homoeopaths should not remain ivory-tower aloof but they do need to be objective observers.

The moral of this is that practitioners themselves need to undergo long-term homoeopathic treatment from a respected colleague so that they are constantly on a path of their own discovery which, as has been said before, is an evolutionary process.

The influence of choice

Choosing a practitioner is a very subjective process. The wrong choice is a sure way of compromising treatment. One needs to build a trusting rapport with the person who is going to spend their creative energy finding out about one's innermost workings. If trust and rapport are not there then the treatment will not be satisfactory. This is not a simple admission that the cure is in the relationship and the pills are nothing but placebo. Distrust and antipathy *create energy* quite strong enough to cause the patient to resist the energy of the remedies.

If you find that you do not respond to a relaxed atmosphere created in the consulting room of a practitioner who is lounging in an armchair, while you sit on a sofa, then your discomfort will help set up barriers. You might be more comfortable with a homoeopath who sits at a desk and interviews you sitting in an upright chair; there are even those who wear white coats. If you feel disturbed by the homoeopath who asks you every detail of your emotional life within the first twenty minutes and seems to ignore the fact that you have come about a stomach ulcer that is playing you up at this moment, then you need to find another practitioner who will address the immediate physical problem with what you feel is the proper sense of priority. Conversely, if you know that your gall bladder problem is the result of persistent levels of stress, the origins of which you feel should be explained, then consulting someone who prescribes only on the physical symptoms is not going to get you further than palliation.

If you are put off by the practitioner who sits opposite you without saying a word, allowing the shade of expectation to darken the room, waiting for you to make the first contribution, then find someone closer to the traditional doctor who will reassuringly lead you down well-worn paths of enquiry. (As long as there are not so many leading questions as to encourage biased information.) If you are exasperated by a practitioner who feeds all the information that he or she is gathering into a computer in order to get a printout of the most indicated remedies, rather than giving you undivided attention, then move on. (Computers are addictive and they frequently disrupt the balance of judgement that should exist between the intellect and the intuition. A machine cannot replace human energy exchange.)

Practitioners can fall short of patients' expectations because they have missed something, they have a bias or prejudice, they have not got the right experience or because they are simply incompatible with their clients. The basis for successful treatment is always a comfortable relationship with the practitioner. Finding the right practitioner for *you* can be a question of trial and error. *Yellow Pages* or one of the homoeopathic umbrella organisations can be a start. Some new patients make a few discreet enquiries of the receptionist, perhaps to get an impression of the personal style of the practitioner they are thinking of seeing. Probably the most satisfactory way of finding your ideal practitioner is to go by a recommendation from someone for whom you have respect and with whom you have something in common.

CHAPTER 8

ANTIDOTES

Can healing energy be cancelled out?

This is something of a 'hot potato'. Controversy simmers in homoeo-pathic circles about what may and may not constitute an antidote remedy. There are various schools of thought: from the hardliners whose injunctions make the taking of remedies a logistical exercise to the lais-sez-faire approach of practitioners who believe that there is no such thing as an antidote. There is no doubt that there *are* occasions when remedies are rendered null and void and there is quite a list of things that can be to blame. It is as well to be aware of these influencing factors, as it is so easy, inadvertently, to spoil the progress of treatment through ignorance.

Radiation

Homoeopathic remedies, when stored correctly, last indefinitely. (They are, after all, nothing less than *nuclear* energy – the nuclear energy of the various substances.) They are usually sold in amber coloured glass phials and bot-tles because experience strongly suggests that direct sunlight obliterates all potentised homoeopathic medicines. Do not expect a remedy to be effective if you have left it in strong light.

Likewise, other things that emit radiation: microwave ovens, CD play-ers, mobile phones, computers and any other source of even small measures of microwave radiation, can render the remedies ineffective. Many patients keep their remedies in the kitchen as it is a convenient place to remember to take regular doses of whatever they have been prescribed. Unfortunately the treatment is unlikely to succeed if the storage space is quite close to a microwave oven that it is in regular use. It is necessary to keep at least five to six feet between medicine and machine. For some extremely sensitive patients healing can also be compromised, if not prevented outright, through the continued *consumption* of food cooked in a microwave.

Electric under-blankets are another consideration. The electrical energy of the blanket can be enough to disturb the process of change that might be otherwise initiated by the remedies. It is unsurprising then, that those who work long hours at their computers might also be among those whose response to the remedies is compromised. (The backs of computers are particularly bad for emitting radiation.) Electrical circuitry and machinery that emit radiation do not affect everyone in the same way or necessarily adversely; they are suspect in some cases however, and need to be investigated in those cases where positive reaction to remedies is limited.

Mobile phone masts are fast becoming a health hazard. There is unofficially recorded evidence of families suffering constitutionally from the microwave radiation emitted by the masts. Homoeopaths are asked quite regularly to offer advice on whether it is a good idea for anyone to buy a house that is within a short distance of one of these structures and the answer is 'probably not'. Not nearly enough is known about the long-term effects of the radiation that is being emitted and the scanty evidence to date is alarming enough to warrant a demand from the 'powers that be' to set up far more rigorous tests to disprove the apparent threat.

For those who travel, there is the thorny question of what happens to remedies on the way through airport security. The short answer is that remedies are either compromised or destroyed by being passed through the X-ray machine. This is contrary to the information given to airport staff by one of Britain's leading homoeopathic pharmacies which has decided that X-ray machines are quite safe. While it is true that some patients have found no apparent detrimental effect on their remedies from the concentrated but brief passage through the machinery, the majority of people complain that their remedies are no longer effective. Airport staff often remark to passengers who insist on having their remedies personally inspected that we are all subjected to far greater concentrations of radiation just by travelling in an aircraft – any pilot flying over the Nevada desert or Winscale and checking his Geiger counter knows that to be true. Nevertheless, most remedies are rendered ineffective by the focused concentration of X-rays emitted by the machines, not by being carried on a plane journey.

There is protective action that one can take that seems to be very effective: wrapping up remedies in aluminium foil protects the remedies in some way. Travellers can be advised to pack their remedies in their main luggage well wrapped in foil while the remedies they might need for the flight should go into their pocket in a loose envelope. The metal detector does not seem to affect remedies and they can be carried through with impunity. Another solution is a lead-lined (photographer's) envelope which would prevent X-ray damage. In fact, it is as well that patients keep their prescriptions and home remedies in a foil-lined box so that there is no risk of damage from the daily threat of mobile phones.

All this is relevant when considering those patients who are obliged, due to their condition, to undergo X-rays or CAT scans. The effect of these diagnostic tests is sometimes to compromise the efficacy of prescribed remedies. Radiation is attracted to the vital energy of the body as iron filings would be to a magnet; it begins 'replacing' our vital energy with its own. People who suffer from radiation 'poisoning' experience what might be described as an 'energy leak'. They feel that energy is draining away from them in the way that water goes down a plughole. Such an energy drain is potentially the worst form of antidoting because it is so insidious. No remedy will ever work satisfactorily if there is a radiation problem.

So extensive is the problem of radiation that it is often viewed as a miasm – a disease-inducing influence. Though there is no incontrovertible proof, it is accepted amongst many practitioners that radiation remedies such as *Radium Bromide*, *Radium Iodatum*, *X-ray* itself and, more recently, *Plutonium* are regularly successful in shifting curative energy positively in those patients who have proved to be unresponsive to other more obviously well-indicated remedies[1]. There are creatures on the planet that can survive large doses of radioactivity, even be apparently oblivious to it. Scorpions and cockroaches are among them. There are some people too who seem impervious to excesses of radiation. Nevertheless, most of us *are* susceptible to it to some degree or other. In fact, there are no 'acceptable safe levels' whatever we may be told by scientists anxious to calm our fears.

An example illustrates this problem well: a woman suffering from frequent bouts of cystitis and recurrent sore throats was given an appointment for a CAT scan. She had recently started to take remedies that had allowed her system to show signs of recovery. Pains and inflammation were reduced by at least 50 per cent and she was pleased to report that she felt better and had more energy than she had had for some years. Immediately after the CAT scan she phoned to say that all her symptoms were back and she felt drained of all energy. She dated the moment of the change to the time she spent in the scanning machine. It was only after she had been given several doses of *X-ray* 30^2 that she began to make a second recovery.

In another example a small boy was brought for treatment for a universal nettle rash that he had developed within minutes of being in the sea near Dungeness power station on the south coast of England. This rash was desperately itchy and he found it impossible not to scratch. He was so restless that he could not stay still for a moment but had to walk round the room continually. He also had a house plant spray filled with water that he sprayed on his limbs to keep them cool. He said that his skin burned and was alive with a sensation of insects crawling. This is a good description of someone who is suffering from radiation burn. He was given *Radium Bromide* 30 to take every two hours. The rash disappeared within twenty-four hours.

Plenty of people who bathe off the coast at Dungeness do not seem to suffer ill effects. However, the nearby power station has had bad press ever since it was first built. It is relevant to note that this little boy was a patient with very fine skin and hair and ginger colouring, a type usually associated with hypersensitivity. Nevertheless, radiation is a relatively common health hazard and should never be underestimated.

Geopathic stress

The ancient art of feng shui is based on arranging living space in a way that reflects and harmonises the earth's natural energies in the environment. It recognises that the earth has dynamic, positively- and negatively-charged areas on its surface that, in juxtaposition, can affect us in ways that are powerful and can influence for good or ill our own dynamic energy. Feng shui is a philosophy that tends to separate strictly rationalist thinkers from the rest, despite its long history in the East and the fact that many Chinese architects simply would not contemplate erecting any building without first consulting a feng shui expert. This philosophy is not exclusive to the East. Ancient man understood the importance of place when siting his permanent structures. His knowledge of ley lines – a network of energy force fields that criss-cross the land surfaces of the earth – enabled him to site structures of ancient mystical and astrological importance such as Stonehenge, Avebury and Silbury so that he could not only make calculations with precision but also enhance the power of his rituals.

Those who practise the art of dowsing or divining using hazel twigs, pendulums or even metal coat hangers adapted for the job, are able to discern where these power lines run. Many of the oldest churches in Britain are built on those places where two or more ley lines cross. Such places can be invigorating to stand on. The energy of ley lines promotes well-being.

There are other earth forces that are not so benevolent. There are other parts of the earth's surface that are cross-hatched with lines of energy that are detrimental to health and we live over them at our risk. The areas where they occur have nothing to do with ley lines. They are rather better described as points of the land surface where the earth emits its waste energy. Living in the environment above them can speed up the process of ailing and prevent any form of healing.

This negative response is known as geopathic stress. It can exist to any degree from the negligible to the malignant. The difference in severity of response is often related to whether there is any other environmental factor to enhance the negative energy. Underground water, streams and wells magnify the negative effects as do the presence of overhead power cables, radio masts and local electricity stations. Concrete buildings tend to exaggerate the influence as well. (They were the origin of sick building syndrome.) Where stress rays are strong, no amount of feng shui will negate them completely and the beneficial effects of homoeopathic remedies are usually dissipated or negated quite quickly. Pets often display telltale signs that a house might be affected. If a dog stays well clear of certain parts of the house or a cat has a favourite spot to sleep in, then these points should be noted. Dogs, like their owners, are adversely affected and avoid the rays.

Cats, on the other hand, will actively seek out a ray to sit in. There are people, too, who are quite impervious to the effects of the rays though there are others who are acutely hypersensitive to them.

The most usual pathological result is fatigue as a consequence of reduced ability to co-ordinate well, to the point of patients being diagnosed with ME, depression, lethargy and loss of motivation, frequent bouts of acute 'flu, colds and accident proneness. Each individual's general condition is governed by his or her susceptibility to producing hereditarily-influenced disease patterns but the geopathic stress will always exacerbate them. So important is the issue that many dowsers and their organisations are now dedicated to investigating the rays and preventing their disastrous effects on peoples' health. These groups can provide an effective answer to what would otherwise be an intractable maintaining cause.

Here is an example:

A couple moved into a bungalow that had been built in the 1930s. The house was in an idyllic setting surrounded by woods and farmland. A stream and a ditch acted as the boundaries to the south and east. A natural spring fed a well on the north side. When they first moved in they had no health problems and felt that the house was perfect. Then they had their children: three in four years. They decided that an extension was necessary. When the extra rooms were completed the couple chose to give their own bedroom to the children and to move into the extension to sleep. While the wife had no difficulty in getting a good night's sleep, the husband began to suffer from restlessness and wakefulness. Within six weeks he felt that his sleep patterns were causing him to feel drained of energy, listless and apathetic and insensitive towards the family. He went to his homoeopath.

Despite a clear indication for the remedy *Phosphoric acid* – to treat exhaustion, weakness, apathy, poor memory, aching soreness of the bones and muscles – his symptoms changed very little. Other remedies were tried but with little success. After some months a friend of the family came to stay. She was a dowser and she suggested that she should investigate. She found that the extension had been built so that a stress ray that had previously only traversed the garden now crossed the corner of the new bedroom. The ray ran right through the husband's side of the bed. The dowser suggested that a 5-foot angle iron should be sunk into the earth at a strategic spot in the garden. She explained that the effect of this would be to divert the ray harmlessly away from the house; it was similar to acupuncture on the earth's surface. Though the husband admitted to being somewhat sceptical he did as he was directed. He had no further difficulty sleeping and his health returned to normal within a very short time.

Some people are so sensitive to the 'vibrations' of a place that they can describe the feelings and sensations that are induced. They are often made to feel foolish or cranky if they explain what they experience to others but we should listen to what they have to say. Even if we make allowances for the tricks of hormones or the vagaries of emotional instability – and it is easy to fall into the trap of being patronising with some people – there are too many others experiencing these occurrences for this curious maintaining cause to be either irrelevant or an eccentricity.

Joanna and Mark and their two children had been living in their house for some years. Since they had moved there none of them had been particularly well, suffering frequent bouts of chest and sinus infections, tonsillitis and earaches. While remedies did help them on each acute occasion, their general constitutional health seemed not to improve; if anything it worsened and their outlook on life seemed to be affected as well. They put the house on the market and felt better for having made a positive decision. Time passed, infections kept recurring, their gloom increased and their energy and positivity diminished proportionately. Nothing seemed to work. Few people came to view the house and if they did then nothing was heard afterwards. After two years someone made an offer but then withdrew. Soon after this happened a second time Joanna found out about a local dowser whom she invited round to check for geopathic stress. A ray was found to go straight through the middle of the house. The dowser recommended putting in an angle iron in a spot some yards from the neighbour's fence which Joanna duly did, temporarily heeling it in so that most of it was visible.

Within a few days all four members of the family had begun to feel brighter and more energetic. The very next person to view the house put in an offer as a cash buyer and went through with the purchase.

In discussing their improved fortunes with the neighbour over the fence, Joanna discovered that things had not gone so well next door. All their machinery – the TV, the washing machine and dishwasher – had packed up; a fox had got in to the hen run and taken all the chickens; the couple themselves were not feeling well. It was at this point in the conversation that Joanna noticed that the angle iron, so carefully and strategically placed, had been moved. It was now much closer to the fence and had been put to use as a washing line: Mark, not realising the importance of its position had decided to put it to better use. The dowser was asked for her opinion and her comment was to the effect that the ray had been diverted too far over and was affecting the neighbour's house. When the angle iron was replaced in its original position the neighbour and her husband both began to feel better. (History does not relate whether their electrical equipment recovered or had to be replaced.)

Geopathic stress may be only a minor maintaining cause in terms of the numbers of people who experience the adverse effects – though there are those who would disagree and say it affects many – but when it is a problem it can be seriously damaging, creating distress, despair and even panic. If and when it reaches such significant levels in anyone's life then it warrants making a thorough investigation.

Noxious substances

One's very livelihood can sometimes be a problem and those who work with strong chemical substances run the risk of preventing homoeopathic remedies from working. Often it is the chemicals that have produced the pathology that has caused the patient to come for treatment in the first place whether they know it or not. Skin symptoms and breathing difficulties are common problems resulting from using epoxy resin or organo-phosphates (and this latter breed of chemicals can also be responsible for causing much worse problems). Poor memory and other symptoms of apparent early senility can result from paint fumes. If the patient is able to stop using the substances then there is every chance that a skilled practitioner may be able to detoxify their system. If the patient is obliged to continue using the substances that are harming him then the chemical effect on the body's energy will continue and be stronger than the effects of the remedies.

There are many farmers (and their neighbours) who suffer health problems related to the herbicides and pesticides that they use on their crops. Most of these are nerve poisons and the effects will appear in the form of an increasingly crippled nervous system and an increased allergic sensitivity. Even if these poisons were not a scourge on wildlife and the countryside, their effects on the human nervous system should be enough to have them outlawed. It is no longer surprising to read in the national press reports of individuals who live on farmland who suffer fatigue-related symptoms: exhaustion, lack of motivation, loss of confidence, muscular weakness, deterioration of the special senses, extreme sensitivity to pollutants, headachest – the list is endless. All the symptoms can be attributed to organo-phosphate poisoning though it is likely that there are other groups of industrial chemicals quite as capable of causing disaster. Though there is much public medical debate about the origins of chronic fatigue syndrome, chemical toxicity should be strongly suspected as a potential cause in a substantial number of cases.

It is worth noting that there is a therapeutic answer to acute industrial chemical toxicity. The remedy *Phosphorus* has proved of great value to those who have inhaled fumes and begun to feel light-headed, ungrounded and hypersensitive. Just as one might give *Arnica* 30 after a minor accident resulting in a bruise, so one might give *Phosphorus* 30 for acute chemical poisoning.

Other substances that are abused

Caffeine

Coffee is another 'hot potato'. The effects of coffee are hotly contested among homoeopaths. Some believe that it does no harm whatever; others believe that it damages incontestably not only the efficacy of remedies but also the body itself. The truth is that homoeopaths are going to continue believing in what seems to work for them. Coffee does not always antidote remedies *directly*. While there *are* patients who are very easily affected by coffee, who quite clearly show signs of having negated the effect of their latest remedy by drinking a cup, there are others who do get and have got better from their ailments while continuing to drink coffee. The former will admit that coffee gives them a 'buzz' and find it immensely difficult to give up; the latter are generally those who wouldn't stop drinking coffee even on medical grounds.

Coffee is a problem for long-term health. Though one might get better from this or that ailment while drinking it, there can be no question that the *full* efficacy of remedies is always compromised. By the 'full efficacy' is meant the remedies' ability to inspire not simply a physical transformation but also emotional and spiritual ones. The *depth of action* of the remedies is compromised. There is not much to smile about if you are a drinker of decaffeinated coffee either. It is different from its unadulterated original state but it can be harmful to remedies none the less.

Coffee is an adrenal stimulant and it is often for this reason that people drink it. Without a surge of adrenalin they feel less able to cope. Coffee is addictive because of the buzz it delivers. If a patient is addicted then he or she is not in control of his or her own system. Adrenalin is an important part of the hormone system and has a profound effect on the way the central nervous system functions. If too much adrenalin floods into the body and is then used up quickly with physical and mental activity then a 'crash' occurs until another cup is downed. While this allows the person to operate at higher than normal levels in the short term, there is always a payback problem. This comes in any number of different forms. There might be insomnia or lowered libido; there might be irritable bowel (prompting the 'porridge' description that signifies that something is amiss in the gut). There could be increased intolerance to minor irritations; there could be heart symptoms such as palpitations or tachycardia (irregular heartbeat).

More subtly but no less disturbing, there can be a shutdown of spiritual awareness with a greater concentration on worldly matters. In esoteric terms coffee gradually can shut off the connection between the head and the heart. 'Higher awareness' can be reduced to starvation levels. This is a contentious point and one that needs a curious qualification. It seems that coffee is far less of a problem for those who live in countries where the plant grows naturally or where it is a national drink. It seems generally to be more problematic for people in northern Europe.

People addicted to coffee will either find every excuse not to comply with an embargo placed on drinking it or simply refuse to believe that it is causing them any harm. This is because they are cut off from their awareness of how deeply their addiction is affecting them. It makes no difference that the practitioner explains the medical reasons for avoiding it; nor that they are told that remedies will not work as well or as deeply as they might; nor that there is a caucus of persistent symptoms that are still there because the coffee is aggravating the organs afflicted. They might even say rather shamefacedly that they have cut the coffee right down… to just one a day. Some people do make a stab at giving up coffee altogether but it often creeps back into the daily routine. Those who do give it up are almost always rewarded eventually with the realisation of how much more significant the remedies are without the interference[3].

Coffee is not the only substance that contains caffeine. Tea also contains high levels of caffeine and its effects on some people can be just as bad as those of coffee. Tea can be addictive, undoubtedly. The effects of tea interfere with kidney function and upset the water balances in the body. (Bear in mind that well over 60 per cent of the body is made up of water.) Generally, those homoeopaths who are concerned about caffeine in tea will put a ban on it only if the kidneys, bladder and circulation are showing signs of distress. There is also good cause, on occasion, for patients to stop drinking tea if they suffer persistent headaches and/or high blood pressure. Tea affects the biochemistry of the body and influences homoeopathic remedies only indirectly. Coffee, being a substance that causes a surge of adrenalin, actually creates a potential curb on the central nervous system's response to the remedy as it goes onto the tongue. (Those anxious to avoid tea but who feel deprived can try Red Bush tea.)

One intriguing case comes to mind that might seem to refute the case against caffeine.

One day a woman came to the clinic attached to the College of Homoeopathy to ask for treatment for her husband. She had been before for herself and for her children. All of them had done well with their treatment and she was fulsome in her praise of homoeopathy. However, on this particular day the woman was very preoccupied. She explained that her husband would never come for treatment himself, as he believed that people were trying to poison him. He was, she went on, suffering from the dementia of tertiary syphilis. He attended a day clinic where he was treated but at home he showed some distinct signs of insanity. He kept his copy of the Koran – for he was a devout Muslim – wrapped up in a polythene bag and submerged in a bowl of water that was, in some way, attached to an electric circuit. He had arranged things in this way as he believed that someone was intent on stealing the book. His wife was concerned that he would do something even more extravagant that might put their children in jeopardy. It was for this reason that she was asking for help.

Having asked her a few questions about his general state of health the students who had been deputed to take the case returned to the supervising clinician and the class. It was generally decided by consensus that the patient should be given *Syphilinum* 10M. This was given to the woman who took it away with much gratitude. She returned in a month, wreathed in smiles. She was overjoyed with the success of the remedy. Within a day of her giving it to him her husband had taken the Koran out of the bowl and restored it to the shelf. He had dismantled the electric trap. He had discharged himself from the clinic saying that he felt different and better than he had for a long time. He was able to take more part in the general family life in a way that he had become unable to over the last few years.

One of the students remembered that the patient had been paranoid about taking anything for fear of being poisoned so she asked the wife how the remedy had been administered. *"I gave it to him in his coffee. He never drinks anything else so I had no choice."*

This anecdote would make a great story if we could leave it there. Unfortunately, the remarkable recovery did not last and he relapsed within three months.

One of the big problems for the patient coming off coffee or tea is that they generally have to go through an aggravation. The usual signs are a crashing headache, tiredness and irritability. There can also be nausea, increase or loss of appetite and increased mucous secretion. This can last up to ten days but more usually continues for only four or five. Those who get through this uncomfortable period of adjustment – where the body's normal functions are restored – generally feel thoroughly cleansed and often remark that they feel much clearer in their thinking .

Fizzy drinks that contain caffeine (or any other noxious substance for that matter) do not receive such bad alternative press as tea and coffee, but perhaps they should. Colas can become addictive and may occasionally be implicated in the undermining of remedies. Most drinks in cans contain preservatives and artificial sweeteners that certainly contribute to the distress of those (particularly children of the last two generations) who are so sensitive that they become hyperactive after a few mouthfuls. Remedies given to children suffering from ADHD (Attention Deficit and Hyperactive Disorder) are almost always compromised if the patient drinks a can of anything that contains aspartame.

Tobacco

Smoking can act as an antidote to remedies. Nicotine suppresses adrenal flow and calms the nervous system artificially. Imagine the confusion in the nervous system if the person both smokes and drinks coffee! If the nervous system is compromised then the remedies which work on it are compromised too. It is as simple as that. Cigarettes are manufactured to contain sugar so that they become *more* addictive. (Sugar speeds up the rate of absorption of nicotine into the body.) Nicotine spoils the purity of the blood; it confuses the function of the pineal, pituitary and thyroid glands, thus undermining the endocrine system as a whole. Without nicotine smokers feel agitated, irritable, depressed and deprived; they can also suddenly develop constipation and heavy mucous production. They often experience a huge increase of appetite and weight gain so, to add to their misery, they suffer from loss of confidence – which was often part of the emotional picture that led them to take up smoking in the first place. These conditions confirm the perverted function of the endocrine glands. The state of withdrawal can be truly distressing but the alternative is to continue with an addiction that slows or stops healing treatment and potentially shortens life.

Those who do give up the habit are often blessed with a really filthy 'cold', which has the benefit of detoxifying the lungs. The mucous membranes that line the bronchus and the tubes in the lungs pour out copious quantities of phlegm that is usually a disgusting brown colour. This is the best possible result. The patient, on seeing what the lungs are producing, is under no illusions as to how serious a hazard smoking really is.

Cannabis

Cannabis is one of the most unfortunate things to have come out of the 1960s. Though it was available before the First World War, it was only in the sixties that it exploded as a major cultural force and a medical menace. Few truly realise that, moral issues aside, cannabis causes profound disturbances to the whole body, mind and spirit. It is *not* harmless. Even for those who use it to relax at the end of a hard day it is potentially damaging. The persistent use of cannabis to relax becomes an addiction in just the same way that a sleepless old lady can become reliant upon diazepam. 'Reliance' is an innocuous term compared with 'addiction' and, as people tend to associate addiction with hard drugs, cannabis has become almost acceptable. Yet if users really understood the health cost they paid for taking cannabis then they might think twice about it.

Physically cannabis has long-term negative effects: bladder, prostate and sexual function can be thoroughly disturbed. Though it can enhance libido to start with, it almost invariably leads to flagging desire and impotence. It can throw menstrual cycles 'out of sync'. The immune system is affected: the white blood-cell count drops. This predisposes people not only to bacterial respiratory infection but also to non-specific urethral infection, to gonorrhoea or chlamydia. This shows that the drug acts as if it were a disease agent causing symptoms that the body would produce if developing its own picture of infection. (It should not surprise us that homoeopathic *cannabis* is a remedy that is used in the treatment of gonorrhoea.) Even more disturbing is the threatened increased risk of developing cancer of the oesophagus or stomach and in the offspring of mothers who smoked during pregnancy there is the risk of leukaemia and birth defects.

Cannabis smokers are likely to become mentally slow and physically inept. Their nervous systems become affected so that they are less able to perform efficiently. Their memories are impaired and their intellects are dulled. They give the appearance of being laid back but this is really a symptom of the distance that the cannabis has fostered between the smoker and reality.

Cannabis also disturbs the delicate balance between the thalamus and hypothalamus and the pineal and pituitary glands. The hormones released by the former glands are responsible for our flight and fight mechanism as well as our appetite, thirst and excretory processes. The trouble is that by the time any of these fundamental areas are showing obvious symptoms the patient is well and truly addicted. Once thoroughly addicted then the understanding of their predicament is denied them as the overall sense of awareness of self is partially or entirely absent. Essentially the ego – which is substantially what is gratified and mollified by the addiction – is unable to access the intuition, that part of oneself that instinctively knows 'when to stop'.

This assessment may be disputed hotly by those who feel that cannabis enhances their intuitive response and releases them from the constraints of everyday life. What these users fail to see is that whatever effects their bodies manifest do not belong to *them* but to the *drug*. They are instruments on which the chemical drug is playing tunes. The effects are no more theirs than they would be if they took antibiotics for a tooth abscess. Any variation in response between two individuals is more to do with variations in bio-chemistry than to do with personal mystical experiences. Users who feel that cannabis enhances their creative processes are under a delusion. It may seem to do this initially, but artistic endeavours are eventually undermined by our inability to produce a creative energy that is stronger than the chemical energy working on us. Drug influenced art is one of the very saddest of illusions; it has a very limited shelf life and cannot compare in quality with anything produced by a drug-free mind. It is one of the great mass delusions of the age we live in to believe otherwise.

Many, many patients who smoke regularly claim that they are not addicted.

Patient: *"I only have a joint once in a while, perhaps once a week at the weekend."*

Homoeopath: *"As it compromises remedies do you think you would be able to stop smoking for the duration of the treatment?"*

Patient: *"I'll try."*

Try they do, for a little while and then fail.

Patient: *"I didn't think that just one would matter."*

However 'just one' does matter – and the effects of remedies given at the last appointment will have been 'zapped'. Much of the early treatment for patients who can't stop themselves from having 'just one' or more than that, has to be based on remedies to deal with addiction and the side effects of the smoking. It is necessary, in other words, to use homoeopathy itself to do the antidoting! It can be just as necessary to detoxify patients from recreational drugs as it is to detoxify them from allopathic ones. Perhaps the most profoundly important of these is *Ayahuasca*, the remedy made from a liana from the jungles of South America. It is itself a hallucinogen of remarkable power and one that seems to encourage the restoration of the integration of *id* and *ego*.

So often the root cause for patients who continue to use cannabis is their lifestyle. A patient might have come for treatment full of determination to 'clean up'. He might then experience a period of thoroughly positive change and arrive at a point where he sees the benefits of his healing force creating opportunities of development. At this point he can so easily fall in with old friends who persuade him out for an evening. The siren call of the nightclub is too strong a pull on his memory. That one-won't-matter 'reefer' leads to the return of all his back pains and headaches or usual gut ache and cystitis may kick back in.

Harder drugs

What do we mean by 'hard' drugs? In reality, any hallucinogenic drug is 'hard' given the potential havoc it can wreak. However, cocaine and opium-based drugs are far worse in their destructive effects on the physical and mental bodies than cannabis. Snorting cocaine not only damages the mucous membranes of the nasal passages and predisposes the addict to polyps; it is also highly likely to be one of the causes of tumours of the pituitary gland. It can destroy regular sleep patterns. It can foul up the immune system. It will, moreover, separate the mind from personal will.

Cocaine may not be as vicious as heroin but it is just as fatal to the efficacy of alternative therapy. While cocaine users do quite often come for treatment and can do relatively well on remedies, very often homoeopathy is powerless to halt the speedy downward spiral of self-destruction experienced by heroin addicts. Certainly, no homoeopathic prescription would survive for very long if the patient persisted in the habit. In fact, treatment of addicts is always painstaking, often frustrating and only rewarding if the practitioner can set aside all prejudice and engender a rapport with the patient where there is deep trust and caring. Seldom is the treatment of drug addicts only to do with the effects on their bodies of the chemicals they use; there is so often a long history of other forms of abuse. Yet it is their dependence on their drugs that prevents healing of the mental and emotional turmoil locked within.

Treatment of hard drug users is extremely time-consuming and frustrating and, it has to be said, unrewarding financially. It is not surprising that the homoeopaths who become involved in this work have infinite patience and great compassion; their reward is the few who make remarkable recoveries. (It is interesting to observe that those who do overcome their addiction to harder drugs invariably discover a life purpose that is beyond any ego-bound limitations.)

Just one example will suffice to illustrate this dark corner of homoeopathy.

A young woman came for treatment with her nine-year-old son. He was extremely aggressive and sullen. He had a tendency to lash out at people. He would shout and scream when asked to do anything. He refused to wash. When spoken to he would remain silent and glare back. His mother was very concerned as he was now refusing to go to school and having him around the home meant that she could never give her full attention to her younger son, now a few months old. She went on to say that she was a heroin addict and so was her husband. They lived in the West Country in a caravan and she was visiting her parents for a fortnight's stay.

She then went on to say that her greatest wish was to give up heroin for good; she knew that it was not doing her children any good. She suspected that her elder boy was angry with both his parents for never 'being there' for him as they had so much of the time been stoked up with drugs. She had not had any heroin for three weeks and was there for treatment so that she could stay 'clean'.

She was given a prescription of homoeopathic remedies (an alternating sequence of *Nux Vomica* and *Sulphur*) that she felt made a remarkable difference within a few days. She felt that her head was clearer and that her energy had lifted. She was less weepy and more optimistic. Her son's prescription (*Hyoscyamus* – henbane) had also made a big difference. She had seen him smile for the first time in many months and he was no longer snarling and snapping. Furthermore, he had had several baths.

Then she had a phone call from her husband telling her that she had to return home to the caravan. She left and did not come back for treatment for two years. When she came for further treatment she confessed that as soon as she returned to her husband he had beaten her up and she went straight back on the heroin. Her son reverted and began to play truant from school and home. She said that she had felt *"all the effects of the remedies ebb away from me"* as soon as she got back into the old routine. Now she wanted to try again.

Sadly, everything happened as before – not just once but twice more over the next four years. Homoeopathic remedies have no power to force choices on people. Furthermore, while drugs may be maintaining causes that damage the efficacy of homoeopathic remedies, it is not a specific addiction that is the problem; it is the addictive personality that is the underlying illness. Treating addictiveness takes time; often longer than an addict is able or prepared to allow.

Aromatherapy oils

Unfortunately, there are some substances that are in common use and that are apparently harmless but which frequently stop remedies from working. These include aromatherapy oils which should be, to all intents and purposes, both efficacious and complementary. However, the essential oils will compromise or antidote remedies even more surely than coffee. Some are worse than others: the stronger or more penetrating the oil's aroma, the more damaging to the remedies it is.

Menthol and eucalyptus are the most frequently quoted as harmful to homoeopathy. Nevertheless, any of the oils should be viewed with circumspection. Lavender oil, when used sparingly, is the one exception to the rule. It is a truly wonderful relaxant when added to a bath. It is gentle and does not seem to have the same dampening effect on homoeopathic remedies as the other oils. Nevertheless, it would always be best, if in doubt, to check with one's practitioner as to whether or not it is advisable to use it whilst on medication.

One of the favourite oils is tea tree. This is advocated as antifungal and antibacterial even by homoeopaths! They should be wary; many patients who use it risk the efficacy of their recent treatment. Clinical observation has shown too often that while local effects may be satisfactory, long-term constitutional results are at risk when tea tree is used. There have also been cases showing that the oil has suppressed necessary discharges of pus from chronic suppurative eruptions which is completely at odds with the curative process. (And why do homoeopaths, trained in natural, empirical philosophy of healing, persist in prescribing tea tree oil for fungal infections and thrush when all they succeed in doing is suppressing the symptoms? Answer: being tempted by a quick fix solution. Fungal infections and thrush can be really persistent problems that put a practitioner on his mettle and may even require help from naturopathy and/or applied kinesiology.)

The message here is that if aromatherapy works well for you then wait for it to take effect before you start homoeopathic treatment. It should be understood that no disparagement of the system of treatment offered by aromatherapists is intended. However, the two therapies are not, strictly speaking, complementary. They are alternatives to one another.

Menthol, eucalyptus and peppermint are often used in toothpaste. Proprietary brands that contain these oils can antidote remedies if the pills or powders are taken too close to the time of cleaning the teeth. The mouth is rich in the nerves that convey the medicines' messages to the central nervous system. If the oils occupy the mouth area then the 'aroma' will be too powerful for the homoeopathic energy to 'get through'. There are alternative toothpastes that do not contain oils that are better from the patient's point of view[4]. If you can bear the taste of those that contain fennel then this is better still; fennel is good for teeth and gums. Peppermint sweets should also be avoided.

One day a patient arrived requiring treatment for an ulcer on the cornea of her eye. This was small and difficult to see but obviously the cause of much pain. She was given *Natrum Muriaticum* 200 for the condition and asked to come back in two weeks. If the symptoms did not clear up within three days then she was instructed to call back much sooner. She returned within the week and complained that her eye had got much better within a few hours but that everything was now just as bad as it had been. She was given a further dose of the medicine. The same thing happened as before. When it then happened a third time a closer inspection of the eye revealed the nature of the problem. In approaching the patient in order to examine the eye it was quite overpoweringly apparent that she had been eating 'Mint Imperials'. She was given a final dose of *Natrum Muriaticum* 200, told about the mint factor and asked to return if need be. The eye cleared of its symptoms within a few hours.

Touching the remedy

One of the common rules laid down by homoeopaths is that patients should not touch their remedies. This is a little misleading. Patients need not fear that they will antidote their own remedies by touching them unless they have hands that have powerful odours or scents on them. Strong soap or chemicals will spoil them. However, taking a pill out of its envelope with the fingers is not damaging.

There is another reason for telling patients not to handle remedies. Anyone giving a medicine to a child by hand might, if in need of the remedy him or herself for their own perhaps undiagnosed reason, take the energy of the remedy in through the skin before the child ever had the benefit of it.

Patients are often advised not to eat half an hour before or after remedies are due to be taken. If this were really a problem then animals given their remedies in their food or drink would not benefit from medication. (It is sometimes easier to disguise a pill in a piece of bread or in a hollowed out piece of carrot or dissolved in a bowl of milk than struggle with clamped jaws. Goats seem particularly reluctant to take things on trust and need some vegetable encouragement!)

There are few foods that are energetically more powerful than homoeopathic energy. Peppermint and spearmint are obvious examples. Some alcoholic drinks such as coffee liqueurs and aniseed are also antidotes. Generally, the 'eating rule' can be relaxed and is usually relevant only to those who are taking frequent doses of a medicine. Most prescriptions are geared to be taken at either end of the day.

Inside out

At this point we move from exterior factors that act as maintaining causes for illness, and focus on the internal reasons for continued illness. These reasons are imperative in the sense that if they are not dealt with either at the beginning of treatment or as soon as they are revealed as a significant problem then success will be negated. Such causes are not always presented unequivocally at the start and they may not, at first, prevent progress or they may be completely absent and therefore unidentifiable and yet prevent any remedy from working at all.

CHAPTER 9

PHYSICAL TRAUMA AND MUSCULOSKELETAL IMBALANCE

Most patients have a postural problem

The human frame is a miracle of nature's architecture but even so it is usual for patients to live in a permanent state of more or less musculoskeletal imbalance. The normal symmetry of the body is based on the way that the spine stems pivotally from the sacrum and pelvis and supports the head, shoulders and ribs. Ligaments of tough fibrous tissue bind these bones together. This tissue enables the structure to move with great elasticity and extraordinary variety while the 'architecture' creates the perfect form to return to.

Fixed structural asymmetry occurs usually as the result of the body's methods of providing compensation after a physical hurt, in which muscles, tendons and ligaments suffer damage, contraction and, often, consequent inflammation. Compensation occurs: the body comes to rely on the undamaged side – either left or right, back or front, upper or lower half – to take the burden of physical structural function to allow the wounded part time to heal. For example, a patient breaks a leg and during convalescence the muscle wastes a little from disuse. Once he is up and about the other leg must compensate while the broken one mends and gains strength. The limping gait of several weeks is enough to throw out the normal symmetry of the spine-centred body. Think of the person with arthritis who spends years putting his or her weight on the knee that does not hurt. Then, when he has an enforced rest from an illness, say, or has anti-arthritis drugs or takes to some alternative therapy, the 'good knee' starts to play up. It has had too much strain for too long from taking the unbalanced weight distribution. Its release from service is enough to cause it to protest for the first time, indicating a chronic imbalance.

If tough tissues such as bones and ligaments were all that we had to consider in the matter, then life might be simpler. Bones are the foundation and scaffolding; ligaments and tendons are the ropes and hawsers for their movement. Bones are living things with blood and nerve supplies; they bleed and feel pain. They are kept informed of all that goes on in the body. How does this happen? A short diversion will provide the answer.

Osteopathy and the reciprocal tension membrane (RTM)

Osteopathy is the practice of manipulating bones, muscles and ligaments back into their correct position to restore good mechanical function. To avoid confusion it is necessary to explain that within the practice of osteopathy there are different approaches to actual treatment. One of them is a refined method of practice that is sometimes referred to as 'cranial osteopathy' though this name implies the predominant importance of the head as the therapeutic focus. This is misleading as all forms of osteopathy, except when used specifically to treat recently injured parts, should be regarded as whole body treatment.

The term cranial osteopathy derives from the discovery of what is called the 'cranial rhythm' or 'involuntary motion' which was first investigated and described by Dr William Sutherland in the early years of the twentieth century. The man who initiated the practice of osteopathy was more interested in the movement of 'fluid energy' throughout the body; he was no bone-cruncher. Osteopaths who follow his lead 'read' this energy – an energy no different from the energy field of the Vital Force – by training to feel with their hands the most subtle of tiny variations in the rhythms of the body. These rhythms of electrical energy emanate from the medulla of the brain (the body's 'battery') and course in a predictable circulatory movement much as if the body were a magnet with north and south poles. When imbalances occur in the system due to physical or emotional trauma or pathological changes then Sutherland-inspired osteopaths are able to detect them by 'reading' the changes away from the norm that are observable in this fluid energy field. This refined system of treatment ranges, in the hands of different practitioners, from gentle and sometimes repetitive physical manipulation of tissues to what appears to be little more than the laying on of hands. (Acupuncture is based on a parallel system with the fluid energy called Qi and the flow of it coursing along meridians, the twelve energy channels and their tributaries. Acupuncturists use needles to effect rebalancing changes while the osteopaths use subtle pressure of their hands.) In referring hereafter to osteopathy it is this subtle form of practice that is to be understood.

Homoeopaths have much to learn from osteopaths and one of the first things to find out is that part of the instrument on which the fluid energy/Vital Force plays its tunes is called the reciprocal tension membrane (RTM). This is made of connective fibrous tissue that is extremely tough but very flexible. We might call it gristle if we found it on the dinner plate but it is perhaps more like the silvery tissue found on the knucklebone of a leg of lamb. It is hard to cut or to tear. It is also contiguous which means that it is a continuum of connective tissue. In the head it is called the dura mater; it surrounds the brain and divides it in two. It extends, posteriorly, down through the neck, surrounding the spinal cord – which is, without the ver-tebrae, a continuation of the brain. It extends, anteriorly, into the thoracic inlet, the area beneath the clavicles at the top of the lungs, and on into the thoracic diaphragm, the huge, dome-shaped sheet of muscle that divides the thorax from the abdomen. It continues through the tissues of the abdo-men and into the diaphragm of the pelvic floor, a double triangle of muscle that supports the function of the organs of the pelvic bowl; then down into the legs in the form of muscle sheath.

The RTM is not lifeless like the gristle that you cut away on your plate with the steak knife, it is as imbued with vital flowing energy as the rest of the body. With the RTM as an integral part of the body's architecture we could be described as being built in the manner of a suspension bridge, the strength of which lies in the flexibility that gives it both stability and move-ment. The physics of its construction mean that storm and stress may rage but where the bridge 'gives' in one place it will make an opposite and compensatory movement in another.

Unfortunately, orthodox medicine does not recognise this. As with everything else in allopathy the RTM is separated into its different parts and not recognised for the whole that it really is. In the head it is known as the tentorium (the floor of the brain) and the falx (the central divider between the two halves of the brain). In the body it is known as myofascial tissue. Between the lungs and the solar plexus it is called the diaphragm. It is seen as vascular, dense fibrous tissue that sheathes skeletal tissues and muscle as well as the supporting nerves and vessels. The protective, supportive role of this tissue is seen by allopathy only in the context of the particular organ or bone or muscle that might be under examination. However, if this tough, elastic tissue is seen as a continuous whole that acts connectively *throughout the body* then it becomes, like any other functional organ, a significant focus of attention in investigating pathology. When viewed as a whole it is immediately evident that it is highly reactive and responsive. Most importantly it registers shock waves right throughout the whole system. A brief and informal look at anatomy will help to underline just how significant the role of the RTM is.

·   The ribs and abdominal cavity are rather like a wardrobe in which the heart, lungs, liver, spleen, stomach, pancreas, kidneys, intestines and reproductive organs all hang. Though these vital organs are all surrounded by protective layers of fascia and fat, they all have room to move and 'breathe'. They need space. Though each constituent part can be given a separate label, it is vitally important to see that functionally there is no such separation between parts thanks to the all encompassing connective tissue. There is a river of 'fluid' electrodynamic energy flowing ceaselessly through them: the physical body behaving as if it were a continuous whole.

This all-through connectivity means, among other things, that the vital organs and their attachments are vulnerable to any long-term alteration in the general musculoskeletal structure. If the skeleton is traumatised and knocked out of symmetry then the soft organs attached via the RTM feel it. Their geography is disturbed. Imagine someone who has been involved in a car crash. The injuries sustained have left him with, say, his left shoulder dropped lower than the right and rotated forward and internally – almost in a protective posture. At the same time the accident has left him with asymmetrical hips; the right is brought forward and higher. This cannot happen unless the left hip is also rotated but twisted in the opposite direction. The new posture has the two sides in opposite but complementary positions even if the degree of difference from the norm is only measurable in millimetres. If you were to ask the patient to stand with his back to you with his feet together and in as relaxed a manner as possible, you would see someone with a drooped and hunched left shoulder and a slightly tilted waistband.

What does this do to the internal organs? The left lung is compressed thus limiting the amount of air that is breathed in. The heart and its protective pericardial sac are also compressed, resulting in pressure on the circulation's pump. The spleen, tucked away beneath the diaphragm below the left lung is forced to follow the rotation set by the shoulder and hip; it is pulled out of shape, fractionally maybe but sufficiently to cause stress. The left kidney's space is also compromised causing possible inefficiency in urine filtration. Lymphatic drainage from the left leg is limited as well; the twist and stretch caused by the body's new posture means that the lymph vessels are marginally narrowed; this can lead to oedema or cellulitis.

The intestines do not appreciate their new position either. If the gut is pulled out of its accustomed position then, depending on its reaction, it can go into overdrive and trigger either diarrhoea, or the opposite so that constipation becomes chronic. Though some of the above might self-correct, the trauma of the accident and any injury will cause the body to seek an altered balance to compensate for the pain felt. If this becomes a chronically held pattern then it can be a significant maintaining cause that will prevent thorough healing taking place.

Flexible the body may be but it works best when everything is in alignment based on symmetrical balance: left and right, top and bottom. Its programme, held within the cells themselves, is to return to this equilibrium. However, if continued pain, shock, fright or grief are added to physical trauma and left unresolved, the net result is usually chronic loss of alignment.

The body first adopts the compensatory posture to mitigate acute pain. Without immediate natural treatment the position will be adopted by the stricken whole and, if it is held for long enough without healing, the original memory of the very cells of the affected parts is superseded by the memory of the trauma imposed on them. Henceforth the tendency will be to hold the out-of-sync posture that was protectively adopted and to return to it in spite of the most assiduous efforts on the part of chiropractors and physiotherapists.

It is common for patients to report that following a visit to the physiotherapist, the chiropractor or the homoeopath they have a short respite from their symptoms only for the benefit to dissipate within a short time. In such circumstances why can't these therapies effect a more permanent change? The compensatory pattern has affected not only the musculoskeletal structure but also the vital organs by dint of the 'seismic' shift in their geography. Once a vital organ has learnt how to function within a compensatory whole-body pattern it will not shift back comfortably through outside intervention. It is as if the organs need to be utterly convinced that 'the Whole' will be able to deal with the return to equilibrium having now learnt how to cope with the trauma pattern.

The Vital Force, even when compromised, will always react according to the health and welfare of the vital organs. It will not respond permanently to being dictated to by having the body's architecture realigned. Patients might spend many years and huge amounts of money on going to therapists – including homoeopaths – for treatment following accidents and traumas and not achieve significantly lasting results. They and their practitioners do not realise this simple fact: that the soft internal vital organs rule even if the cell-energy that keeps them functioning is stuck in a pattern far from the norm. However hard we try we will never get a traumatised body to return permanently to a normal symmetrical position while the soft organs continue to be informed by the memory of the trauma (physical or mental). In such circumstances the only therapies that create the opportunity for curative healing are those that remind the body of the trauma ('like with like') thus putting the Vital Force back in touch with its original programme for self-adjustment.

The energy of the body's memory

To summarise so far, the tissues of the body, being made up of living cells informed by the Vital Force, have memory: this is the 'black box' flight recorder. These cells remember three things:

> Firstly, their programme for function depends on correct nerve conduction, nourishment and maintenance.
> Secondly, injuries.
> Lastly, and rather more controversially, they remember emotions associated with traumatic events.

Here's a hypothetical example:

> Suppose that a patient falls in the street and, in trying to avoid dropping his lunch, he twists his torso to bring the left forearm round to break his fall while his right arm remains raised with sandwich aloft. As he falls he knocks his head on the wing mirror of the car standing next to him and is dazed. As he lands on the ground he fails to finish swallowing his mouthful properly and he chokes. The net result is acute shock on two levels: from the pain and from choking.
>
> After treatment for bruising and abrasions he soon gets back on form. Then one day while sitting at the computer in his office he makes a movement that sends his cup of tea to the floor. He lurches forward in a similar rightward twisting movement in order to save the cup. Suddenly his heart rate quickens and his throat tightens up. He feels more shaken and irritable than the minor incident should warrant and he goes home that evening feeling more than usually tired, somewhat aggressive and emotionally out of sorts. His body is reliving the accident but without knowing how to use the opportunity to restore its original integrity. The memory of the accident, never thoroughly dealt with, has been woken and it has superseded that of the Vital Force.

Whiplash is a common injury that results in a jar to the cervical vertebrae (usually C5) causing the head suddenly to be thrust forward (and sometimes to one side as well) and back and then forward again. This usually causes tightening of the tissues at the top of the chest and consequent compression of lung space due to the tremendous shock pattern sustained on impact and to the sudden postural change. The shock of the accident is often enough to·cause the tissues involved to sustain their new mode. This leads to reduced intake of breath, increased adrenalin (triggered by shallow breathing), the characteristic neck pains and headaches, strain on the pericardium (the membranous sac surrounding the heart), poor liver function and digestive problems. Treating the neck with painkillers, collars and physiotherapy is usually insufficient.

> A woman aged fifty came to the clinic without an appointment on the off chance that someone would be able to give her advice. She had just come out of hospital after a short stay following exhaustive tests to find why she had suddenly had an attack of low blood pressure, nausea, numbness, headache, vertigo and fainting. She had thought that she was dying. In hospital she underwent blood and urine tests, scans and X-rays. Nothing amiss was found and she was discharged. The patient wanted to know whether there was any explanation, as she had been offered none by the doctors. She was asked to take off her shoes and coat, to stand in as relaxed manner as possible and with her arms down by her sides. It was immediately evident that her head was poked forward from what should have been its normal position. This was in a manner that suggested her first cervical vertebra was not in alignment. The shoulders generally were rounded with an incipient hump in the other cervical vertebrae. She was asked if she had suffered whiplash at any time. Yes, she had: some five years before. She was then asked if she had been coughing recently – her voice was a little hoarse and she could not stop sniffing. Yes, violently, was the answer and that had stopped only when she was in the hospital.

If the first cervical vertebra is out of position one can expect just such a range of symptoms. The violent spasms of coughing had triggered off some of the symptoms familiar to those who have suffered whiplash. When this was pointed out she agreed that though her original injury five years previously had not caused such extreme symptoms, she did remember feeling dizzy, nauseous and faint with numbness and tingling down the arms. She also said that she had never fully recovered her energy levels since the whiplash; since being taken into hospital this time she had felt just as exhausted as she had been after her accident. Her RTM had held the 'shock posture' for five years and coughing had exaggerated it sufficiently to cause aggravations. She took up the suggestion of undergoing treatment with the osteopath; she quickly re-established her energy, normal circulation and heart rate.

Combining osteopathy and homoeopathy with a common purpose

Immediate osteopathic treatment that successfully realigns the physical body is not necessarily sufficient to restore emotional balance. If an injury is serious enough then dealing with the physical picture alone can be worse than useless. If other circumstances surrounding the accident impinge on deeper, pre-existing psychological matters then these too must be involved in the healing process. Therefore, if a patient was already fairly near to emotional dysfunction prior to the accident or if the accident affected tissues and emotions at the same moment then the therapist must take a whole view for the treatment to be successful. Strange as it may seem, in cases where the patient is already in a delicate emotional state it could be argued that an accident is potentially a blessing in disguise. In seeking alternative treatment for the effects of the accident the patient would also have the opportunity to address the other issues, dormant or suppressed until now. Nevertheless, the longer appropriate treatment is left the harder it is for the Vital Force to re-establish physical and emotional equilibrium. Here is a short example of what frequently occurs:

> Doris, a buxom woman of fifty-four, had wrenched her left shoulder during a house move some five weeks previously. She had also bashed her right knee and both were causing her some pain. She wanted urgent treatment as she had to make a long car journey to visit relatives in Scotland and was aware that driving would make things worse.
>
> The shoulder was out of alignment being forward and rotated inwards. The tissues of the area were somewhat inflamed and the left side of her chest felt compressed and tense. In osteopathic terms this indicated that the heart area was under pressure; confirmation of this was that her blood pressure was slightly raised and her pulse rate was a bit higher than usual. She was given a dose of *Rose Quartz* 200 while she underwent osteopathic treatment. Within a few seconds Doris began weeping silently. At the end of the treatment she thanked the practitioners and apologised for her display of emotions. She explained that she had not

wanted to move house as she would miss all her close friends; her husband had insisted that they do so and he had been completely unsympathetic to her feelings. She felt much better for having cried. On examination it was obvious that her shoulder was now back in its proper place, pain-free. The tissues were showing no sign of inflammation and she said that she could breathe much deeper now. Her blood pressure and pulse rate were back to normal.

Rose quartz is a remedy that has an affinity for the tissues of the pericardium, the protective sac round the heart. It is also a remedy that in its broader, general picture covers that kind of incommunicable grief that is accompanied by a strong desire to go home. It was Doris' wrenched shoulder that obliged her to seek treatment for a condition far more serious.

The following is a description of a rather more extreme example of physical trauma highlighting an emotional one.

Josh, a man in his early forties, came for treatment having been referred by a cranio-sacral osteopath. He had been in a car accident when he was twenty-four and had never felt well since. He had been driving to the cinema with his fiancée when a drunk driver had shot out of a side road, veered out of control and struck them on the passenger side. Josh's fiancée had been so severely injured that she had died later in hospital. Josh had sustained severe injuries to his head and legs which had become trapped in the wreckage of the crash. He had received hospital treatment and physiotherapy. For years afterwards he went for conventional osteopathic treatment but always felt that whatever good it did the results would fade within a few days.

Finally he had started with biodynamic osteopathy and found that though his legs and back responded for only short periods his head was a lot clearer and he felt generally fitter. He was encouraged by the slim results to pursue it. He also noticed that he felt *"quite emotional"* when he was undergoing the treatment. It was when he told the practitioner about this that he was referred to homoeopathy.

It was obvious that there had been a very powerful emotional element involved, beyond the appalling tragedy of the accident. Just before the fatal day Josh had realised that he no longer wanted to marry his fiancée. On the night before she died he had decided to take her to the cinema and tell her how he felt. He had not met anyone else; he simply knew that *"it wouldn't work"*. Ever since her death he had felt guilt and remorse and a fear that he had committed some terrible sin. He explained that he had never had a satisfactory relationship since. His girlfriends either dumped him or he chose girls who only wanted a *"good time"*. He had now been living for six years with a girl who never made demands on his time or attention, who hardly ever spoke to him and who more or less used the house as a hotel room. He was irked by this but did not know how to change the status quo. He was stuck.

Several years on Josh was still receiving treatment and a pattern was discernible: when the emotional aspect was considered as the focus of remedial action his physical body would throw up old symptoms related to the accident – his legs would suddenly collapse, his back would go into spasm, he would have pins and needles with numbness all down his right side. When the physical symptoms were seen as needing attention because he seemed so much better emotionally he would become thick-headed, confused, diffident, fearful, and nervy. Though he reported that he felt better overall for going through with both therapies it was evident that the devastating experience he had suffered was deeply locked in despite, at one time or another and when indicated, being given all those remedies best known for such circumstances (and, it must be said, a good few lesser ones rather out of desperation!)

Josh felt that everyone had done something positive for him. He said that he never felt as bad now as he had before he started. He said much the same about the osteopathic work. Yet his life was still crippled. The extensive physical damage matched the emotional damage. His physical body did not seem strong enough to be able to manifest the emotional expression needed to get to the heart of the matter. For him, to be emotional meant that he would become shaky and uncoordinated. His job got in the way of letting that happen too often. His emotional body did not feel strong enough to enable him to make a decisive move and ask his partner to leave or to change his dull job that carried more responsibility than he really wished to cope with.

However, a conference between the osteopath and the homoeopath and a study of all the notes that had been taken over the years of treatment revealed that, though painfully slow, progress had been made. Josh's immune system was far stronger and he no longer succumbed to frequent colds and 'flu as he used to. His back was much stronger in spite of throwing acute crises of spasms whenever he lifted something awkwardly or felt depressed about work or when it was nearing his birthday. Most importantly, Josh wanted to continue his treatments. His disabilities were the result of two maintaining causes that were inseparable and dynamically linked. There is seldom a 'happy ending' in treatment for people like Josh; it is all hard slog and takes many years. Not everyone has the extraordinary patience and determination that he has always shown. For those without these qualities it is usually a question of trailing from one therapist to another and switching between alternative and orthodox practitioners desperately looking for 'the answer'.

The body is a two-way street

Homoeopaths are notoriously fond of discovering psychosomatic causes for ailments they have been asked to treat. There are times when this just does not work though. The body is a two-way street in that emotional disturbance and even troubles of the spirit can arise from physical distress just as much as the other way round. Psychiatrists should sometimes consider this before prescribing antidepressants.

Many depressed people may find considerable mental relief from radically altering their chronic bad posture, developed following a physical trauma perhaps long forgotten. Alexander technique, t'ai chi or yoga can often release stress and tension held in the physical body that inhibit fluent movement; in chronically held patterns these disciplines can be very useful complementary therapies.

A fall downstairs is a common enough accident that can create a twist in the spine and torsion in the diaphragm and solar plexus. Such tension can easily tighten up the sac that surrounds the liver and cause the cœliac plexus of nerves (the gut's private nervous system) to 'misfire'. In turn this creates problems associated with poor drainage of toxicity from the liver and less efficient elimination through the bowels, not to mention restriction of air space in the lungs and reduced oxygenation of the blood. It can also mean that the whole balance of nutrition is upset. Physical trauma can lead to faulty chemistry in the system.

If the enzyme balance of the digestive system is upset as a result of all this then depression can result from the reduction in the levels of serotonin, a vital neurotransmitter that is essential to feeling good about oneself and that is partially dependent on what happens in the gut. (It is interesting how many victims of serious injury turn to cannabis for pain relief. Cannabis acts as a replacement for the missing serotonin. It also means incidentally that the patients seldom come out of their injury pattern.)

If there has been shock, fear and injury after an accident then the risk of developing depression can be even greater. In life-threatening situations the Vital Force can actually seem to withdraw from the physical body altogether in much the same way that it does under general anaesthetic. This leaves the patient 'ungrounded', 'not on this planet', 'far away'. The attachment of spirit to body becomes tenuous. The patient becomes vague and unattached, slower in response and sometimes less emotionally involved with those dear to them. The connective tissues of the body then remain 'stuck' in the protective physical mode they went into on the instant of the trauma while, as it were, the spirit begins to divest itself of its physical vessel and slip 'out of focus'. The only way out of this is through matching the out-of-body-ness with a similar remedial energy or, strange as it may seem, another accident that matches the intensity of the first. (Many accident victims go on to have other accidents and their stories often show a theme of repeated similar traumas that are imitations of the original.)

> Marilyn was a case in point. She had been thrown through the front window of her car during an accident and had sustained concussion, a broken nose and lacerations. Her sinuses plagued her as they constantly poured mucus. There was compression of the cervical spine and she suffered severe headaches. She was referred to the homoeopath by her osteopath after most of the physical trauma had been dealt with. She no longer had the headaches and her sinuses remained clear but she complained of feeling blank. She felt little or no emotion. She seemed to have no interest in her family and simply *"went through the motions"* of being wife and mother. She also felt vague and *"unattached"*.

> *"I just don't feel that I'm in my body at all. I watch myself doing things and saying things and it's really like someone else. If I see myself in a shop window it's really weird. I have to remind myself that it's me there. I drift from one thing to another. If there weren't a routine to follow then I would float away, I think. It's not even really like daydreaming because I don't feel imaginative or anything. I'm just not there. And my memory is appalling!"*

Apart from this curious mental/emotional state she did have one or two pertinent physical symptoms. She felt hot a lot of the time; she felt waves of heat come over her as if she were having hot flushes (she was only thirty-six). She felt that her bowels were sluggish: she only managed to pass a motion once in four or five days even though she had no discomfort. Such a picture is covered by *Opium* which she was given in the 1M potency. Within forty-eight hours, *"I felt I'd got back in my body!"*

Opium is a drug said to be taken by those who wish to forget; it takes them out of themselves. The remedy is often needed by those whose memories have been severely affected by a traumatic incident and who subsequently feel as if stuck in limbo. What was interesting in this case was that Marilyn had received great benefit from the osteopathy in all aspects of her physical trauma but had not been able to *'come back into'* her body. It took the 'like' remedy to allow her psyche to feel comfortable about its physical suit.

It makes some people feel distinctly uncomfortable to think one's spirit is able to come out of the body at any time before death but one only has to be around patients like Marilyn for a little while to realise that their language alone explains much of how things can be. (Whether or not it is a delusional state due to altered chemistry in the system is probably irrelevant when considering what the indicated remedies need to do.)

Before looking into other typical accident patterns that become common maintaining causes we should look at 'accidents' of birth as these have a life-long influence on health. It is here that we find stuck energy patterns that are frequently impossible to detect from the homoeopathic point of view. Discovery of such patterns is usually the work of the osteopaths and their 'hands on' energy-detecting treatment. For this reason alone homoeopaths should cultivate good working relationships with osteopaths. Combining the two therapies is one of the most professionally satisfying healing activities that one could imagine.

Patterns altered in childbirth

Troubles can start early in life. The birth process can be the origin of all sorts of problems. A selection of typical hazards will serve to illustrate.

Poor contractions and delayed widening of the cervix can lead to a forceps or ventouse delivery. Forceps are applied to the sides of the baby's head in order to pull the baby free. The consequence is that the temples are crushed – however careful the handling. Though the baby's head is constructed so that overlapping 'plates', which keep the cranium small enough to pass through the birth canal, can open out gradually after birth, the effect of firm and sustained pressure on the temples or occiput and forehead can be enough to leave the head traumatised. The tissues in the area are bruised and the overall effect can be that the shape and rate of growth of the head is fundamentally altered. This is not necessarily manifest straight away. Sometimes the distress that the baby shows is put down to the emotional trauma of a difficult birth. However, intercranial irritation of the meninges (brain covering) as a result of the external application of pressure can result in distress often manifest as furious crying and general restlessness. This can continue for many weeks and months when left untreated.

The ventouse system is different in that suction is used rather than mechanical force. The effect can be similar in that the procedure can pull the tissues of the cranium out of their normal shape. Though the body can usually cope with the subsequent considerable bruising, it may not be able to deal with the physical shock which leaves its mark on the young cells not programmed to deal with being pulled so far out of their normal place. Persistent headaches in children can be attributed to this kind of trauma. So too can postural problems. The head, balanced as it should be on the atlas bone at the top of the spine, can sometimes be pulled forward or backward by intervention at the birth. This leads to strain and pressure on the spine itself and compression on the chest or the dorsal area of the back; both predispose the person to pathology such as frequent ear and sinus infections, conjunctivitis, coughing and a tendency to wheezy breathing.

As before, the RTM stretched out of alignment shows the strain: mucous membranes attached to tissues that are pulled out of place (by even a small amount) register their discomfort by pouring mucus from their 'goblet cells'. Because the vessels of the lymphatic system in these same tissues are also stretched they are less efficient at draining the area of waste. This leads to the local build-up of toxic material; hence the ear infection, the 'claggy' throat or the mucky eye. The throat and upper reaches of the lungs can suffer from the opposite problem: not enough fluid. If the blood vessels to this area are stretched out of alignment then dryness of the mucous membranes can happen; a chronic cough pattern is the result. This often leads to a misdiagnosis of asthma.

Feet first is a bad move

Malpresentation at birth is another problem. The baby can get into a difficult position in which the head – or any part of the body, for that matter – is awkwardly placed. If the head is forced into a place where pressure is put on one side or the other then the baby may be delivered with a skewed face, a conical cranium or a flattened brow. Either situation is going to cause intercranial compression, distortion of tissues and consequent irritation of them. A skewed face will lead to dentition problems and sinus difficulties. A distorted head will mean that the function of the endocrine glands in the brain can be compromised and the central nervous system might be less responsive than usual. If the meninges are irritated they tighten up which means that compression of the brain itself occurs. This restricts the activity of the pituitary and the pineal glands. If this happens then there can be delayed growth, poor reactivity and some types of learning difficulties. Such children often suffer very high *Belladonna* fevers.

Breech birth is often a hidden maintaining cause. A breech baby is commonly one that is not yet ready to be born, who may need longer in the womb than the hospital considers appropriate. (Paediatricians do prefer to go by the due dates of their own reckoning and these do not always coincide with the mothers'.) Some babies – especially first babies – just naturally need longer to 'cook'. There might, however, be some early emotional reason why a baby does not turn to be head down. Babies are quite capable of feeling sufficient fear about their own imminent birth that they obstinately refuse to arrive. Very often a dose of *Pulsatilla* can give them the courage to change their minds. (Frequently the mother of a breech delivery is already in a state needing *Pulsatilla* herself, neatly matching the baby's condition.) Another reason for a breech presentation is that the umbilical cord may be twisted around the baby's neck. Nothing is going to change this except for mechanical intervention. (Interestingly, if a mother is given a *Pulsatilla* in this circumstance then the baby usually attempts to turn but then realises that it cannot go the whole way so reverses its decision and goes back to its original position.) Whether a breech baby is delivered vaginally or by Caesarean a trauma pattern is set up.

With vaginal delivery there is the risk of the baby's shoulders becoming stuck in the birth canal thus causing a traumatic compression of the thorax or a twist to the shoulder girdle as the baby is pulled out speedily. If this happens then overproduction of mucus, breathing problems and glandular swellings are often the result. If the hips have suffered a similar twisting then one might expect severe colic problems. If a Caesarean is necessary then the results are likely to be more on the emotional side. Bonding between mother and baby is a frequent, buried maintaining cause. Sometimes the baby is never able to sleep soundly and suffers nightmares full of terror. *Stramonium*, known as datura or the thorn apple to gardeners, is a very powerful hallucinogenic plant that reproduces an energy similar to the terror that might be felt by a baby going through a Caesarean – or any kind of difficult birth. It is therefore very commonly useful for very young children especially those who suffer fear of and have nightmares about the dark, of monsters and long dark tunnels.

Menstrual difficulties long after a breech birth

A young woman, Jackie, came for treatment for her painful periods and premenstrual tension. She had severe pain every other month on the left side of her abdomen in the ovarian region. She would feel swollen with intolerable internal pressure – as if she were a pressure cooker – and could not wear clothing that was in the least bit tight. The pain was bursting and hot. Her temper matched the physical pain. She felt weepy and furiously angry by turns. She became "*paranoid*" about the people around her and felt that she had to "*creep away*" and yet she hated not knowing what her boyfriend and family were up to. For a week before the period she would feel the build up of all these symptoms. When the period flow arrived she would feel instant relief. She felt that all this was an odd contrast to her usual self. She described herself as fun loving and humorous, a bit shy and very much a "*people person*".

Essentially, from the first interview, it was apparent that the period state that she went into once every month (the PMT was monthly even if the severe pains were bi-monthly) was typical of *Lachesis*. *Pulsatilla* answered the general picture of her as a whole when the period problems were not in evidence. These two remedies may, in the *Materia Medica* descriptions, be poles apart but they are related in the sense that *Pulsatilla* is known to follow on well and is a common enough prescription after the fearsome snake venom. Jackie found that *Lachesis* did help but only if she started to take it early enough in the cycle. *Pulsatilla*, when she took it in high potency during a different time in the month, gave her a little more energy and boosted her libido. These remedies were allowed plenty of time to do their work but despite this there was no real overall shift out of the pattern that had been set up. During the first interview Jackie had mentioned that her birth had been difficult; she had got "*stuck*". She had been a breech presentation and the doctors had tried to turn her. They had not managed it and she had been born feet first. She had been pulled out "*one leg and arm at a time!*" This and the fact that the indicated remedies were affording only partial relief were enough reason to refer her to the osteopath for an examination and treatment.

The osteopath did indeed find that both her hips and her shoulder girdle were out of alignment. There was compression of the left ovary and the left fallopian tube was narrow and stretched. At the time of her period this was enough to create poor drainage of the whole pelvic floor and lower abdomen. The extraordinary degree of relief felt when the menstrual blood began to flow demonstrated that internal drainage was a significant problem. As a result of the displaced hips and shoulder there was a 'twist' in the spine – a tendency to want to corkscrew. This and the increase of pressure in the head from altered blood flow (that is typical of *Lachesis* patients) in turn set up a cranial pattern that disturbed the hormone system causing Jackie to feel, as she put it, "*evil*". The combination of osteopathic and homoeopathic treatment gradually relieved this situation and within six months Jackie's periods were entirely normal as her RTM no longer held the pattern it had been in since her birth.

Apart from the osteopath's very necessary input the remedy that was used to relieve the physiological stress of the birth pattern was *Ayahuasca*, the liana from the South American jungle. It is interesting to note that not only does this remedy have an affinity for patients whose spines are held in a twist by their RTM but it is also of great value in treating people for the shock and fear that a difficult birth can cause. Not only that but it comes from the very same jungles that are home to the lachesis snake.

When the umbilical cord is related to asthmatic breathing

A baby born with the umbilical cord around its neck is at risk of developing breathing difficulties. Cutting away the cord and handing the baby to the mother does not relieve the trauma of being throttled as it is being born. The body remembers what happened to it and whenever there is an instance of I-can't-handle-this stress, the memory (held in the RTM) can return and the body can go into its acquired trauma pattern of distressed breathing centring on the throat and upper chest. A sense of restricted breathing causes panic anyway so in the body of someone who acquired the panic response so early it is not difficult to understand how hard it is for them to handle stress well. A significant number of adults with asthma might well find that the origin of their complaint either lies in just this situation or contributes to it. The following case is illustrative of just this problem.

An asthma patient came presenting a picture of *Arsenicum*, a very common remedy for this complaint. He had nightly attacks of asthmatic breathing that kept him from sleeping between midnight and 2 or 3 a.m. He could not stay in bed but had to pace up and down. He would feel restless and very anxious. He would go downstairs to make a cup of tea. He would run a bath which would make him feel better in himself but would make him feel tight and hot in the head. Exhaustion would eventually cause him to relax and he would feel his upper chest and throat become less restricted. In the morning he would be congested with quantities of catarrh which he would have to cough up. He felt that *Arsenicum* gave him some relief. He took it whenever he had an attack and he claimed that it always shortened the length of the attack and lessened the severity. But he did not get better enough for the attacks to cease altogether.

He was given *Tuberculinum*, a complementary remedy to *Arsenicum*, and he quickly reported that he had far more energy and that the mucus that he was inclined to produce was not nearly so coloured. However, the attacks persisted though still with less fierceness. One day he hurt his back through lifting something heavy and this led him to go to an osteopath. After two or three sessions of osteopathy his back felt much better but the osteopath reported that there was a traumatic pattern in the neck. This had led him to ask the patient what his birth had been like. He had to ask his mother who told him that he had been born with the cord round his neck and that he was blue on delivery. The doctors had had to resuscitate him and then extract mucus from his airways. Armed with this information the patient was asked to come for a further osteopathic session at which homoeopathic treatment would also be administered. Concentrating on the neck/throat trauma 'held' since birth the osteopath, with the assistance of a remedy called *Laurocerasus*, was able to address this maintaining cause. The patient promptly fell asleep on the osteopath's bench. On waking he felt light-headed and rather giggly. He went home and slept almost solidly for three days.

What is significant about the remedy *Laurocerasus* (laurel) here is that it is not only well known as a remedy that is often indicated in restoring 'blue babies' to normality but it is also one that is called for in the treatment of certain cases of asthma.

Laurocerasus asthma is characterised by symptoms of acute breathing difficulties with gasping and blueness of the face and chest with sudden sinking of all physical strength – and a sense of constriction or contraction around the throat! What was peculiar about the particular patient was that he did not describe his asthma attacks in this way. This is not uncommon in those who have been obliged to use drugs over a long time. Chemotherapy adds a layer of negative energy, so to speak, on top of a patient's general condition thus changing the symptom picture of the original problem. Though the drugs had saved this man's life and he was grateful for that, the patient realised after his osteopathic treatment with the aid of the *Laurocerasus* that he could now change the status quo. Within eighteen months he was able to manage his asthmatic breathing with homoeopathic remedies alone.

Without the information about the birth pattern this patient might never have received *Laurocerasus*. The conditions that call for it were not evident in the patient's symptom picture; the *Laurocerasus* energy had remained well and truly buried in his tissue memory, covered up by years of being in an *Arsenicum* state. He would have continued to take the *Arsenicum*, quite contentedly it must be said, because he felt that there was no true cure for his condition. His careless lifting of a heavy object had profound ramifications for the rest of his life.

The risks of hasty diagnosis

From these examples it is easy to see how pathology that manifests any time from soon after birth to middle age and even beyond might well have its origins in a birth trauma. No allopathic doctor (or homoeopath for that matter) could be expected to judge whether this is so, given that he or she is not trained to see patients from the 'tissue memory' point of view. If a patient walks in with a hydrocele (a water filled swelling) of the left testicle or persistent, crippling sciatica down the right leg it would seldom occur to the practitioner to ask whether the birth had been traumatic. Few asthma patients are asked for their birth history. Very often initial treatment for the specific symptoms of such conditions (as are likely to occur from birth trauma) is successful to some degree. More often than not the success is short lived; the patient is back in the consulting room asking for more pain relief or for a reappraisal. For practitioners prepared to re-study anatomy and physiology in the light of 'tissue memory' the rewards are great. For homoeopaths this often means understanding remedies they know well from a new perspective and learning of new remedies such as the extraordinary energy of *Ayahuasca*, the hallucinogenic liana that has such a powerful affinity for anything that can be attributed to a difficult birth and fear of life. It can also mean learning to adjust prescribing techniques to suit patients who may be presenting the energy picture of one remedy but who need the addition of another to address the tissue memory of trauma long suppressed or forgotten.

Just imagine how many prescriptions are made based on incomplete case notes because the practitioner did not realise that the history of birth trauma was in some way either essential then or would become so. Birth trauma can be part of the root of many chronic conditions; anything from menstrual disorders (including infertility), asthma or headaches to a variety of digestive problems, sciatica and spinal pains.

The vulnerability of the spine

Mention of the spine brings us to the next group of mechanical maintaining causes: injuries to the spinal column. Twenty-four separate vertebrae, the sacrum and the coccyx make up the spine. The latter two are fused vertebrae and incapable of the extraordinary flexibility of the other vertebrae. The coccyx is a 'vestigial tail' but is not as unimportant as this makes it sound. The sacrum is a shield-shaped structure of 5 fused vertebrae that, together with the hips, provides an arch of considerable strength to support the weight of the body. Through the sacrum run both nerve tissue and blood vessels. Attached to it are ligaments and muscles that support internal organs and operate the legs. The 7 cervical, 12 thoracic and 5 lumbar vertebrae are separate bones but attached one to another by muscles and ligaments and the RTM. From between each vertebra, on both sides, nerve ganglia (groups) extend into the body laterally. The greater number of these goes to form the sympathetic and parasympathetic nervous system. (The sympathetics are basically the nerves that cause things to happen and the parasympathetics are the nerves that are required in vegetative states. The former operate the responses to the 'flight or fight' signal, increased blood flow to muscles and organs, pupillary dilation and increased heart and respiratory rates. The latter are involved in secretory processes of the bowel and bladder and glands.) Other nerves serve to operate the arms and legs.

It therefore stands to reason that if the spine is traumatised at any point along its length then there can be long-term consequences. Furthermore, skilled practitioners can tell just what is likely to be symptomatically wrong with the body once they know precisely where the injury happened in the spine. Conversely, it is often easy to judge which vertebrae have been damaged by asking the patient for his symptoms. This is because the nerve 'stations' that come out of the spinal column at the separate vertebrae each have a particular and individual target function that they serve. So someone who has had a history of whiplash that has damaged the area of the sixth and seventh cervical (neck) vertebrae might be asked by the osteopath if they suffered from pains in the shoulders and upper arms, frequent colds with swollen tonsils, dramatic loss of energy with a gradual weight gain due to thyroid insufficiency or pains in the elbows. Another patient with a history of lumbago (with damage to the L1 vertebra) might be asked if they had trouble with constipation or abdominal cramping.

Banging a drum makes the floor vibrate

If you fall off a horse and land on your coccyx then your pelvic floor muscles will tighten up in shock. If the fall is not too bad then all that is suffered is a bruise. If it is bad then there will be more to know. The diaphragm (sheet of muscle) that opens or locks the rectal and urethral apertures is geographically very close to the coccyx and attached to the same bony structure (the sacrum). Why does the thoracic diaphragm also tighten up? There are two reasons:

i) the shock of the pain causes an emotional response with a sharp, sudden intake of breath;

ii) more importantly, whatever causes a trauma to any one of the diaphragms of the body is reflected in the other diaphragms. Just as the velum stretched across the bottom of a side drum resonates when the top velum is struck so too will the other diaphragms resonate in sympathy with any one that is traumatised.

There are five diaphragms to consider:

1. the floor of the brain otherwise known as the tentorium;
2. the thoracic inlet, the ligamentous tissues that gather at the top of the lungs and lead into the base of the throat;
3. the thoracic diaphragm, that huge dome of muscle that separates thorax from abdomen;
4. the pelvic diaphragm, diamond shaped and divided into two – the front half to control the urethral opening and the back half to control rectal movement;
5. the muscles and tendons that form the sole of the foot.

Each one, remember, has individualised local function but is ultimately connected to the rest of the body's flexible tissues via the RTM. No surprise then when a patient fails to improve permanently from any one of a host of varying conditions (possibly even those unrelated to the spine) if an old injury pattern is left unresolved.

The coccyx

One of the most common injuries to the spine is a trauma to the coccyx and it is often more serious than most give it credit for. It is a favourite of riders, sports people and those who go playing about in the snow on toboggans. If you land on your coccyx, quite apart from the pain, you will jar the whole length of the spine. You may go into shock. The shock wave can cause all the muscles and ligaments of the spine to tense up; this will inhibit some vital nerve responses. It will also cause the RTM generally to go into tension which means that the diaphragms can go into spasm. The consequences of all this are not necessarily long-term but nevertheless headaches, diminished eyesight, profuse mucus production from the sinus behind the bridge of the nose, raised blood pressure, irregular heart beats, restricted breathing, indigestion, slowed bowel function and difficulty walking (and more) may follow.

The pain can be so intense – and for a very long time after the event – that the sufferer will often adopt a compensatory posture. The patient will sit askew in the chair in order to accommodate the pain. This in turn means that the spine is put under a certain amount of instruction to maintain the crooked bias. A bad habit is formed. A telltale sign is when a patient shifts uneasily in the chair but consistently adopts a cross-legged posture.

Once the traumatised coccyx has been recognised as a factor in the chronic health picture then prescriptions can be made that address this problem. While it is usually a good idea to refer patients to an osteopath there are a number of remedies that should be used to resolve the injury pattern. One of the most important of these is *Arnica*. When indicated by its characteristic bruised pain a high potency dose of *Arnica* to complement the osteopath's hands-on treatment can set a sequence of healing in motion that completely stops the habit of returning old symptom patterns. Another well-known remedy for this injury is *Hypericum*, St John's wort. This has different indications: the characteristics are of nerve pains in the neck and down the limbs with twitching of parts of the limbs.

The sacrum

Injuries to the sacrum are equally likely to cause long-term consequences. The hips can be knocked out of alignment for one thing. If this happens then a twist with a left or right bias will develop because hips cannot move away from their normal position without causing a rotation in the whole pelvic floor. This, in turn, will put a slewing pressure on the spinal column and bring about a twist there too. Once again the diaphragms will respond by tightening up. With all this there is likely to be a compromised blood supply to the organs of the pelvis causing trouble in the reproductive system, the urinary system and the vascular and lymphatic drainage of the whole area. This latter problem means that the lymphatic system cannot remove body fluids that need to be recycled or excreted. Tissues swell as a consequence. Venous blood on its way back to the liver and lungs also tends to become sluggish. When this occurs then haemorrhoids will follow. In addition, there can also be nerve pain. Many nerve lines are fed through the sacral area. If there is any malpositioning of the bone and its related structures then the nerves will complain or scream. Sciatica is a condition that causes patients to stop in their tracks and demand instant attention. In how many cases does this become intermittent with frequent relapses? In as many as there are patients with hips that are out of alignment.

Though it is not usually regarded as an injury, giving birth is possibly the most common reason for the hips to go out of alignment. There are many women whose physical structure simply never returns to its original state, and it is the sacrum that is most often the part that has been displaced. If the sacrum is forced forwards and down (through the circumstances of delivery) then the internal organs associated with it will fall too. It is for this reason that so many women suffer from prolapse. The bony sacrum is in the wrong place, lower than it should be, and the ligamentous attachments that are also forced downwards in turn pull the soft organs (bladder and uterus) with them. The same problem may affect the bowels too. This is the condition so often described by the one word: sag. Sag does not only affect the tissues though. Through the consequent effects on the ovaries and their relationship to the rest of the hormone system it can also lead to feeling depressed. Women who have suffered from long-running post-natal depression, asthmatic breathing or severe indigestion would do better not to take Prozac or steroid inhalers or antacids; they need to investigate the possibility (or probability) that their physical bodies are out of alignment due to an unresolved displacement of the sacrum.

Above the sacrum

The story is the same all the way up the spine. If there is an injury anywhere along its length that is neglected and the consequences are allowed to become chronic then symptoms will tell the tale. It will also be a possible cause for the failure of treatment for something else seemingly quite unrelated. Patients are notorious for not making connections between causes and results. The mind so often forgets what it does not want to know about. The all-important cause – important because it can lead to the appropriate treatment – gets lost in history. Who would necessarily realise that their frequent colds and chest infections were due to an old injury at the level of the eighth thoracic vertebra? Yet this is not at all uncommon. It can happen like this: there is a fall on the stairs. As the person falls he lands on the eighth vertebra and reacts by twisting round and down to the left at waist level. It is a protective reaction. As a result the spleen – one of the neglected organs of the body – becomes suddenly compressed and traumatised. It is an organ that likes plenty of flexibility and 'room to move' for it can readily change size. It is active in providing new blood cells and lymphocytes for the immune process. If it is both traumatised and restricted then the immune response is hampered. The net result is that the patient suffers from the inability to ward off infection; the susceptibility to illness is increased.

Treatment for this condition might well, at first, address only the lowered immune system. Many remedies might be indicated so the practitioner would need to ask for more generalised symptoms than the characteristics of the infections themselves. This would help to define what the body is 'describing' with its symptom picture. What makes the case confusing is that the patient might not mention that he has aching in the left side at the level of and just below his lower ribs – pains like these are easily overlooked because they can come and go and may not be so debilitating as the persistent colds. Only when the selected remedy helped just temporarily, marginally or not at all does a deeper cause such as the injury pattern have to be found. Such a situation could be tackled in a number of ways but they would all need to involve cajoling the body back to its original physical posture so that the spleen was no longer compressed and the spine and ribs that sustained the injury (however many years ago) would feel comfortable.

The spinal column is so important a structure that it is usually a very good plan for a homoeopath to ask any new patient to stand without shoes or loose clothing so that even a cursory examination of front, back and profile might reveal whether any part of the body is out of alignment. The range of postures held by patients is remarkable. They can be extreme enough that it is impossible for the patient to stand up with his feet together without falling over. It is usual to find that a person who performs the exercise with confidence may become distressingly unsteady when asked to close his eyes. This leads to the conclusion that the person's spine is no longer in balance and that being able to stand up steadily depends heavily on his vision and not, as should be the case, on the fluid within the inner ear. Any obvious lack of symmetry will have a history and this should be thoroughly investigated. Without the information – even if it is not immediately relevant – one of the edge pieces to the jigsaw of the case will be missing.

CHAPTER 10

GENERAL ANAESTHESIA AND SURGICAL OPERATIONS

A temporary state of death

A woman, Greta, was referred to the homoeopath by her cranio-sacral osteopath for treatment. She was aged forty-two and had twin girls. She suffered from mild arthritic pains in her fingers, the occasional headache and a very poor memory. It was her memory that caused her the most distress. She complained that she felt vague and far away all the time. She was unable to remember what she had gone into another room to do; she could not recall what she had said to her husband at breakfast. She was known to have gone into town to do the shopping and to be unaware of what she should buy as well as unable to remember why she had got into the car. Her deepest concern was that she might forget something really important to do with the children who were still very young. She became distressed when explaining her symptoms, in a quiet and introspective way. She explained that she felt that she was unworthy to have two children because she felt unable to carry the burden of responsibility; she saw herself as a liability.

She had been going to the osteopath for some eight or nine months. Her visits had been regular because she had experienced a certain amount of trauma to do with the birth of the twins. Following their birth Greta had had to have an operation for the removal of her wisdom teeth. The operation had been planned originally before the twins were conceived but had been put off till after the birth. The operation was performed with a general anaesthetic. When Greta awoke from it she felt *"distinctly peculiar"*. She felt that her temperature had gone up to an abnormally high level even though the thermometer read 'normal' or below whenever she took it. She had flushes of heat that swept up over her from time to time as if she were having hot flushes. (She had asked the doctor for a blood test to check whether she was going through an early menopause.) She felt *"out of my body"* all the time. *"This is just not 'me'!"*

Osteopathic therapy helped a little but the osteopath felt that any achievement was negligible – even though the twins had been treated and had responded beautifully to treatment. Having been small, underdeveloped and miserable for their first two or three months they were now putting on weight, growing apace and becoming very bright. The doctor had told her that she was suffering from post-natal 'blues' and that Prozac might be a good short-term solution.

We have met the answer to this problem before in an earlier case: *Opium* (see p.189). Greta was struggling to live with the after effects of anaesthesia and her health would never improve until this had been lifted. These effects often resemble the intended effects of smoking opium: loss of memory, impaired perception of reality; but with this come sluggish torpor and a curious sensation of heat that washes over one in waves but is only subjective as the body is actually cold. General anaesthetics also resemble a 'death'; life goes into an unreal suspension. If the person cannot come back from that odd state fully then they will also feel considerable fear. It is a fear that is often left unexpressed as the sluggishness of mind and body prevents the patient from thinking clearly enough to describe such feelings. Though Greta was aware enough to be concerned about her children's welfare it was only afterwards that she was able to say how frightened for herself she had really been. She described it as living a nightmare – which is again a typical symptom of the *Opium* patient. Opium, after all, is used to avoid living in the here and now because for those who use it reality is the nightmare.

Greta was given *Opium* 10M after which she became well. She was able to hold a reasonable conversation again. She no longer felt that she was living in a fog and that her body and mind were not connected. She felt that something profoundly heavy had been lifted from her. Now she felt that she was quite capable of dealing with the children, the house, her husband's business and his colleagues and all the other things that she had felt so inadequate to cope with. Further, in the following months the treatment from the osteopath was more noticeably effective and remained permanently so. Her jaw pains and back pains were resolved; her arthritic fingers improved; her 'clicky' neck vanished.

The general anaesthetic had been a maintaining cause. It had imposed on her whole being an energy profoundly at odds with her normal vitality. Not until this energy was removed with a similar and superior force did Greta start to feel well again. Not only that but it resolved a situation that would sooner or later have required specialists to prescribe drugs.

Not everyone is so lucky. Another woman had a very different experience.

Joan came to the clinic with an underactive thyroid for which she was on medication – *"for life"*. She had been in hospital two years earlier for what she thought would be a minor gynaecological operation. When she came round from the anaesthetic she felt far from well. After several weeks she was diagnosed as having myxoedema: underfunctioning of the thyroid gland. She also had a swelling of the gland known as a goitre. Joan's symptom picture was very similar to Greta's though the two women were very different personalities. Where Greta was naturally outgoing and gregarious, Joan was quiet, easily cowed and given to weeping easily. She was also rather under the thumb of her husband and daughter to both of whom she deferred when it came to all major decisions. She confessed that she was not very comfortable in seeking alternative help as she had consulted neither of them but had come on the recommendation of a friend.

Joan also explained that she had had a severe shock when she came round from the anaesthesia because they told her that she had had a hysterectomy because her womb had been in such a poor state. She was deeply affected by the fact that she had not been given any choice in the matter even though she realised that something had had to be done. She felt that the situation rather typified the way her life was generally characterised.

Joan was given *Opium* 1M and over the next few weeks had greater vitality and less mental confusion. She was aware of wanting to do things again that she had simply given up thinking about: sewing, making cakes and writing to her sister in Canada. She also went to the medical surgery for a check-up on her thyroid levels and was astonished when she was told that the readings had changed for the better. (She was not told to reduce her Thyroxin.) She continued to improve in these ways but increasingly felt speeded up, sweaty, anxious and irritable. She had begun to show the typical signs of hyperthyroidism, the very opposite condition from that which she was supposed to suffer. She was now taking too much Thyroxin as her own thyroid was attempting to re-establish its normal functioning. At the surgery she was told in no uncertain terms that she should do nothing about her prescription.

She returned for her homoeopathic treatment in an understandable quandary. What should she do? She knew she was taking too much Thyroxin but she was afraid of going against expert advice – even though it had been the clinic nurse and not the doctor who had given her the last instruction. She eventually made an appointment with the doctor who told her that it was unusual for thyroid levels to change so noticeably for the better. He did not want to change anything too rashly; she should return for another blood test in four weeks' time. This she did and the readings were now apparently near normal; they appeared to suggest that she was only slightly underactive.

"I don't understand it because I feel so racy and anxious all the time! I thought that's how you feel when you've got too much of the stuff."

Joan was right. She may have had readings to suggest a near normal thyroid activity but her body demonstrated otherwise. Thyroid dysfunction is notoriously difficult to monitor. Hormone levels to and from the gland do change, seemingly without much rhyme or reason. Very little is straightforward in most thyroid cases; even the textbook descriptions of under- and overactive thyroid cannot be relied upon. Some people have typical symptoms of both at the same time.

Joan eventually decided to try cutting down her Thyroxin by herself. Though the homoeopath could offer support and medication it was quite outside his brief to instruct her do anything but discuss the situation with her doctor. The result was that she began to feel better. She found that she was more motivated and energetic but without the attendant feelings of near panic. She even began to lose weight. Unfortunately, her daughter began to disrupt her newly found well-being. She came to live at home as her relationship with her boyfriend had deteriorated beyond repair. Joan phoned the clinic in distress to say that she felt that her old symptoms of torpor, lethargy, depression and confusion were returning. She explained that her daughter had told her that she should go back on the medication and that she should never come off it. As her husband agreed with her daughter she now felt obliged to go back to taking her original dosage and that trying to do things the homoeopathic way was really too difficult and *"thank you very much"*.

Joan's habitual deference to her immediate family was stronger than her will to get better. Yet her initial success suggested that she did have the capacity to achieve something near normality. She was in no doubt that the general anaesthesia and the shock of discovering that she had lost her womb were the original triggers for what became a serious and lifelong threat to the stability of her health. Whether she would ever have quite the courage to admit to herself that her daughter's influence was the decisive negative factor in her life was another matter. As we shall see later on, relationships can be the most difficult maintaining causes of all.

Scar tissue and adhesions

The effects of anaesthesia are not the only trouble to arise from having an operation. The surgery itself, however necessary it might undoubtedly be, can cause major and even irreparable harm. The primary problem resulting from experiencing 'the knife' is probably adhesions. Adhesions occur when tissue that has been cut in surgery heals and, in reaction to the injury, does so by reinforcing the area with more flesh than was there before and 'anchoring' the new tissue to adjacent organs. It is no more than a protective mechanism but one that sometimes over-responds. Take this example.

> Helen had had an operation to remove her gall bladder. When she came for treatment some two years later she was still complaining of symptoms similar to those for which she had had the operation in the first place: bloating, flatulence, discomfort high up in the stomach area, nausea and a filthy taste in her mouth. In addition she had a stitching pain between the bottom of her ribs and her navel and it was associated with the enormous scar from the operation. She said that she could still conjure up the image of the surgeon's knife slicing through her flesh. She felt that she had been through the operation for no reason as she still felt the same but now she had the extra pain of the scar tissue. "*If I ever met that doctor I'd not be able to stop myself being rude to him!*"
>
> She was given *Staphysagria* (delphinium) which covers that curious imagined sense of the knife wound. This did remove the squeamish feeling about the scar. She was also given *Chelidonium* for the symptoms of her gall bladder condition – even though she no longer had a gall bladder. This did help to remove the digestive distress but it did nothing for the actual pain of the scar tissue. This she felt came from inside and not the surface skin. She felt not only the sharp pain but also a pulling

from within as if tissue was being stretched out of place. It restricted her movement, making it difficult to bend or stretch comfortably – she always felt that something would tear inside if she made any swift or awkward movements. For this she was put on *Thiosinaminum*, a remedy made from the oil of mustard seed, which has a reputation for encouraging the body to restore scar tissue to its former integrity.

As the cells damaged by trauma die off they are replaced by new cells, encouraged to work to the old, pre-trauma 'programme' by the remedy's influence. The process of repair can be long and painstaking but very satisfactory when the remedy is indicated. Helen returned after a month on the remedy and reported that she had had no pains from the scar for over a fortnight – a remarkably short time.

The shock of the surgeon's invasive surgery had been enough to lock Helen's body into the pattern of symptoms that persisted, despite the removal of the offending organ. On top of that the scar tissue threatened to make the rest of her life uncomfortable – an intolerable situation for someone of only forty-three and otherwise reasonably healthy. The operation and its immediate results were no solution to her gall bladder problem even though the surgeon had been right to perform it. The problem was not so much the surgery but the way the patient's body coped with it. Helen's system was one that tended to make scar tissue too readily and in excess. Not everyone reacts in this way but when it does happen it can be a serious maintaining cause.

Scars from inguinal hernia operations can also be a real trial. Patients complain of drawing and pulling sensations in their groins. They can feel tugging sensations in the abdominal area. In deep scarring this can even lead to shortness of breath because the pulling from the scar on the abdominal viscera leads to a sympathetic tightening of the diaphragm. As we have seen, if the diaphragm contracts then the lung capacity is limited; all of which can lead further to a chronic irritating cough and even to frontal headaches as the whole frontal fascia (the soft fibrous tissue of the anterior abdomen and thorax) reacts in sympathy to the tightening of the local scarred tissue. The drawing tension of all the tissues involved may be measured only in fractions of a millimetre but the effect is nevertheless far-reaching and contributes to apparently unrelated symptoms. Who might have guessed that the patient complaining of headaches in the forehead was actually suffering from the drag created in his gut by scar tissue that had been continuing to form slowly ever since the operation for a hernia repair five years before?

The procedure common today for the repair of a hernia is to insert a neat piece of gauze over the weakened muscle wall so that muscle from below cannot protrude. It acts like a local mini truss. Unfortunately this piece of gauze, being a foreign body, is sometimes enough to encourage the formation of bulky tissue around it. This in turn can create a pull on local tissues including those around or near the prostate gland. This leads to the gland being pulled out of alignment and the restriction of the urethra that passes through it. The consequence is prostate trouble with difficult urination.

Who would have thought that a man suffering from bowel pains and haemorrhoids was actually getting symptoms from adhesions that had formed after an operation to remove his prostate gland? Prostate removal can cause the adjacent part of the bowel to adhere to the remaining local tissue. This can be the bladder in some cases. Stress incontinence is usually the result. Constipation and piles are not uncommon and nor is pain in the testicle of the affected side.

Similar things can happen after an appendectomy. Scar tissue can begin to form around the site of the surgeon's incision and this can lead to poor lymphatic drainage from the area, liver congestion and toxicity of the blood. The psoas muscles, large and powerful, run from top to bottom of the abdominal cavity joining the mid-spine to the pelvis, left and right. If either are involved with adhesions as a result of an abdominal operation then not only will there be poor flexibility of movement in the midriff, low back pain and a tendency to stoop but also chronic tiredness, poor liver function due to congestion and blood toxicity from a generally sluggish system. For some reason the psoas is particularly prone to harbouring toxic waste.

The operation to remove ovarian cysts can result in adhesions too. It can cause a fallopian tube to become blocked as it is dragged infinitesimally towards repairing tissue. This can result in anything from menstrual pains to infertility. It can also bring on the secondary symptoms of a distressed liver or spleen depending on which side was involved. So the woman who consults the practitioner for aching in the right side below the ribs, recurrent indigestion which is worse for lying on her back at night in bed (i.e. stretched out), frequent calls to pass water and water retention (especially in the ankle) might well be asking for help to recover from an operation to remove a benign cyst.

Adhesions are often a problem for those who have had glands stripped out after cancer operations. The most usual situation is that following breast cancer when the glands under the arm are removed. This often leaves the patient with tightening tissues from the armpit and across the whole chest. It also can cause considerable difficulty with nerve conduction – so feeling is altered – and lymph drainage. There is often swelling and puffiness from retained fluids even down into the hand. Not only scar tissue but also flesh that begins to adhere to damaged tissue, as part of the repair mechanism, can become a troublesome maintaining cause. Though there are remedies, like *Thiosinaminum*, that can help to restore the integrity of damaged tissue, sometimes the problem is too far gone or too old for a satisfactory homoeopathic solution on its own. This may mean that further surgery is the only answer.

Not everyone has a system that will manufacture excessive scar tissue but others suffer torture as a result. One condition not given very much publicity is the scar tissue that forms after sewing up an episiotomy, the incision made to facilitate delivery. Some women simply do not return to the same shape despite retaining the usual elasticity of the skin in the vaginal area. Many put up with discomfort and pain, others opt for further surgery. Those who have homoeopathic treatment and who are looked after throughout the time of pregnancy and delivery and have after-birth care do have a greater chance of avoiding the problem. *Graphites*, the remedy made from the black lead of drawing pencils, is just one of the remedies well known for their power to initiate positive changes in surface scar tissue and adhesions.

It is when symptoms resulting from the presence of scars and adhesions are not traced to their hidden source that it becomes obvious why this maintaining cause should be examined. Imagine going to your practitioner with constipation, griping pains in the bowels, lethargy and headaches. The physician might well be led to suppose that you were suffering the ubiquitous irritable bowel syndrome (IBS), which is a much abused and fairly meaningless term. You would be advised to look at your diet, to take a mild laxative and increase your exercise or, if the healer were a homoeopath, you might be given remedies to address such a picture. The advice and prescriptions would probably be of no lasting avail – unless the general picture indicated a remedy that also covered scar formation; not, unfortunately, always the case by any means. Osteopaths are generally the first to 'pick up on' the causative nature of scarring when it is present. Otherwise, it is often left to specialists who can read scans and X-rays to find the real underlying reason. Unfortunately, most practitioners – alternative as well as allopathic – are simply not sufficiently aware of the significance and frequent incidence of this problem.

CHAPTER 11

ALLOPATHIC DRUGS

Many patients choose to consult their doctors as well as their homoeopaths about their conditions; they like to keep a foot in both camps. A cynic would say that they are hedging their bets but this is often not the case. There are many conditions that do require allopathic medication either because the problem is no longer entirely susceptible to alternative treatment or because the patient feels that the particular condition is beyond the scope of a natural therapy, needing drugs and careful monitoring by those best placed to do it. Obvious examples would be the treatment of asthma, high blood pressure, angina, depression or breast lumps. (Those with heart conditions are often especially wary of putting themselves exclusively in the hands of any except the most obviously well-qualified health professional.) This means that homoeopaths are often asked to treat patients who are already on prescription drugs, some for life.

Purist homoeopaths do not like treating patients who are on allopathic medication. Some refuse to do so feeling that their efforts would be compromised by the effects of the drugs; this can even extend to women who take the contraceptive pill. This attitude seems rather high-minded. It is certainly unnecessary as much can be done to support patients who have made this particular choice. It is up to the practitioners to make the therapies as complementary as possible whatever compromise of philosophical approach might need to be made. The alternative treatment is still worthwhile. It is important to avoid the patient feeling confused or developing a sense of divided loyalties – as this can complicate treatment unnecessarily.

Patients with chronic illnesses that need permanent drug treatment – even for something as relatively unthreatening as, say, a peptic ulcer – seldom have any idea of how much help they can expect from alternative therapies. They have a vague notion that they can be made to feel more comfortable but any thought of thoroughly healing themselves is beyond their horizon of expectation. This means that the allopathic treatment is, as far as the homoeopath is concerned, not negotiable. Whatever remedies might be indicated and prescribed must do their work on the patient whose natural symptom picture is being suppressed. The suppression of natural symptoms does not preclude all success.

It is not uncommon for the mothers of children who suffer from asthmatic breathing to insist that steroid inhalers continue to be part of the treatment. The reason is not only fear of an acute attack of asthma but also to avoid time being taken off school for recuperation. There is frequently a lack of knowledge that homoeopathic remedies are usually quite capable of dealing with acute attacks. In nearly all but the most severe cases the result is that the treatment continues for a lot longer; this is because any acute episode, which is really an aggravation set up by the body to teach itself to eliminate properly (if rather dramatically), fails to complete its purpose. Nevertheless, in time parent and patient come to trust the remedies to do their work and there comes a moment when the steroids and antibiotics become negotiable. It is noticeable that as soon as the careful weaning process begins the general health of the patient starts to improve markedly and the body eliminates far more efficiently.

Even in those whose history of and dependence on orthodox treatment is as long as their arm and therefore very unlikely to become a subject of any negotiation, there is every reason to use remedies, as the general health of these people can be supported and improved if not thoroughly redeemed. Many asthma, ulcer and heart patients become grateful for the knowledge of how to use remedies in acute crises even if the practitioners, clearly playing second fiddle to medical practitioners' prescriptions, are left feeling vaguely cheated of any more obvious spectacular success.

This is to look on the positive side of a situation that can cause despair. Drugs do interfere with remedies by compromising the healing process. Part of the homoeopath's work is find ways round that. However, first of all it is necessary to assess just what benefit the drug is affording. On some occasions patients may complain of a condition that is actually imposed on them by taking inappropriate drugs. This is an iatrogenic maintaining cause: one caused by inappropriate medication.

An elderly gentleman, Sidney, came into the teaching clinic (where acute problems were handled) and asked advice about his latest symptoms. He complained of frequent headaches and tiredness, dizziness and an inability to think clearly. He was also constipated which he claimed he had never been before and he had noticed that he felt nausea every morning when he woke up. This continued until he had been moving about for a while and had taken the dogs out for their morning constitutional. He explained that he had had these symptoms for about three weeks. When asked if anything had changed in his life that might have brought on the symptoms he had difficulty in identifying anything unusual. He was asked if he had any other health problems that perhaps preceded the present acute situation. No, he said that he was otherwise well. Not entirely convinced that the whole picture was revealed the homoeopath gave Sidney some *Pulsatilla* as this was the most indicated of the possible remedies.

On his return after four weeks Sidney said that at first he had felt that the remedy had been making a difference. He had felt a little more energetic and had less nausea and dizziness. However, within a few days these symptoms had returned and he was now *"back to square one"*. This report provoked a few more questions about his general health; questions that had not been appropriate in the 'acutes clinic'. It transpired that he had been on medication for high blood pressure and angina for some time. For this condition he had always taken a drug called Verapamil which is prescribed to slow the heart rate and reduce the output of the heart. This drug had never caused him any side effects that he was aware of. However, just before the onset of his acute symptoms he had been to the doctor who, for a reason that did not seem clear to Sidney, decided to change the Verapamil for another drug called Istin. It was this drug that he was now taking.

It was clear that all Sydney's current symptoms were side effects of Istin. In the *British National Formulary (BNF)*, the doctors' *Materia Medica*, each of the symptoms is listed specifically as such. When he was shown the description of the drug in the book Sidney declared that he would *"tackle my doctor about that!"* He rang the doctor who promptly told him to halve the dose. (He had been given 10mg once a day, the maximum dose.) This he did but the symptoms did not seem to abate very much unless he took daily doses of *Pulsatilla* as well. (*Pulsatilla* is known to influence the body to eliminate some side effects of drugs.) When he rang the doctor again he was told that his symptoms were probably psychosomatic and that he should now go back up to the full dose: two

5mg tablets each day. Sidney was very reluctant to do so. When he did he found that the *Pulsatilla* had no effect whatever. All the nausea, dizziness and confusion with the headaches came back. He was convinced that the Istin was doing him harm but was reluctant to cross swords with his doctor.

He asked the doctor if he could go back on his previous drug and if he could be referred to the cardiologist he had seen before at the hospital. He was told that Istin was a superior drug for the heart condition that he had and that seeing the specialist would not serve any purpose. Sidney felt blocked and put down. He was very cross. This distress added to his symptom picture. Not only was he emotionally upset at having his request denied and at being, as he put it, stymied but also he was fearful for his general health and the condition of his heart.

He chose a day when he knew his own doctor was not on duty in the surgery and saw the locum. The result was that he was given his old drug but with the instruction that he should make the earliest appointment to see his doctor to report on the situation. This gave Sidney a temporary reprieve. By the time he went to see his own doctor he was back to his old state of health. All the dizziness and nausea, confusion and lethargy had gone quickly when he was given *Pulsatilla* again but without the interference of the Istin. He had also recovered his self-respect and was able to take charge of the interview. With admirable restraint he insisted on remaining on the original medication, declared that he would take nothing else and if he had a heart attack as a result he knew what would have caused it.

This case illustrates several things. The first is that it is always important to take into consideration the side effects of allopathic medication that impose symptoms on top of any that might be the patient's own. The second is that homoeopathic remedies can be given without detriment to those who are on allopathic drugs. Sometimes they will be reduced in efficacy by the dominant chemistry of the drug setting up its own symptom energy. (The daily dose of *Pulsatilla* was able to work to help reduce the side effects of the Istin, albeit marginally, when Sidney was taking the half dose.) The third thing illustrated is that homoeopathic remedies can be effective in removing the side effects gently and promptly once the offending drug has been eliminated. Drugs can be a maintaining cause if they do more than they are intended to do either because of a misjudgement of the dosage or because they are selected inappropriately. A well-chosen drug given in the right amount should do no more than maintain a chemical status quo which is intended to correct the biochemical shortcomings of the patient's own system. For Sidney, the Verapamil was fulfilling just this role. The Istin changed his body chemistry inappropriately and his system protested. Had he remained on it, not only would his health have been compromised but homoeopathic treatment would have been valueless for him.

Antibiotics and steroids

Sometimes drugs can be a maintaining cause long after they should have been eliminated from the body by its waste-disposal unit. The two chief culprits here are antibiotics and steroids. Antibiotics can be a particularly vicious influence. Their 'scorched earth' effect on the intestines – even if their target is elsewhere in the body – is the most usual result. The naturally occurring bowel flora that should be there to aid the digestive process are severely decimated. While some people can take them even quite frequently and show no long-term ill effects, there are many who cannot tolerate the side and after effects. Children are especially susceptible. Those who have regular ear, tonsil and chest infections for which they are given one or other of the penicillin group often develop persistent diarrhoea or the opposite, obstinate constipation. It can sometimes take weeks for the bowel to improve sufficiently for the regrowth of the friendly bacteria.

Some patients so afflicted are also susceptible to food allergies that surface and become an obvious health problem only after a prolonged dosage of antibiotics. The antibiotics render the intestinal walls sensitive to anything that can cause inflammation. The most usual threat is from wheat and gluten and not far behind are the mucus-forming dairy products, milk and cheese. (Indeed, it is frequently the case that dairy products predispose patients to the infections in the first place.)

Normally a healthy, resilient system can cope with such foodstuffs that the human gut finds hard to digest. With the liver prevented from exercising one of its functions – stoking fevers to 'burn off' infection – and the bowel flora having been killed off along with the bacterial infection, the system is no longer so able to create or restore its own biochemical balance.

Following an antibiotic blitz the body becomes unable to remember what the system should be like. The result is that alternative treatment often needs to focus first on this drug-instigated condition rather than any more obvious symptom picture. As the gut is a primary organ of elimination and the whole effect of alternative treatment is intended to encourage elimination it is necessary to restore the integrity of the digestive system as soon as possible. A damaged gut can be a strong maintaining cause requiring supplementary assistance as well as remedies. (Acidophilus either in pill form or as live yoghurt is well known to encourage the growth of bowel flora. *Nux Vomica, Sulphur* and *Pulsatilla* are the best-known remedies to encourage the liver to speed up elimination of toxic drug waste.)

Steroids have been mentioned before in some of the illustrative cases particularly to do with eczema and asthma. They are very versatile and come in four forms: as creams, in tablets, as injections and as inhalers. Topically they are used for eczema, psoriasis and pruritis. The *BNF* instructs doctors to avoid the stronger steroids in cases of infantile eczema and most cases of psoriasis as the side effects of stronger applications are well known (i.e. interference with the endocrine system). After long use, however, hydrocortisone – the most common topical steroid – will cause thinning of the skin, depigmentation, spontaneous bruising and even adrenal suppression (i.e. the suppression of adrenalin): all this without curing the condition for which it is prescribed.

What is not mentioned in the *BNF* is that the suppression of eczema and psoriasis leads to the manifestation of the condition in another part of the body and eventually another form. The alternative treatment of these skin conditions depends on encouraging the body to use the skin as an eliminative organ. There is no other way that eczema can be permanently removed; it will not go through the bowels or bladder nor will it be sweated away through parts of the skin untouched by the cream. The use of topical steroids is a very serious maintaining cause.

"What happens though when the skin flares up and my daughter can't stop scratching?"
Sadly it is often the case that the patient has already had so much steroid cream that the first thing the body wants to do is excrete all the excess

steroid that it has been obliged to absorb through its skin. This means that the treatment must involve a time of eliminating highly irritating chemical toxicity back through the surface. Parents and child must suffer what is sometimes a torment as the thin, sticky, serous fluid exudes. However, to see the patient's state as only of the skin is a mistake. Most children in this position will willingly put up with it as, in themselves, energetically and emotionally, they are aware of their *general* improvement. It is usually the adults (parents or practitioners) who spoil the progress of such cases as they cannot bear to look on.

It is for emotional and cosmetic reasons that many eczema patients do not see their treatment through. Yet in the case of the prescription of steroid creams the homoeopath can be considered justified in interfering with another practitioner's prescription and discouraging the patient from using them. Steroid creams are one of the few prescription drugs where this is the case. The result is not threatening in any way except cosmetically. The results speak for themselves: the patient's skin shows a reaction – even violent on occasion – but always eliminative. If a skin infection also follows with inflammation and pus then this too is natural. It provides an opportunity for the body to relearn a lost skill. Remedies such as *Belladonna*, *Apis*, *Mercury* and *Graphites* all have the ability to match such an acute condition.

When steroids are given internally for breathing troubles or for inflammatory processes then the waters are muddied. We produce our own corticosteroids from the cortex of our adrenal glands. The body uses them for various purposes: such as maintaining sodium levels, assisting in metabolising fats, reducing inflammation and compensating for high levels of adrenalin in the system. People with asthma or an inflammatory condition such as severe ulcerative colitis do not have sufficient quantities of their own hormone to deal with the symptoms and are therefore given the chemical equivalent. Unfortunately, if synthetic steroids are used for long enough the adrenal cortex gets the message to switch off its own supply as too much of the stuff is as bad as too little. Worse still the adrenal cortex does not just switch off but can begin to atrophy so that there is no way that, once better, the patient could go back to producing his or her own steroids. For this reason the amount of steroids is always carefully monitored.

The following case suggests that despite suppressive drugs homoeopathic remedies can work; it is not necessary for the homoeopath to retire once orthodox specialists come on the scene.

Kevin, a man of forty-eight, suddenly developed severe abdominal pains and bleeding from the rectum. His intestines felt inflamed and hot. He developed a fever and headache. He was taken to hospital after several hours and was kept in for tests. They quickly suspected ulcerative colitis (where ulcers form on the inside of the colon and cause the blood vessels that feed the gut to haemorrhage). He was kept in hospital for several days and put on steroids to reduce the inflammation. When he went home he was told to stay on the drug for ten days, maintain a strict diet and then to see his doctor.

His doctor suggested that he should start to reduce the steroids gradually. However, the bleeding came back as soon as he had got down to half his original dose. At this point he saw the homoeopath who found that his *"moods were very up and down"*, that he felt very restless one moment and then suddenly exhausted and sleepy the next. He also found that the pains were still burning and *"stinging"* as well as griping and that the bowel was still haemorrhaging. He gave *Apis* 30 twice a day for two weeks.

When Kevin reported back three weeks later he said that he had had a difficult time for two weeks and then suddenly felt very much better *"in myself"*. He had developed lots of large pustular spots all over his back. His stools had become more solid and less frequent and he had no further bleeding. He said that he had stopped taking the *Apis* as soon as he began to feel a sense of well-being. (He was still taking the steroids *"because I don't feel quite safe yet without them"*.) Now what he wanted was to concentrate on clearing up his skin: *"I still feel a bit toxic."* He was given *Calendula* 6 twice per day for a month. At his next appointment he said that the spots were now all coming to heads and discharging, that he no longer felt so toxic but that all that sense of well-being had gone. Instead he felt apprehensive, withdrawn and dispirited; he could not tell quite why, though he now complained about having to take the steroids. He was given *Natrum Sulphuricum* 100, one to be taken every week for four weeks. (This remedy matches those who feel withdrawn and tense, have a sluggish liver, feel hot a lot of the time and who incidentally produce yellow pus from the eyes.)

When Kevin returned he had a story to tell. He had decided to wean himself off the steroids and see how things developed. He had no further symptoms of ulcerative colitis. However, what was now very obvious to him was that he had been *"festering with rage for years"* about his father who had left home when Kevin was twelve. Now, he said, he realised just what a pathetic, weak man his father had been. *"He had bowel cancer in the end. If I hadn't been through all the hospital business with the steroids I wonder if I'd have ended up the same way. I feel that in some way I had to do all this. It was something eating away at me and I'd never given it any time before."*

Kevin, in common with many others, felt that he needed the experience of going into a crisis that was treated allopathically as it had contributed to an insight into a slice of his own history. The steroids had not inhibited his body's energetic response to the remedies but had maintained a status quo in the intestines while he worked through to the end what it was that his body meant to do. It is a moot point whether he would have had such a satisfactory result if he had only come to take homoeopathic medicines much later in treatment; ulcerative colitis is a condition that can have intermittent flare-ups for years. Those who start taking remedies after a long time on drugs find it very much harder to improve.

Hitting the drug wall

From these various illustrations you will gather that though treatment can be compromised unless the problem of drugging is taken into account as soon as possible, it nevertheless remains perfectly feasible to pursue alternative healing even if the patient is quite unable to do without the potentially troublesome but supporting drug or drugs. However, there are some drugs that are so powerful in their effects on the body or mind that very little natural healing could ever take place while they are being taken. Some are even so altering to the biochemistry that, even if the patient has been off them for some time, few if any homoeopathic remedies would ever succeed completely in 'cutting through' the drug layer.

Particularly unfortunate in this respect are the drugs for epilepsy, for schizophrenia and for psychoses. While it is true that comparatively very few patients with such conditions would consult a homoeopath, it is worth mentioning that for those who do there is often considerable frustration and disappointment. The drugs they are obliged to take are not curative even if they seem to make life tolerable. Lithium (an anti-mania drug) or haloperidol (an anti-psychotic drug) may have saved many from asylums, suicide or homicide but they are so suppressive that they alter the very spirit of the patients to whom they are given.

An Australian woman in her thirties came for a consultation. She had been treated previously by various homoeopaths and explained that for one reason or another she had become dissatisfied with their efforts. She spoke rationally about her several years of frustration with homoeopathy and other alternative therapies. She was particularly scathing about one practitioner who had given her a dose of *Silica*. This, she declared, had all but killed her. The rest of the interview was taken up with a straightforward 'case taking' to establish a general, overall picture. This included such ordinary symptoms as sweating on the face, a tendency to suffer from the cold, sensitivity to the light and deteriorating vision. It also revealed that she had, *"many, many years ago"*, taken a range of hallucinatory drugs including LSD which had caused her to have such a severe reaction that she was sectioned and put into a psychiatric hospital. Even though she denied that this episode had anything to do with the treatment she was required to take over the following few years – haloperidol and rehabilitation – the evidence suggested otherwise. She no longer took any mind-bending drugs. What she wanted treatment for was to re-establish her constitutional health.

If it had not been for her rather aggressive antipathy towards the practitioner who had given her the *Silica* it might have been hard to tell that she was a psychotic patient. However, as she left she said, *"Please don't ever post any remedies to me. I must insist on that. The postman always checks my mail and he would replace the pills with something poisonous."*

It turned out on enquiry that Sheila, as she was known in the practice, was a source of some entertainment to various other practices in the area. This was hardly a generous or humanitarian view but nevertheless an unfortunate reality. All the other practitioners contacted had a supply of bizarre anecdotes to tell about Sheila's antics as a patient. For one thing she believed that she was being pursued by surfers from Melbourne. She would be hanging out her washing – at 11 o'clock at night – and find wet-suited young men lying in wait for her. She would ring up her homoeopath for instant advice. The delusion that people were trying to poison her meant that she never ate food prepared by anyone but herself and this she would only eat at night.

In the three years she came for treatment it was obvious that the only remedies that ever made any curative difference were those for the common cold. Even this was uncertain as she might have recovered from her colds without any assistance. No remedies ever touched her psychosis. In fact, as time went on it became apparent that her sickness seemed to grow in confidence and produce an insidiously increasing aggression.

"If I thought for one moment that you would give me Silica *I'd smash this over your head."* Her hands were gripping the table lamp. She described how this or that prescription would make her sweat or give her spots on the chin. Another would relieve her indigestion for a while. Despite the best indications for certain remedies her mental state seemed completely out of reach of homoeopathy. It was comforting to know that others, with all their combined experience, had had the same result. Sheila's mind was fixed into a mode of bizarre psychosis by first the LSD and then by the haloperidol. Not only did she have delusions of being pursued and being poisoned – which might well have stemmed from her LSD trips – but she also had too many symptoms known to be side effects of the haloperidol: poor spatial awareness, drowsiness, insomnia, depressiveness, constipation, irregular menstruation, irregular heart beats and contact dermatitis. Sheila's maintaining causes were historical but unremitting. Despite the rather black humour of some of her exploits her case remains one of deep and unresolved tragedy.

The nearest that most homoeopaths come to treating this stratum of patients with any regularity is when they are consulted by those on antidepressants. If a patient has been on a drug such as Prozac for only a relatively short time then homoeopathic remedies can contribute to the restoration of health. Nevertheless, sooner or later the patient who has been on Prozac or one of its type will need to deal with exactly those mental or emotional problems that the drug had temporarily made less disturbing. It is unlikely that anyone who has suppressed such issues for a while would not find them coming up again to be resolved. Mind-altering drugs do not actually make the problems disappear; there can be no sleight of hand in medicine.

Problems really occur in those who have been on antidepressants for years. This is commonly true for those who have been prescribed, against the pharmaceutical industry's express advice, anxiolytic drugs such as diazepam. This is a group of drugs that is designed for short-term use to help patients through an anxious period or a prolonged bout of insomnia. However, it is easy to see how patients with mild depression, whose symptoms include anxiety and insomnia, might well come to rely on a drug that would 'knock them out' for the night, the most anxious part of the day. For homoeopathy to work well in circumstances such as these the patient would need to go through a period of sleepless anxiety as a natural aggravation; they would need to go 'cold turkey' on their sleeping pill. The maintaining cause here is as much the patient's reluctance to face this dragon as the psychological damage imposed by the drug.

Isopathy: 'same cures same'?

The fact is that drugs that affect the mind and the central nervous system compromise or prevent the curative effects of homoeopathic remedies because they alter and suppress the very vehicle needed by the curative energy. There are some homoeopaths who use isopathy with patients who present such intractable difficulties. Isopathy is prescribing the homoeopathic preparation of the offending drug and giving it to the patient regularly. This is carrying 'like cures like' to its extreme. The idea is that the patient is given a homoeopathically prepared dose of the selfsame drug that is causing the problem of 'block'. Thus, someone who has been on Lithium or who is in the long process of being weaned off it, is given *Lithium* 30 or 200 fairly regularly. Not just 'like cures like' but 'same cures same'.

Patients who are or have been on steroids have been known to do well when given *Cortisone* 30 weekly. Cancer patients on heavy-duty chemotherapy have been given their allopathic drugs in potency at the same time so that, while the drugs do what they are intended to do, the potentised version limits the chemical side effects. This method seems to work often enough for some practitioners to keep using it. All too often, though, it tends to fall short of expectations. It is a practice that sets a frown on the purists' faces but it is a tactic that is worth trying when all other, better-indicated avenues are closed off[1].

CHAPTER 12

HORMONE DRUGS

The Pill

The contraceptive pill has been one of the most commercially successful medical enterprises of all time. For this very reason it is highly unlikely that criticism of its efficacy will be allowed to undermine its reputation, certainly not without torrents of refutation of the alternative view written by chemists with axes to grind. Criticism there *has* been and much of it based on serious studies by scientists. For every study that has shown statistically how risky 'the Pill' really is, there are others that show how relatively safe it is. (Note the word 'relatively'.) The Pill, more than any other drug, is subjected to the literary machinations of those most adept at playing the statistics game. The unembellished truth about this drug cannot be found by comparing x number of women with y. It is only possible by beginning with the anatomy and physiology of the human body and looking at the potential for short- and long-term effects that the drug has on our biochemistry. The result of this exercise will not suit those who see the Pill as the banner of the liberated female or those who see it as a practical humanitarian answer to the vast overpopulation of the world. It certainly would not be acceptable to the drugs companies that manufacture the Pill who base their continuing sales on the assumption that there is such a thing as a female universal norm.

A brief history of chemical birth control

Much of the history of medical biochemistry began in the last twenty years or so of the nineteenth century. It was at that time that it was first realised that the yellowish corpus luteum, a glandular mass found on the ovary from which an egg has been released, secretes something that switches off egg production temporarily thus ensuring that if fertilisation takes place it will be singular. In the 1920s the secretions were identified as the hormones oestrogen and progesterone. It was postulated that these two chemicals might be synthesised and used as contraceptives.

The earliest experiments were with animal sex hormones. Both the horse and the pig were thought initially to be suitable subjects for experimentation, but were quickly excluded from consideration as the production costs were prohibitive. (The issue never got as far as sparking any ethical or moral debate.) It was then discovered that wild yam was a source of natural progesterone. At first this avenue of research proved to be a dead end too as progesterone is destroyed by stomach acids and material doses of wild yam cause severe and agonising symptoms in the gut[1]. While it had been known for some time that progesterone could be injected into the blood stream (to help maintain pregnancy in women who had little of their own progesterone), chemists in Mexico determined to discover a way of synthesising the chemical compound they had found so that it could be used orally. Their purpose was not yet part of the search for a contraceptive but to promote the very opposite in those who would otherwise miscarry every pregnancy. What they produced was a synthesised variant of the male hormone, testosterone, still used today as an integral part of the contraceptive compound.

Early oestrogen trials (in the 1930s) had caused mammary cancers in test animals (as oestrogen promotes cell growth) and progesterone trials had caused unacceptably heavy haemorrhaging. Then the indomitable Margaret Sanger, America's answer to Marie Stopes and founder of the International Planned Parenthood Federation, swept onto the scene with money and a commission. She held a dinner party in New York in 1951 to which she invited a biologist, Gregory Pincus, who had already spent time studying the effects of progestins on rabbits and people. (In one study on poor Puerto Rican women there were three fatalities.) Sanger wanted scientists to produce a cheap, effective and simple-to-use pill that all women could swallow that would effectively prevent pregnancy.

It was quickly realised that the body had the right idea in the first place by combining the two hormones in varying proportions according to the time of the month. Early efforts seemed less than encouraging. The first trial tested on a group of Harvard University volunteers and another group of mentally ill patients demonstrated the effectiveness of the approach: the women stopped ovulating altogether and the men stopped producing sperm. One of the men was found to have shrunken testicles as a result of the trial.

With his laboratory resources and the research already done on the Mexican yam, Pincus eventually produced a synthesised combined pill that in due course (though, as it turned out, too soon) was given a licence under the name Enovid. This proved to be a mixed blessing to the many hopeful women who first took it in the early 1960s. After reports of fatalities due to thrombosis, embolism, strokes and high blood pressure Enovid was seen to be far too high a dose of the combined oestrogen and progesterone. The search began for the minimum dose. It was soon discovered that Enovid was some ten times stronger in its effects than it needed to have been.

Today there are a wide variety of contraceptive pills, the most common and widely used being those that have comparatively small doses of the two hormones. Mercifully, in the context of the history of medicine, it took a relatively short time (some twenty years) for scientists to experiment to the point where they found a viable and apparently 'safe' method of chemical contraception. Side effects are minimised and, in many cases, apparently eradicated. Though most women are familiar with the threat of certain side effects of taking the Pill they are content to believe the information sheets that describe any risks as acceptable in comparison with the benefits. Before looking at the nature of the Pill itself and the way it is presented to us we should make a short detour into the intricate mechanism that controls all the hormones of the body to see just what is being tampered with by the drug.

The endocrine system

The body has rhythm; it has a clock that is self-regulating. It is an almost unfathomably complex system that is responsive not only to its own inner physical, emotional and spiritual workings but also to external circumstances such as the seasons and geographical environment. The clock must have an engine: a system of chemical telegraphy that is capable of adjusting the body to adapt to any circumstances whatever might be happening within. This engine is the endocrine system and its ignition is the pituitary gland.

The pituitary gland is a pea-sized organ hidden deep within the head. It hangs down from the floor of the brain on a stalk, like a stalactite. It is protectively cradled in a saddle of bone (the sella turcica, or Turkish saddle) which has two wing-like bones that spread out on either side. We have already come across this apparatus, the sphenoid bone, in the case of the little boy with the asymmetrical head. As noted before, it is designed to move rhythmically back and forth though we are completely unaware of its tiny rocking motion. This motion is essential as it creates a pump action that keeps cerebro-spinal fluid (CSF) washing continuously past the pituitary. CSF is blood without the red cells. Blood entering the endocrine mechanism of the brain is divested of the oxygen-carrying red blood cells so that hormones may be released into the colourless fluid by the hormone factories: the hypothalamus and the thalamus. All the hormonal messages from these (which, along with the pineal gland, substantially make up the primitive brain) must pass the pituitary gland that reacts by sending out the appropriate hormonal signals to the other organs of the endocrine system: the thyroid, thymus, pancreas, liver, spleen, ovaries, testicles, kidneys and adrenal glands.

The hypothalamus deals with hunger, thirst, temperature and defence (i.e. fear and rage, flight or fight).

The thalamus receives and interprets crude sensations from the central nervous system and causes the motor nerves to react (for example, if you knock your mug of tea off the table you lurch forward to save it); it also integrates sensory input with emotional reactions – thus a baby cries when it feels hunger. It has the further vital function of maintaining consciousness and awareness.

The pineal gland produces melatonin which influences sexual maturation though even today the rest of the precise role of the gland is not clear. Medical opinion favours the idea that the gland 'switches off' at puberty as its physical function has been accomplished by then. However, as the pineal stores and releases serotonin, the neurotransmitter essential for the 'feel good factor', it would seem that this gland has a far more significant role that awaits further research.

The pituitary gland has two parts to it: an anterior and a posterior lobe. Between them is a cleft that is connected by its stalk of nerve fibres and blood vessels to the hypothalamus and thus to the rest of the brain. The anterior lobe sends out hormones that stimulate growth, regulate the sex hormones, cause the thyroid to maintain control of the metabolic rate, cause the breast tissue to produce milk and keep the kidneys filtrating and secreting urine. The posterior lobe is concerned with storing and causing the release of hormones that stimulate uterine contractions and milk secretion as well as one that causes the kidneys to slow down the production of urine. During pregnancy and the menopause the gland quite naturally enlarges.

The pituitary message system is not a one-way street. There are negative and positive feedback mechanisms within each one of the endocrine glands. This means that whatever hormone the pituitary sends out, the recipient organ sends a hormonal message back to say when it has had enough. The delicacy of the fine-tuning and balance of this sophisticated system is not to be underestimated. Positive and negative emotions affect it and vice versa because there is an intimate relationship between emotions and the secretion of hormones. Nor should it be forgotten that the system works automatically without any external stimulation beyond the intake of food and water, the sensations of heat and cold and the influence of the seasons. Anything that is artificially introduced into the body to affect the hormone system is registered as alien to it. Hormone-altering drugs are necessarily powerful enough to *impose* their chemistry on the system; this means that any pre-existing state is masked. As with every other area of chemotherapy, hormone therapy causes the natural status quo to be overridden or suppressed. For those who take the Pill to suppress the symptoms created by difficult periods this would seem a blessing though even here there is a price to pay.

Oestrogen and progesterone

Oestrogen and progesterone are the hormones related specifically to gynaecology and are synthesised naturally by the body from cholesterol, a form of fatty steroid alcohol that occurs naturally in various parts of the body. They are steroidal sex hormones though they are of wider importance than this description would suggest. To understand their individual purpose in the body is to begin to see how the artificial introduction of industrially and artificially synthesised versions might affect the system adversely and how the results of taking them would become a maintaining cause of illness.

Oestrogen is secreted by ovarian egg follicles in response to follicle stimulating hormone (FSM) sent out by the hypothalamus. It is involved in the development of the female reproductive organs and the growth of hair and tissue characteristic of the feminine form. It helps to prevent skin from drying out and becoming wrinkly. It keeps the walls of the vagina elastic and receptive and allows it to expand during pregnancy. It raises libido around the time of ovulation and alters the mucus secreted by the vaginal walls so that sperm find it an easy medium through which to swim. Without oestrogen eggs would not be able to pass down the Fallopian tubes towards the uterus as the muscles of the tube walls would not be stimulated to contract; nor would the endometrium – the mucous membrane lining the womb – be able to develop into a suitably nourishing place for any fertilised egg to become implanted.

Oestrogen also has a role to play in maintaining the structure of bones, in the workings of the liver, in fat metabolism and in keeping blood vessels free from becoming clogged with heavy lipoproteins that would cause atherosclerosis (hardening of the arteries) or an embolism (a blocked blood vessel due to a clot). It also is involved in breaking down excesses of testosterone (male hormone) and progestogens (hormones that promote gestation). When we come to cite the acknowledged potential side effects of the Pill it will be seen that every facet of oestrogen's body purpose is affected.

If oestrogen is vital to the promotion of a cyclical, fertile period in the first half of the menstrual cycle then progesterone is equally important in preparing the body for pregnancy during the second half. Progesterone tones down the action of oestrogen so that the ovaries switch off from preparing their follicles for the release of further eggs and the corpus luteum, the egg pod, becomes the foetus's hormone reservoir for the first three months of pregnancy. Progesterone also thickens up the mucus in the vagina so that sperm remain sealed in the nurturing environment of the uterus.

Oestrogen and progesterone are not mutually exclusive. When progesterone is secreted by about day twenty-one of the cycle a new chemical balance is struck between them and the two hormones prepare the endometrium for its development into the placenta. In addition progesterone is needed in combination with prolactin to stimulate milk production. When there is no pregnancy to prepare for then the levels of progesterone and oestrogen drop and 'starve' the endometrium. This leads to its breakdown and dissolution resulting in the menstrual bleed. The whole cycle should take twenty-eight days and, because we are made up of around 70 per cent water, should be subject to the phases of the moon. Such is the textbook norm.

So finely tuned is this biofeedback mechanism that it is hardly surprising that much can go wrong with it when there are predisposing factors. Smoking, alcohol, excessive amounts of sugar, junk food and inappropriate dieting (especially amongst teenagers) can all upset the hormone levels. Frequent antibiotics, steroid drugs and hallucinogens will do the same as will emotional disturbances such as grief and fury. Even flying and jet lag will disturb the balance just as synthesised oestrogens that are bled into our environment in the water supply, in plastic utensils and even some pesticides can do. This is even before we look at the specific side effects of the Pill, let alone heredity or any other internal predisposing illness[2].

What's in the packet?

The Pill ranges from combined oral contraceptives in low, standard or high strength to progesterone-only contraceptives which come in the shape of pills, injections or intra-uterine devices which release the drug directly into the area of the endometrium. Though all are intended to prevent pregnancy they have different ways of effecting this: the combined pill prevents the ovaries from producing eggs in the first place and the progesterone-based pill thickens the cervical mucus to become a hostile environment for sperm. The chemists have had to come up with ever more sophisticated tailoring to suit the needs of the enormously varied types of women who demand contraception. The side effects that have been logged and registered since the 1960s have dictated the need to diversify the range.

The low-strength Pill is prescribed for obese or older women; the high-strength is prescribed for those on long-term drugs for conditions such as epilepsy because the medication that is necessary to prevent the symptoms of their pathology will cancel out the effectiveness of the low-dosage Pill. There are at least twenty-four varieties of the standard strength. Without exception all of them carry cautionary advice about the possible side effect of venous thrombosis: developing a blood clot in the leg. Thrombosis is potentially an extremely serious acute condition. In *The British National Formulary* (BNF) there is half a column entitled 'The risk of thromboembolism' giving the statistics of the number of women out of 100,000 actually at risk from particular types of the drug.

For thromboembolism to be a risk factor at all it is evident that in those unfortunate few who suffer this condition the Pill is capable of reaching beyond its biochemical effect on the sex hormones. To cause problems with the circulatory system it must also affect other hormone functions of the pituitary gland. At the end of its cautionary essay the *BNF* gives a list of reasons to stop taking the Pill immediately.

These are:

  (i)   sudden severe chest pain
 (ii)   sudden breathlessness (or cough with blood stained sputum)
(iii)   severe pain in the calf of one leg
 (iv)   unusual severe, prolonged headache
  (v)   hepatitis, jaundice, generalised itching, liver enlargement
 (vi)   severe depression
(vii)   blood pressure above 160/100
(viii)   detection of a risk factor.

All of which suggest that not only can the circulation and pituitary be affected but also the liver, the heart, the lungs and the psyche. Factors (a), (b), (c), (d) and (g) all have to do with the blood and circulation. Factor (e) is to do with the damage that the Pill can cause to the liver. Factor (f) is to do with the effects on the pituitary and very probably the pineal gland.

To help a doctor make his prescription of a contraceptive the *BNF* also gives advice in the form of two lists. The first advises caution if any of the following factors are present in the patient:

(i)   family history of venous thromboembolism

(ii)   obesity

(iii)   long-term immobilisation (e.g. being reliant on use of a wheelchair)

(iv)   varicose veins.

The second list suggests that oral contraceptives should be avoided if two or more factors are present:

(i)   family history of arterial disease (in a relative aged under forty-five)

(ii)   diabetes mellitus

(iii)   hypertension (blood pressure of more than 140/90)

(iv)   smoking (avoid if smoking more than 40 daily)

(v)   obesity

(vi)   migraine.

Having listed this information the *BNF* then lists the side effects of the drugs, some of which you will see are not mentioned in the previous information: nausea, vomiting, headache, breast tenderness, changes in body weight, fluid retention, thrombosis (more common in those with blood group A, B, or AB[3]), changes in libido, depression, chorea, skin reactions, chloasma, hypertension, contact lenses may irritate, impairment of liver function, hepatic tumours, reduced menstrual loss, spotting in early cycles, absence of withdrawal bleeding, rarely photosensitivity[4].

There then follows a paragraph about the 'small increase in the risk of breast cancer diagnosed in women taking the combined oral contraceptive pill'. It says that if tumours do occur they are likely to be confined to the breast tissue (i.e. there is virtually no risk of it spreading[5]). It further mentions that women are most at risk after coming off the Pill but that the risk lessens gradually over the ten-year period following. A small additional note is made that running the risk of breast cancer should be weighed against the benefits and evidence of the protective effect against cancer of the ovaries and womb. The rather peculiar, twisted logic behind this statement is clearly lost on its authors. When the statisticians did their maths they did not take into account that before the Pill was introduced cancer of the ovaries and uterus were far more likely to occur in women over the age of childbearing.

The *BNF* draws on the results of clinical experience as well as laboratory-run research. Empirical observation has dictated just which groups of women are most at risk. Neatly, where there are still risks they are minimised by drawing attention to benefits that might not actually be of any value to the user. So much for what the blurb says. What does it not say?

What else does the Pill do that you would rather it didn't?

See what happens when the chemist starts juggling? Pills that contain:

(i) high progestogen and high oestrogen stop the menstrual flow altogether

(ii) high progestogen but low oestrogen cause irregular, scanty withdrawal bleeding

(iii) low progestogen and low oestrogen bring a significantly higher risk of pregnancy and irregular bleeding

(iv) low progestogen and high oestrogen leads to tissue changes in veins

(v) progestogen on its own has been associated with arterial disease.

Add to this the known effects of excessive amounts of either one of the two hormones.

Oestrogen:

(i) migraines (often the result of liver malfunction) and headaches often associated with blood pressure or low levels of vitamin B6.

(ii) dizziness

(iii) nausea

(iv) water retention with attendant weight gain and high blood pressure

(v) bloating

(vi) increased vaginal discharge

(vii) aching in the legs (incipient varicosity)

(viii) development of gall stones

(ix) lowered tolerance of glucose (incipient diabetes)

(x) endometrial cancer.

Progesterone:

(i)   predisposes users to chronic weight gain
(ii)   tiredness and lethargy
(iii)   lowered libido
(iv)   vaginal dryness
(v)   acne vulgaris and acne rosacea; greasy skin
(vi)   anaemia
(vii)   depressive illness, including pre-menstrual tension (PMT)
(viii) breast cancer.

Bearing in mind that a healthy body produces just the required amount of these two hormones in the correct balance and that any pill that delivers an extra and (from the body's point of view) an untimely quantity is creating a new and artificial biochemical balance, does it make good medical sense to use the Pill? If we look at the side effects a little more closely then we begin to see how the Pill should be considered a prime reason for users' health to remain below par.

Nausea and vomiting
The combined Pill sets off a false pregnancy and the nausea can, like morning sickness, be associated with the hormonal changes that affect the stomach and gut. Tension build-up in reaction to the increased presence of hormones can tighten the diaphragm, raise blood pressure and cause the autonomic nervous system to register the symptom.

Headache and migraine
Blood vessels are affected by chemicals triggered by hormones. The same chemicals are responsible for altering mood, behaviour and diet. Raised intercranial pressure caused by the decreased oestrogen and increased progesterone levels just before the period means that too much blood is circulating in the head without good enough drainage. There is greater pressure in the head, then there is tension in the neck and shoulder muscles. Hence some women succumb to tension headaches at this time in the month. This is often aggravated by consumption of alcohol, cheese and chocolate and sometimes by acid fruits. If the liver is overloaded with toxicity anyway then the headaches become bilious, accompanied by nausea and

vomiting. Sometimes the characteristic visual disturbances of migraines are present. The incidence of migraine or tension headaches rises considerably amongst Pill users. If these people also smoke then the risk of these symptoms increases.

Breast tenderness
Some women have a tendency towards 'lumpy breasts' and this is often exaggerated while on the Pill. It is not uncommon for this condition to become chronic; the breasts enlarge and the lumps become permanent. Even if these women do not have a history of breast cancer in the family (and are therefore not considered to be at particular risk) they are some four times more likely to require treatment for suspicious or malignant growths – see the paragraph on liver impairment below.

Changes in body weight
Changes in body weight may be due to water retention (short-term) or to putting down more adipose (fatty) tissue (long-term). If water retention is the problem, it is an indication that the kidneys, which maintain the balance of essential minerals in the body, are not functioning normally. This leads to the characteristic bloating of the abdomen and can cause an increased tendency to wheat/gluten intolerance with all the attendant problems of an irritable bowel.

Where there is a build-up of fatty tissue it suggests that the thyroid gland is being disturbed, as it is this gland above all others that orchestrates the metabolism. The parathyroid glands, tiny organs situated just above the thyroid, are not to be interfered with lightly as they are the organs chiefly responsible for the calcium levels in bone – unfortunately, another of the potential side effects of the Pill is increased risk of osteoporotic changes, a condition where bone density is reduced. In other cases women can lose their appetites and become anorexic.

Water retention
This might not seem to be much of a problem if it is temporary; however, the retention of water in the body can put a strain on the kidneys and increase blood pressure. It also contributes to lethargy and is often a concomitant symptom of depression.

235

Thrombosis

Comparatively few (60 in 100,000 say the statistics) produce the symptoms of thrombosis or stroke. Very many more produce symptoms of the early warning signs – aching legs, breathlessness, overheating, sweat and head-ache. Even if these symptoms are very mild the body is putting out signals of abnormal levels of physical stress. Continuation of the cause inevitably leads to worsening symptoms. Women who notice nothing more than a tendency to ache in the lower legs while standing in queues and the devel-opment of thread veins on the calf or thigh do well to learn to read the writing on the wall.

Changes in libido

Many women suffer a considerable loss of interest in sex once they start tak-ing the Pill (with high progesterone and low oestrogen). This is not due to the fact that they know that they cannot become pregnant while taking the Pill but to the overdose of progesterone. They are, in effect, switched off. (The glee and triumph of sexual freedom has for many a nasty aftertaste and was, in any case, largely a myth established by journalists.)

Depression

The high progesterone/low oestrogen pill will block a woman's own oestro-gen production and contains too little oestrogen to maintain the 'feel good factor'. The production of serotonin (which is the 'happy hormone') is cur-tailed towards the end of the menstrual cycle (hence the irritability of PMT). This is because there is a rise in the level of monoamine oxidase (MAO), an enzyme found in the gut that is essential in the breakdown of food stuffs. MAO renders serotonin inactive. False levels of progesterone can have the effect of promoting MAO production and activity and interfering with the biofeedback system between the gut and the pituitary. It is possible that the Pill also prevents the body from synthesising L-tyrosine, an amino acid that is important to the functioning of the nervous system and the thyroid gland. The depressive symptoms are quite likely to be phobias, hysterical out-bursts and hypochondriasis (fear of disease). (Vegetarians may be more prone to this if they are found to be deficient in vitamin B12.)

Coming off the Pill can be difficult for some women. They find that they 'go cold turkey' for the first month and suffer anxiety, neuroses or black moods. Suicide has also been recorded in some cases of women on the Pill – though would only occur in those with a peculiar predisposition (see Part III: Syphilis). This is ascribed to the fact that copper levels can be significantly higher in certain women while they are taking the Pill. Copper is toxic in high quantities and causes depression, psychosis and even schizophrenia.

Chorea
Chorea manifests as involuntary jerky movements that can affect the limbs or the whole body. Many women experience 'jumpy leg syndrome' when they sit in the evening or lie in bed; their legs become restless and jerky to the point of disturbing sleep. This can be due to vitamin and mineral deficiency. Vitamin B6 is known to prevent convulsive movements but the Pill reduces its level in the body. It is interesting to note that zinc levels are reduced through taking the Pill and *Zinc* (in homoeopathic potency) is well known as a remedy often indicated in conditions of weakness and restlessness of the body.

Skin reactions
Skin reactions may include acne, acne rosacea, 'liver spots' and itching. Each of these also indicates that the liver function is disturbed. Acne rosacea is usually considered to be a condition related to the menopause but excessive progesterone can cause the problem to come on too early. Chloasma is associated with both the liver, and melanin production (a function of the pituitary gland). Rashes also may occur but they may not arise until some time after starting taking the Pill, even years. Rashes may be due to increased susceptibility to fungal infection as a result of lowered immunity known to be caused by the Pill or due to allergic reactions to ingested substances in the gut.

Hypertension
High blood pressure develops due to the thickening of blood vessel walls. This occurs most commonly in the pelvic area causing local congestion and poor drainage from the lower half of the body. If the uterus and ovaries are affected then fertility is impaired. In an American study conducted of

women who had just had hysterectomies in 1977 it was found that all the subjects had moderate to severe thickening of the inner layer of the main artery that fed the womb; the length of time taking the Pill determined the severity of the thickening. In subjects taking the combined Pill such changes are more common and can occur anywhere in the body.

Hypertension can also be the result of increased viscosity of the blood causing the formation of clots on the walls of the arteries leading away from the heart. High levels of oestrogen in the body such as occurs in pregnancy, increase the clotting factor, though the body counters this by producing antithrombim III to prevent the clumping together of sticky blood cells. No such failsafe mechanism works when the oestrogen levels are higher due to taking the artificial Pill. The Pill can also cause a disturbance of the secretion by the pituitary gland of vasopressin (an antidiuretic hormone) which is necessary for maintaining the water balances of the body. It does this by causing blood vessels to constrict and influencing the rate at which water is reabsorbed and minerals retained in the kidneys. If this balancing act is upset then high blood pressure can result.

Dry eyes
Contact lens users can find their lenses cause trouble due to a drop in the flow of tears from the lachrymal gland. This is a common problem in menopausal women and is usually the result of progesterone and liver dysfunction.

Impairment of liver function
Enzymes in the liver that are necessary for the breakdown of toxins are inhibited by progesterone in the Pill. In the absence of the normal levels of these enzymes, proteins will not be broken down by the normal process. This leads to abnormal balances of the essential minerals in the body. Zinc and vitamin B6 are depleted which alters carbohydrate metabolism and cellular metabolism. Copper levels rise in some women and this, combined with the loss of zinc, leads to food intolerance and appetite changes: anorexia and bulimia may even result. In addition, the normal levels of iron, chromium, iodine, magnesium and manganese can all be altered. Between them these minerals affect just about every aspect of biochemistry in the body.

Gall bladder disease

The Pill interferes with cholesterol levels in the body and this can cause stones to form in the gall bladder. If this occurs the person is likely to become far more irritable. If the liver is affected then it becomes far less efficient at processing and eliminating toxins; this creates a predisposition to jaundice. One of the early warning signs is itching of the skin without any eruption or the telltale yellowing of the cornea of the eye.

Hepatic tumours

Tumours in the liver are not necessarily cancerous or malignant. However, they should be regarded as precancerous whether they tend in that direction or not. Cystic tumours of any soft organ can remain indolent and benign for years but then change to become something more sinister. The reason for this is that the cells that form a tumour are abnormal and though the body can tolerate this the affected area remains weak. Any functional, biochemical or emotional trigger can put the abnormal cells into a potentially more aggressive mode. If the liver function is also affected by changes brought about by the Pill then the likelihood of malignancy increases.

Reduced menstrual loss

A reduction in menstrual loss means the loss of a valuable eliminative process. Despite the theory (popular among some gynaecologists and medical journalists) that women do not need to bleed or even to ovulate unless they wish to become pregnant, it is important to realise that women are able to use their menstrual bleed to eliminate toxins that would otherwise circulate for a lot longer in the bloodstream until they found their way out through the bowels and urine – a process that is impaired in those who take the Pill. To put it in plumber's language: the uterus becomes a sump to the overloaded liver. Sometimes the liver's dependence on the uterus's ability to take its overflow contributes to symptoms that require treatment: clotted blood that causes pain, excessive blood loss that causes debility. The orthodox answer to these symptoms is often the Pill. This effectively prevents the elimination process but does not help the body to find another route thus creating an internal build-up of the toxicity leading to headaches, gall bladder disease, blood disorders and a lowered immune system.

Breast cancer

Breast cancer just won't go away. The statistics relating to the incidence of breast cancer as a result of taking the Pill simply are not reliable as most of the early testing was done in such a haphazard way that the results would not bear the scrutiny of modern laboratory technicians. In most cases the tests were carried out using false controls i.e. women who claimed never to have been exposed to hormone treatments had in fact at some time been given oestrogen or progesterone. As part of the whole debate has to do with the long-term consequences of taking these hormones this is an absurdity.

The number of women who have stopped taking the drug and have later developed cancer has been used as a statistic to show that the Pill can *protect* against cancer. The incidence of cancers in Western women has neatly kept pace with the introduction into the culture of hormone treatment. While breast cancer was certainly well enough known before the advent of the Pill, the drug is quite the most likely agent implicated in the extraordinarily dramatic rise in malignant disease. This suggests something else: that taking heredity into consideration when prescribing hormonal contraceptives is an insufficient strategy. There are many cases of breast and cervical cancers that occur in women with a less than average incidence in the family history. A study published in *The Lancet* in 1983 (Prof. M. Pike) demonstrated that high-progesterone pills are likely to create a higher risk of breast cancer. It also showed that women who had taken the Pill for five to six years before the age of twenty-five were considerably more likely to develop cancer than those who began later. This was the third such study to prove that women who started the Pill young and before their first pregnancy were far more likely to develop cancer and that the risk increased with prolonged use of the drug. There have been many more studies since and ones that directly contradict these findings. Nevertheless, it appears that those who are particularly susceptible to the carcinogenic state (i.e. those who do have a strong hereditary link with cancer – see Part III: Cancer) tend to produce their symptoms relatively quickly while others, who take the Pill for considerably longer with no apparent side effects, are lulled into a false sense of security. Their constitutions are strong enough to maintain a status quo despite the external influence of the drug. They continue to take the Pill, sometimes for fifteen years or more, gradually increasing the risk. What too few realise is that such women develop cancer after they reach the meno-pause and when they have stopped taking the drug which is why the finger of blame is not pointed at the Pill.

Cervical cancer
The story of cervical cancer is much the same as that of breast cancer. Oes-trogen is the miscreant here and causes predisposing pathology such as pelvic inflammatory disease, endometriosis, fibroids and adenomyosis (a benign ingrowth of the endometrium into the muscle of the womb). With the suppression of such conditions cancer of the womb becomes signifi-cantly more likely. Ovarian cancer, one of the most feared, used to be more common in older women. Today 80 per cent of those who develop the symptoms have taken the Pill. As oestrogen and progesterone are sex hor-mones specifically targeted at the generative organs by the drug it is hardly surprising that they should bear the brunt of the ultimate disease condition, where cells lose their integrity and turn rogue.

Metabolising carbohydrates

Glucose is the end product of carbohydrate metabolism and its purpose is to provide energy. If there is more in the system than is immediately neces-sary then it is stored in the liver and muscles as glycogen for use as needed. It is also converted to fat that is stored as adipose tissue. What controls the utilisation of glucose is insulin, a protein hormone that is secreted by the pancreas. If there is too much glucose in the system for the insulin to cope with then the risk of developing late onset diabetes is considerably increased. (This form of diabetes is characterised by extreme thirst, hunger, progressive weakness, emaciation, frequent urination, breathlessness, aci-dosis and a tendency for the skin not to heal. It is not necessarily severe or dangerous and is often controlled by diet when it is mild.)

Progesterone can raise blood sugar and cause a resistance to insulin. It is not surprising to learn of a study carried out at St Mary's Hospital in 1966[6] which showed that as many as one in five women who were taking different versions of the Pill had abnormally high levels of blood sugar, nor that it had been observed that late onset diabetes had been caused by the Pill in a proportion of women. Yet diabetes is not mentioned in the *BNF* as either a side effect of or a contraindication against taking the Pill. This is important because there are no guidelines to help judge whether a woman is susceptible to developing this condition or not. Furthermore, diabetes can be associated with diseases of the blood vessels which have already been mentioned above as one of the major side effects. Women who have a family history of diabetes or whose mothers had diabetes of pregnancy should be given cautionary advice if they are determined to go on the Pill.

Women who have taken the Pill before becoming pregnant may go on to develop diabetes of pregnancy and menopausal women who used to take the Pill might produce late onset diabetes as a chronic result of the contraceptive, even long after the chemicals themselves have been excreted.

Smoking and the Pill

Don't smoke and take the Pill! Those who both smoke and take the Pill do run a greater risk of either vascular disease or cancer, particularly of the cervix – and the risks vastly increase, the earlier one started and the longer one continues. Studies in Britain and America[7] have shown that nicotine in the bloodstream will more than double any risks run by taking oral contraceptives. It becomes unimaginably hard for a natural therapy practitioner to treat the patient in whom the two maintaining causes exist together. As we shall see when we look at some cases, treating a patient who is on the Pill or who has taken the Pill can be accomplished relatively easily but when the addiction to nicotine is thrown into the works things become far more complicated. This is not necessarily to do with attempting to correct the altered biochemistry – though that is without doubt a factor – but with addiction per se which is one of the hardest conditions to treat in anyone. (See Part III The Miasms – Sycosis.)

Allergies, intolerance and the Pill

Just as our bodies can adapt to injuries that create slight (or greater) imbalances in the musculoskeletal structure, so too they can adjust when potentially harmful substances are introduced into the body. For example, if you drink enough alcohol each day your system will tolerate it to the extent that eventually you would need quite a lot more to make you drunk. If you drink coffee every day you will notice that it no longer provides the buzz it once gave you. The body arrives at a biochemical status quo. What are missing are the warning symptoms. All is apparently well in the house but the cellar might be flooding.

Women taking the Pill often feel comparatively well for some years. They don't associate with the Pill acute episodes that begin to happen: perhaps fits of sneezing and cold symptoms that never quite go away or recurrent sinusitis. It is frequently the case that women taking oral contraceptives start to produce allergic reactions to a variety of different things – depending on their biochemical and hereditary make-up. (See Part III on the miasms for a fuller study of hereditary influences.)

Oestrogen tends to increase the presence of antibodies. For this reason many suffer from morning sickness in the form of food intolerance for the first three months of pregnancy. Progesterone lowers antibody levels so, when there is an abundance of both hormones towards the end of pregnancy, food should no longer present such a problem. Levels of both hormones drop sharply after giving birth which is a prime time for women to produce the first signs of allergic reactions. The most common are rhinitis, sinusitis or hay fever. Reactions are far more likely to happen in women who have taken the Pill as the body has to adjust to both the post-partum state and to the absence of the Pill (which is not recommended to be taken while breast feeding). The body has to remember what it should be doing to cope biochemically but with the handicap that the pituitary had been accustomed to being instructed to produce pregnancy reactions on a monthly basis.

Other allergies include vaginal thrush, cystitis or more generalised candida – a condition caused by the presence of a fungal type infection that can invade any part of the body though it is most often associated with the pelvic organs. As progesterone tends to dry up mucous secretions, the vulnerable membranes of the vagina and mouth become hospitable places for viral and bacterial infection to develop. Chlamydia, trichomonas and other sexually transmitted diseases become greater hazards – though manifestation of any of these does depend on the individual's susceptibility. (See Part III on the miasms.)

Many women taking the Pill complain of more frequent bouts of colds or 'flu or even that they have persistent symptoms of a cold that will not 'come out'. Others complain of becoming intolerant of acid fruit. Some can no longer take dairy products without feeling unwell. Yet others begin to complain of heartburn and acidity. Alcohol starts to become a problem for some and they suffer from biliousness and headaches if they have more than a glass of wine. There are those who show no greater sign of distress than an intolerance to their usual hot cups of tea (which now leave a nasty taste in the mouth and cause frequent calls to the bathroom) and there are those who suffer intolerably from the slightest overindulgence in rich food. It cannot be known how anyone who does not fall into the very obvious categories listed by the *BNF* would react to taking the Pill; at least, not without an extensive case study of every aspect of constitution and heredity.

Who suffers?

The point is that every woman who takes hormone therapy is affected and her hormone system is being changed either subtly or grossly and, more often than not, permanently. The stronger and more efficient her constitution, the better able is her system to cope with the imposed divergence from her own norm. The weaker and therefore more susceptible the person, the more of a threat to the natural status quo the Pill becomes. The strong ones may have an enviable ability to adapt but they are often lulled into a false sense of security by their own strength. They do not realise that their bodies do a magnificent job of adaptation but at a price: these are the women who might well have a very prolonged menopause – sometimes as many as ten years of hot flushes and mood swings; if these stop it is often because the body has found this, energetically, to be too expensive a way of manifesting symptoms and now begins to produce disease of the heart and circulation or possibly even cancer. The women on the Pill who are best off are those who realise that the drug is causing some bodily malfunction and decide to drop it.

Would that we could leave it there. The least-known potential side effects of the oral contraceptive and yet the most serious of all are those that might be affecting the gene pool of each successive generation. If the administration of artificial hormones can affect the genetic blueprint of any child born to a mother who has taken the Pill then the genetic predisposition to produce serious and potentially fatal diseases becomes a familial pattern of pathology. Not only that but any new pathological patterns, having been imposed from outside the body, would have no immediate internal self-healing answer. It would need possibly several generations of children to be kept off allopathic medicine for the self-healing mechanism to find a way of undoing such negative patterns. This would be unlikely as heavy-duty pathology is usually (through fear) taken to allopaths for suppression which in turn sends the wrong message to be stored in the genes: what is left unresolved by one generation will, in one way or another, be repeated in the next until either an internal solution is established or the line dies out.

Why should we consider this? Few if any are suggesting that we face such a genetic Armageddon. For homoeopaths the answer must be that they need to be aware of drug reactions in the children of those who took them, in order to see as whole a picture as possible on which to prescribe. Another reason for looking at this is that scientists are, despite their vociferous demands that everything should be tested under the strictest conditions, notoriously lax about their own rules when they have a 'eureka' moment. Their excitement of discovery throws them into a frenzy of experimentation and they tend, historically, to rush into the market place to sell their wares before they are ready to be sold. The Pill itself was a prime example. Thalidomide was another; the Salk polio vaccine yet another.

A less well-known one was the synthetic oestrogen, diethylstilbestrol – DES for short. This was an early hormone drug used to prevent miscarriage. Introduced in the 1940s it was shown to be unable to prevent miscarriage by 1953 but was still administered for this purpose till the 1970s. Then in 1971 an American doctor published a paper[8] showing that DES was directly related to cancer of the vagina in teenage girls born to mothers who had taken the drug earlier in life. (Foetuses exposed to drugs that divert the course of natural growth patterns are at considerable risk of later pathology.) Some one million women had taken DES before the discovery that a rare cancer of the glandular tissue of the walls of the vagina was becoming more common. It was shown that 60 per cent of women exposed to DES in early foetal life had increased vaginal gland tissue. Such tissue was regarded as precancerous even though it was benign because it is common to find it around tumours. Eventually it was revealed that early foetal exposure to DES caused miscarriage, stillbirth, premature labour and sterility in women and genital malformation, abnormal semen, sterility and cancer of the testes in men[9].

This horror story serves to remind us that none of us really knows what we are doing to future generations of children by the continued use of synthetic oral contraceptives. Even though the dosages of oestrogen and progesterone are minimal these days it is still more than the body would ever need and it is still given to trick the body into believing something that is unnatural. Furthermore, women are not taking a human secretion when they ingest the progestogen in the Pill. They are taking an artificially produced chemical derived from plant fats: an ersatz hormone. As its first chemical effect in the body is to block the natural progesterone receptors there are none of the body's phenomenally subtle failsafe mechanisms to help if and when the synthetic drug starts to rock the boat.

What more is there to add?

The above goes some way to explain those side effects that should be common knowledge and to identify potential conditions that any homoeopath might be asked to treat. Many women who consult their health practitioners (orthodox or alternative) may not realise that they are complaining about the direct or indirect effects of the synthetic hormones they take daily. There are yet more who do not realise that they are suffering from a complaint that arose because they *used to* take the Pill. The patient does not make the connection between cause and effect and, if the causative agent has been removed, it is even less likely that they do so.

It behoves all practitioners to familiarise themselves with every aspect of the abuse of the hormone system caused by the Pill because without doing so they will be unable to effect positive changes in their women patients and will be reduced to palliating or suppressing symptoms. It is so often necessary to focus homoeopathic treatment directly towards antidoting the side effects of the Pill when dealing with the resulting pathology because although the body creates symptoms that may well indicate this or that remedy quite clearly, it is the *shock* of the assault on the system created by the drug that prevents any long-term rebalancing of health.

Antidoting the effects of the Pill

None of the foregoing information would be of much use in a book such as this unless it could be followed by clinical (and therefore empirical) evidence that showed that homoeopathy was capable of relieving patients from the distress that had its aetiology in taking the Pill.

Eliza, a woman of forty-three, came for treatment. She said that she had never really been well since she took the Pill when she was nineteen. She had taken it for a few months only before becoming aware that she felt it was harming her. Although she had flirted with homoeopathy for some time and had learnt how to use remedies such as *Sepia* and *Pulsatilla* for PMT she had decided to take her treatment more seriously now as she was worried about her general health.

There were times, she said, when she *"could kill"*. For this she took *Sepia*, which relieved the worst of the symptom but it never prevented it from coming back from time to time. For two days before each period – which came every three weeks – she felt as if she *"was not on this planet"*. A headache, a brown bloody discharge and clots sometimes accompanied this feeling. The period lasted seven days and was invariably painful. The flow of menstrual blood was always intermittent but at least when it came the symptoms of the otherwise ever-present candida stopped. (These included itching and a white discharge like cottage cheese.) She also said that she had become allergic to antibiotics and certain food additives.

She was worried about her memory: she had little recall of anything that she had just said or done and found it very hard to bring out quite simple words and expressions. Another problem she found distressing was that she was agoraphobic. This was also something that she could relate back to her short time on the Pill, she explained. When she started taking it she soon felt *"uneasy going about in the street"*; she had felt this way ever since though she was fine if she was with a companion. She had had two nervous breakdowns, one in her twenties and the other in her late thirties. Both, she felt, were to do with her *"appalling lack of confidence"*. (As a child she had not lacked confidence being one of several siblings that enjoyed a normal and gregarious upbringing in a country community.)

Eliza was given *Oopherinum*. This is a remedy made from the trituration of the expressed fluid of a sheep's ovary. Repellent though this sounds it is recognised as a remedy that, when other indications are there, has the power to cause the Vital Force of the patient to reverse the negative process begun by taking the Pill. It is not the only remedy to do this. In this case it was prescribed partly on the basis (and this might seem ridiculously fanciful) of the fact that Eliza was a very suggestible person in her present state, one that had existed since she started the Pill – which she had done at the prompting of her then boyfriend. (Sheep are amongst the most easily cowed of animals.) The results spoke for themselves.

When she returned she had had a period at four weeks and had felt as if her uterus contracted. There were no clots or brown discharge. The palms of her hands were itching and *"I'm shedding skin all over!"* (Often a very positive sign of a remedy working.)

She now complained that her body temperature had risen and that she often felt hot in the head. This brought on copious amounts of catarrh in her sinuses. In addition she had become more aware of her *"creaky joints"* and a lower backache that previously had been a background problem. She was given *Thuja*, a remedy that is often called for in cases where the endocrine system is out of balance and where there are arthritic tendencies.

At her third visit she mentioned that the period symptoms had reverted somewhat to their old pattern and that all her joints hurt, especially her lower back. Nevertheless, what she spent most of her time talking about was her job. She wanted to give up teaching. She hated the preparation work that she nevertheless did overconscientiously as she dreaded getting anything wrong. She felt that she was failing all the time, not just herself but also her pupils. She was then given *Lycopodium*. This is a remedy that covers a sense of imminent failure, a perpetual anticipation or even dread of not doing things the right way or well enough. When she returned for the fourth appointment she had changed: she was feeling very well and had had no return of any of the symptoms that she complained of at the first consultation. None of her joints hurt and she felt that she was no longer inarticulate in a conversation. Her friends had noticed that she was far better company and more lively. She had arranged to go on holiday to Egypt. *"I'd never have dared go on my own before!"*

In this second case the aetiology of the complaint was just as indisputable.

> Sally suffered from cluster migraines. They came on every day of her life and every third one was so severe that she would vomit and faint. The pain *"comes in waves like an electrical pulse and it makes me terribly panicky"*. She would become very hot and photophobic. She had found that both chocolate and prawns would aggravate her condition. This had all begun fourteen years before when she had been prescribed the Pill and had taken the first dose. She never took another as the headaches had started that same day.
>
> Sally took *Pulsatilla*. This prescription was not based on the fact that she had never been well since the Pill but on her general state and the acute symptoms of the migraines. This was a case where the constitution and the complaint were covered by the same remedy – not always so in those who suffer the consequences of taking hormone therapy but more likely to be so in those with very good constitutions.
>
> After the remedy Sally had a ten-day respite from the migraine, something she had not experienced for fourteen years. Then the head pain returned but it did not last as long as it had before. She said that, *"when I took that remedy I just got in the car and I went round all the lanes screaming and screaming. I just screamed my head off and I cried and cried. It was such a relief!"*
>
> She was given *Pulsatilla* to take once per week. It seemed that she had run out of steam on the first dose. When she returned she said, *"It seems so unreal but I feel well. So well that I'm almost scared of feeling like this."*
>
> Nevertheless, she did still have some symptoms of hormonal imbalance. She was sweating an unusual amount (for her) – a good sign – and her stools were extremely foul smelling. Her moods were fickle and *"I can't stop feeling randy"*. She repeated that things seemed so unreal. This meagre symptom picture suggested *Thuja*. The result was that she was left without any of the symptoms that she had started to suffer from the Pill and now felt *"at peace with myself"*. She has remained well since.

The third case illustrates more specific pathology in a case in which the Pill predominates as a maintaining cause.

> Frances had been diagnosed with fibroids. She had gone to her doctor because her menstrual cycle was short, heavy and exhausting. Following tests, she was told that she had several fibroids; one the size of an orange

on the left side of the uterus and at least three others that were much smaller. It was the large fibroid that was causing the heavy blood loss and the dragging pains that she experienced before each period. She also suffered cramping pains with sharp twinges in the region of her left ovary every other month.

Frances had other symptoms that distressed her: the menstrual flow was characterised by bright red blood with large dark clots *"that look like bits of chopped liver"*. These tended to frighten her and added to her general fear of disease. In addition, Frances found that intercourse was very painful: she would feel contractions and stabbing sensations. There were two other physical symptoms significant in the choice of prescription because they were 'strange, rare and peculiar'. The first was that her menstrual flow all but stopped when she stood up and moved about and flowed more at night when she was lying down. The second was that she had a persistent pain in her sacrum that felt as if it penetrated right through to her pubic bone.

With the physical 'picture' of her symptoms there was an emotional state that confirmed the only possible choice of remedy: only *Sabina,* the juniper tree, covers these peculiar pains and a psychological state of chronic apprehension and dejection. She was given *Sabina* 30 to be taken three times each week for a month after which she was to return for a follow-up appointment.

At her second interview Frances seemed brighter and more animated. She volunteered more information about herself than she had been willing to do on the first visit. She felt that the remedy had been *"doing something but I'm not sure quite what"*. Her period was just as heavy but there were fewer clots: *"I'm pleased about that!"*. The pains were the same but *"I didn't feel nearly so washed out afterwards"*. She asked why she had been prescribed the *Sabina*; on being told that it was a remedy that might influence her system to restore hormone balance and eliminate the fibroids, she declared her determination to continue treatment despite the fact that progress was not particularly marked. As she was gathering up her belongings before leaving, she said in an offhand way,

"Of course, you know, I've never really felt well since I went on the Pill. I can't think why I did really but then we all did in those days, didn't we? It's what was normal."

She was invited to sit down again and explain further.

"There's nothing else to say really. It just made me feel so unwell. I had bad leg aches and headaches and I put on weight. I couldn't control my moods; they swung about all over the place. I wasn't me, if you know what I mean. And I haven't had anywhere like the same energy I used to have. A bit sad really when you think about it."

At the first interview, the practitioner had assumed that because the symptom picture was so obviously covered by *Sabina*, it was not necessary to look further. By hearing what Frances had to say about the origins of her problem, another facet of her condition had been revealed; here was the true maintaining cause and one that had to be addressed remedially before the *Sabina* could be expected to effect full healing. Frances went home with more *Sabina* and a packet of 3 doses of *Folliculinum* 1M.

Folliculinum is made from the natural secretion of a human ovarian follicle. It has become a major addition to the homoeopath's tool kit ever since it was introduced in the 1970s having been studied first only as recently as the 1950s. Why it is so important is that it is probably the first remedy to consider in treating women who have suffered as a result of hormone therapy. In many respects it is very similar to *Oopherinum* though the latter is less widely used and seems to be of more service in post-menopausal women – though this may prove to be a matter of preference on the part of different practitioners.

When Frances returned in approximately six weeks she had a lot to tell. Her periods were far less painful; the bleeding was less profuse and much less clotted; her mood swings were almost non-existent – her partner had noticed that she was far less disagreeable and had maintained her sense of humour. She still felt that there was more work to be done. The dragging sensation and pain on intercourse were still ongoing though not quite as marked. She still felt tired though less often.

"The main thing, though, is that I feel hopeful. Something is happening and I can really feel it. I want to go and do things; I don't want to crash out every night. I used to be a 'doer'. Well, now I feel more like that again. And something else, I really like my husband; I was always nit-picking and I hate that about myself. I don't know if that's got anything to do with the remedies but I know I don't want to go back to how it was."

251

Over the course of the next year Frances made steady progress, at first with the *Sabina* 30 and then with the 200th potency. She decided to go for a check-up and a cervical smear test at her doctor's surgery. She quizzed the nurse about the fibroids but they were not detectable on palpation of the abdomen. Frances decided not to go back for an ultrasound scan. She is content with how well she feels now that none of the symptoms she first came with exist.

Folliculinum

What is most striking about *Folliculinum* is that the mental/emotional aspect of the remedy should be so close to the state that many women feel themselves to be in after having taken oral contraceptives for any length of time. This emotional state, which has several facets to it, has never been considered by allopathy in any of the major studies that have been used to support the efficacy and safety of the Pill. This is partly because popular journalism has maintained the myth that oral contraception for women has given them freedom commensurate with men's. This is patently not true except, it can still be argued, in the early years of sexual activity before any long-term partnership becomes a serious consideration – precisely the years when they are at their most vulnerable to disease as a result of having frequent sexual partners.

So what does this state look like? How do we recognise someone (homoeopathically speaking) who needs this remedy? There are a number of themes that make up this condition. The first is that the woman does not feel in control of her cycle or of the natural rhythms of her body. She feels that something has been suppressed. This can first be evident in her lack of libido. Many women on the Pill describe their conjugal relationship in the following terms, *"I love my husband very much but I just don't get turned on as I did. Sex is a chore now but I don't know why; it never used to be. All I want to do when I get to bed is to sleep."*

She notices that she has less energy, sometimes far less. As it can happen gradually the process is insidious. She may not relate the lethargy to the altered hormone cycle. This leads to a feeling that though she has to continue working at the same rate as before she has fewer reserves. By the end of each day she is too tired to do more than slump in front of the television or go to bed early. Yet she recognises that others continue to expect the same of her as she was achieving before. Most women who continue to take the Pill or who go back to it once they have had a child also have jobs. Our patient goes out to work and comes home to work as well. Very soon – and this might be within four or five years of settling into a partnership or marriage – she begins to lose her self-respect. She begins to feel less sure of her confidence and her ability to make even quite ordinary decisions. She saves her dwindling energy for the chores: shopping, cooking, washing and making sure the children are organised. She no longer puts herself first in any situation. Even if she becomes angry about things she quickly backtracks, feeling guilty and apologetic. She feels, by now, colourless and drained. Sometimes there is a variation on the theme: she might become addicted to putting others first. She does not stop at making sure that her husband and children are all organised but begins to do the same for needy friends or relatives. Anything to put off the time when she might have a moment to look at herself. As this road gets harder to travel so she feels more and more like a 'doormat'. No longer is her life her own but it seems to belong to everybody else. Husband, children and friends can seem like emotional parasites feeding off her.

Another variation is of the businesswoman who does not have the same domestic picture. She pours all her considerable energies into the aggression of the marketplace. She becomes less feeling in a feminine sense – more yang than yin. She puts herself at the disposal of the forces of commerce, of institutions or corporations. The Pill affords her the security of knowing that pregnancy would never interfere with the pattern and, as children do not come into the picture, sex becomes an enjoyable end in itself; but this can make her feel increasingly less of a woman and more of an object. Though she may not lose her sense of identity in business she can and often does feel that personally. Her appearance may well become more androgynous and her temper more aggressive. Her manner might become harder, more masculine. Her creative life belongs to the boss or to the school or the bank. As she approaches the menopause she begins to avoid looking at the gaps in her life. Eventually, it is a series of minor illnesses that oblige her to begin to take stock. While none of this might affect a woman with a genuinely corporate or commercial mind, it certainly does those who have found their way into the marketplace through following trends and parental influences.

Any woman who fits these generalised descriptions will have their individual differences but they will all eventually agree in feeling less than they once were in terms of energy and creative potential. The major thing that most of them have in common is that they take or have taken synthetic hormones. The feelings of being out of control of one's body, of living according to the expectations of others, of living life on an energy overdraft, of losing one's sense of individuality are all common to those who have taken the Pill. None of this would be news to practising homoeopaths who are asked to deal with such cases many times in a year. *Folliculinum* is called upon to put into effect the patients' self-healing in a significant proportion of them.

As if to confirm the value of this remedy in reversing the negative effects of oral contraceptives, *Folliculinum* also covers almost all the expected physical symptoms. There are not only the typical, recurrent gynaecological symptoms such as abdominal pains at ovulation, at the period and even between, pains in the breast with swelling, clots and dark, unpleasant (even rank smelling) blood but also chronic ones such as fibroids, cysts on the ovaries, endometriosis and breast lumps. Not only this but also *Folliculinum* is a wonderfully effective remedy for those going through the menopause – it has proved itself of the greatest value in cases of persistent hot flushes, flooding, debility, irregular bleeds and loss of libido, hair and skin tone. It has also been successfully used in cases in which women have developed the early signs of osteoporosis when other indications have been present.

Folliculinum, then, is a major reason for now stating unequivocally just how damaging the Pill is. By association, hormone replacement therapy (HRT) for perimenopausal (those who are showing early signs of the change) and menopausal women should come under a similar degree of scrutiny. Almost everything that has been said about the negative effects of the Pill can also be levelled at HRT. *Folliculinum* is also useful, when indicated, as a remedy for the relief of symptoms that derive from this interference in the natural and necessary process of the menopause. It seems to have passed the medical profession by that the menopause is as important a stage of life as puberty. Pre-empting it with medication is cosmetic at best; foolhardy and dangerous at worst. *Folliculinum* is a cause for celebration among homoeopaths as it is a remedy that unquestionably can be used when other indicated remedies fail, in cases where there is a block to cure of hormonal origin – especially when that block was one imposed by hormone-related drugs.

Finally, one other aspect of *Folliculinum* is worthy of note: it is invaluable in treating women who have felt obliged to take the 'morning-after' pill. This drug can leave a wake of very unpleasant side effects. To meet women who have been relieved of the suffering and of the concern for their long-term health from this vicious drug is to realise that some of the worst effects of medical chemistry can be successfully self-healed.

CHAPTER 13

DENTAL AMALGAM

Mixed metal fillings in your teeth

Sooner or later, most of us develop tooth decay that needs surgical intervention. The cause of the decay is usually ignored or blamed on poor diet or too many sweets or occasionally on heredity. The decay is drilled out and a filling is used to stop up the hole. The filling material that is used more often than not is of a metal compound known as amalgam. It consists of 50 per cent mercury, 35 per cent silver, 9 per cent tin, 6 per cent copper and a trace of zinc. (These proportions can vary.) In Britain amalgam is considered both safe and effective by dentists adhering to the advice of the British Dental Association. It is relatively cheap and easy to use.

Conventional dentists say that amalgam has been used for over a century and has been used successfully to fill the teeth of millions of patients who would otherwise have suffered considerable pain and loss of teeth. In the United States alone some 100 million fillings are put in place annually. It is this long-term use and the durability of the material that recommends it to the dental profession. There is no need to change what has worked so well for so long when so little evidence of any harmful side effects has been brought to light. Furthermore, the alternatives that are available are far more difficult to use, more expensive and last less time.

If it is so failsafe, why are there dentists who refuse to use amalgam? Why are there patients who are demanding to have their old fillings replaced with the new alternatives? Why do alternative health practitioners all agree that amalgam fillings are not only injurious to health but also a major reason why their patients might not get better? More sinisterly, why do those whose jobs it is to remove the amalgam waste from dentists' surgeries wear such elaborate protective clothing? Why are there posters in doctors' surgeries of some European countries forbidding the use of amalgam in pregnant women?

A potted history of mercury fillings

Of the five metals in the compound it is mercury that causes the debate. A little history sheds some light on this extraordinary metal. Mercury has been used in medicine for centuries. The silver liquid metal was extracted by alchemists from cinnabar ore as early as the Middle Ages. It interested them particularly as it had curious properties: it would disappear into vapour if warmed and it would dissolve the powders of other metals if heated to room temperature. It was also discovered that it would expand when warmed within a vacuum. The Chinese were the first to use mercury mixed into a paste to fill decayed teeth as early as the seventh century.

In Europe, gold and silver were often employed as filling materials but these were expensive and beyond the pockets of a lot of patients. Lead, tin and cement were also used. However, by the early 1800s a composite of mercury, silver and copper was increasingly more popular. The most serious problems that were noticed were that the fillings would expand after being placed and would crack the filled teeth. Patients would complain that their 'bite' was altered by the enlarged filling. Fillings would also fall out as mercury can contract as readily as it expands. It was discovered in the mid 1800s that the addition of tin to the composition prevented the mercury from being as volatile as it would normally be. This ensured its ascendancy as the material of choice. This was not without controversy.

Amalgam was first introduced into North America in the 1830s. By 1845 there was considerable concern that the mercury in the compound, long known as a dangerous poison if ingested, was too much of a hazard to health. Amalgam was swiftly proscribed in a resolution of the American Society of Dental Surgeons. This situation was short lived and the newly formed American Dental Association declared amalgam safe and by the late 1800s the formula that is still in use today was being widely used. Some ten generations of patients have now experienced the dubious benefits of this potentially dangerous compound.

Doubts and scepticism have arisen periodically in one country or another but so successful and commercially viable is amalgam that it wasn't until the 1980s and 1990s that its safety was seriously challenged. Now, by the early twenty-first century, the days of amalgam are numbered even though the majority of dentists in Britain and America still advocate its use. There is, though, a growing body of evidence that the mercury in fillings contributes significantly and in a number of different ways to the steady and insidious undermining of health. It is also becoming clear that it is capable of causing serious damage to children through its influence on foetal development.

Is it safe?

A dental assistant came for treatment. Tracy was twenty-six and she had been suffering her symptoms for some two and a half years. The list of ailments was daunting: extreme swings of temperature, profuse sweating (particularly at night), heartburn, persistent gastric disturbance with nausea and vomiting of foul, acid tasting mucus, mouth ulcers, extreme thirst, headaches and progressive weakness and emaciation. She said that she would go to bed freezing cold only to wake up within half an hour with sweats and feverish hot flushes. This would quickly pass when she flung the covers off and she would start to shiver. She would have to change her nightwear and the bottom sheet as they would be soaked. What was more was that the linen would be stained slightly yellow and be stiff as if overly starched. She suffered constantly from acid rising from her stomach and this would burn her throat and make her feel sick. The mouth ulcers were large, painful and caused her breath to smell cadaverous. She dribbled at night and complained that she always had a profuse amount of saliva in her mouth. This was strange when considered along with the extreme thirst. (She also mentioned that she always wanted to put ice in the water – another strange symptom given that she so often felt miserably cold.) She had lost a lot of weight and appeared gaunt in the face. Her arms were thin and her fingers excessively bony. She was constantly tired and her headaches came on a daily basis. Tracy also suffered from eczema which she had had as a child. This had gone away completely by the time she was thirteen but it had returned with a vengeance in the last six months.

She was asked what she thought had triggered her problems. She replied that she could not be sure but that she felt that the symptoms had gradually increased since she began working with her present employer some three and a half years before. As part of her job she was required to prepare the dental amalgam for patients who had come in for a filling. She had never done this for her two previous employers. She was also asked if she had any fillings herself. *"No, my teeth were always really good but since I've been ill I feel that they have been very sensitive. I sometimes find it agony to eat."*

Tracy's symptoms are a veritable compendium of what one might expect from mercury poisoning. Though the toxic effects of the poison can cause many other symptoms her description is a perfect match and it is shared to some lesser or greater degree by many. The likely cause was explained to her and she felt vindicated even though her employer had ridiculed her suggestion. (He had never suffered such symptoms and he had always prepared the amalgam for himself before she had come to his practice.) She continued to prepare the amalgam but insisted that she wore protective rubber gloves from then on. She also took *Mercurius Solubilis*, the homoeopathically prepared remedy of the metal. She gradually began to improve over the next four months with an abatement of all the symptoms with the exception of the eczema which continued to weep and crust – her skin became the organ of elimination. (For someone suffering from mercury poisoning four months was a remarkably short time to show such improvement.)

Jolie was an art student with a bad history of teeth problems. Every double tooth in her head had a large amalgam filling in it. Her symptom picture was slightly different from Tracy's: she vomited after every meal (though she suffered no nausea), she was becoming progressively more and more emaciated being quite unable to put on any weight. She had recurrent mouth ulcers and tooth abscesses. She had been on antibiotics too frequently to count. Her thirst was prodigious and her night sweats were just as bad. She also suffered from foul breath, an unpleasant metallic taste in her mouth and profuse salivation. She felt that there was a permanent slime around her teeth which she was unable to remove however often she brushed her teeth. She always felt much worse at night and this meant that her sleep was disturbed. By morning she felt exhausted.

She was rarely free of what felt like a 'fluey' cold. She had mood swings: one moment she might feel pathetically feeble and the next she would be ready to go out and have fun. She could be snappy or she could be childish by turns. The mouth ulcers were large and grey coloured and sometimes bled. What concerned her most were the abscesses. Whenever she developed an abscess her tonsils would swell enormously and threaten to close her throat. They would go dark red and become so painful that she could not swallow despite her strong thirst. Her glands – even those of the abdomen, the mesenteric glands – would always be swollen and painful. Her tongue would thicken and become stiff and the indentation marks from her teeth would be imprinted along its edge.

This is another typical picture of mercury poisoning. Though such a case might present itself without the aetiology of amalgam fillings, these days it is far more common than not for the patient to have a head full of them.

Jolie took some three and a half years to begin to show improvement that was convincing and it was only after she had had all the amalgams removed that any remedies worked at all satisfactorily. Throughout that time she was given varying doses of *Mercury* at frequent intervals. Sometimes she would need the remedy in one of its several variants: *Mercurius Iodatus Flavus* or *Mercurius Iodatus Ruber*. (These two have affinities for symptoms that favour one or other side of the throat.) She would always have an acute flare-up after one of the fillings was removed – she had them taken out one at a time with at least two-month intervals between and under the strictest protocol.

After four years homoeopathic hard work she no longer had tooth abscesses or mouth ulcers. She no longer had a foul taste in her mouth and nor did she have night sweats that made her feel debilitated. She slept better and she could eat well though she still had an inclination to vomit after eating a main meal. Her immune system worked better and she did not fall foul of every virus going the rounds at work. She put on weight and her cheeks filled out and her colouring changed from coffin lead to a normal pink though when tired she could have dark rings beneath the eyes as she had had permanently before.

A third case is necessary because this one illustrates that the older a filling gets the more dangerous it becomes.

Mary, a farmer's wife, was approaching the change of life and was worried about her periods. She felt that they went on for too long, were too irregular for someone who had always been used to a monthly cycle and *"not right"* in the sense that she passed a lot of very dark, foul smelling clotted blood. It was not immediately apparent that she needed *Mercury*, the remedy, or that it was her fillings that were the maintaining cause of her ill health. There was no neat package of symptoms as there had been in the other two cases. Only gradually, over several interviews did it become evident that she too had night sweats and variations of temperature. Then she mentioned that she had heartburn and, worst of all, intolerable vaginal itching especially once she had become warm in bed. This was so bad that intercourse was painful due to the rawness of the skin where she had not been able to stop scratching. Eight months after her first appointment it was obvious that the indicated remedies did little or no good and that the amalgams were the probable cause of the signal lack of success.

Mary went to her dentist and asked him to remove all her metal fillings. He advised her strongly not to do this and told her that her fillings could not possibly be responsible for her health problems. He also said that indiscriminate removal of the amalgams could be more dangerous than leaving them in; the odd logic of which he signally failed to see. So strong was his manner that she felt obliged to change to a more sympathetic practitioner. Her fillings were removed over the period of a year. At the end of it she claimed to have felt some benefit in spite of still suffering most of the symptoms albeit less fiercely.

In her case she needed another remedy that antidotes the effects of mercury poisoning: *Hepar Sulphuricum*. Patients who need this remedy are extremely sensitive to the cold, the wind and noise in general. They become irritable and intolerant of any fuss. They prefer to be left alone so that they can sit quietly and without any movement. They appreciate warming drinks and lots of blankets. They feel that any pain that they suffer is ten times worse than was ever suffered by anyone else. They become peevish, anxious and truculent by turns. This was how Mary described herself when she was tired and down at the end of each day. With a daily dose of this remedy in a liquid form she gradually got better. The itching disappeared. The periods cleared up and became regular again. She had no more heartburn.

Mary's fillings had been in place for over twenty-five years. Her health problems had not started to manifest until some three years before she came for homoeopathic treatment. It was only after she had had all the fillings removed that she had the thought that her symptoms had begun after she had broken a tooth on a nut. She had gone to the dentist who had drilled out the filling and done a repair job on what was left of the tooth. This too is typical of many patients who have amalgam trouble: they only begin to suffer symptoms after a trauma – which does not necessarily have to be over a tooth. It is as if the trauma triggers the more obvious activity of the poison.

Is mercury safe? No.

How does mercury poison us?

Mercury is an unstable metal. It reacts according to its environment and its reactions occur in two different ways. It reacts to heat and cold and when mixed with other metals. The first result is that when warmed tiny toxic particles are released into its environment in the form of vapour. The second is that there is a galvanic reaction to other metals. This means that when mercury interacts chemically with other metals it behaves like a battery, discharging electricity. As amalgam fillings are a compound of five different metals it goes without saying that those with filled teeth are poisoned by both means: chemically and electrically. While it is easy to understand how chemical poisoning should be avoided, electrical 'poisoning' is rather harder to swallow.

If one has a 'battery' of amalgam in one's teeth, emitting a small but significant current, then the electrical circuit of the body's nervous system can be interrupted. The body produces a natural average of around 3 microamps of electricity to run itself efficiently. The recorded range of electrical output from amalgam fillings is between 0.1 and 10 microamps. If the body's own circuitry is inhibited or 'fused' then every function of the whole is likely to be affected. The source of the body's natural electricity is the medulla at the base of the brain. The amalgam is within a very few centimetres range. If the patient has gold fillings as well the reactions are usually worse.

The combined effects of this electrical and chemical toxicity on the body are truly appalling and it beggars belief that amalgam is still not only in use but advocated by professional bodies.

What does mercury poisoning do?[1]

There is not a single part of the body unaffected by mercury poisoning. What is confusing to researchers is that not everyone shows a textbook reaction. Some will suffer in the way illustrated by the three cases cited. Others will have quite different symptomatic reactions. Many will appear to have no reactions whatever. The following is a resumé of some of the effects, any one of which might well make mercury a maintaining cause.

Mercury and the bacteria harvest

Bacteria normally resident in bowel and mouth are increasingly resistant to amalgam toxicity and to antibiotics. This means that as well as suffering the effects of amalgam fillings one might be playing host to superbugs that do not respond to antibiotic treatment and the destructiveness of mercury. Studies have shown that oral streptococci, enterobacteria and enterococci can all flourish quite well in such a toxic environment despite the use of quite powerful antibiotics. (Perhaps it is not simply *overuse* of antibiotics that has led to their increasing failure rate.) Though homoeopathy eschews the use of antibiotics it is easy to see that if mercury is affecting the body then the electrical if not the chemical toxicity might be powerful enough to prevent remedies from working well or at all. (Bear in mind that homoeopathic remedies are not material in effect but electrical.) While such bacteria are often to be found in the body without giving cause for treatment, once they adapt to a toxic environment generated by the patient's reaction to a poison, the bacteria are unlikely to remain dormant. Streptococcus is often evident in diseases of not just the gums and throat but also in acute kidney disease and lung disease. There are various forms of it and it can also arise as a result of meningitis, mastitis and bowel problems.

Kidney damage

Amalgam toxicity impairs kidney function. The kidneys process the fluids of the body; they filtrate urine in their tiny tubules in order that valuable minerals are retained while waste products are excreted. Mercury interferes with the filtration. It does this by altering the electrolyte balance. This has to do with the way atoms and molecules become positively or negatively charged electrically and whether they bind together or remain free flowing. Mercury toxicity can be responsible for poor response to treatment of kidney disease. It has been estimated that two thirds of the mercury excreted by the kidneys is from amalgam. Other sources of mercury poisoning are fish that have lived in polluted waters, and pesticides. Some cosmetics are also suspect as mercury is sometimes added as a form of preservative. Even more controversial is the fact that mercury is put into certain inoculations so that it is introduced directly into the blood stream[2].

Mercury at home in the brain

Amalgam has been shown to be a potential cause of neurological disorders. This is to be expected as it has long been accepted that the brain absorbs mercury very readily (as do the kidneys and liver.) Studies[3] have shown that traces of mercury and other heavy metals have been found in brain tissue of patients who have died after developing Alzheimer's disease. It was noted that mercury reduces the level of tubulin (a protein essential for the maintenance of tubules that carry nerve tissue) in the brain. It was concluded that mercury toxicity was a contributing factor to the manifestation of the illness. Certainly there have been anecdotal reports that patients showing the early but typical signs of Alzheimer's disease who then had all their amalgam fillings removed went on to recover their mental faculties. What the scientists were unable to tell was whether mercury was the causative factor or a secondary event. As far as homoeopaths would be concerned the latter is the more likely. Not everyone with high readings of mercury in their systems would necessarily develop Alzheimer's. Comparatively small numbers would be likely to do this. However, if there is an inherited predisposition to produce disease with characteristic nerve tissue destruction then the likelihood is that mercury becomes a far more significant threat.

Multiple sclerosis (MS) is another disease in which nerve tissue is progressively damaged. Hal Huggins, author of a well-known book about mercury fillings called *It's All In Your Head*, has treated many cases of MS and records that the majority of them have high levels of mercury poisoning. There have been recorded cases of patients going into more or less permanent remission from the symptoms once they have had their amalgam fillings taken out. In most cases, however, the patients continue to consider themselves as MS patients and do show signs from time to time – particularly when under stress – of the disease. (To understand why this should be see the chapter on the syphilitic miasm in Part III.)

Mercury and infertility

There have been studies[4] done to show the connection between infertility and heavy metals in the body. In one such, by looking at the medical profiles of some 500 infertile women, it was seen that not only was there a relation between the presence of heavy metals and the inability to conceive but also with the pathological conditions that existed among the women, including uterine fibroids, history of miscarriages and other hormonal disorders. What emerged as a result of the tests was the understanding that by introducing a chelating agent (a chemical that binds metal ions to it for the purposes of excretion) the rate of conception was significantly improved.

Whether the heavy metal burden was primarily mercury would be determined by the symptom picture of each individual. This part of the test was not carried out but it is possible that a significant number of women with pathological influences that precluded their ability to conceive would be found to have mercury toxicity. The characteristic reactions of the human body to mercury may be many, varied and confusing, sometimes even hidden to all but those who know what to search for, but the core symptoms sooner or later make themselves manifest.

Mercury can cross the placental barrier and pollute breast milk

Mercury is readily absorbed and stored in the soft organs and the highest amounts are to be found in the liver and kidneys. In tests carried out on sheep and rats it was found that mercury toxicity is passed on to the foetus through the placenta. This causes changes to normal growth patterns of nerve tissue and to behaviour. When this is linked with information on the abnormally high levels of measurable mercury in the blood stream of humans with amalgam fillings, then it is not unreasonable to conclude that mercury poisoning can be implicated in foetal malformations, motor nerve dysfunction, deficiencies in spatial awareness, dyslexia, attention deficit disorder (ADD) and attention deficit and hyperactive disorder (ADHD). It is now well known that there are an increasing number of children with all these problems.

It might be said that the number has not actually increased but our awareness of the problems has greatly improved. Yet it is the character of the results of these problems that tells us that this is not entirely so. Children with dyslexia, dyspraxia (poor physical co-ordination) and attention deficit hyperactivity disorder (and there are many who have all three problems at once) often become highly frustrated and disruptive. They become antisocial in their behaviour patterns. They are unable to relate to others in the usual accepted sense. They become the despair of their parents and their teachers. Such behaviour is far more commonplace now than it was in the middle of the twentieth century. The number of such afflicted children in any classroom continued to rise dramatically in the late 1990s. (No doubt there will soon be studies to show that the rate of the increase was commensurate with that of the number of children suffering from allergies and asthma.)

Another revelation was that breast milk can be polluted by mercury from the mother's fillings. As the baby ingests milk the mercury passes into the digestive system and thence to the blood stream, liver and kidneys. Not only is the foetus affected but the poisoning continues beyond birth into the earliest years of the child's development. As many of the children who are measurably affected by mercury toxicity are also inclined to suffer from intolerance to certain foods and additives, allergies and hay fever or eczema, the symptom picture of most of these patients is likely to be very confused and difficult to diagnose. In homoeopathic terms such patients are difficult to treat because there are so many facets of dyscrasia (pathological condition) that as soon as one aspect is being addressed another comes up to muddy the waters.

It is certainly very common to have to use the *Mercury* remedies for acute conditions in children very frequently – particularly for mouth, gum, throat, ear and gland conditions. Many children have repeated acute bouts of diseases that are characterised by exuding pus (greenish) and blood especially of the ear, nose and skin. This is typical of one type of reaction to mercury poisoning. If the conditions persist and if they are concomitant or in alternation with bouts of mood swings, irritability, unreasonably babyish behaviour, mischievousness and secretiveness then underlying mercury toxicity has to be suspected.

Mercury gets to the heart as well

Reports from tests[5] carried out on patients who have suffered fatal conditions of the heart muscle have shown that the concentration of mercury in the tissue was as much as 22,000 times higher than in those with no heart pathology. Treating patients with cardiomyopathy (disease of the heart muscle) is difficult for any practitioner, orthodox or alternative. If there were to be an underlying maintaining cause like mercury then the situation would become virtually impossible without first eliminating the toxicity.

Testing for Mercury

When the first suspicion occurs that mercury is a maintaining cause it is usually advisable to seek confirmation. This is done in a number of ways with varying degrees of success. Blood tests can show up the toxicity well but you need to have either a doctor who is willing to carry out the tests or private means to pay for them at a specialist clinic. This second option can be expensive.

Hair analysis
Some people prefer to go for hair analysis. Hair samples are sent to a laboratory to find traces of minerals and metals. This is not always accurate as the hair may not necessarily have any trace of mercury. There are computerised machines called Vega testing machines to which one can be wired up that measure every imaginable toxicity. The results, on a printout, provide all

the data one would want on toxicity, allergies, deficiencies and intolerance. There are even more sophisticated 'biofeedback' machines available which tell you not only about the presence of poisons but also suggest and provide prescriptive treatment. Another and usually more accurate method of detecting the presence of the metal is through applied kinesiology.

Kinesiology

Kinesiology is a system of diagnosis through 'muscle testing' which does not rely on machinery. Every part of the body is made up of cells that, though they may be of different shape, size, location or function, possess the same genetic information and whole-body electrodynamic reactivity to negative influences. When a potentially toxic substance is placed within the electrodynamic field of a chosen muscle then the cells that make up that muscle will react by becoming weak if there is toxicity already within the body to which no effective internal positive response has been found. If the challenge has no effect then the muscle remains strong. In other words, if you are being poisoned by mercury and your body has found no internal answer to the problem then your muscles will show weak when the kinesiologist challenges them with mercury. The only time when this might not be a satisfactory test is if there were a stronger toxicity going on. The muscle might react marginally to the mercury but it would show most weakness to whatever is the greatest negative influence. Mercury, if it is there, is usually uppermost but occasionally some other poison such as cadmium or copper can register as a stronger negative influence.

The kinesiologist can give an invaluable second opinion in cases where the diagnosis of mercury poisoning is dubious. It is not, as has been intimated already, always precisely clear that amalgam is responsible for maintaining the ill health of a patient. To advise a patient to have all his or her fillings out without confirmation might be foolhardy. Kinesiologists have another role as well. Just as they can uncover such poisoning, so too can they advise on mineral supplements to be taken in preparation for the removal of the amalgams and suggest dietary changes and supplements that would encourage the swiftest elimination of the toxicity afterwards. This is not an area of expertise that many homoeopaths know about. They are not usually trained in naturopathy and, in general, only have a comparatively sketchy idea of nutrition and biochemistry. Though it would add to the patients' expenses it is worthwhile referring them to kinesiologists who could complement whatever homoeopathic treatment might be indicated.

There are some dentists equipped with milliamp-meters that can detect the tiny electrical charges given off by affected filled teeth. To get a reading can be a useful confirmation of the mercury factor.

Removing dental amalgams

Every time you chew your food you are increasing the amount of leakage of the mercury. The interaction of your saliva with the amalgam and the raised temperature inside your mouth conspire to pour out the vapour at an alarming rate. If a dentist changes one of the fillings then the process of drilling will cause even more toxicity to rush into the system. High-speed drills cause the amalgams to fragment into an infinitesimal number of tiny particles that embed themselves into the gums, soft palate and tongue from where they will migrate to soft organs of the body; and this is not to mention the heavier lumps that chip off and get swallowed. If you keep the amalgams you're damned and if you lose them you're damned – or so it would seem.

All the experts on the removal of amalgam are agreed: if you have the fillings removed then you have to have it done under the strictest protocol to minimise the danger of greatly increased toxicity. To begin with they say that no-one who is pregnant should contemplate such a procedure. (Some suggest that a woman who has mercury poisoning who also wants to conceive should not become pregnant within one year of the removal of her amalgams.) Even before you have any amalgam removed you are usually advised to take nutritional supplements in order to start the process of chelation. The usual recipe includes vitamins A, C and E and selenium; also zinc and magnesium. (It is worth thinking about going to a kinesiologist/nutritionist who would advise on the amounts required for the individual. It can be easy to fail because the dosage is incorrect.)

The removal procedure should include the use of a rubber dam. This is a small sheet of thin rubber that isolates the tooth from the rest of the mouth. The tooth protrudes through the rubber which is stretched over a wire frame that completely covers the mouth. Any particles of mercury become embedded in the rubber. An air suction tube is used to remove saliva so that it cannot be swallowed – in case any vapour penetrates the latex. (Dentists who adhere to the strictest protocol insist that it is not enough to use just the super-efficient suction tube.) The dentist is recommended to remove the filling in as large pieces as possible. The drilling should be carried out with high volume evacuation equipment.

Other precautions that are also recommended by some include the removal of no more than two fillings (and preferably just one) at each appointment; that appointments should be made at intervals of no less than one month apart; that vitamin C should be administered before the operation. (This last is recommended as vitamin C and mercury have an affinity for each other. The most satisfactory way for this to be administered in this circumstance is intravenously as vitamin C in the muscles is far less effective at binding with mercury than it is when it is in the bloodstream.) It is also reasonable to expect an appointment for the removal of fillings to last considerably longer than it would take to put in an amalgam; it takes skill and care to replace old fillings with the white or porcelain ones.

Some specialist dentists would think that these precautions were insufficient. They would recommend a far more stringent approach. They would insist on whole-body protective clothing, a special ventilation system, anti-allergenic wallpaper and floor covering. This might well be needed by those who have an ultra-sensitive reaction to the amalgam but the cost of removal can become prohibitive. (For those who can afford it this is rightly not a deciding factor.) For most people it is probably sufficient to follow the simpler protocol advocated by dentists who are broad-minded enough to see that amalgams are dangerous and require very careful handling.

The dentist would normally begin by assessing which fillings are causing the most trouble. It is interesting to note that not all the fillings in a person's mouth have the same amount of leakage. Usually there is one particular offending one – often the largest or the oldest. It is as if this one is the core of the 'battery' effect and the milliamp-meter can pick it out. It is this one that the dentist will start with. If it is particularly large and awkward he may well deal only with the one. Once this is removed there is a wait of up to three months before tackling any others – the time depends on the urgency, sensitivity and pocket of the patient. By the next appointment another tooth will have taken over as the major active source of toxicity and it is this one that has to be removed next. Usually it will be a tooth in the same quadrant as the first or it will be its pair on the opposite side of the mouth.

While this process is continuing it is important for the homoeopath to be giving remedies to help. *Mercurius* itself might be called for or *Hepar Sulphuricum. Arnica* is always useful for dental operations, not simply to help with the trauma of having one's mouth and jaw pulled about but also because it is a good remedy for toxic shock. (Occasionally, in the case of really difficult teeth in very awkward positions *Emerald* – a wonderful remedy for extractions of any sort – or *Amethyst* can afford considerable relief depending on the indications.)

Once all the amalgams are removed it can be some time before the patient feels the benefits. Some will respond immediately saying that they feel relieved of a burden but this might be psychosomatic. Others will notice a gradual abatement of their physical symptoms. Those who did not have much in the way of physical symptoms but whose brain tissue was affected might find it took them longer to notice that they were able to use their mental faculties with greater facility (especially short-term memory and the ability to summon up words in a conversation). Those with allergies that are the result of a beleaguered immune system might take a while for their T-lymphocyte[6] count to rise. Sometimes it is a question of the longer standing the toxicity, the longer time it will take for healing, but strong constitutions with good bowel elimination will take the shortest time to recover. It is through the bowels that mercury is removed most speedily.

Whatever any patient's individual susceptibilities might be, the rate of recovery might be speeded up considerably by taking a professional kinesiologist's measured recommended dosage of mineral supplements. The supplementary treatment would in no way alter the effectiveness of any homoeopathic remedies – would, in fact, enhance and promote the patient's response. For any patient of homoeopathy mercury is one of the most serious and threatening potential maintaining causes of chronic ill health. Even for the strongest constitutions it is dangerous. One might not be at all aware of the danger because of the absence of recognisable symptoms but sooner or later it is likely that even the toughest person succumbs in one way or another to the insidious effects.

Let this case speak for many others:

> George, suffering for many years from arthritis and rheumatism, came for treatment for the pains in his hips, shoulders and feet. He said that he had to keep moving about slowly all the time because, if he sat down for more than a few minutes, his body would start to seize up with stiffness. He got some relief from hot baths and greatly appreciated the odd unprofessional massage he had from his wife. He could never get a good night's sleep because the pains and leg-cramps kept waking him up. This is a typical picture of *Rhus Toxicodendron*. He was given this remedy in the 30th potency with the instruction to take it twice per day. It did nothing – though when he returned for the next appointment he said that he was sweating profusely at night, had burning hot feet which he had to stick out of bed and was drinking water at the rate that made him think that he was following his mother towards diabetes. The *Rhus Tox.* picture was still there in his limbs but now he showed signs of needing *Sulphur*, a remedy that answered not only the new chief symptoms but also his constitutional bearing: built like Henry VIII, rubicund, hearty and hot with a penchant for spices and wine. *Sulphur* did nothing at all – unless it was responsible for uncovering the lurking problem beneath.
>
> Now George mentioned that he felt as if he was cracking up; he still had the insatiable thirst but now he had a strong metallic taste in his mouth. He dribbled at night and the room smelled foetid when he woke in the morning. His sweat was clammy and oily and rank. His digestion was bad and he now had heartburn after his evening meals. He felt depressed and morose. His rheumatism was much worse and quite frequently he felt feverish with shivers which came and went for no apparent reason. George was asked to open his mouth. Inside, every one of his molars was filled. The grey fillings of two of them had gone black – a sign that the filling had become highly suspect. He was told about mercury and its dangers and he agreed to go to a specialist dentist for an investigation. The result was that he decided to have all his fillings changed in a gradual process over the next eight months. At the same time he was given remedies to support the procedure and supplements recommended by the dentist. Within a year George was able to say that he not only had been relieved of all the symptoms except those of arthritis but that he was much more energetic and that he was thinking so much more clearly – something that he had not complained about before. What

was more was that he now felt that the *Rhus Tox.* was beginning to help him with his original symptoms.

The alternatives to mercury amalgams

There are two alternatives to mercury amalgams: one is made of acrylic, a petroleum-based product and the other is made of porcelain which originates from clay. The acrylic filling – known as 'white fillings' – is the more common and the cheaper material. Dentists slower to fall in with the rapidly expanding numbers of 'anti-amalgamists' say that white fillings are more difficult to put in, require longer to set and do not last so long. They do require more time and care to fit because they are put in in layers and each layer must be set and dried. The improvements made to the material since it first was produced however make it very durable. The one drawback that anyone with an alternative view of medicine would take as potentially serious – though it is comparatively rare – is that some patients are particularly sensitive to petroleum products.

Porcelain is more expensive and requires the same amount of expertise as white fillings. It would be a useful alternative to anyone who has a petroleum allergy. However, porcelain is made of clay, a substance that attracts and holds radiation. It is possibly worth considering that porcelain fillings might attract the radiation emitted during routine X-rays. It might be as well to take the advice of your homoeopath or kinesiologist before going to the dentist or, better still, to seek out a dentist who specialises in alternative dentistry.

We cannot leave the dentist's surgery quite yet. The next chapter explores the effects of another kind of filling procedure that is on the list of maintaining causes; one that is far less likely to call attention to itself than the use of a poisonous material. Comparatively few voices have been raised against it – with notable exceptions[7] – and yet it is one of the signals that there is something rotten in the state of the body.

CHAPTER 14

ROOT CANAL FILLINGS

Teeth are not simply flat outcrops from our jaws used for chewing. They are living tissue and have an integral relationship with the rest of the body. Though we would rather our teeth were not connected to the nervous system when we are suffering from toothache, it remains a fact of body geography that they are.

Strange as it may seem, each tooth has an affinity for one or other part of the anatomy. The energy lines that course through the body – called meridians in acupuncture and Chinese medicine – do not leave out the teeth. Hence the incisors run on the same energy pathways as the kidneys and bladder; the canines on those of the liver and gall bladder; the upper molars and premolars on those of the stomach, spleen and pancreas; the lower molars and premolars on those of the lungs, bronchi and trachea. You can see this at work in children's teething problems. Babies cutting their incisors often have very acid urine that causes severe nappy rash. When they cut their upper premolars they might well have thick mucous congestion of the chest or even a bout of croup. When they cut their canines they sometimes throw a *Belladonna*-type fever which is stoked up by the liver.

These connections are given scant attention in western medicine but they become useful to know when symptoms arise in the teeth of those who have chronic health problems. This is particularly true in the case of tooth abscesses. An abscess under a tooth can suggest whether there is cause for further investigation in the rest of the body to see if there is any underlying dysfunction in a related organ. For example, a patient with a chronic abscess in the socket of an upper canine which flares every so often and who has a constant post-nasal drip of thick, yellow mucus is most likely to have a toxic overload in the liver and very possibly a potential problem in the gall bladder. The treatment for this is not just to have the abscess drained or even the tooth removed but to deal with the fundamental sickness of the liver so that there is no need for the body to use the tooth socket as a vent for the expression of toxicity.

How does all this have any bearing on root canal fillings? To understand this we need to look at dental anatomy. A tooth is made up of three different types of tissue. The outer layer is enamel. This is the protective covering for dentine, the main body of the tooth. Dentine is not solid matter but porous tissue with a myriad of tiny tubules. Encased within these two layers is the central pulp, soft tissue which houses the tooth's nerve and blood supply. The socket into which the tooth fits should best be seen as a joint, like any other in the body. If decay sets in it is the enamel that begins to break down. If the enamel is breached then the decay gets through to the dentine. Sensitivity to hot or cold or chewing becomes excruciating pain once the decay lays bare the nerve within the pulp. This is damage that a dentist cannot repair. He may well have stemmed the tide by filling the tooth but if there are any bacteria lurking within the dentine's tubules then the decay will march on.

How can bacteria get into the dentine if the decay was drilled out and a filling put in to plug the hole? The answer is that bacteria can arrive in the blood supply from elsewhere in the body. While the system's immune processes are working well the bacteria may be little more than sitting tenants. If the body's immune responses are lowered by disease, tiredness, shock or trauma of any kind then these squatters may start making a nuisance of themselves and create an abscess. The usual medical procedure is to suppress the abscess with antibiotics, to drill out the old filling, expose the diseased root and remove it. Once the root canal is cleaned of all debris it is filled and the tooth is pronounced dead. Unfortunately it is not always allowed to rest in peace. The reason for this is that the dentist did not fill in the tubules of the dentine – there is no way of doing this – so the bacteria lost only their front door in the assault on the decay. They are still able to cause havoc – which they do by altering their composition and lifestyle to suit the new anaerobic (oxygen-less) conditions. Once this adaptation is underway the bacteria start producing toxins that leak into the mouth.

275

Molars, the double teeth that are most often affected, can often have more than one canal away from the root. Extra canals are not often detected and are quite frequently missed on X-rays. It is these other root canals that can become the site of the returned abscess. What can also occur is that the tooth next door starts to develop symptoms – sometimes with no apparent objective evidence.

The abscess never really went away because abscesses are never simply local problems; they are whole-body events which are meant to occur when the body is ready to deal with some toxicity that it wants to eliminate. The origin of the problem is not that our mouths are home to countless millions of bacteria all the time – which they are; the most toxic animal bite of all is that of a human. A healthy person has ample means of self-protection from the apparent depredations of opportunist bacteria. The core of the disease is that the body needs to express its susceptibility to infection by producing the characteristic symptoms. This means the raising of a local or a general fever, the flooding of the area with white blood cells that eat up the resident bacteria and the consequent formation of pus. The pus is harmless to the patient though it is disgusting material. The infected area becomes a vent for the whole system – a drain hole which is meant to continue pouring out pus until the body has expressed it all.

The problem with this kind of recurrent abscess is that it is seldom treated as a process of elimination but as a cause for suppression. What is more, dentists are reluctant to undo their root canal treatment because they regard the offending tooth as dead and, therefore, as no further cause for disease. Rather more sinister is the fact that the *suppressed* abscess may never develop in the same form again. The problem may return as a completely different pathology altogether. Evidence shows that people with a history of root canal fillings that harbour toxin-emitting bacteria may go on to suffer from heart disease and kidney disease. This should not be surprising as streptococcus, the bacteria involved, has a well-known affinity for the heart and the kidneys once it has got past the usual defence mechanisms of the body.

Who suffers most from root canal fillings? The research[1] so far shows that it is those who have a significant number of forebears who suffered from degenerative diseases. To homoeopaths this is easily translated into those with a strongly syphilitic miasmatic family history – which is true also of those who suffer most readily from mercury poisoning; syphilis and mercury have a long-standing mutual relationship in history and the threads of it are extraordinarily pervasive, even today. To understand the miasmatic (hereditary) aspect to these two maintaining causes see Part III: The hierarchy of the miasms.

To illustrate the importance of avoiding root canal treatment here is a case study:

Janet was thirty-four when she first started homoeopathic treatment. She had many different symptoms not all of which could be related easily to her general state of health. She was permanently tired and suffered headaches. She often felt rather nauseous. She had frequent bouts of either colds or 'flu. She had a plethora of gynaecological symptoms with painful, messy periods which were notable for the excessively vitriolic mood that preceded them and for the quantity of blood and clots that she passed. She had had four children and now had a prolapse which caused her considerable discomfort in the second half of her cycle and stress incontinence as the relaxed womb pulled the bladder out of its position. This is not an uncommon state and one that is often treated successfully with *Sepia*. Janet did respond to an initial dose of this remedy but all the symptoms returned within a short while. A repeat of the prescription made no impression on her health at all.

For some years Janet returned regularly for remedies. She came persistently because her children did so well as a result of their treatment that she was convinced that homoeopathy might sooner or later offer her a solution. Some of the prescriptions had worked well, particularly those for infections of the throat, ears and teeth, but these were for acute episodes. Remedies given for the chronic complaints were never more than partially curative. It was only when it dawned on the practitioner just how strong a feature of her case were the frequent throat and tooth infections that Janet was asked if she had any root canal fillings. She had two, both on the left side of her jaw. *"All my pains are on my left side,"* she had always said. *"It's always my left tonsil or my left ear. And it's my left bloody ovary that gives so much pain."*

She went to the dentist who told her that there was nothing at all the matter with her teeth. He took an X-ray to prove it. When she told him that she had so much sensitivity on the left side of her jaw she was told that it was psychosomatic; that she had grown to accept that that side would be painful, so it was. She went to an alternative dentist who agreed that her root canals could well be the seat of her problem and that the solution was to remove the two dead teeth and fillings and some of the bone of the cavity. For cosmetic reasons she declined any treatment. Two years went by before the repeated infections in her mouth, throat and then the bladder and kidneys, forced her to have the drastic treatment carried out. Once the fillings were out and the teeth and affected bone removed, Janet's health began to improve. Now the remedies for her constitution had far deeper and longer lasting effect. Despite the prolapse, her moods and the period pains improved considerably. She was no longer so tired. She did not feel that she was brewing 'flu all the time. She no longer had what amounted to a permanent cold and all the stiffness began to go out of the muscles of her limbs and chest. (Streptococcus is often associated with rheumatic pains when found in a chronic state.) Though she is careful how she smiles she is relieved that so much illness is behind her.

The best possible way to avoid the whole question of root canal fillings is to see your dentist every six months, brush your teeth *gently* (not by scrubbing them with hard bristles) and to use floss *and* an inter-dental brush. If you have dental caries in spite of such efforts then there will be a constitutional reason for the decay which is causing it from within – and that suggests the need for constitutional treatment from the homoeopath.

CHAPTER 15

DEFECTIVE NUTRITION

Throughout this book physics is viewed as taking precedence over chemistry – energy before matter. In this section we consider how chemistry can upstage physics. Normally, the energy of the body (physics) is inspired by creative purpose, driven by the will and put into action by the central nervous system. For the central nervous system (CNS) to operate it must make use of chemistry.

When body biochemistry goes awry then the physics of the system should set the imbalance right. All it may require is a simple change of habit: stop drinking so much alcohol or stop smoking; book the weekend away for two in Paris. You might need to avoid fats for a while or cut out bread and pasta from your diet. Maybe the balance might need to be adjusted by suffering a cold which floors the system for forty-eight hours while a copious amount of mucus eliminates unwanted matter. Then again, being advised to eliminate all dairy products, coffee and sugar may be a more efficacious and considerably cheaper solution than paying regular visits to the health food shop. Avoiding an excess of substances that the body does not actually need can often relieve an overtaxed Vital Force from having to work harder on its waste-disposal unit.

Common sense and moderation pay considerable dividends: take more exercise, eat more healthily, take time off and stop feeling guilty for needing time to yourself. Pain can be deleterious to the nutritional balance as well: go and see the osteopath to do something about that chronic backache or the homoeopath about those persistent period pains. Suppose, though, that there were conditions in which the depletion of minerals or vitamins was so severe that the CNS was unable to function properly until the missing chemistry could be restored and maintained, until such a time as the Vital

Force could get back in the driving seat – conditions, for example, that arise from having mercury poisoning or from smoking cannabis for too long, from taking the Pill or going on HRT.

There is a host of causes for mineral deficiencies in the body: specific illnesses which affect particular minerals, autoimmune disease, allergies, heavy metal toxicity, radiation, parasites, blood loss, dehydration, poor diet, uncongenial climatic conditions, pollution and more. This is not to mention traumatic emotions that can so easily cause a slump in vital body chemistry. While patients can often improve their biochemistry by restoring the activity of the Vital Force through the use of alternatives such as homoeopathy or acupuncture or by taking dietary advice, there are occasions when taking supplements becomes a necessary part of treatment. There are cases where a Vital Force, stricken by toxic or emotional overload and suffering from the lack of one or more minerals, is so poorly that there is not sufficient energy for homoeopathic remedies, an osteopathic therapist's hands or the acupuncturist's needles to galvanise that Vital Force to maintain its self-healing momentum. In such cases there is always a hidden maintaining cause that must be investigated.

A caveat

This is not the same scenario as that in which patients, otherwise quite well, seek preventative or protective cover from supplements off the shelves of the local health food shop. Chewing quantities of vitamin C tablets to prevent colds or downing bottles of echinacea tincture to ward off winter lurgies is either an exercise in putting off the inevitable or a waste of money in pursuit of a bug-free break. This is mild (sometimes not so mild) hypochondriasis. Colds are necessary eliminative processes that unfortunately seem to happen at inconvenient moments – usually as soon as the sufferer has got off his particular treadmill and is about to relax into a well earned holiday! Influenza, glandular or gastric, is also eliminative and an unpleasant episode that should have positive results. To allow these conditions to happen with infrequent occurrence is good biochemical housekeeping. Those who use supplements as a means of perpetual prevention delude themselves that they are maintaining their health. Those who feel the need to do this because they are forever succumbing to infections are using supplements as sandbags. They are locked into an intolerable state with the tide of ill health constantly rising. Where cold and 'flu prevention does make sense is in the old and infirm but here supplementary vitamin, mineral and herbal medicines need to be complemented by constitutional treatment from one of the other major therapies.

Supplements must be respected

From the point of view of homoeopathy it is necessary to sound a note of caution before looking further into the use of supplements. Contrary to the way we are encouraged[1] to think about the biochemistry of the body we are not constantly in need of supplies of supplements as a car requires petrol. The body is its own chemical factory and capable of synthesising and balancing its own mineral requirement – as long as the diet is relatively well balanced and *suited to the individual* and as long as the individual is not beset by stress, trauma or accident. We synthesise and store minerals readily as long as the body's own natural resources are chemically relatively well balanced[2] and this need not even depend on a consistent diet. A perfect balance 100 per cent of the time would be unrealistic so the body is built to adapt to all sorts of changes that disturb that equilibrium – not least by calling on reserves when there is either a dearth or an excessive use of one mineral or another due to a crisis. (One way the body deals with a lack of a vital chemical component is to cause a temporary craving – a few days of wanting to add salt or of eating a couple of bananas, perhaps.)

Quite often it is not that we are not taking enough of this or that mineral or vitamin as part of our diet but that the body 'factory' that processes what we ingest is defective and cannot handle them properly. Taking in more vitamins and minerals simply means that there are more to excrete. It is not the absence of fuel that is the problem: it is the temporary inability of the engine to make use of it.

Despite perfectly legitimate claims, taking calcium tablets does not automatically protect women from osteoporosis[3] or lower anyone's cholesterol levels. Taking magnesium does not necessarily raise your energy levels or prevent premenstrual tension. Selenium does not improve sex drive or protect against cancer in everyone who is told that it does. Zinc is not going to boost the immune system, prevent cancer, improve male libido, eliminate acne and reduce the pains of rheumatism in everyone who suffers from any of these conditions. For all these conditions to respond curatively to the introduction into the system of these minerals there must be an individualised reason for each patient to take them. There also needs to be a careful assessment as to whether there is an underlying reason for the system being unable to utilise any of the essential vitamins or minerals – which there always is. What is more, minerals need to be introduced into the system in a sequence that the body can deal with. Because mineral metabolism is a very complicated string of chemical events based on a biofeedback mechanism it is always necessary to see just what mineral is particularly needed at any moment to complete the cycle.

Taking blunderbuss prescriptions of mineral supplements takes no account of the fact that a reasonably healthy body can re-establish its mineral equilibrium; nor that a distressed body needs supplementary help in the form of a *sequenced* introduction of supplements. Most of the minerals bought are simply excreted by millions of bowels and twice as many kidneys because the requirement has not been specifically individualised. The amounts actually necessary for healthy functioning are relatively small. The scale of the folly of trying to improve on biochemical balances (as if we were debating what kind of petrol the car needed) is illustrated neatly by vitamin E: it has been pointed out that one capsule contains sufficient vitamin E to supply the population of the British Isles for a day – and some patients are advised to take this dosage daily. Fortunately it is relatively difficult to harm oneself from overdoses of supplements because the body is so good – even in illness – at throwing out what it does not need or cannot process. So, what are these substances that make so much vital difference to our lives even if they are needed only in the tiniest amounts?

Vitamins, minerals and trace elements

Vitamins are a miscellany of organic nutrients that act as chemical catalysts in normal metabolism. They work at a cellular level. The body does not synthesise vitamins in great enough quantity without the need to obtain them from external sources. Vitamins A,D,E and K are all fat soluble and therefore can be stored in the body. Vitamin C and the B vitamins are water soluble so cannot be stored in the body and are readily excreted. They all contain carbon. 'A' is found in fish oils and meat – especially liver. It is also found in carrots, broccoli and spinach, tomatoes and lettuce. 'C' is found in fresh fruit and vegetables. 'E' is found in cereals, grains, vegetables and eggs. 'K' is found in vegetables and live yoghurt. The various 'B' vitamins are found in plant and animal products as well as dairy produce. Brewer's yeast is particularly rich in 'B6'.

Minerals and trace elements are inorganic and are not carbon compounds. Though the amounts required of these minerals are measured in infinitesimal quantities they are each essential to the health of the body. The difference between minerals and trace elements is simply that the latter are required in amounts of less than 100 milligrams per day.

The vitamin content of foodstuffs is fairly constant wherever one lives. The mineral content of plant foods can vary widely depending on geography and the quality of a region's soil. For this reason, from a biochemical viewpoint, it is often considered more likely for patients to suffer from mineral deficiency than it is from vitamin deficiency. Though today in Britain, with so much import and export of foodstuffs, deficiency is more likely to be due to eating processed forms of foods rather than eating foods that are grown on soil deficient in the required minerals.

The minerals most essential to the body's functioning are calcium, phosphorus, sodium, magnesium, potassium and sulphur. Trace elements regarded as vital include iron, copper, manganese, zinc, selenium and chromium.

The difference between homoeopathic minerals and their material origin

It is interesting to note that every one of these minerals is a homoeopathic remedy in its own right yet they are seldom prescribed homoeopathically on the evidence of biochemical deficiency in the body. If one of them is indicated as the remedy similar to a patient's whole symptom picture, the analysis of the choice is unlikely to rest on the typical signs of that mineral's absence. This is because each of the *energy* medicines developed from its material dose, while having aspects identical to symptoms caused by its *material* absence, has a unique picture that is underpinned by its very characteristic signature which is evident not so much on the cellular level but on the general, emotional and mental levels.

The absence of magnesium – one of the most common deficiencies – can cause the dysfunction of every biochemical process in the body from the electrical regulation of the heartbeat to maintaining muscle tone. To a homoeopath the most typical biochemical signal of magnesium deficiency is 'spasm' – in the muscles, especially of the abdomen – though this would never be enough of a reason on its own to prescribe it in potency. There are many other remedies that also cover this symptom. As a homoeopathic remedy *Magnesium* is prescribed on a broad picture of someone suffering easily from nervous strain, hypersensitivity, anxiety and irritability, weakness, spasms, gastrointestinal disturbance and acidity. Yet a patient with this homoeopathic symptom picture may not necessarily be suffering primarily from a serious deficiency of mineral magnesium. Conversely, alcoholism does not feature in the description of anyone needing the remedy *Magnesium* even though alcoholics almost always suffer from a depletion of this mineral.

What this illustrates so well is that there is a significant difference between the *atomic* energy of a substance and its *chemical* energy. It points up the difference between homoeopathy and naturopathy – the study of nutritional therapy – and shows how they should be viewed as complementary. It also gives us our first example of a patient who might not get better without mineral supplements: an alcoholic is not likely to do well unless given magnesium supplements because the quantities of alcohol consumed, even after homoeopathic treatment has commenced, will be enough to continue blocking the mineral from being used. The alcohol, in other words, is in competition with the remedies prescribed and the restoration of the body's normal functioning. Even if the patient genuinely went on the wagon, the appalling state of the liver would probably prevent the fullest use of the mineral – which is necessary, among other things, for the conversion of blood sugars into usable energy (often missing in alcoholics) and in maintaining an emotionally balanced view of the world (always missing in alcoholics).

We can look at this from the other way round: a patient on a diuretic due to high blood pressure may well be losing too much potassium from the body as the drug encourages the excessive excretion of this mineral in the urine. Yet this is not a good basis for considering any of the homoeopathic potassium remedies as indicated by the general condition. If potassium loss continues despite homoeopathically indicated remedies then it is time to consider the use of a potassium-rich diet to support the system naturopathically or to visit the doctor for a potassium prescription.

> John suffered from high blood pressure, excessive body heat, swollen feet and ankles, persistent diarrhoea, profuse night sweats and breathlessness and was put on a diuretic by his doctor. He found, as a result, that he passed more water at night so his sleep was disturbed. Though his blood pressure stabilised his breathlessness increased and he felt more lethargic, more easily confused and had slower reflexes. Despite taking *Sulphur*, the remedy that most matched his general state, he found that any improvement he made did not last for long. Once he was given a diet rich in potassium – raw vegetable salad, avocados and bananas – he began to maintain his steady improvement. He was able to cut down and eventually phase out his diuretics gradually. The *Sulphur* was only able to 'hold' once the diet was changed in order to cater for the negative effects of the diuretic.

What could prevent the body from utilising essential minerals?

Toxicity, infection, infestation, chronic pain, suppressive drugs, hallucinogens, pollutants and long-held emotional trauma, most readily answer this question. All of them interfere directly or indirectly with the delicate biochemical feedback system. Usually patients come for treatment with a combination of at least two or three of these factors and sometimes more. (It takes so long for people to realise that they do not have to put up with symptoms that compromise their lives.)

Heavy metal toxicity

While homoeopathy is capable of dealing with a variety of different kinds of toxicity there are some that remain hidden for long enough and deeply enough and in such quantity to frustrate the practitioner's best efforts. While *Sulphur*, *Nux Vomica* and *Pulsatilla* are all remedies well known for encouraging the system to flush out the poisonous effects of antibiotics and steroids, they may not do so well at making an impression on a system storing heavy metals such as lead, aluminium and cadmium (a metal found in bread made from refined wheat). Any one of these can bring out specific characteristic symptom pictures of poisoning if present in sufficient quantities though generally they cause mineral and vitamin deficiencies that impose functional limitations on the body. So powerful is the chemical energy of these metals and so different is the atomic energy of the homoeopathic remedies made from them that it is not likely that a patient suffering from the specific toxicity of any one of them would find much benefit from antidoting their toxic effects with their homoeopathic counterparts.

A patient with lead poisoning (as a result, perhaps, of having lived through one's childhood in a house with lead pipes) seldom responds deeply to being dosed with *Plumbum* in potency. While the body is primed to deal with relatively minor deposits of chemical toxicity there are insufficient internal self-healing resources for organising the removal of such quantities of alien toxic waste from the system[4].

Insidiously seeping toxicity is often hidden competition for other maintaining causes such as a widespread yeast infection or troubled emotions. If the practitioner is prescribing, perhaps, on a general picture of long-held grief with a history of antidepressant suppression at the same time as there is also aluminium poisoning present, then the results of homoeopathic medication are going to be very meagre. Each time the Vital Force is prodded into working on the psyche, the physical body proves too weak to match the effort. The chronic toxicity keeps seeping out and yet there may be no apparent significant symptomatic reason to give priority to, say, metal poisoning above grief or a history of never being well since antidepressants or the Pill.

A referral to a kinesiologist who would carry out an exhaustive muscle test could well reveal the underlying maintaining cause of a long-held metal toxicity – the only symptom of which might be the failure of well-indicated homoeopathic remedies not inspiring the curative changes expected.

Drug trouble

In the last illustrative case it was seen that a diuretic given on perfectly reasonable grounds was capable of upsetting potassium levels to the detriment of the patient. Not only are all drugs suppressive but they also cause chemical imbalances and therefore have to be considered as more or less toxic despite the good intentions behind their prescription. This is especially true of repeat prescription drugs. (Herbal medicines, though some can be toxic if given in excessive doses, are biochemical in action but generally neither suppressive nor toxic as the intention behind their prescription is eliminative.) The best-known drugs to cause chemical imbalances are the antibiotics.

Both acute and chronic infection can cause chemical depletion. Where there is a state of chronic infection – such as bronchiectasis, a condition in which the lungs are cough-damaged with the result of pus-filled holes in the lungs or, say, Crohn's disease, the toxic inflammatory condition of the intestines – then the constant recruitment of lymphocytes to combat bacteria is very debilitating and mineral-depleting. Magnesium, zinc and iron can all be seriously lacking and the body's use of vitamins would be seriously compromised. The longer held the state of infection, the more difficult it is for the body to 'remember' how to start up its correct biofeedback system. The more drug-suppressed that state is, the more likely it is that supplements would be required to support the Vital Force in re-establishing itself.

Parasites

Infestation is something that most of us would not contemplate being a problem these days unless we were discussing worms, nits or fleas. Such high profile parasites rarely present the homoeopath with too much difficulty though it is often hard for scrupulous parents to accept that worms are usually present as a means of mopping up unwanted gut rubbish and that the successful treatment of head lice almost always marks a significant development stage in a child's life – see Part III, Psora. Yet there are smaller fry that present us with quite a different challenge. Microbial parasites that find a congenial home in the liver or the gut, the bladder or the kidneys are capable of gathering sufficient strength of numbers in a weakened or susceptible body to cause an infestation.

Candida, that almost universal fungal growth that can affect any organ of the body, should be seen in the same light. It is not uncommon for parasites or yeast infections to be maintained by the body at such a level that the host continues unaware that there is much amiss beyond a drop in available energy, some loose stools from time to time and a desperate urge for some antisocial scratching. Yet it costs the host energy to entertain guests and the general fabric of the house is weakened. Bacterial or fungal parasites create their own list of demands and dictate their terms of tenancy ruthlessly. Their requirements can eventually conflict so strongly with the host's own needs that the net result is that the normal biochemical balance is lost. When the invaders' energy becomes stronger than the host's Vital Force then supplementary chemical reinforcements can become indispensable.

Here is a typical case where homoeopathy was insufficient on its own.

Kathryn, a mother of two young children, had suffered from candida for some years. It most obviously caused vaginal and anal itching. She also had digestive problems and period abnormalities. She was tired and listless yet found enough energy to keep going both as a mother and at her job. She was so exhausted, though, by the end of the day that she would fall asleep in front of the television every evening. She was snappy with her husband and intolerant of any mischief perpetrated by the children. She looked pale and had dark circles under her eyes. She was consumed by a feeling of gloom as her period approached each month. She felt that a black cloud descended over her. Though she would normally be constipated, at the time of her period she would have diarrhoea with cramps in the gut. This was accompanied by period pains, particularly severe on the left side in the ovarian region. During the menstrual flow the blood would be dark and clotted and then profuse and bright red. She had been told that she had small fibroids in the uterus and that sooner or later they would grow and need to be removed; she

288

might possibly need a hysterectomy. Her periods always made her feel weak and drained. She would hardly recover from one before the next was upon her. The only positive aspect of her period was that the thick, white cottage cheesy discharge that was the result of the candida would stop – only to start again by the fifth day of the cycle.

Kathryn said that she had not felt well since she had had her last child and that she thought that she had profoundly damaged herself when she had taken the 'morning-after' Pill some three years ago. From the homoeopathic point of view the most significant aspect of Kathryn's story was the impact that her deranged hormones had on her daily life. Yet the candida was also important as it was a constant drain on her energy and her nutritional resources: candida is greedy and will cause people to change their appetites to suit it. Kathryn had the typical candida urges: a strong desire for sweet foods, carbohydrates and chocolate. What made things even worse for her was that her diet, dictated by the candida, was inimical to her system. She did not tolerate gluten (which is ever present in our wheat based diet) or dairy products well. The net result was that she suffered bloating, flatulence and abdominal pains as well as frequent headaches and occasions of feeling nausea.

She was given several prescriptions of remedies before it became apparent that as soon as she showed a little improvement in one area another became worse. *Cimicifuga*, from the black cohosh plant, a favourite North American Indian remedy for gynaecology, certainly helped some of her mood change before the period and softened the severity of the ovarian pain. *Lycopodium*, a remedy well known for its effect on those who suffer from wheat intolerance, made a small effect on the gut symptoms that then got worse. After *Folliculinum* Kathryn said that she felt that she had definitely turned a corner with her gynaecological symptoms even though she still 'flooded' at the period.

Kathryn was then asked to go for a blood test at her local surgery and to see a nutritional therapist who would test her system for deficiencies and allergies. The blood test showed that she was slightly anaemic and the nutritionist found that she lacked iron, magnesium, vitamins B1 and B6 as well as zinc and copper. As a consequence Kathryn was advised to cut out all dairy products, all gluten products (wheat, pasta, etc.) and all sugars. She was also asked to eat more protein food such as fish, lamb and offal: particularly liver[5]. Liver is a rich source of iron. Also on her shopping list were acidophilus tablets, which were to restore the beneficial bowel flora that had been so upset by the candida; vitamin B complex tablets and magnesium tablets. She was not given an iron supplement as iron deficiency had not been particularly strongly marked in the muscle testing. Too much iron in the system can cause problems, particularly with the spleen, the organ partly responsible for the production and deployment of new blood cells.

Kathryn's life took a decided turn for the better. The periods became far less traumatic as the blood loss reduced, the black moods (eased though they had been by *Cimicifuga* and *Folliculinum*) ceased altogether and the pains became far more manageable. Her energy levels no longer troubled her as she was able to maintain them throughout the day. The digestive symptoms calmed down though they did not leave her entirely. She still suffered from wind and bloating if she ate a packet vegetarian meal. She also lost weight and showed off her slimmed down ankles; she had complained of water retention before which had *"offended my vanity"*, she said. She also said that she now felt that whatever homoeopathic remedy she took worked far more swiftly and deeply. Before she had had to search for things to say that might be ascribed to the effects of the prescriptions. Now she had no such doubts.

Kathryn's story is not unusual. Her system was so affected by a combination of different conditions that her Vital Force simply did not have the resources to conjure up the requisite biochemistry to effect the changes needed. With the assistance of additional minerals she was able to reverse the negative chemistry of candida and recurrent blood loss. She did not need to keep taking the supplements ad infinitum but only for two and a half months. By then her system was able to cope with the remains of the candida which gradually faded over the following three months.

Pain

Chronic pain is astonishingly common. Patients put up with debilitating pain for years. They may have tried to do something – or everything – about it but drawn a blank. Gradually they accustom themselves to it and they fail to remember what life was like without it. Probably the commonest site of chronic pain is the lower back though that is chiefly because correcting such common skeletal structural problems requires a far subtler approach than orthodox treatment can offer – see Chapter 9: Physical Trauma and Musculoskeletal Imbalance. There are almost as many patients who put up with chronic pain in the gut or long-held neuralgia in almost any part of the body.

A common side effect and a maintaining cause of pain is the loss of minerals. One or more of magnesium, calcium, potassium, silicon and sodium might well be depleted. The quality and modality of the pain suffered could point to the deficiency. With magnesium the pains would be neuralgic and spasmodic; they are more likely to be worse while resting and better for moving gently about; they are often exaggerated by triggering irritability in the highly sensitised patient. Where calcium is lacking the pains are often associated with bones, teeth, tendons, glands and nerves in a system that is slowing down and stiffening up. Where potassium is lacking the pains are likely to appear in a patient who suffers from nervous disorders exaggerated by stress, hypersensitivity and anxiety; where there is congestion or stricture of a part. With silicon the pains are violent and intensified by sudden movement or jarring; they are often associated with the tubes of the body (ear, gut etc.) and occur in patients who lack stamina and 'grit', have a tendency towards glandular disorders and becoming malnourished. With sodium the pains are likely to be rheumatic, gouty, throbbing or aching; when there is acidity of the system generally.

If a constitution has had to bear with pain for so long and has had to devise compensatory measures (postural, behavioural or medicinal) to afford even a small amount of relief, then the system will have become locked into a fixed habit that is often very difficult to break with only one means of therapy. A combined approach works well and even better if the various practitioners are able to confer. In a patient whose history includes a traumatic childhood, several surgical procedures, a number of injuries, a gradually increasing degree of intolerance to certain foods and a list of various suppressive treatments then, finances permitting, combining homoeopathy, osteopathy and naturopathy would be advisable.

Amino acids, lipids and nucleic acids

Amino acids, lipids and their derivatives and the nucleic acids are also vital components of the biochemistry of the body. Homoeopaths are generally not well versed in this particular area, not least perhaps because none of the twenty amino acids are proven homoeopathic remedies. We do not know in what way the nuclear energy of these chemicals might be 'like' the sickened energy of a patient. Of the lipids only cholesterol, oestrogen and progesterone have been potentised while deoxyribonucleic acid and ribonucleic acid (DNA and RNA for short) are both available in homoeopathic potency and have been proved; though the 'pictures' that they present are too sketchy for them to be of general interest and there has been little follow-up literature on cases benefited by these remedies. None of them is particularly widely used and none of them could yet be genuinely regarded as 'constitutional' remedies in the same sense as *Sulphur*, *Calcium*, *Silica* or *Phosphorus*. (When they are prescribed it is more as 'drainage' or support remedies rather than constitutionally.)

The twenty amino acids are like building blocks that in different combinations create all the various proteins required for sustaining life. The compounds are principally made up of carbon, oxygen, nitrogen and hydrogen while others include vital minerals: sulphur, zinc, phosphorus, iron and copper. Proteins are used for the building and repair of body tissue, to form enzymes, hormones and antibodies and to combine with other chemicals to keep the neurological engine running: neurotransmitters and neuroinhibiters keep the sympathetic and parasympathetic nervous systems functioning. (The sympathetic system is proactive and causes events, such as peristalsis, to happen in the body while the parasympathetic system inhibits them so that for every functional activity there is an oppositional resting mode.)

Of the twenty, eight of them are known as 'essential' and the rest are 'nonessential'. These terms refer to the fact that the essential amino acids are not manufactured by the body and have to be obtained through diet. The rest are synthesised within the body's own chemical factory.

Nucleic acids are divided into two categories: deoxyribonucleic acid (DNA) and ribonucleic acid (RNA). They are arrangements of strings of molecules that provide the genetic instructions for the whole individual.

DNA consists of a backbone of phosphate and a sugar with a spiral staircase of rungs branching from it. This structure is composed of just four chemicals: adenine, thymine, guanine and cytosine. It has the unique ability to synthesise itself – perhaps the most basic mystery of them all – and it is present in all animate forms of life. The inexplicable physics of DNA has purpose in perpetual recreation: it instigates the production of proteins. The work of differentiating the DNA's genetically coded messages and then putting the resulting proteins into production is carried out by RNA which orders the twenty amino acids into specific sequences to create particular proteins. Proteins are the regulators of the body's chemistry.

DNA and RNA have become a small part of the biochemical health revolution for the man in the street (or, rather, the person about to go into the health food shop) because the rate of replication and repair of DNA and its interaction with RNA have been noted as significant factors in the ageing process. As a result there has been a steep rise in the sales of such products as folic acid and zinc, both of which are reputed to maintain DNA/RNA activity. That nature requires these chemicals for cell replication is undisputed but whether mass-produced pills of them are able to affect DNA and RNA directly is a moot point.

These supplements may well be successful but the evidence of the need for either folic acid or zinc is likely to appear in the symptom picture for other reasons than simply faulty DNA; neither folic acid nor zinc ever did a great deal for halting the reality of ageing, a process that is far more strongly determined by the potentially terminal combination of heredity, emotional baggage and continual stress than simply missing minerals.

What homoeopaths bear in mind is that it is most likely that *the genetic code that carries the susceptibilities of the patient* determines ageing. It is as much an inherent part of the patient to have a tendency to heart disease or chilblains, chest infections or boils as it is to have red hair or a Roman nose. These susceptibilities towards disease patterns are a vital part of arriving at a homoeopathic prescription. By employing remedies according to those clearly expressed tendencies and patterns that can be objectively observed, DNA/RNA activity is being promoted – and not simply as far as the ageing process goes but more importantly, if controversially, at the level of the susceptibilities themselves. The reason for making this assumption is that, in terms of homoeopathic philosophy and generations' worth of circumstantial clinical evidence, it is the Vital Force that inspires the perpetual self-synthesis of DNA. (For a deeper appreciation of this whole aspect see Part III.)

Lipids have been the subject of fierce scrutiny and debate since the 1980s when people's consciousness of the 'fat' problem ballooned out of proportion. Chiefly this happened because cholesterol began to be targeted by the medical press as being responsible for so much circulatory and heart disease. Having thoroughly scared the public and given rise to that most disastrous and absurd institution, the fat-free diet, journalists belatedly admitted that cholesterol had, in fact, a vital role to play in the body's economy. What had been missing was an overview of the 'how', 'what', 'when' and 'why'. Sadly the damage was done and we now have hosts of patients who are routinely prescribed anti-cholesterol drugs which, because they are aimed at just one aspect of the body's biochemical process, do not take account of any individual's needs. The result is that there are many who take the drugs to reduce their cholesterol levels but suffer unnecessary and damaging side effects such as constipation and acidity of the gastrointestinal tract, tendency to form gall stones, inflammation of muscles, fatigue, dizziness, nausea, irritability and impotence. Furthermore, these drugs can precipitate in those who would be susceptible to heart disease anyway the very problem that they are trying to prevent – coronary heart disease. What a pity it is that the underlying causes of abnormally raised cholesterol levels are not investigated with each patient – for each one will have their own particular reason, biochemical and/or emotional. (Causes can also include the taking of other drugs such as the Pill, beta blockers and diuretics.)[6]

The fats in the body are all compounds that include carbon, hydrogen and oxygen. The compounds include triglycerides, phospholipids, cholesterol, steroids and fatty acids. The normal interplay between these lipids results in the quality and integrity of cell membranes being maintained. The degree of fluidity and permeability is important for cells of all the structures of the body. The balance between oil (fats) and water is struck here and is constantly being regulated. If the balance is out then the way the patient describes his symptoms would lead the homoeopath to ferret after evidence that would answer certain disparate but key questions. Is the patient's whole system drying out or becoming waterlogged? Is the patient inclined to rheumatics and hypertension? Does the body deal with inflammation and pain well? Does the patient have a healthy immune response? Does his blood carry enough oxygen around the body or does he get breathless on exertion? Is there a suspicious hint of stickiness of the blood that might be causing plaque to form on the artery walls somewhere?

This approach may seem rather unscientific given the availability elsewhere of sophisticated laboratory testing equipment but this is the sort of questioning that helps homoeopaths to arrive at a whole-body picture of symptoms and to assess whether the patient needs additional support and advice outside homoeopathy. Nevertheless, what even the naturopathically untrained homoeopath knows is that it is really important for those patients who do suffer from either high cholesterol, or any other aspect of disordered fat chemistry, to realise that diet plays a key role. For those who are scared by any diagnosis that suggests potential heart disease there is little difficulty in adhering to quite strict dietary advice[7]. Others, who do not feel the imminence of the threat, find it really hard to discipline themselves. It is common to find patients who need to be given a salutary shock before they will listen to their bodies. Eating rich food and fast food, smoking, drinking far too much alcohol and drinking coffee, added to a stressful daily work routine, are bound to be a major maintaining cause and one that can quite easily overwhelm homoeopathic remedies. It is sometimes shocking to find just how wedded to their dangerous lifestyles people can be.

One of the main problems here is that people become hooked on their adrenal-driven roller coaster; their material success is far too exciting a stimulus or their duty-bound work ethic far too well entrenched to be given up without good reason. So often that reason is provided by pathology or the threat of it. It is not until they have been referred to a consultant in a hospital with worryingly long corridors, rooms full of sinister equipment and had to wait while busy nurses swish to and fro on squeaky linoleum floors that they really sit up and take notice.

Summing up nutritional support

Patients may present relatively straightforward symptom pictures of remedies that can reset their biochemical balance even when such basic chemical problems as amino acid deficiency, excessive viscosity of cell walls or even cosmetic signs of *Anno Domini* are in question. It remains true that if there is a flaw in the ergonomics and ecology of the body then it is the engine that must be addressed and not just the fuel – even if it would not go amiss to improve the fuel on occasion. The ergonomics and ecology of our bodies is to do with the whole body; they are aspects of holism – which is what homoeopathic philosophy is all about. Too many flaws in the system, though, can mean that remedies on their own, without naturopathic assistance, would be hard pressed to deal with all the biochemical maintaining causes.

CHAPTER 16

ARTIFICIAL IMMUNISATION
AND VACCINE DAMAGE

O f all the contentious medical issues, artificial immunisation is the one that inspires by far the most passion. Those who see the use of vaccines as a cornerstone of preventative medicine consider any questioning of the reasoning or results to be anathema. In contrast, those who have seen or have been patients damaged by the vaccination process believe there is no question that any immunisation programme is either suspect or the greatest folly.

Those against tend to see immunologists as anything from misguided and blind to arrogant, interested only in the broad canvas of disease eradication. They are accused (with some justification) of manipulating statistics for their own scientific ends and of not accepting empirical evidence that individuals can be and have been permanently damaged. In short they are casuists determined to win their own endgame.

Those in favour do not see the David and Goliath aspect of the debate and believe genuinely in the humanitarian good that can be done by making it impossible for potentially threatening and fatal viruses and bacteria to prey on us. Two sides implacably opposed with almost no common ground. Between them, in no man's land, stands the patient, basically ignorant and certainly confused (if he is interested to listen) by the slanging match that frequently erupts around him.

What the enquiring patient will have noticed is that the debate will not go away, that it is increasingly newsworthy and that the numbers of people who have made up their minds to side with the 'antis' are swelling. As more and more begin to question accepted wisdom, so the medical scientists underline the breadth of scope of their intentions and the extraordinary dangers of not following their lead. Doctors seek to educate the general public by explaining the fatal threat that measles and whooping cough and rubella can present – and, incidentally, by doing so vastly overplay their hand. We are told that even mumps and chickenpox can have dire consequences. They exhort us to see the appalling effects of meningitis and tuberculosis in an effort to scare us into protecting our children with the vaccines. They remind us of the extraordinary triumph that the smallpox vaccination has been. The net result is that many of us are made to feel positively antisocial if we consider the option of not putting our children through the immunisation programme; unvaccinated children are *ipso facto* a health hazard, harbourers of malignant disease and capable of initiating epidemics.

What is the line that homoeopaths take? After all, practitioners thoroughly versed in the philosophy of natural healing know categorically that vaccines of any description are maintaining causes: that a patient with whatever condition may well not get better because the Vital Force has been compromised by *artificial* immunisation. Homoeopaths learn and experience through practice that the insidious effects can be as hidden and pervasive as mercury toxicity or hormone treatment. So, what might you expect as advice from a homoeopath about the whole question?

The official line of the registration bodies is that patients must be allowed to decide for themselves whether or not to go along with orthodox medicine and that it is beyond a practitioner's brief to persuade anyone otherwise. While some are content with this approach, others find the implicit constraint hard to bear. (This is, to them, political correctness obliging them to go against their better judgement.) Doctors practising homoeopathy who have studied the philosophy in depth and had sufficient clinical experience have a tougher time: the homoeopathic hospitals are decidedly pro-immunisation.

Patients can (and almost always do) ask alternative practitioners for their opinions and the reasons for them. As a result, patients are frequently left with an even stronger dilemma. They tend to be given a cocktail of different reasons for action and non-action, each of which may have its origins in powerful clinical and empirical experience but which to the patients is a jumble of indigestible facts. The problem is that the variety of reasons why artificial immunisation is bad medical practice cannot be explained briefly – they are worse, in fact, than the vast majority could contemplate. So important is the whole question, and so rational does the premise for carrying out mass immunisation appear to be, that to arrive at a comprehensive understanding needs time, patience and courage – and a willingness to suspend faith in some of the most firmly established precepts of medical orthodoxy. Perhaps the best place to begin to explore this behemoth is with history.

A brief history of vaccination

Cowpox is a disease that affects the udders and teats of cows and is very similar – though a great deal milder – to smallpox in its symptom picture. It can affect humans; those infected by it recover and are immune to the worse disease. Vaccination was a term coined to name the process of using cowpox infected serum taken from cows to protect people from smallpox, the first disease to be singled out for eradication. The first examples of artificial immunisation were not developed, as is commonly thought, from Edward Jenner's experiments with cowpox serum. Jenner came onto the field to bat rather late in the day.

Smallpox is believed to have appeared first some 10,000 years ago in north-eastern Africa. From there it is thought to have been spread by merchants to India and then along trade routes to China and elsewhere. The evidence of the disease is first seen on Egyptian mummies 3,500 years old. The first recorded epidemic occurred in 1350 BC.

The first recorded observation that those who had already suffered and survived the disease became immune, came from the quill of Thucydides in Athens in 430 BC. He it was who first expounded the theory of acquired immunity: if one suffers a disease and survives then the body will never suffer the same condition again. The Greeks, too, were amongst the first to take the next logical step and induce immunity by giving a dose of smallpox to otherwise healthy and unaffected people, in the form of a pustule scab from the skin of a sufferer. This extremely risky procedure has become known as variolation after the virus variola that is found to proliferate in smallpox sufferers. Other cultures have had different ways of carrying out the same procedure. In China, powdered scabs were blown down a tube into the nostrils of healthy people; in India scabs or pus were applied to skin which had been scratched. In the late 1600s, one hundred years before Jenner, the Chinese took pills made from fleas collected from cows – the first recorded example of vaccination.

The Sultans of the Ottoman Empire had a penchant for women from the Caucasus mountains. Young girls destined for the harems of Istanbul would be variolated in places where scars did not show so that the disease would not impede their social progress. The Royal Society in London had the first reports of variolation in 1714, eighty years before Edward Jenner began his work. The eighteenth-century English medical establishment did not take up the idea of variolation though country people and the royal family did, relying as so often on their own keen observation. Several of their number had already suffered, notably Queen Mary II and Queen Anne.

It began to be noted that, though there were side effects to the process of variolation, the incidence of infection among those immunised fell markedly. This was in addition to the side effects that included developing smallpox, syphilis or tuberculosis as a result of taking on the infected serum of the donors. In fact, it was noted that variolation could set off a new wave of epidemic.

It was observed officially in 1722 that amongst the unvariolated the death rate was some fourteen times higher than amongst those who had been artificially immunised. With such statistics it is no wonder that the technique of giving smallpox scabs or pus as a means of preventing the appearance of the disease became quite widespread by the 1740s. However, by the 1920s other, rather more sceptical opinions were appearing in print that showed how the death rate among smallpox sufferers who *had* been vaccinated was higher by some fourteen times. It seems that the great game of statistics played to different rules is not exclusive to our own times.

In spite of this spreading acceptance of variolation many frowned on the idea of vaccination – the use of cowpox material – which was preferred amongst rural communities. A Dorset farmer was much vilified for dosing his wife and children with scabs from a cow's udder. Like most rural dwellers he was aware that having a bout of cowpox gave permanent immunity to the worse disease. His children never developed smallpox despite local epidemics but his wife nearly lost her arm from severe inflammation caused by the vaccination. In the 1790s Jenner, having come across this rustic revolution, began routinely vaccinating children and the practice mushroomed from then on despite grave doubts from those who observed the gravity of side effects that some people developed. None of this took any account whatever of the fact that there was more than one type of smallpox. There was the lethal variety called variola haemorrhagica or purpura. There was the benign form (variola minor) and there was the variety that seemed to be produced most commonly amongst those who had been vaccinated. In addition there was a variety that was endemic to Africa and South America called Kaffir-pox which was very mild.

It is now believed that smallpox has been eradicated from the world as a result of vaccination. The Russians and Americans keep samples of the virus in high-security laboratory conditions; both sides believing the other might use the disease as the basis of biological warfare. However, the question remains: was smallpox eradicated or has it changed its shape? While the disease has undoubtedly disappeared, it is not so easy to be categorical about its absolute demise. One only has to look on the internet in search of articles about smallpox to see photographs of African children with a disease called monkeypox that looks and behaves extraordinarily like smallpox, that kills at least 20 per cent of sufferers and only appeared in the middle of the twentieth century. This disease originally appears to have developed in those who had been vaccinated against smallpox. Furthermore, smallpox is a viral disease and, by now, we all know how viruses are prodigiously capable of mutating.

Once the microscope was developed in the nineteenth century it did not take medical science long to believe that other diseases could be dealt with in the same way as smallpox. The most obvious candidate was tuberculosis (TB). The first efforts ended in tragedy when thousands died in an experiment conducted in 1900 by the German, Robert Koch, that involved introducing into willing patients tuberculous material gathered from guinea pigs and cultured in ox bile and glycerine. The subsequent search for a vaccine against TB was long and tortuous – and still involved cows. They discovered that human TB might help to keep cows immune from their own version of the disease but there was an unpleasant offshoot: the human form of the bacillus could happily live on in the cow and multiply in the milk

301

which was then transmissible back to us. Eventually, through a process of attenuation – the culturing of increasingly weaker strains of the bacteria – the BCG serum was developed. By 1921 the BCG vaccine was ready to be launched and its use spread quickly in the hope that the disease would become history. As we now know, the hope was vain.

It was in 1913 that an immunisation for diphtheria was first discovered though it was too toxic for use. In the 1920s the addition of formaldehyde, itself a toxic chemical with preserving properties, rendered the vaccine 'safe' for general use. It has been seen since as the cause for the steep decline in the incidence of diphtheria even though the disease was on the wane anyway. Whooping cough followed with a vaccine in the mid 1920s though it was not until the 1950s that its use was nationwide.

Two polio vaccines were developed. The first, the Salk vaccine, was highly controversial and seen to be the cause of severe side effects which tragically included death. The other is still in use today. This vaccine is attenuated through the use of monkey kidney cells on which the bacillus is readily cultured. In 1963 measles, and in 1970 mumps, each had their own vaccines. Rubella was also developed by using the kidney cells of green monkeys. (Green Monkeys feature famously in articles on AIDS as they have been indicted *in absentia* with being the origin of the disease. What is not so commonly known is that these benighted creatures are kidney donors on a spectacular scale for the furtherance of medical science.)

The vaccine programme

In the 1950s it was recommended that children should be vaccinated for whooping cough, diphtheria and polio by the time they reached three years old. They were then expected to have boosters at the ages of five and seven. The BCG was recommended at twelve or thirteen years old. Nowadays this policy has changed so that children are routinely immunised with DPT, polio and HiB (the haemophilus influenza bacteria that is present in meningitis) at two, three and four months old, and with MMR (measles, mumps and rubella) at twelve months old. Both these vaccines are then given again at pre-school age though the pertussis (medical term for whooping cough) is usually left out. At the end of secondary education adults are recommended to have a further booster of the diphtheria and tetanus vaccine. The meningitis C vaccine is also recommended as it is the seventeen to twenty age group that most readily contracts this variety of the disease. There are variations to this schedule across the country.

What is in the syringe?

In the hypodermic syringe is a cocktail; not only of live, attenuated or detoxified extracts of the viruses and bacteria, but also of preservatives such as formaldehyde, antibiotics (such as streptomycin), mercury, aluminium and a range of far from innocuous chemicals such as hydrochloric acid. Any reports of side effects are seen to be caused by the bacteria or viruses used. This may be an inaccurate premise as any chemical or metal foreign to the body is capable of causing biochemical reactions within the organism. Formaldehyde can cause tissue damage; antibiotics can cause disturbance to the digestion and to the hormone cycle; mercury causes toxic reactions such as have already been discussed; aluminium can cause paralysis.

Furthermore, in an effort to encourage a broad-spectrum immunity to several diseases early on in life, the syringe contains the material of several diseases at once. The two-month-old body is asked to cope with the introduction directly into the bloodstream of five differing diseases: whooping cough, that affects the respiratory system; diphtheria, which attacks the lymphatic tissue of the throat; tetanus, which affects the entire central nervous system; haemophilus, which is an influenza virus that can cause meningitis; and polio, which affects the gut, the musculature and central nervous system, and which is introduced orally. Amongst these five, only whooping cough is actually a recognised childhood disease. Meningitis C is given separately but is nevertheless expected to be taken on by the infant body at the same time as the others.

The measles, mumps and rubella vaccine is a shot that is intended to protect against three childhood diseases that are usually of short duration and without any lasting side effects. The MMR and, most recently, meningitis C and the pre-school boosters are all given before puberty sets in. This means that children are immunised against nine different diseases before their own natural immune system's defence mechanism has matured. In addition, this toxic brew is introduced *directly into the bloodstream*, a situation that does not happen in nature *at all*. (Though tetanus is the result of a wound, it is the nervous system that is affected and not the circulatory system or the lymphatics.)

The role of the thymus gland

The history of epidemic diseases has caused such deep fear in us that our rational minds seek the security of anything that promises to prevent the diseases from occurring. It is our rationalising about disease – believing in effect that we live in a hostile environment in which there are potentially lethal pathogens waiting to prey on us – that has led us to accept that the body is incapable of putting up a sufficiently reliable defence. Yet we do have an effective immune system which is automatic and it starts working from the beginning of life. One of the main organs involved in developing the immune system is the thymus gland.

The thymus gland is a pinkish grey, two-lobed organ that lies under the mediastinal area of the chest, a little above the heart and below the thyroid. It is situated in front of the aortic arch and trachea. It has been referred to in literature since the ancient Greeks but it is an organ still of some mystery as science has not yet discovered all of its secrets. In animals it is known as the sweetbreads and is considered a culinary delicacy.

The origin of the word 'thymus' is from the Greek *thymos* which etymologically derived from an earlier European root word *dheu* that had the meaning 'to rise in a cloud'; 'to burst into flames'; 'to smoke'; 'to fume'. The word *thymos* denoted 'life force' or 'soul', though it originally referred more directly to 'the breath' or the 'breath of life' – upon which depended energy and courage.

It was discovered only as recently as the 1960s that the thymus gland plays the central role in creating and maintaining the immune system. It was at one time believed that the thymus was useless rather in the same way that the appendix is usually viewed today. Then it was considered that it was an organ of childhood only because post-mortems revealed so many shrivelled or atrophied thymuses. At one time, it was believed that an intact thymus was a sign of illness as children who died from sudden cot death illnesses were found to have 'enlarged' thymuses. This led to the belief that radiation treatment on the thymus would limit disease in children. Yet, more recently, injections of thymus extract have been given to children suffering from severe, life-threatening infections with very satisfactory results. It was also once thought that the thymus was only active during childhood and that with puberty it atrophied. It was seen as an integral part of the maturation process but of no consequence in the adult.

The thymus gland is at its most active from birth to puberty in the sense that it is central to the creation and maintenance of the mature immune system. Not only does it produce lymphocytes that are essential in the elimination of viruses and bacteria but also other cells that are specialised in seeking out, neutralising and eliminating cancer cells and foreign tissue.

White blood cells originate in the bone marrow and about 50 per cent of them go straight into the bloodstream for immediate deployment while the rest are carried via the bloodstream to the thymus gland where they are further processed into T-lymphocytes. These T-cells have three major functions:

i)   they stimulate the production of more antibodies by other lymphocytes;

ii) they stimulate the growth and activity of phagocytes which are specialised to surround and engulf bacteria and viruses;

iii) they themselves are designed to recognise and destroy foreign and abnormal tissue.

The gland also secretes thymopoietin which impairs the transmission of post-synaptic neuromuscular signals; without this the body would be in a constant state of overstimulation -- which occurs in myasthenia gravis, a condition that leads to muscle weakness. Interestingly, some four out of ten cases of thymoma, cancer of the thymus gland, occur in those who suffer from myasthenia gravis.

Without the thymus we are in danger of succumbing to even the least infection. The removal of the thymus causes tremor, weight loss, easily broken bones, weakness and susceptibility to infection and the early development of cancer. The gland acts like a thermostat to create the right balance of immunity. It increases the output of lymphocytes to fight infection and cancer but it turns down its activity to prevent an autoimmune disease. Its role is therefore vital in the body's ability to deal with infection, allergies, cancer and autoimmune diseases in general, and tissue rejection in the case of transplants in particular. Anything that interferes with the process of developing the thymus's full potential is likely to threaten the body's defence system.

Any of the following can lessen the effectiveness of the thymus gland: smoking, alcohol, prescription drugs, recreational drug use, high levels of cholesterol, excessive sugar consumption, food additives, mental, emotional or physical stress and chronic ill health especially where that includes a lot of pain or depletion of the body's resources. It is not surprising that early post-mortems discovered that the thymus glands of the deceased were withered: disease and malnutrition had had the effect of reducing the thymus to a size and function level that was inadequate for survival.

Puberty does not begin until the thymus has done its initial work for the immune system. It secretes a hormone that signals the initiation of sex hormone activity and the end of its own expansive activity of contributing to the general process of maturation; or it should do. Problems arise when it does not do this. Enlargement of the thymus can, due to its anatomical location and structure, cause interference with the return blood to the heart from the brain; thus it can also interfere with the cerebrospinal fluid and thus hormone output. It can also put pressure on the heart and lungs.

There appear to be two types of children who are, so to speak, thymus dominated and they are relatively easy to spot. Those whose thymus is damaged through illness, malnutrition or any other factor are fragile, pale and have porcelain-like skin that is laced with blue veins or, at least, rather mottled. They are prone to conditions most readily associated with TB: infections of the lungs, ears and mucosa; they have weakened bones that break easily and may be accident prone (see the chapter on tuberculosis in Part III).

If the thymus is enlarged, continues to be pro-active and yet there is also sexual maturation developing there is a different picture. The subject appears completely out of touch with any finer feelings (and later with any idea of spirituality) and is entirely physically orientated. There is very early interest in sexuality and later excessive libido with a tendency to violence and aggression. Criminality may be part of this unattractive picture. There is little refinement and right-brain activity is limited to physical sensation while cultural and artistic sensitivities remain out of reach. There is a gross quality overlaid by negativity. Facial expressions (or none) might be permanently set. There is suspiciousness, and humour may be evident only through grinning with downturned corners of the mouth.

Damage to the thymus can be caused by thymoma, a tumour of the gland, but this is comparatively rare. More often, though, damage is caused by severe trauma, mechanical accident and artificial immunisation. Drug intervention (particularly antibiotics and steroids) is also detrimental to the gland. Childhood fevers with opisthotonos (arching of the back) should also be considered suspect. Emotional trauma, especially if sustained for any length of time, is certain to affect this gland: fearfulness that induces emotional dependency is a prime indication. (In adults this often becomes a fear of disease with a dependency on medical intervention.) The thymus is an organ with a vital role to play in our survival but which is under threat from the very beginning.

What most concerns us here though is how artificial immunisation adversely affects the thymus gland. Consider how this organ must play in tune with the body's whole orchestra. It is programmed with a specific function that is part of the evolution of humanity: to prepare the defence mechanism to deal with the toxic results of disease; not just acute diseases but also chronic and even, by toning down its activities, autoimmune processes. Yet the jabs are given at an age when the thymus has hardly begun its work of preparing the body to deal with future disease and while the recipient is still being protected (hopefully) by its mother's breast milk and antibodies. The jabs, in effect, deliver a two-sided chemical message that tells the body that it is under attack from several diseases at once and that its immune system is inadequate in the first place.

Do scientists really know what happens within the body when a mixture of childhood diseases, epidemic diseases, neurotoxic disease and a cocktail of toxic preservative is delivered directly into the bloodstream of a two-month-old baby? The fact that *the body never produces the symptoms of more than one acute disease at a time* seems to have completely passed by the collective scientific mind. What is also left unsaid is that children have a purpose in developing their childhood diseases – as you will see in the third part of this book.

Side effects of the specific vaccines

Diphtheria, pertussin, tetanus (DPT)
Children with glue ear are often pale, weak and susceptible to infections of the ears, nose and throat and lungs. They don't have good powers of recovery and frequently need to resort to antibiotics. They have little stamina and poor appetites. They can be shy and alternately pathetic and aggressive or stubborn. They often have sluggish bowels as well. This is usually all put down to the fact that the child cannot hear with all the mucus in the Eustachian tube but it is also a good picture of a child with a damaged thymus gland. This picture is common and very familiar to homoeopaths. It is the typical picture of a child who has been damaged by the vaccine containing *pertussin* – the whooping cough vaccine.

Pertussin
Pertussin has been linked to side effects such as: high fever, skin rashes, disturbed sleep patterns, chronic rhinitis and sinusitis, recurrent bouts of vomiting of post-nasal mucus, disorders of appetite and thirst, susceptibility to chest infections, croup and asthma, behavioural disorders (withdrawal and aggression), epileptic fits (both petit mal and grand mal) and sudden infant death syndrome (SIDS)[1]. Often, in treating children with any of these conditions, it is beneficial to give the homoeopathic remedy made from thymus gland itself in order to effect a lasting and thorough result[2]. The physical symptoms may well retreat under other more common remedies but sometimes the mental/emotional symptoms only improve on a fundamental level when the body receives the energy of thymus gland. Though there is no proof, this might suggest that patients with these conditions have a damaged thymus; certainly it is an area of study that demands research.

It is very common for babies of two, three or four months to spike a fever whether they have been vaccinated or not. A naturally occurring fever will often resolve itself by being expressed as a cold or as diarrhoea or a skin rash. The same is true of fevers that occur after vaccination. Such apparently minor incidents do not necessarily occur at a predictable interval after vaccination; some babies will produce a fever within hours, some within days and others within weeks; all of which means that it has been very difficult to secure reliable statistics and data about the incidents of side effects. Any reactions that happen much beyond a week after vaccination can be dismissed easily as the result of an infection. Yet there is a discernible pattern in a significant proportion of those immunised: fever, restlessness, swollen glands, profuse mucous discharge and loss of appetite and slowed development. It is this last symptom that is telltale. The pattern is followed by recurrent fever, sore throats and/or ear infections when the eardrum swells, bursts and releases quantities of pus and mucus. This is not permitted to continue: antibiotics are routinely given and a cycle is then begun which results in the addition of respiratory disease, buccal and intestinal thrush and increased sensitivity to allergens such as wheat, gluten, sugar and preservatives. The last thirty years of the twentieth century saw an alarmingly steep rise in the occurrence of these conditions, a trend which continues today. It is therefore appropriate to consider the impact of the mass vaccination programme at least as a major factor in this trend – if not as the whole cause.

In worse cases the affected children become asthmatic. They do not actually have asthma but bronchospasm. They produce quantities of thick mucus in the throat that is swallowed and more in the lungs that is difficult to cough out. This leads to acute bouts of croup and bronchiolitis. Antibiotic and steroid treatment is then employed and the situation quickly becomes chronic. Before long these children are labelled as asthmatic on their medical records and the inevitable long-term treatment of steroid inhalers is instituted.

If a body reacts to a vaccine it is attempting to initiate a process of elimination: it wants to rid itself of toxicity by generating a fever or mucus. Frequently the body is unable to eliminate satisfactorily for a number of reasons, including shock at the introduction of so many disease factors at once and, as we shall come to in the discussion of the miasms in Part III, hereditary disease taints. (For those with a family history that contains evidence of tuberculosis there is a far higher risk of negative reaction to the DPT vaccine.)

Vaccines and other suppressive treatments administered in response to the pathological reactions that follow are so often the reason for the state of chronic pathology in the very young: eczema, asthma, irritable bowel conditions, permanently enlarged tonsils, allergic rhinitis, catarrhal deafness that requires grommets, bladder and kidney conditions. This lists only the physical effects. Behavioural disorders, sleep disorders and learning difficulties must also be considered because clinical evidence of successful homoeopathic treatment in such cases bears this out.

Yet, despite the fact that pertussin has been used for over 50 years and has been pumped into the arms of four generations of children, whooping cough has not been eradicated. It is still with us though it is sometimes difficult to diagnose as the symptom picture may no longer conform to the traditional textbook definition. It is not uncommon to hear of reports of epidemics of persistent, croupy coughs among vaccinated children. It is also true that many who have been vaccinated and do not contract the disease, develop a chronic cough that can continue for months on end, even sounding like whooping cough. Many of these cases result in the diagnosis of asthma for which the patient is put on steroid inhalers; it does not take long for the jab to be entirely forgotten, and therefore never considered as the original culprit[3].

Tetanus
The side effects of the tetanus vaccine are harder to gauge as they take so long to appear. This is not surprising when one thinks how the bacterial spore that causes the disease is capable of lying dormant for many years until introduced into the local dying flesh, deep within a wound. The main effects of the vaccine include scoliosis, lordosis and kyphosis all of which are conditions of curvature of the spine. The most common is kyphosis of the upper thoracic spine with consequent unremitting tension of the associated musculature. It has also been suggested that it is responsible for weakness of the bladder sphincter muscles.

Diphtheria

The diphtheria vaccine has not had much publicity, partly because it is regarded as being such a success. Nevertheless, since the introduction of the vaccine increasing numbers of children have grown up with chronically enlarged tonsils that fail to perform their prime function of being the first line of internal defence of the body. So swollen and full of toxic material can they be that they are unable to react defensively for the system in the face of infection.

Polio

Polio has received less attention in the press since the Salk vaccine was replaced due to so many reports of severe and even fatal side effects. The current vaccine, nevertheless, can cause its own problems. It is possibly responsible for slowed rate of growth, cramps, digestive disturbances including food intolerance, behavioural changes (especially phases of dis-orientation and anxiety states), loss of balance, vertigo and low-grade fevers.

There is more to the story though. Reports of paralysis occurring after the diphtheria injection were not uncommon from 1942 onwards when the inoculation became widespread. (Paralysis was also reported after the per-tussis vaccine.) Polio was seen as a threat from the late 1940s onwards when there was an apparent outbreak following World War II. In fact, there have been many reported cases of polio following the diphtheria jab from several different countries. In the USA it is widely accepted that the inci-dence of polio is the result of handling the nappies of recently immunised babies.

Would that this were all there is to say about polio[4]. The vaccine con-tains not one but three different strains of the virus cultured on the kidney cells donated by monkeys. In the early days of culturing the vaccines, in the 1950s and 1960s, monkeys that had been infected with SV40 monkey virus were used. The SV40 virus is one that causes the growth of tumours. The most common form of cancer that is associated with the administration of the vaccine during those two decades is brain tumour. Leukaemia and bone cancers follow on the list. As SV40 has also been found in semen samples of healthy men it is quite possible that the virus is transmissible hereditarily in some way.

HiB

The haemophilus influenzae B bacterium is commonly found on people without any symptoms being manifest. It can nevertheless be harmful as it is associated with complications that can lead to chronic after-effects and even death. The chronic diseases linked with it include pneumonia, meningitis, septic arthritis and septicaemia. Though it should be borne in mind that all these conditions would result only in those people with strong hereditary disease taints, they are all serious and potentially life-threatening in those with a weakened immune system.

Perhaps the most curious feature of this vaccine is that it is based on a disease cultured on the brains of a cow. This would put the vaccine right out of court for any family that is dedicated to a vegan way of life. It also raises the spectre of CJD, Creutzfeldt-Jakob disease (the human form of BSE).

As the vaccine is combined with the DPT it is harder to implicate it in major side effects. However, it is quite likely that the DPT shot weakens the immune system generally and sufficiently for the normally harmless HiB to become a serious toxic invader for which the body may have no effective means of elimination. Amongst the side effects recorded are vomiting, diarrhoea, fever, allergic reactions, HiB influenza, joint pains and fitting. In some of the trials of this vaccine, carried out in conjunction with DPT, there were cases of death[5].

In the autumn of 2004 a new combined 'five-in-one' vaccine was introduced with the intention of replacing the DPT and HiB inoculation. The new vaccine was announced as being 'cleaner and safer' than the old version. (This official quote is tantamount to an acknowledgement that the old vaccine was not fit for use.)

The three main advantages of this shot are that thiomersal, the mercury-based preservative, is removed; the 'whole cell' whooping cough vaccine 'has been changed for a cleaner version' and 'the polio element is a safer, deactivated vaccine replacing the live, oral vaccine'[6]. While we should be grateful that it has at last been recognised that mercury and live whooping cough virus are too harmful to inject into infants' bloodstreams, we should be cautious about the new vaccine for a number of reasons. *Five different diseases are being injected at once into immature immune systems.* There has been precious little time to run extensive trials of this vaccine, let alone to discover the long-term effects of injecting the disease material of five different viruses directly into the bloodstream. It requires many years to test vaccines adequately; the side effects last for years, even a lifetime and in some cases – as appears to occur with tetanus and measles – the effects can lie dormant until another trigger (such as an acute illness or a trauma) sparks them into activity.

Meningitis C
Meningitis C becomes a serious problem in those who are susceptible when the bacterium that is normally found harmlessly in the mucus of the nose and throat proliferates in the bloodstream *as a result* of the typical symptoms of inflammation of the brain, headache and fever. The injection is often responsible for any of these symptoms as well as rheumatic muscle pains, diarrhoea and vomiting and blackouts.

Measles, Mumps and Rubella
Of the three other childhood diseases, measles is seen as the most threatening because of the potential damage to the eyes and because it is associated with viral meningitis. Otherwise it is a reasonably innocuous disease in spite of its reputation these days (much exaggerated by the medical profession). Measles *can* cause severe and tragic consequences however in those whose inherited familial disease patterns are connected with what, in homoeopathic terms, are called syphilitic conditions: autoimmune disease, hectic inflammatory states of the brain, tissue destructive processes, rapid terminal cancers, alcoholism, suicide and degenerative diseases. Mumps is normally no trouble unless the sufferer is adult and the gonads may be involved. In rare cases however, meningitis can be a complication. German measles is regarded as a problem only in relation to women who have conceived recently as it can be so detrimental to the health of the unborn child. The potential threat from side effects of the vaccines far exceeds in significance the distress of suffering the common symptoms.

313

Side effects include:

Measles: Fever, vomiting, swollen glands (including the mesenteric glands and the reproductive glands), pneumonia with atypical measles, rashes, febrile convulsions, emotional distress with prolonged periods of screaming, respiratory problems, loss of hearing, paralysis, lack of co-ordination, tremor and violent head shaking, behavioural changes, irritable bowel syndrome, Crohn's disease, food intolerance and allergies, encephalitis, meningitis, Kawasaki syndrome, thrombocytopenia (decrease in the number of platelets) and death.

Mumps: Encephalitis, febrile convulsions, seizures, meningitis, epilepsy and insulin-dependant diabetes.

Rubella: Nerve pains, numbness, meningitis, encephalitis, paralysis, ME, thrombocytopenia, rheumatoid arthritis.

The triple vaccine was introduced in 1988. It was following its introduction that viral meningitis became so much more prevalent; so much so that scientists were obliged to find vaccines for the various strains that began to develop. They had to do this so quickly that there have been reports that the research work to ensure their safety was grossly inadequate. What is more, anyone with vegetarian leanings should know that the vaccine contains both chick embryo cells and cells from a human foetus.

One of the most common complaints of this triple vaccine is behavioural change with increased susceptibility to viral infection and learning or behavioural difficulties. It is not unusual for a mother to bring her child for treatment complaining that ever since the child was about a year old, he or she has had tantrums, frequent colds, ear infections and difficulty in some way with communicating, maintaining eye contact or learning relatively simple tasks that require hand-eye co-ordination. The mother does not necessarily associate the symptom picture with the MMR vaccine until she is asked directly *"Do you think that your child was making average or good progress up until the period in which the MMR was given?"* It is more usual than not for the mother to say that she had never noticed anything untoward before that time, or words to that effect.

Many children who are being diagnosed as ADHD (Attention Deficit Hyperactivity Disorder) or autistic may also have immune systems or nervous systems that are damaged following the administration of the MMR vaccine. They frequently suffer infections that require antibiotic treatment or have problems of hypersensitivity or spatial awareness that result in clumsiness. (*What Doctors Don't Tell You*, a magazine dedicated to open debate about contemporary medical practice, has pursued the link with autism with enthusiasm, and has come down firmly on the side of those scientists who have shown statistical evidence, from their own studies as well as those used by government sources, that there is a link between the MMR and autism.[7])

Another area of consistent complaint is in the digestive system. Increasingly large numbers of children are complaining of food intolerance and allergies with Crohn's disease and celiac disease (wheat intolerance[8]) being the result at the worst end of the scale. It is recognised that the measles virus can affect the normal balance of bowel flora in the gut; it has been the subject of enormous controversy that the virus has been identified in the bowels of autistic children. If the range of resultant symptoms were consistent it would be less difficult to point the finger at one cause. It is no surprise to most homoeopaths that when indicated remedies, supported by homoeopathically prepared medicines made from the MMR vaccine itself, are used, the symptoms begin to retreat and something near to a normal balance is restored in the body.

It seems incongruous in the light of so much controversy that the British medical authorities should continue to protest the safety of the MMR when, for example, Japan has taken the results of government surveys so seriously that this vaccine has been banned (though the individual vaccines are recommended).

Many parents feel strongly that even if their children should be allowed to have measles and mumps naturally, there should be protection against rubella because of the risk of damage to unborn children from the disease in pregnant women. Research in the USA has demonstrated that vaccinating children before puberty has meant that the age at which this disease is naturally developed has changed and is now more prevalent in those over fifteen years old. This has increased the risk of contracting the disease at a time when it is likely to cause the most concern. It is also recognised that by allowing people to develop rubella earlier in life, permanent immunity is conferred while it is widely recognised that the vaccine has relatively short-term efficacy.

BCG

The most common long-term side effect would seem to be (from unofficially recorded clinical evidence) rheumatoid arthritis which makes itself apparent only some time, years even, after the vaccine is given. However, it is also implicated in the incidence of intermittent fevers with sweats, respiratory difficulties including asthmatic breathing, susceptibility to throat and sinus infections, persistent dry cough, hay fever symptoms and skin reactions. More seriously it is implicated in causing ulceration and abscesses, chronic swelling of glands and anaphylactic shock.

Death has been recorded in various countries as a result of the immunisation. (It is interesting to note that Holland does not have a BCG programme of vaccination and has the lowest incidence of TB death rate in Europe. It is also revealing that *The Lancet*, in March 2002, published the findings on a study of 83,000 people who had been vaccinated against TB. The conclusion was that no statistically proven protection against TB was given by the BCG injection.)

Hepatitis B

This inoculation is commonly given to people in the health professions who might be at risk of infection from the patients they care for, or from instruments (such as needles or scalpels) used by or on those who were likely to be infected. Those likely to be carriers include drug users and those assumed to follow a promiscuous sex life such as prostitutes and homosexuals. It is now de rigueur for nurses and care workers in hospitals and clinics to have the inoculation; the management insist on it and it is a requirement of employment.

The list of side effects for this jab is long and given that it is mostly those in the medical caring profession that suffer them it is extraordinary that the vaccine is still in current use. The side effects include all the usual immediate problems: swelling and pain in the arm with fever and tiredness. There are also headache, itching, sore throat, diarrhoea, vomiting, profuse sweating, rheumatic pains, respiratory tract infection, cramps and abdominal pains. The bladder and kidneys can be affected as can the central nervous system and the hormone system. Hepatitis is a disease that affects the liver and the function of this organ is almost always compromised; sometimes it causes jaundice. As a result there is a tendency to more frequent infections and to overactive lymph glands. It is also common for those seriously and chronically affected to develop the symptoms of myalgic encephalomyelitis, otherwise know as ME.

Cases to illustrate the vaccine problem

To support all this data a few cases might illustrate the extent of the problems created by artificial immunisation.

Case 1

A mother brought in her twelve-year-old son, Brian, who was suffering from eczema. The skin was universally affected though the worst areas were in the usual places: the backs of his hands, his wrists, inner elbows and backs of the knees. He had phases of getting better when only these areas showed any sign of the condition; they were always red, sore and itchy and after he scratched they would bleed. At other times his whole body seemed to be affected and he would not know where to scratch for relief. The symptoms were always worse when he was in bed at night. By the morning his bed would be littered with flaky skin and the sheets would be spotted with blood.

Everything about the case indicated that Brian needed *Sulphur*, probably the most common remedy for eczema. He was given a daily dose and asked to report back in three weeks. When he called he said that his skin had got very bad and had wept thick yellowish serum for several days. (This had been predicted as Brian had used steroid ointments for years. He had been told to expect his body to throw them out.) Then things had gradually improved so that he had two days where his skin was bad only on the knees and elbows. After this he had gone downhill again. Furthermore he was tired, listless and apathetic. He was also surly towards his mother. She also reported that he seemed to be running a low-grade temperature all the time.

Brian's eczema had begun when he was six months old. His mother was not sure whether he had had any reactions to the DPT injection – *"possibly a slight fever."* He was given *DPT 30*, one each night for five nights with a dose of *Thuja* 200 to follow immediately. The result was speedy: he developed a streaming cold with mucus that poured thick and yellow from his nose and throat, his ears seemed to fill up as well and his eyes watered profusely. He nevertheless felt much better in himself, he was far more energetic and the slight fever left him. His mood and behaviour changed so that his mother reported that she had *"the old Brian back"*.

DPT is a remedy made from the inoculation serum of the diphtheria, tetanus and whooping cough vaccine. It is regarded by homoeopaths as a direct antidote to the poisoning effects of the immunisation. *Thuja* has long been viewed as the most important remedy to restore integrity to a vaccine damaged immune system. Hahnemann first discovered its profound effect in vaccinosis (the state of being poisoned by the smallpox vaccination) and homoeopaths have since used it successfully in dealing with the effects of other inoculations; so its record goes back over two hundred years.

Case 2

A little girl, Wendy, was brought for treatment of her tonsils and ears. She had suffered from constant throat and ear infections since she was four months old. She had grommets in both ears and her tonsils were permanently enlarged. Her mother was anxious to avoid any further doses of antibiotics and hasty trips to the hospital with high fevers. Wendy was plump and pale, whinging and clingy. She never wanted to eat anything except crisps and raw carrot and never drank anything but milk. Her nose was perpetually seeping green mucus and she often brought up the very phlegmy contents of her stomach. Her breathing was laboured and rattling and at night she snored, wheezed and coughed.

Wendy was a good example of the *Pulsatilla* archetype. She was given the remedy over three days in a relatively high potency, the 1M. Milk was also removed from her meagre diet as it was highly likely that it contributed to the heavy mucus production. The mother reported that Wendy responded immediately. After the first dose she had fallen into a deep sleep that lasted for twelve hours much to her parents' anxiety. Then her left ear had poured pus-laden debris for forty-eight hours and she began to have diarrhoea. This lasted for a week though she did not show any signs of weakness or dehydration. She began to get colour into her cheeks and she added toast and porridge to her small repertoire of foods.

On examination it was apparent that the grommet in the left ear was now missing and the one in the right ear was dislodged and only held in by thick wax. Her tonsils remained as large as ever.

Within six weeks Wendy went down with another ear infection – though it was not as bad as usual and it responded to a further dose of *Pulsatilla*. There was no need for antibiotics. However, she then developed a very high fever and presented an acute picture of *Belladonna*. She was given a high potency of this and the fever reduced promptly. She seemed well again and in record time for her. Yet the same thing happened again after another eight weeks and then again six weeks later. It was clear that the constitutional remedies were insufficient to restore Wendy's health to its original state.

She was given *DPT* 200, once a day for three days and *Silica* 1M to follow[9]. The result was that she had no further ear infections but her tonsils became active. They almost closed over her throat, caused her breath to smell rank and exuded white matter, mostly from the left side. She had no fever and appeared well in herself. This situation continued for well over two weeks with Wendy showing no particular general ill effects. She was cheerful, more independent and very active. Eventually the tonsils reduced in size and stopped producing the white matter. She remained well until the next winter when she had a cold. Her mother reported that it was the first cold that Wendy had had which did not bring on the ear and throat infection. It lasted for two days and left her well.

Case 3

A young man of sixteen, Michael, developed quinsy – a severely swollen throat with enormously enlarged tonsils and a fever. He was too ill to come in to the clinic and the treatment was carried out over the phone. Michael had already undergone constitutional treatment for some time and had not needed any remedies recently though in the past he had a history of eczema and debilitating acute sore throats.

He was suddenly very ill. The tonsils were dark red, almost purple. His throat was covered in a thick membrane of almost milky mucus. He could not move his neck for stiffness; he could not swallow for the pain. The bones of his cheeks were excruciating and he had rheumatic pains all over his body. He could not speak as his tongue was so swollen. This is the picture of *Mercurius Iodatus Ruber*, the red iodide of mercury. He was given the remedy in the 200th potency, to be taken every two hours. It did very little. In this circumstance, because the symptom picture was both clearly indicative of the remedy and also a good example of nature imitating a specific disease, Michael was given *Diphtherinum* 200, the nosode of diphtheria. This is what made the difference. He quickly recovered from the worst symptoms. He was left with weakness, poor appetite, a constantly runny nose and nausea – and these symptoms persisted. Despite remedies that might have been expected to get him back to full strength, little further changed. He was eventually given *DPT* 30 and the effect was evident within two days. Not only did he feel much better from the whole acute throat episode but he said that he felt generally better in himself and this despite a fresh flare-up of his eczema. He has remained well since except that it his eczema that now flares up when he feels below par.

In this case it is reasonable to say that the effects of the DPT vaccine had lain hidden but active right up to the quinsy crisis. He had never known the full potential of his energy. The quinsy was not simply an infection. It was an expression of a family pattern of the disease; he did not 'catch' it, he developed it. With the link between heredity and the diphtheria vaccine being made in the acute, Michael's stricken Vital Force could not throw off all the effects until the vaccine influence was overpowered.

Case 4

Martin, a lad of ten, was brought by his mother for treatment for persistent attacks of unsteadiness, clumsiness and disorientation. There was no special indication for any remedy other than *Silica*: he was short for his age but thin and gangly. He was always chilly and had a tendency to have swollen glands in his neck. *Silica* did improve his constitution so that he no longer had frequent colds but it did not do anything for the transient attacks that seemed to stem from a dysfunctional nervous system.

He came to the clinic one day during one of these episodes. He was asked to stand upright with his feet together in a relaxed manner. He was quite unable to do it. He needed to prop himself up against the wall as he felt that one or other leg would give way and that dizziness would make him fall backwards. When these sensations came on he would begin to

feel very hot and sweaty, his stomach would churn and he would go
deathly pale. He was given *Polio* 30 there and then. He never had another
attack.

Case 5

Tracy, who was sixteen at the time, complained of tension in the back.
The muscles across her shoulders and shoulder blades were very hard,
stiff and painful to move. She said that she had noticed the gradual
increase of tension and lack of mobility over several months. She had had
a lot of osteopathic treatment and cranio-sacral therapy but to little lasting
avail. What was also evident was that scoliosis (curvature of the spine)
was developing and kyphosis as well (the formation of a hump). After
several well-indicated remedies failed to make any impression at all, Tracy
was given *Tetanus* 30. She noticed a virtually instant reaction and within
twenty-four hours her back was 50 per cent improved. Over the following
months the symptoms gradually faded. She was advised never to have
another tetanus injection.

Case 6

An anxious woman phoned the clinic to say that she was on holiday in
the area and, though she was another homoeopath's patient, she could
not contact her practitioner and her little boy needed urgent treatment.
She brought him in her arms. He was unable to move voluntarily. His left
hand and right foot twitched. His eyes were rolled up showing almost
nothing but the white. He had shallow breathing and he was a deathly
pale grey. He responded not at all to his name or to the offer of food or
drink. The mother explained that he had been like this for twelve hours
but that it had had a gradual build-up over the two previous days. After
close questioning there seemed no clear picture. To observe, his state was
most similar to the remedy *Helleborus*, the Christmas rose. Yet there was
an indefinable suspicion that amounted to little more than intuition that
there was more to the case.

The mother was asked to go back over the days before her son had
fallen ill. At first she could think of nothing unusual except that the
family had been preparing to leave London to come down into the
country for their holiday. Then, in quite a matter-of-fact and offhand
manner, she said that on the previous Wednesday (it was now Monday)
she had taken him to the surgery to have his MMR jab. The boy was given

a dose of *MMR* 30 at once. The effect was both dramatic and shocking. His face turned puce within twenty seconds and he began to 'burn up' with a high fever. He began to whimper and stir. His mother looked on astonished and cried out, *"What have you done to my son? Oh my God! This can't be happening!"* She fled from the room and the clinic.

The next day the mother phoned again and asked to bring her son in. Again she carried him in but this time he was able to cling on to her, he was looking round him and he was no longer feverish. She explained that the fever had not lasted long and little by little he had become more alert and more mobile. He still did not want to get off his mother's lap or off the sofa; it was as if he did not quite trust his legs. His shoes were removed and some gentle massage was applied to the area of the feet that corresponds to the spine in reflexology. Within half a minute the boy got off the sofa, walked round the room and asked his mother for something to eat – the first time he had spoken words in three days. Because the boy was now thirsty, generally rather hot (though not feverish) and wanting to eat salty things (he had asked for bacon and Marmite sandwiches) he was sent off with a dose of *Sulphur* 30. Their family homoeopath rang to say that the boy remained well.

Case 7

Lilly, a little girl of four years old, was brought by her mother for treatment because of hyperactivity. Her mother explained that the child's behaviour had changed some twelve months before when she had stopped talking, had become anxious and tearful when left with the childminder (to whom she was usually very attached) and inclined to scream and hide from anyone who visited the house. The health visitor had suggested that Lilly should be taken to the paediatrician. After various appointments and tests Lilly was diagnosed as autistic. Despite improvements in her general health from being taken off wheat and gluten products Lilly still continued to be hyperactive. She would become extremely easily frustrated. She would destroy whatever it was she was trying to do. She could not concentrate on what she was doing for more than a few moments. She walked round rooms aimlessly touching things and picking them up. She would make unintelligible noises instead of using words. She would become spitefully aggressive especially if she had eaten sweets. Everything was exaggerated when she was with anyone: her movements were impulsive and the more of an audience she had the more flurried and aggressive she became. If she was in a room on her own then the behaviour would be a lot less frantic. The mother was absolutely certain that her daughter had been perfectly well up to the time she had been inoculated with MMR.

The homoeopathic remedy that is most similar to Lilly's symptoms is *Tarentula Hispanica*, the spider. Her mother was given a packet of this remedy so that she could administer it to Lilly every time she had a strong outburst of the difficult behaviour. She was asked to use the remedy, in other words, if Lilly went into acute episodes – like using *Belladonna* for a fever, or *Pulsatilla* for an ear pain, this remedy was for the manic activity. The effect was satisfactory up to a point. The mother reported that she could now control the attacks to a large extent though she would have to use the remedy at least once a day. It was also obvious that after a few days Lilly seemed to be aware of the distress within her self. She would ask her mother to give her a *Tarentula* pill (which she could only do by pointing to the shelf on which the packet was kept). It was clear that *Tarentula* was not the only remedy needed.

Lilly was then given *MMR* 30 for five consecutive nights, with a *Thuja* 100 to follow. The first noticeable result was that Lilly did not need many *Tarentula* tablets. She herself would now refuse them on most occasions when the mother suggested taking one – and it was obvious that Lilly now knew best. She was generally calmer and happier. She began to speak again after a week, using a few words when she wanted to ask for anything. She no longer showed the same inclination for sweets and she began to eat more than just the meat on her plate. Her fluid intake dropped to the point of concerning her mother. Nevertheless, she was also inclined to cling to her mother and to remain indoors if she possibly could. This was unusual as she had always enjoyed being outside. She also developed a very mucus-filled nose. At this point Lilly was given a *Pulsatilla* 1M and a weekly dose of *Thymus Gland* 30. She grew rapidly, her speech returned to what it had been, she became cheerful and outgoing.

It would be dishonest to claim this success for homoeopathy alone. Lilly's mother also took her to an osteopath, a nutritionist and an educational specialist. She also devoted an inordinate amount of time to Lilly to the point where she drove herself to near exhaustion. The family as a whole was particularly loving and united. There is no doubt that all these things played their parts in Lilly's recovery; but what is indisputable is that the process of healing had been blocked until Lilly had received the MMR antidote.

Case 8

Kevin was six years old when he was brought to the clinic. He suffered from cerebral palsy and had been recently diagnosed as autistic. He was hyperactive: he was constantly restless, grabbed at things or people if they were near and he shrieked and giggled in turn. He picked things up and then dropped them shortly after as soon as his attention was seized by something else. He had overactive bowels and frequent bouts of diarrhoea.

The pregnancy had been normal though the mother reported that he had been a 'footballer' in the womb. The birth was fast but he was normal and no-one suggested that there was anything the matter with him. He did suffer from a lot of mucus and was given nursery medicines for this: Calpol included. What was also significant was that there were cases of leukaemia, cancer, schizophrenia, hypothyroidism and heart disease in the close family.

Suddenly at four and a half months Kevin had a screaming fit. He was given antibiotics as the doctor felt that he was suffering from delirium – even though his temperature was not high enough to suggest that fever might have been the cause. This first bout happened three weeks after the first DPT injection. He had three further bouts over the next twelve months.

At fifteen months old he was given his first MMR jab. His mother said that from then on Kevin began *"to slow down"*. He continued to have screaming fits, his development virtually stopped and from two years old he started *"head banging"*. By two and a half he had constant diarrhoea. It was also increasingly apparent that he was intolerant of foods that contained colourings and preservatives. He never slept through the night and needed little sleep anyway. His nose perpetually ran with mucus, his chest was always rattly and he was unable to control the copious amounts of saliva from his mouth. What should also be added was that tests were carried out on Kevin and it had been shown that the measles virus was alive and well in his gut – one of the hotly disputed signs of the side effects of the MMR vaccine.

This is the kind of case that seems to defy the practitioner. Not only is the patient in a state of biochemical and emotional turmoil but the character itself has been perverted. The physics and chemistry are so far out of sync and the child's developing personality so hobbled with negative experience that it is improbable that one therapy alone would be able to make much significant difference – let alone a single prescription. Nevertheless, remedies did, over the period of treatment, make some small but notable changes.

It became apparent that *Mercury* was useful for his throat and chest infections. After the first doses he developed a cough that had a 'whoop' to it. He was given *Drosera* (a very common whooping cough remedy that is characterised by a deep cough started off by a persistent tickle in the pit of the throat that is worse for lying down) and then *Pertussin* 30. After this a rash *"from head to foot"* that looked like measles came out though he had no temperature with it. Following this there was a period of fewer infections and calmer behaviour.

Kevin's mother, being thoroughly versed in alternative medical thinking and keenly observant of any little signs of change, was able to report on progress made. She noted how Kevin responded to osteopathy, to music therapy and supplementary nutritional therapy. He began to increase his vocabulary very slowly. He was brighter in himself. The control of his saliva was easier and the diarrhoea lessened. In a period when he was comparatively physically well he was given *MMR* 30, *Silica* 1M and then *Thuja* 1M in succession. After this his sleep improved, his impetuous reactions slowed down and he was more reflective and he began to increase his vocabulary of signs. However, the underlying state of cerebral palsy and autism persisted.

There followed swinging episodes of lapses and upturns. Sometimes he would have a return of diarrhoea and at other times he would be constipated. He might have good bladder control or he might wet the bed every night. He had long periods of walking on tiptoe and then he would walk on the whole foot.

There came a moment when his symptom picture indicated the need for *Pulsatilla*. He had become floppy, pale and tearful. He wanted a lot more attention and responded well to being cuddled. He also stopped drinking and appeared to have pains in his kidney area. Though his gut had quietened down he seemed distressed by being too hot for comfort. He was given a *Pulsatilla* 1M. His mother reported that this remedy seemed to go very deep emotionally: he wailed and wept all day. Following this he had an episode of severe kidney pain which gave way to his feeling much calmer. He was able to participate in activities far more readily and seemed happier in himself than he had previously been. A few months later his mother was able to say that he was much more *"with it"* than before and that he was now able to be cross, something that she had not really seen. Before he had only been able to express frustration; now he was able to direct his anger. She also said that he would go into a depressive state if he was missing someone particular.

Treatment continued on a sporadic basis – partly because he went away to school – though Kevin continued to have support from all the other therapies that his extremely conscientious mother had found beneficial. What was nevertheless apparent was that he continued on a merry-go-round of symptom rotation. When his bowel problem calmed down then some aspect of his behaviour might lapse; when a chest infection needed remedies then his gut would flare up again. Furthermore, when it was realised that the severe intestinal infestation of measles virus was chronically impeding his general progress he was put on a 'bug-killing' sulphur drug. Despite this, which might have been seen as a way of coping with the intestinal trouble while the other therapies worked on the rest, Kevin continued to be in a delicate balance where progress was frequently countered by relapse. He remains cerebrally palsied and autistic despite all the positive developmental changes that he has managed to make. The question as to whether the two childhood vaccines had anything to do with his condition will always stand. He is one of what now amounts to thousands of cases.

What is the difference between the MMR and the separate vaccines?

Britain's policy of abandoning the single vaccines – the early ones being implicated in the spread of meningitis – in favour of the triple one, has complicated the debate. While the real question should be *"Would Kevin have suffered in the way he did if he had not been artificially immunised?"*, most people these days would ask other questions. Would Kevin have suffered in the way he did if he had been immunised by three separate injections? Is there a better and less commercial reason for the triple vaccine to be regarded as superior to the separate jabs than simply the increased cost of administration? 'No' is possibly the answer to both questions.

While there are children who have undoubtedly suffered from having been given the single measles, mumps and rubella injections they are far fewer than the number that suffer from the triple vaccine. It was not so very unusual for homoeopaths practising in the 1970s, 1980s and 1990s to have to antidote the effects of the measles vaccine with the use of the nosode, *Morbillinum* or the potentised version of the vaccine itself. This was particularly true of those who developed atypical measles shortly after having the jab or even suffered meningitis or related symptoms. The same applies to the mumps and the rubella vaccines – though it was measles that caused the worst damage, probably as it is potentially a far more serious disease – the reason for which is explained in Part III in the chapter on the syphilitic miasm.

As has been said already, to inject a person with three live viruses each of which are associated with three separate characteristic symptom pictures is begging for trouble. Viruses are capable not only of mutating very rapidly but they also have a habit of lying dormant until a propitious moment when the host's guard is down or weakened. For the body to have to register that three different disease products have been introduced into the system and in a way that is utterly alien to it (directly into the bloodstream) gives us cause to realise that the collective medical mind is focused on the diseases and not on the human body at all – except in a very generalised socio-ethical way. There is no truly perceptive understanding of the fact that if a patient contracts mumps and then, very shortly after, measles, there is no possibility that the body will develop symptoms of both diseases together. The patient may start to show signs of glandular swelling and the typical neck pains but if the measles state of the patient is the stronger (which it usually is) then the mumps will disappear for the familiar mottled red measles rash to spread across the body. Only when the stronger of the two conditions is dealt with by the body's healing mechanism will the secondary problem return. (Measles usually takes precedence over mumps in the rare cases where they appear simultaneously.) The body, in other words, deals with one thing at a time in acute viral illness and, left to nature, will only do any of it when ready. In the triple jab, however, there is not necessarily any wakened susceptibility (i.e. that occurs in a body ready to express such acute ailments) that would give rise to any of these three viral diseases.

327

So how does the body recognise what to do when it is in such an unprepared state? The shock to a system that is already compromised hereditarily with any or all of those conditions associated with the childhood diseases can be so profound and confusing that any part or all of the system may be affected, sometimes irreparably (see Part III on the hierarchy of the miasms in which the relationships of acute diseases and chronic, inheritable disease taints are discussed in full).

When the patient's body has damage to the central nervous system along with maintaining causes such as chronic inflammatory bowel disease then there is little likelihood of the restoration of the body's full functioning. Kevin's was just such a case.

Following are a few further illustrative cases:

Case 9

> Marcus was eight years old when he was brought for treatment. He had been suffering from headaches, abdominal pains, flatulence and constipation for several months. His headaches were characteristic of someone with a dysfunctional liver: the pains centred on the forehead, especially over the right eye. An acupuncturist would specifically identify this as a gall-bladder headache. His abdominal pains were periodic and spasmodic. They caused him to bend double for a while and then to need to lie down on his bed. They were worse after school when he had got home and had something to eat – invariably something sweet. Sometimes the pains would continue into the night hours and prevent him from sleeping.
>
> The interview turned into comedy as soon as Marcus had to talk about his bowels and their habits. His sense of humour was tickled into activity by being asked if he passed smelly wind – and there were hoots of merry agreement and mock disgust from his brother and sister who were also present. He said that he was never able to finish a meal as he became full up very quickly. His stools were often very hard to pass but once the first efforts had been made then he passed very loose motions that smelled rotten. His mother remarked that he became very sleepy and incoherent if he ate too much bread or pasta – she had become aware through reading articles that he might be allergic to wheat. He was often irritable and crotchety, never suffered fools gladly and was quickly angered and became spiteful if interfered with by his siblings. Originally the parents

had thought that there was something emotional going on as a result of some undisclosed happening at school. They had investigated this but had drawn a blank. The family doctor diagnosed 'abdominal migraine' while a cousin who was a doctor said that Marcus had irritable bowel syndrome.

Marcus presented a symptom picture most similar to the remedy *Lycopodium*. This he was given in the form of drops that were to be taken daily. When he returned in four weeks there had been some minor changes. He did have a bit more energy. His bowels had become a bit more regular: he was 'going' every day rather than every third day. He was *"marginally less tiresome"* according to his mother. The aggravation from sweets and gluten products suggested that Marcus suffered from candida in the gut. When the mother heard that this was a possibility she volunteered that she felt that Marcus had never really recovered his appetite since he had a fever after his pre-school boosters. He was given *MMR* 30 to be taken each night for five days followed by *Thuja* 200. This was then followed by *DPT* 30 to be taken at the same dosage with a *Silica* 200 to conclude the prescription – one that was not strictly speaking homoeopathic but one that was aimed at ridding the body as quickly as possible of the effects of vaccine damage. Marcus was also told to avoid all wheat, dairy and sugary products as far as possible. This was essential as candida, a condition in which the gut is colonised by a yeast, is fed by this combination.

Marcus gradually made progress. The headaches went first. Then his appetite returned. He had a cold with a slight fever after which his energy surged. He had a growth spurt, having been stuck at below average height for his age. He became more outgoing as well and no longer complained about the teachers at school – he had said that they were 'down' on him all the time and always gave him low marks. He had mentioned that he had had a persistent dry cough *"for ever"* at the first appointment. He now said that he no longer had this cough at all and his mother added that she thought he could hear better as well – she no longer had to shout at him to turn the television down.

Marcus's bowel symptoms and headaches were almost certainly the result of the MMR injection. The cough and chronic catarrhal ears were far more likely due to the DPT inoculation. When he came back for a further assessment he appeared cheerful, bright, happy and in good health. He was full of bubbly good humour. As he had other characteristics of a healthy *Phosphorus* picture he had a dose of this remedy to keep him well – which it has done to date.

Case 10

Charlotte, a woman of forty, came to the clinic complaining of aches and pains in her hands and feet. She was much put out by this as her business was making curtains and other soft furnishings. She needed her hands for her work. She had tried to relieve the problem by changing her diet and she had been to see osteopaths for a long time, always with general benefit but none that would affect the worsening condition of her fingers. They were swollen, puffy and reddened and the joints of her fingers were becoming disfigured.

In the past she had also had homoeopathic treatment for various ailments and had had all her amalgam fillings removed as it had been evident that they were causing her some toxicity. Since then her energy had been excellent and she no longer suffered the mouth ulcers and sore throats that had plagued her. On the day that she came to the clinic she was also due to go for her regular appointment to see the osteopath who had kept in touch with the homoeopath about Charlotte's progress. She was given a remedy to take with her which she was instructed to take once the osteopath had made her overall assessment of Charlotte's present energy state. When this was done Charlotte took the remedy and the treatment continued. Within twenty seconds of the dose her arm began to swell and become very hot, hard and red. Within two minutes it was twice its normal size. By the end of the treatment Charlotte's arm was less swollen, less red and hot and much softer but she was desperate to pass water. She went to the lavatory and passed quantities of urine which had a dark yellow colour and a faintly rank smell. Her fingers were no longer puffy or swollen though the joints were knobbly. To this day she continues to sew as much as ever and there is no further sign of rheumatoid arthritis – a condition she was on the point of going to the doctor about and the suppression of which often eventually leads to heart pathology. The remedy she was given was *BCG* 30.

Why do people react differently to the vaccines?

Why is it that one child should develop asthma and hay fever after the DPT jab and others produce 'glue ear'. Why do some have behavioural disorders and others develop chronic gut problems after the MMR? Why do many people seem not to react at all to any of the inoculations? Why do some have no reaction at the time of the immunisation but then, months or years later, produce symptoms that no one associates with the jabs? The answer lies in the hereditary disposition and susceptibilities of the individual. It is impossible to grasp the whole of the homoeopathic view of artificial immunisation without taking heredity into account. From this it might seem that homoeopathy is attempting to climb on the bandwagon of the latest scientific research into genetics; but this is not the case at all.

Homoeopathy has known about the importance of heredity since Samuel Hahnemann wrote *The Organon*[10] and his other works on inheritable disease taints – two hundred years ago and more. Those who have studied these books and all the literature that has followed have accepted and worked according to the principle that the childhood illnesses are linked to inherited chronic disease patterns and that to suffer them in childhood is a positive step in a child's development. This would be a difficult statement to support if it were not for the fact that homoeopathy is unsurpassed in the treatment of these childhood complaints. Chickenpox, measles, mumps, whooping cough, German measles and even scarlet fever are a necessary part of our lives (see Part III on the hierarchy of the miasms). What is more, all of them are covered by well-known homoeopathic remedies that can easily form part of any home first-aid kit – though treatment of these diseases is best overseen by a qualified practitioner.

Eradication of disease?

Man and his own epidemic diseases are inseparable; they are not simply virulent bacteria and noxious viruses. First and foremost they are *energies* that are no more than genetic echoes until it comes time for each individual to express them; because it is common for others to *recognise energetically* when a vital acute disease is being expressed it is normal that these diseases should appear in epidemic form. 'Catching' a disease is no more than picking up on the energy of it as it is being expressed in another person at a moment when one is particularly and peculiarly susceptible to the same energy. Without that susceptibility there is no reason for the body to produce symptoms; therefore there is no illness. A child who is brewing chickenpox or measles will not necessarily infect all the other children at his best friend's birthday party; only those who, being in close proximity to a child who is expressing a necessary eliminative disease that will promote the further development of the immune system, are 'reminded' energetically of the body's purpose of 'house clearing'. The roots of constitutional susceptibility in terms of disease are buried deep in heredity. It is only possible to eradicate disease by eradicating the individual's susceptibility – someone who has had an epidemic disease becomes non-susceptible to it and, into the bargain, gains a stronger general immunity. Indeed this is the purpose of epidemic illnesses. The only way for disease to be eradicated in a general social context is for each individual to express their susceptibility through symptoms that teach the body how to react, from within. Then the information for this success is transmissible to the following generations.

All attempts at eradication of the acute childhood or epidemic diseases by artificial immunisation are doomed to failure and worse. Humanity will have to find an alternative expression for the diseases and in a suppressed body that will ultimately mean a more dangerous expression. Hence it is that we now have vastly increased numbers of children with asthma and hay fever, multiple allergies and chronic debilitating symptoms that defy any known diagnosis. More recently we have a steep rise in the incidence of meningitis, a viral or bacterial disease that has many forms, which has manifestly been more widespread since the introduction of the MMR vaccine in the 1990s. It is well known that measles can have meningitis as a major complication. The incidence of autoimmune diseases is on the march. We also have a catastrophic explosion in the variety of viral diseases that now have their own brand new diagnoses: Kawasaki syndrome, Reye's Syndrome, AIDS, the various atypical forms of hepatitis (non-A and non-B) and the even more alarming Ebola virus – at present only in Africa.

Unfortunately it is easy in our polluted world to blame quite a few other things for the mushrooming ill health of children. A lot of time and energy is poured into researching the effects of chemical pollutants in the atmosphere, in the water and in our food but comparatively little is done about the pollutants that are pumped into children's arms.

Does 'like cure like' in a material world?

This question gives us the opportunity to summarise the salient points of the alternative and specifically homoeopathic view of the most important of all current medical debates. It is also the point at which we must answer the most common question that homoeopaths are asked in relation to the vaccination debate: 'If homoeopathy treats according to the philosophy of "like cures like" then why should homoeopaths object to the prevention of disease by injecting a small amount of the pathogen?' After all, isn't that using 'like with like'? A little of what causes a problem sent in to make sure the problem doesn't arise; like setting a thief to catch a thief.

The answer to this lies in the difference between physics and chemistry. The alternative view of the human body is that it is firstly an energy system; the orthodox view is that it is firstly a physical form organised by biochemistry – biochemistry is not the servant but the master. Homoeopathy, osteopathy, acupuncture and the rest treat the source of energy; allopathy treats the biochemistry and in acute disease that includes killing off pathogens that appear to destabilise and threaten the 'machine'.

In homoeopathy we do not view pathogens in acute disease as *the cause* of the symptoms but as *the result* of the expression of disease. Though we may catch measles or mumps from others in an epidemic, we are not reacting to the introduction of the virus but to the *energy* of a disease that has found an echo or resonance within our own system and that needs a physical expression to resolve the condition.

As we have intimated, it is the result of a susceptibility to a particular disease state that is the cause of our illness. *Only* if we have inherent within us that susceptibility will we produce the disease symptoms. Our gene pool carries the hereditary susceptibility to the acute diseases and when the time is right the body will express its need to produce a specific set of symptoms in order to teach itself how to recognise the underlying chronic state that is related to the acute condition; the purpose of which is to strengthen the immune system. This is also why any of the childhood diseases might come up either in an epidemic where there is a local collective response to the disease energy or in an isolated case where there was no other case to blame as the carrier.

Orthodox medicine, by introducing *material* disease toxins directly into the bloodstream takes no account of the fact that the body initiates a reaction to them *as if it were being poisoned* not as if it needed to express a condition genetically inherent. Nor does it take into account any individual body's timetable for dealing with its own inherent weaknesses, or the fact that to suffer measles or whooping cough might have some lasting benefit for the immune system.

Why, after all, should we be the only animals on the planet to suffer these childhood diseases? Why should it be that after chickenpox or mumps children often have a growth spurt or their baby teeth start to fall out more easily? Why do those rare children who suffer several episodes of measles seem to be so poor in health and to be the result of a long family history of appalling pathology? Could there be a relation between those who suffer severe asthma and bronchiectasis as a result of whooping cough and their forebears who had a history of tuberculosis?

Allopathy views bacteria and viruses as if they were parasites looking for a host to prey on. We should view them as if they were the *by-products of a process of elimination that is inspired by and starts with the Vital Force working to clean up the gene pool.*

Any danger we fall into as a result of that process is not to do with the pathogen but with our body's inability to express the disease safely and eliminate the toxic waste. If we have meningitis with a bout of measles it is because there is, somewhere in the gene pool, a kink inherited from a forebear that has diverted the self-healing mechanism from its usual path. If we suffer orchitis as a result of mumps then it is due to the body needing to express an inherited pattern of chronic disease to find a way of resolving it. *Though it stands rational medical philosophy on its head, it needs to be seen that one of the prime intentions of the energy system is to imitate chronic disease in the form of acute diseases in order to reverse inheritable trends set up through suppression or neglect in previous generations.*

Here is the real 'like cures like': the body's ability to imitate patterns of inherited chronic disease so that the self-healing mechanism can recognise what to do to prevent that chronic pattern either being passed on to future generations or causing pathology in the present expression of life. *Disease comes from within.*

Despite the well-meaning intentions of orthodoxy, artificial immunisation is one of the most indiscriminate and deleterious medical practices ever undertaken. In terms of the history of western medicine it has risen to its present dominant significance in no more time (comparatively) than it takes to bat an eyelid. There has been no time at all to take an honest look at the appalling harm that is being perpetrated on future generations of humanity – just enough to see the immediate apparent changes as the threatened diseases seem to withdraw beneath the onslaught. There has not been enough time to witness in what ways those diseases will need to be expressed in the future.

For a disease to be truly eradicated it is not enough to be able to say that no-one suffers the diagnosable and characteristic symptoms of it any more. For a disease to be genuinely eradicated there must be no susceptibility to producing those symptoms. This means that no disease has ever been eradicated by human intervention, not even smallpox – despite the claims. If the last remaining stocks of this disease were released onto an unsuspecting population then there is no doubt that many would produce the symptoms and some would perish. So how is it that neither diphtheria nor bubonic plague feature so largely in our consciousness any more? Diphtheria was already on the wane before determined vaccination began. Our collective gene pool had begun to learn how to deal with it. Bubonic plague had its day years before systematic immunisation was ever thought of. Both diseases still exist but cases of them are very limited and certainly not nearly as newsworthy as they once were; not in the face of the return of diseases like TB or the steady and implacable escalation of AIDS.

It takes courage to refuse to have one's children immunised; it seems that one is flying in the face of all reason. It helps to remember that for all its sophistication, orthodox medicine is still very much a science of discovery. It is based more on the logical, rational world of chemistry and less on the genuine empiricism of observing clinical, whole-body reactions in individuals or populations. However, in spite of the dangers of misjudgement through personal emotional involvement, observation is still the only way to witness nature at work. The truth is that scientists are too ready to bend statistics to support what are, in humanitarian terms, praiseworthy theories. The little incidences of negative and even tragic reactions in individuals are not enough to demonstrate the reality of artificially suppressing epidemic diseases: the general undermining of natural immunity that is a vital component of our survival.

An unusual way to make up one's mind on the vaccination debate

Chloë was an aspiring actress of twenty-two when she came not so much for treatment as to investigate what homoeopathy could do for her. She was curious and she was healthy. So well was she that it was hard to make a case at all out of the information she gave. She was bright, chatty and happy with her life. She seemed never to have a day's illness with the odd exceptional day of a cold every so often; no more than one day in six months perhaps. She had a good home background with loving parents and she was very much attached to her boyfriend who was also an actor. Both of them were appearing in a play that their theatre group was touring with and performing in local schools. She ate a good diet, drank enough water, slept enough hours and had plenty of energy.

There really was nothing current on which to base a prescription. The one possible blip anywhere in her health biography was the fact that she had been immunised against diphtheria, pertussin and tetanus as a child. She had no recollection that she had reacted in any way to it, on any of the occasions it had been administered. She was, nevertheless, given *DPT* 200 for no better reason than it might have acted as a block to other remedies. The main idea was that when she returned for a follow-up consultation she would be given *Phosphorus* as this was the remedy that was most similar to her general state of constitutional wellness. She had no idea as to what the remedy was that she took away.

Chloë came back in six weeks. She was just the same as before: well, confident, warm and smiling. She said that she had *"not truthfully noticed any difference from the remedy"*. She apologised for not being able to be more positive. She had hoped so much that *"something extraordinary would happen"*. There was a pause in the interview; she started to look pensive and she frowned for the first time.

"Actually something has changed. I am not really enjoying my work any more. It's not the acting; I love that. But I am not comfortable about the play I'm in. I play a mother who is really worried about taking her child to the clinic for vaccination – the DPT triple jab. I have scenes where various people – the nurse, the health visitor, the doctor – all persuade me that it is safe and better for my child and how it is better for the long-term health of society and so on. I keep thinking about how the play is sponsored by one of the big chemical firms and how I am performing to children – children, for heaven's sake! – in schools. It all seems so calculated and propaganda-ish."

She paused and then added, *"Anyway, I don't really believe in the words I have to say. I can't tell you why but I feel uncomfortable saying what seems false."*

When she was told the name of the remedy she had been given she was amazed. She found it hard to believe that circumstance had offered her such a serendipitous experience. It also made her feel that she had been intuitively right in her feelings.

CHAPTER 17

ALLERGENS

Allergens can be virtually anything that will provoke a hypersensitive reaction. They range from the sun to tomatoes, from mobile phones to horsehair, from the scent of a particular flower to plain water. Reactions may be mild or life-threatening or anywhere in between. Whatever the individual's response to the allergen, it is certain that the body's biochemistry will be triggered into making abnormal changes. The changes can range from little more than indigestion or a mild itching of reddened skin, to anaphylactic shock or asphyxia. It is the degree of the reaction that determines whether it should be labelled an 'intolerance' or an 'allergy'. However severe the person's response is and whatever the manner of symptomatic expression, it is the individual's hypersensitivity to the trigger or triggers that is the real maintaining cause and not the allergens themselves. The usual practice in the treatment of allergies is to screen the patient for responses to particular allergens. This can be done in a number of ways via blood tests, skin sensitivity allergy tests (both favoured by physicians), hair analysis tests, kinesiology (muscle testing) or tests carried out by attaching the patient to a computerised machine minutely sensitive to the body's biochemical changes (Vega and Bio-resonance testing). The purpose is always the same: to find the symptom-provoking allergen. The sense of this lies in the patient coming to know what to avoid. This is extremely important in the case of food allergies: wheat, gluten, eggs, nuts and shellfish are some of those substances that can create severe and even fatal consequences. Those who suffer from a sensitivity to animal fur usually know what it is that affects them while those who suffer from hay fever (a misnomer as it covers so many different types of allergy) can often tell which plants cause them trouble. Mothers of hyperactive children usually realise quite early on that colourings and preservatives in foods (especially sweets) are potential hazards.

The homoeopathic approach to allergy

There are two different aspects to the treatment of allergies. The first is the strictly therapeutic one: when a patient comes for treatment because he or she has acute symptoms then the appropriate remedy, most similar to the condition, is selected. The second is the need for long-term constitutional treatment to eradicate the tendency to be overreactive to substances that the body should normally be able to deal with.

A man came into the clinic covered from head to toe with hives. He said that it felt as if he had fallen into a bed of nettles – he looked as if he had. He said the pains were stinging and that he felt as if he had ants crawling under his skin all over his body. He also felt nauseous and looked faintly yellow. These latter symptoms suggested that his liver was affected and this in turn meant that he had probably eaten something that his system did not know how to deal with. This was the case for he had eaten lobster the night before. He had woken up in the very early hours feeling ill and with the skin in its present state. When asked if this had happened before he said that whenever he had anything with either crab or lobster he tended to suffer in this way.

This is not a difficult situation to treat as it is simply a question of selecting the remedy that would cause the same degree of suffering in someone else with a similar sensitivity. The remedy he was given was *Astacus Fluviatilis*, the common crawfish. He sat a while in the clinic waiting room and watched the skin gradually go back to its normal state.

On another occasion a small boy was brought in suffering from an acute allergic reaction to egg. He had eaten a piece of cake that had been made with eggs and now had a livid red ring around his mouth so that he appeared to have been playing with his mother's lipstick and his breathing was laboured. He was extremely thirsty, very hot and as limp as a rag doll. All these symptoms suggested that *Sulphur* would make an impression on the condition. He was able to go home within half an hour with no symptoms. Since then his mother has used this remedy several times whenever her son has inadvertently eaten anything with egg in it.

Another anxious parent reported that whenever her son visited his friend's house he was tempted to eat sweets, especially a particular brand of brightly coated chocolate buttons. His reaction after eating them was to become cheeky, rude and very loud. He would become manic. He would make very lewd jokes and laugh in a high-pitched hysterical way. If reproved he would throw a tantrum and then the furniture. He had been known to take a knife out of the kitchen drawer and chase his elder brother round the house screaming curses and imprecations at him. The whole episode would last until he exhausted himself and fell asleep on the floor somewhere. In the morning he would be morose to start with and utterly exhausted. His mother had learnt to leave him in bed and not force him to go to school. When he did emerge from his room he would be pathetically contrite and tearful.

Such a state is answered by *Hyoscyamus*, (henbane – a weed long known to ancient witchcraft). The mother was given a 4 gram bottle of this remedy in the 200th potency so that she could administer it whenever her son was tempted to indulge in anything that contained colourings that were toxic to him. She also brought him for constitutional treatment so that after some eight months the need to use *Hyoscyamus* became part of the boy's history. How extraordinary it is that a plant that has hallucinatory powers and has always been known as the preferred poison of that witch of legend, Hecate, should also provide us with a twenty-first century remedy for the manic hysteria engendered in a sensitive body by superfluous artificial colourings in sweets.

Such cases are commonplace but none of them tells us the whole story by any means. For true healing each one of these patients needed to be treated constitutionally to eradicate the underlying sensitivity from which their allergic reactions derived.

Histamine reactions

Histamine is a derivative of histadine which is found in all body tissues. Histamine causes capillary walls to become more permeable so that more antibodies and nutrients can reach a stricken area. The local result is inflammation and contraction of the involuntary smooth muscle. The general result is of lowered blood pressure. However, in allergic reactions the heart rate can rise dramatically and the muscles of the chest can contract to cause shortness of breath, while mucous membranes can become severely swollen – all of which causes the characteristic signs of allergic asthma. This is histamine gone rampant and the usual medical answer is antihistamine. So prevalent is the use of this class of drugs that the names are part of our everyday medical vocabulary. Even so, and despite all the immediate relief they give patients, these drugs can be a nuisance, as they can mask the true symptoms of an allergy picture. Suppressing allergic reactions prevents the selection of indicated remedies and can confuse the general constitution. This is what often happens with hay fever sufferers.

Acute hay fever

Hay fever is never as straightforward as it may seem. It is quite common for those who had eczema earlier in life (now suppressed) to have all the typical symptoms of itching, sneezing, crawling, watering and wheezing. Those patients whose parents had the symptoms are highly likely to inherit the same. Though it is less common, it is still usual enough to find patients who develop the signs 'out of the blue' with no apparent exciting cause. What all of them have in common is extreme sensitivity. In the mind of the homoeopath the hunt is on at once for not only the acute symptoms but also the hereditary background and the preceding circumstances that may have resulted in the attacks.

The immediate circumstances can be many and varied: a period of extreme stress, a stretch of taking steroids for some inflammatory problem, a long drawn-out emotional saga, going on or (paradoxically) coming off the Pill, a minor accident that has given rise to a period of continual pain – any of these and more can be implicated. If nothing like these is evident then it may be necessary to look further into the past and see if there is the suppression of eczema and/or asthma that is so common. If this is absent then it is possible that as a child the patient went through a long spate of high fevers sometimes accompanied by measly skin rashes.

Untreated history can be – must be – mined for information. Often, a variety of dormant maintaining causes are turned up; ranging from neglected or suppressed childhood respiratory ailments to vaccinations, from subdued eczema to intolerance of dairy products. Whatever time of life the acute hay fever begins, all these events hidden in history would need to be addressed sooner or later. The tissue memory of the body must express itself and hay fever is one way to do it.

How do we know this? Because the treatment of hay fever often requires several years to reach a satisfactory conclusion and encompasses en route the elimination of exciting historical causes such as have been mentioned. It is not enough to give the remedy for the acute symptoms as, even if the patient is very satisfied with the results of it for this year, the problem is very likely to occur next year. If the acute symptoms are not seasonal but perpetual then the chosen acute remedy is likely to become redundant after a while; though it may have worked well to start with, it becomes less and less effective with time. What's more, the next remedy chosen for the acute may well not be as effective as the first one was initially – suggesting that there is missing underlying information that, unless it is addressed, will continue to compromise the Vital Force's ability to respond.

A case to illustrate the history behind hay fever

Chuck, an irritable man in his early twenties and very much in a hurry, came for treatment for hay fever. He was brusque in manner and clipped in speech. His nose was red and swollen and he frequently blew it noisily. This alone was almost sufficient to prescribe *Nux Vomica*, a nut that contains strychnine. However, the patient had all the other characteristic signs: his nose blocked up at night so that he could not sleep and then ran profusely in the daytime so that he could not think. His nose was raw from the mucus being so acrid. The sneezing attacks that came on as soon as he got up and lasted till mid morning were shattering. His eyes were dry and red-rimmed. His ears itched mercilessly. He could not taste his food and his teeth were extremely sensitive. *Nux Vomica* did the trick nicely: he quickly ran out of his first bottle of pills and came back for more. This sufficed for the first season.

The next year came round and the symptoms began again. His wife said that he no longer believed homoeopathy worked as his condition was all the same and he was too busy to waste any time but she persuaded him to return for further treatment. He was extremely sceptical (not unusual in a *Nux Vomica* patient) but went away with his new prescription. The result of this was that his symptoms did improve but

that he had a violent bout of diarrhoea and a face full of spots. *Sulphur* was the second prescription as he had had a long course of antibiotics a few years before for persistent acne – and nothing effects the elimination of the memory of antibiotic suppression like *Sulphur*. Though he was not best pleased he did find that the *Nux Vomica* now worked well again and that he did not need to take it so often anyway. The same thing happened the following year though he was more willing to participate.
Nevertheless, he said threateningly that he wanted an assurance that he would not have any further physical reactions like the ones he had with *Sulphur*.

He went off with a new prescription but this time only reacted by having a temperature for twelve hours. He said that he felt very peculiar for a while: light-headed, faintly sick, hot and sweaty and lacking in any energy. By the time he woke the next morning he felt perfectly well and his hay fever symptoms were nowhere near so aggravating. He had been given *DPT* 30.

In the following year he came without persuasion 'for an MOT', he said. He had some of the minor symptoms he used to have but he could cope as he was able to sleep so much better. He was also very much less impatient, less hectoring, more measured in his attitude. He had a persistent cough though, and he wanted to get rid of that to feel really well. As his uncle and his grandfather had both had tuberculosis he was given *Tuberculinum* 1M. He required no further treatment for hay fever – or anything else.

Heredity in hay fever and other allergies

This case illustrates the need for medical archaeology: to dig with remedies. When the patient's own experience is no longer a source of maintaining causes then heredity must be looked into. Actually, heredity usually comes into play far earlier in the treatment of allergies than Chuck's case suggests. Inherited disease patterns are always present and are the main reason for the extreme sensitivity that is common to all allergy sufferers. In Chuck's case tuberculosis was obvious in the family but sometimes it is not so clear. Some patients can present extremely complex and convoluted family histories which have to be teased out layer by layer using remedies sequentially with the patient's changeable condition dictating the pace and direction.

For a far more comprehensive view of this see Part III where it will become clear that TB is never the only inherited causation of disease, just the one that is most immediately associated with hay fever.

It is these underlying maintaining causes of history and heredity that make both seasonal and perpetual hay fever symptoms so complex to treat. It is why nutritional supplements are so rarely sufficient on their own and why orthodox treatments simply provide relief at best and suppression at worst.

Allergy vaccines

Any treatment aimed at desensitising patients towards their particular allergens is a very questionable approach. It can, and usually does, complicate the genuine holistic healing process. The practice of allergenic inoculation (usually restricted to defusing reactions to pollens, spores and chemicals) is as unwise a procedure as artificial immunisation because it takes no account of the background cause of the susceptibility of the individual. Those who start off by being desensitised towards horses often go on to being acutely sensitive to dogs, then cats. The same happens in the case of people who have their sensitivity to grass pollens deactivated; soon they become allergic to flower and tree pollens. It is the age-old story of suppressing rather than eliminating the cause. In this case desensitisation is not the suppression of symptoms but the 'blowing of a fuse': the body, inoculated with a bombardment of weakened allergens, finds its usual reaction to the toxins overloaded and 'blown'. To express its hypersensitivity it must find something else to react to.

A case of multiple allergies

A woman phoned the clinic to arrange for a phone consultation. This is not normal practice but proved to be necessary as the patient could not leave her house. She said that her name was Eithwen and that she suffered from so many allergies that unless she stayed within her own four walls she could not cope with her physical reactions. She suffered headaches from sitting inside a car as she was acutely aware of the petrol.

She was poisoned, she claimed, by traffic fumes, scent, all factory chemical odours, pollens in general, most foods and any electrical interference. She could not have a television on for long and even the telephone caused her some problems. She was able to eat a very limited range of foods: pears, rice crackers, avocados and peas were her staple diet. She was a virtual prisoner.

She explained that the only time that she dared to go out was to allow a friend to drive her to a clinic many miles distant where she would stay for two weeks and receive anti-allergenic inoculations. The first few days would be needed to recover from the effects of the journey, the remainder being needed for the regular injections. She had made this excursion only three times in some six years as she could not afford to go more often. It became apparent that, despite the initial relief that she felt which could last up to six or eight weeks, the effects of the inoculations were not lasting. Indeed, it was obvious that over the years her condition had deteriorated disastrously. She had not been housebound at the start of her illness.

There are plenty of people who have been through a desensitisation programme who have not reacted so badly but they were unlikely to have had the same emotional history as this patient. Missing so far from the description of this woman's misery is the fact that she had suffered cruelly from a disappointing and, at times, violent marriage. Underlying everything that she said that was not directly related to her physical symptoms was a passionate and undying grief and hatred for her husband. She said that he had been uncaring; he was always far too busy for any domesticity. All he wanted was 'bed and board'. When she fed him he would disappear off to work and if she ever refused sex he would rape her. What was curious was that, despite divorce and her natural feelings of humiliation, disgust and fury, she still worked for him and did his accounts. What was even odder was that the husband was sufficiently solicitous to come and fetch the remedies for his ex-wife. What could explain such a situation?

It gradually came out that the woman had married to get away from home. 'Home' to her meant a place of earlier misery and degradation where her father ruled the roost with an implacable rod of iron. Her father had always shown favouritism to a younger, spoilt brother. 'Mother' had been feckless and cowed. Eithwen was the intellectual and outshone the rest of the family. She had been destined for university – or so she had fondly thought. Father had had other notions.

Though Eithwen persisted for some years with remedies, very little progress was ever truly made. She had some remedies in the house that she relied on 'to keep me going'; they included *Arnica* but this was the only one that might remotely have made any sense as a prescription of a remedy similar to her condition – but even then, only partially. It was as if she imagined that her self-prescribing was doing her good – the placebo effect. Even this was better than nothing. It is likely that she was never really able to let go of the emotional ropes that bound her and confused her recent and past histories. Even if it had been possible for her to afford all the naturopathic treatment she needed to regulate her biochemistry – sufficient at least to assist the homoeopathy – and to undo all the suppressive anti-allergenic inoculations, it is questionable whether she would have been able to undo the years of victim programming. Despite several years of quite regular prescriptions that covered every conceivable aspect of her case, Eithwen's allergies remained obstinately entrenched. She kept spinning round on an emotional hamster wheel; in her extreme state of loneliness and apparent rejection of the world she never relinquished her hold on the negative emotional ties with her husband and her father. Eithwen's is an extreme case but it does illustrate that some people continue to suffer allergies because of emotional undertows.

The emotional element

Lorraine, loquacious and ebullient, erupted into the clinic to ask for help with her allergy. She would inexplicably come out in red weals all over her arms and legs. She was rather worried as she was now beginning to have the symptoms on her throat. Her limbs would become puffy and swollen, red and stinging with pain. Recently her neck would swell and feel as if it threatened to restrict her breathing. She would become very tired and listless and overcome with a desire to sleep. This was very unlike her as she was always on the go. She had the remnants of an attack still on her arms. The reddened area, when pressed with a hand, would go white for while and show an imprint of the fingers.

She had no idea what might have been the trigger. Close questioning revealed no food problem, no chemical culprit and no possible link with anything suspicious from a foreign country. What eventually emerged was that her histamine reaction was due to her unabated revulsion for her new boss. He repelled her physically and emotionally and she suspected him of being *"a dirty old man with one idea in his head"*. She said that she got *"the creeps whenever he walks into the room"*. She also felt that he picked on her to do all the awkward, tricky jobs in the office. He watched her and leered at her and made her feel very uncomfortable. He was not in the office all the time but when he was she would always feel tremendous anger which was followed by an exaggeration of these symptoms – she had just not put two and two together.

Lorraine took *Apis*, made from the common honeybee. The weals never returned. They did not need to because she went over her boss's head to the department chief, an understanding woman, who agreed to transfer her out of the secretarial pool and into accounts, *"Which is where I wanted to be anyway, so that was alright!"*

CHAPTER 18

FAMILY POLITICS

The idea that a loved one might be a maintaining cause of illness seems perverse. Yet hidden deep within the walls of family relationships can be extraordinary Machiavellian mischief and downright wickedness. When the tortuous emotional ties between people who live together or who have lived together become so tightly twisted that they threaten to crush the creative life force of one of them, then those bonds should be seen as a maintaining cause.

For a patient to have an appointment during which he or she might feel comfortable enough to speak confidentially about the terrible hold that someone has over his or her life, to receive a prescription that most similarly matches the general and particular health state and to book in another meeting with the idea of continuing treatment, all counts for very little if the patient must return to the situation which makes him or her suffer. Most of us know someone who is held negatively in the thrall of another person; perhaps it might be a spinster daughter under her mother's thumb or a twenty-something man trying to live up to his exacting father's expectations. It could be a nervy wife cowed by her vicious, disappointed husband, he, in his time, a victim of his father's vitriol; or it might be an older sister, duty-bound by upbringing, unable to cope with her wily younger sister's careful manipulation of their older parents. We might be able to see all this and yet we do not notice how the relationship is stealthily undermining the victim's health. It is only when we hear that cancer has been diagnosed that we say with conviction: *"Well, I'm really not surprised."* But all the signs were there before if only we could have read them.

Leonard and Margaret

Leonard was an old soldier. He had led an extraordinary life during World War II. Though he did not crow of his achievements or of any bravery, he certainly loved telling some of the stories of his exploits. He had been in Special Operations Overseas and had served in France and Italy. He always spoke in the first person plural and seldom mentioned what he did on his own. His other great passion was Italian opera about which he was extremely well informed. *"If I hadn't been a soldier I would have been a tenor."* At which point he burst out with *La Donna E Mobile* from *Rigoletto.* At most of his appointments he would open the conversation with what to others overhearing would have been inconsequential chat about music he had recently been listening to. To him, in his retirement, it was life's blood. The nearest thing he could get to it was singing in the church choir. Those who knew him well said that he had a very good voice.

Leonard suffered from headaches. They were frequent and debilitating. The pain always occurred in the same place: beneath a scar that began on his forehead and extended back over his skull – a legacy of his wartime activities. He had had these headaches for some ten years but they had gradually become worse and worse. They usually came on when he was indoors or in the car. He agreed that they were probably worse for his being in an enclosed space. Otherwise he appeared a fit man, extremely well for a man in his late seventies, and still powerful. But this was not the whole story.

Margaret was Leonard's wife. She was buxom and freckled, had a beaming smile and a booming laugh. They had been married some thirty years. She had married him soon after his first wife divorced him. She was at least ten years younger than Leonard and was extremely well in herself. She never seemed to suffer any ailments at all. What was a little unusual about these two was that when she was present – and she insisted that she attend every appointment – he was never allowed to speak without interruption or reproof. She would correct him or tell him not to exaggerate details. She would answer questions directed at him. She would keep notes on his state of health and the frequency of his headaches. She would explain what the pains were like and how many paracetamol he had needed. She would relay what the osteopath had said about his treatment. She would sit in the patient's chair herself, leaving him with an upright plastic one. If he began to describe any of his recent doings she would become restless and impatient. If he spoke about his war days she would tell him not to be so boring as everyone had heard him tell those stories so often.

He had been to see a homoeopath before but after a while the practitioner had insisted on seeing Leonard on his own. He went for one solo appointment only; the next one was cancelled. It seemed that there was a handicap to his treatment from the start. So it proved. Leonard received remedies for some six years. In all honesty, very few of them had much impact. The most successful were those that were intended to affect the acute pain when it came on. At different times *Aconite, Belladonna* and *Hepar Sulphuricum* were all able to give him a certain amount of relief.

Sometimes he would come into the room before his wife. He would manage a few minutes talking before she finished dealing with the receptionist. During these few moments he would hint at the strain he lived under. *"Well, you know, it can be a bit difficult living with someone with such a strong character. Hard to get round. She doesn't like it if I don't do as I'm told, you know. That comes from being a soldier…you get into the habit of following orders!"*

It became apparent that his headaches always came on when he was in an enclosed space with Margaret. He never had them if he was on his own or out for a walk; nor would they occur when he was at choir practice. Margaret was his maintaining cause.

What Margaret's motivation was can only be guessed at. She would make odd little comments such as *"You silly old thing, I'll just have to put you out to grass."* She would blurt out irritably that his memory was going if he could not remember something at once – he often took a long time to answer a question (after it had been repeated for his benefit) and it seemed as if he would go into a reverie. He might just have been enjoying the silence. Very gradually it became obvious that Leonard's memory was impaired; he may even have suffered a minor stroke as his speech became a little indistinct and he would become disorientated. The more confused he became the more intolerant Margaret was. Then his mother-in-law was brought into the house – a withered shell of a woman who had already embarked on her decline into senility. Margaret set him to babysit the old woman while she went off to sort out the Women's Institute or the parish council. Now when Leonard came for his appointments he was silent and his face was a picture of doom. Remedies for the most profound depression did nothing. Remedies for the descent into second childhood failed as thoroughly.

Then, one day, Leonard came to his appointment alone. Someone had damaged the car as they parked it and Margaret had had to sort out the exchange of names and addresses for the insurance. He made good use of his time. He poured out an avalanche of grief and humiliation in a long, rambling saga of degradation. So powerful was his feeling that it seemed as if the remedies might have at last begun to get through and were giving him the strength to express himself. He even spoke of having rung up his first wife to ask her if he could go and live with her.

It was the last time Leonard ever appeared at the clinic. He quickly deteriorated into complete senility, became quite violent, according to rumour, and within a few months he was dead.

Roger, Geraldine and their daughter

Roger and Geraldine had been married for twenty-four years. He was a male nurse and his wife was a teacher. Their lives were apparently uneventful and it is unlikely that even the few good friends that they had knew anything worth gossiping about. The pair were grey and colourless and admitted as much, wondering if they could cope with anything that would upset the routine of their daily existence.

Roger was a gentle person; some would have described him as feminine though he was not at all effeminate. He was softly spoken and had a perpetual, nervous smile hovering about his lower face. He never criticised anyone or anything; the nearest he would get to making a judgemental comment was when he used the word *"difficult"* to describe someone. He would invariably qualify this with *"rather"* or *"quite"*. He used to enjoy his work at the local hospital and he had been popular amongst his colleagues.

Geraldine had a flat, monotonous tone of voice which betrayed as much emotion as a cold pancake. It seemed that she wore the same clothing – of a uniform dun colour – to every one of her many appointments. She sported no make-up and only one item of jewellery: a Victorian cairngorm brooch that might have belonged to a long-deceased maiden aunt. She taught geography and must have been singularly uninspiring in the classroom. The most animated part of her was her digestive system – which plagued and embarrassed her. She suffered from food intolerance; she reacted to dairy food, sugar and sweet stuff and all things made of wheat. Despite avoiding all these things she could still not rid herself of pain, discomfort, flatulence and the cadaverous smell of breath and flatus. So scrupulous and acutely aware of her symptoms was she that she had banished herself from the conjugal bedroom. Roger's comment on this was that it was sad but that it made no difference to their physical relationship – *"Neither of us has any inclination any more."*

Roger had his own problems: he suffered from chronic fatigue. He had no idea how it crept up on him; he had *"suffered from tiredness for at least five or ten years"*. He could not think of any event that had set it off though he suspected that it had probably been the result of a number of different things: a history of chronic backache, annual bouts of 'flu some years before, a period of working night duty – all may have played their parts in his present condition. The fatigue could be so bad at times that he could hardly lift himself from his chair. He was certainly unable to work for any length of time. He was on sick leave but had little hope of returning to his job.

Geraldine was very willing to follow naturopathic suggestions. She maintained a strict watch on her diet. She always made sure that she ate her main meal before 7p.m. and she had discovered for herself that she responded well to 'food combining' – not mixing protein and carbohydrate foods at the same meal. She stuck to this regime – for the most part. It transpired, with time, that she was not absolutely honest about what she would eat. Though all her meals were carefully balanced, she did treat herself to iced buns and hot cross buns in between. She could not resist them.

Over the years this couple received a lot of treatment. They had many hours of homoeopathic consultation; they went to remedial massage; they visited a naturopath who used sophisticated computer equipment to diagnose their conditions. They took the alternative route seriously and spent a lot of their little spare money on trying to heal themselves. They did find that homoeopathic remedies would help but they seldom made long-term changes. They were impressed with the masseur who found that they both suffered from tremendous muscle tension especially in the upper back and neck. Geraldine also had such tension around the vertebrae of the mid-back (T5 to T10) that it was impossible not to see this as part of the digestive condition. (If this area of the back is rigid then the nerve messages that operate the organs of the solar plexus and the gut are compromised.)

The hunt for maintaining causes turned up various possible problems: amalgam fillings, the Pill, physical traumas and vaccine damage – both had reacted badly to a typhoid jab they were given before going to Goa some years previously. There might also have been the question of emotional trauma had their forebears been other than ordinary: Roger's parents had been quiet and unassuming and his two older sisters had

been academically bright but more interested in domesticity while
Geraldine had been the only child of doting parents. Geraldine had had a
domineering paternal grandmother who managed to make her father
spend more time with her than with his wife and daughter but Roger
never knew his grandparents as they had all died relatively young. So
what could have been preventing the long-term healing process?

Roger and Geraldine had two children: a boy of eighteen and a
daughter of twenty. Mark was into sport and wanted to become a physical
training instructor. He spent much of his time at the local sports centre or
on the various local games pitches. He had a group of very close friends
all of whom had grown up through school together. His parents hardly
ever mentioned him though when they did it was with obvious pride.
They had no concerns for his welfare and he never had a day's illness. He
appeared in the evenings for a meal; otherwise they hardly saw him. They
did go so far as to say that he preferred to do his schoolwork at one of his
friend's houses. *"We speak to him more often on the phone than we do to his
face,"* was one of Roger's most critical remarks.

Louise was their daughter. She was training to be a primary school
teacher and she took her studies very seriously – so seriously that
Geraldine suspected that they had an effect on her physical condition.
Louise suffered from asthma. She had officially suffered from asthma from
the age of thirteen though it had crept up on her as she approached
puberty. Her mother mentioned that she had been highly strung ever
since she was born but her early periods had seemed to make matters
more difficult. As her GCSE mock exams approached she started to
demand absolute quiet in the house for her revision. If she felt that there
was any disturbance then she would start to hyperventilate. On several
occasions during the mocks and then with the GCSEs themselves she had
to be driven to the hospital in status asthmaticus where she had stayed in
overnight on a nebuliser and after which she was sent home with steroids.

When she was eighteen, Louise came for treatment. She presented a
very clear picture of the remedy *Arsenicum*. She was a thin girl with the
slightly hunched shoulders of an asthmatic. She was very precise with her
words and described herself exactly and how her asthma affected her. She
said that she was the sort of person who never left anything to chance;
she always felt the need to be ready for any eventuality. She never went to
school without checking her bag and making sure that she had all the
right books for the day. In the evening she would prepare her room for
work by setting out all the necessary stationery and by making a
sandwich and a hot drink of milk. She had special home clothes that she

would wear as they made her feel more comfortable and before she settled down to do prep she would take all the day's clothing to be put in the wash.

She was mostly well in the daytime but by the evening she would often feel pressure build up in her chest. She became anxious and restless just at the time that she would want to settle down to do her homework. If there were any noise in the house she would have to put a stop to it. She could not work unless there was complete silence. She forbade the use of the television or the radio. Even though she would work upstairs in her own room with the door closed she could not tolerate the sound of the vacuum cleaner if her mother started cleaning. She would not allow her parents to go out in the evening during the week. They had to stay at home in case she needed to ask them for help with her work. If Roger and Geraldine wanted to go out at the weekend then they had to be back by 6 o'clock because Louise would work on Saturday and Sunday evening as well.

Arsenicum did a lot for Louise. She found that it took away most of the symptoms of pressure in her chest and that she could sleep through the night. She no longer needed to rely on her inhalers so much. She was able to eat a little more at mealtimes and she put on weight so that she looked less gamine. When she had a cold – a typical herald of an asthma attack – she was able to cope with it well by taking *Pulsatilla* and *Antimonium Tartaricum*[1]. Her periods became regular as well with the use of other remedies such as *Medorrhinum* (see Part III: Sycosis for a full appraisal of this remedy) which, incidentally, helped her to cope with the nerve-shredding build-up to her A level exams.

None of these remedies did anything to mitigate the tyranny Louise operated within the home however. In fact, on the last occasion Louise came for treatment she said that she was not at all comfortable with the way homoeopathy affected the psyche. She specifically and categorically declared that she only wanted treatment for her breathing difficulties.

Where their daughter was concerned both Roger and Geraldine were smitten like a rabbit caught in the headlights. They were utterly incapable of mentioning that they felt that her demands were a burden and that they saw their lives as curtailed by her routines and her vicious temper. Though they knew that it was Louise's intolerance and hypersensitivity that kept Mark from the house, they could not see how to alter the situation. If either her mother or father said anything that could be interpreted as even the mildest criticism, Louise would throw a tantrum and collapse into asthma. On the rare occasions that they had made a bid for independence Louise had finished up in hospital in intensive care for a week. This situation continued up until the time came for her to go to college.

Louise chose a college that was within driving distance of home. She rang her parents every weekday and at the weekend she came home with mountains of preparation work to complete. Roger and Geraldine began to feel the relief of being held accountable only to the phone from Monday to Friday. They could now watch television or listen to a play on the radio. Mark began to come back into the home a little more often; Roger's symptoms began to ease a bit and he felt a little more energetic; Geraldine's gut became slightly less irritable.

Then everything went wrong. Louise decided that it was too difficult to travel between the college and home so she asked her parents for help in setting herself up in a flat. They sold a small plot at the bottom of their garden to make the money available and Louise moved in. Not more than a month later she asked her mother to move in with her – and her mother decided to go.

What followed was difficult to assess. Roger, as ever not wishing to be judgemental, said very little though he did say that he thought that Louise had been *"working on Geraldine"*. Whatever the truth, Geraldine went to her solicitor and sued for divorce; the case was bitter and acrimonious. Two years later she remarried. She had never returned for further treatment – and more than likely did not need to as she had found a solution to the stalemate of her former existence. History doesn't relate what Louise thought of her stepfather. Mark began to stay at home for longer and now brought his friends round on the odd occasion. Roger, still easily fatigued, took a part-time job in a newsagent's.

The temptation is to judge this peculiar set of circumstances as an indictment of a paranoid young woman or perhaps as the result of a marriage that did not quite work. But it makes no medical sense to take a moral stand. What is medically important is to see just how patients can be so affected by the negative energy of those who live with them that their pathology is not only exacerbated or even caused by it but also maintained. It is not as simple as to say that Louise was to blame for her parents' predicament.

For Louise to have had such a negative hold over her parents suggests that they must have played their own part in the situation. Many people simply would not have tolerated such behaviour, asthma or no asthma. Louise found some response in her parents to her chosen method of getting what she wanted.

People who need *Arsenicum* are often possessed of powerful personalities; they make things happen around them and they thus either attract or repulse people. Louise not only held her parents in her emotional grip but she also deliberately repelled those who would not fit in with her needs. Roger, happiest when he had time to sit listening to and caring for geriatric patients, wanted a quiet and uneventful life. With hindsight, it might be said that Geraldine used her symptoms to free herself from a marriage that had long since died – Louise being the catalyst in a long drawn-out separation. Whatever the truth, Louise was, for better or worse, a maintaining cause.

There are many such cases of apparently self-seeking and even wicked people imposing their willpower on others. There is the daughter with a duodenal ulcer whose mother phoned her six times a day to complain that she did not have any sympathy for anyone who was ill or dying, least of all her own parent. There is the man racked with arthritis and humiliated by impotence whose family of sick, aged parents and maiden aunts, all living in a gothic pile with Victorian plumbing and medieval hygiene, exerted such a malignant, festering hold on him that he almost never ate a meal in his own home, neglected his wife and children and spent his life wishing himself back into a period that Dickens would have wanted to describe. There is the woman with high blood pressure whose husband obliged her and their growing number of children to move house thirty-five times in twenty-five years of marriage because of his restless nature and who never would consider settling anywhere near where she felt her roots to be. There is the teenage schoolgirl smothered with acne, brought by her domineering mother who negatively qualified every tentative answer to each question, who vetted every prescription made and dismissed any idea that there might be any emotional symptoms to be considered in this case – or in any other. There is the confused and frightened fourteen-year-old anorexic whose stepfather would say goodnight by whispering into her ear each night that she should never trust what her mother said as she was a liar and a witch with evil powers.

The list in every homoeopath's casebook is long. All practitioners face the prospect of attempting to find healing in victims of the effects of the malign force of their aggressors. It is all too often a frustrating task as the negative power of the manipulators is usually either more persistent or greater than the healing power of the patients' reaction to their indicated remedies. What commonly determines whether a patient is successful or not is when there remains alive a spark of the creative fire, a sense of purpose that is enough to promise a continual process of personal development through endeavour and achievement. When this is a reality then it is not too fanciful to describe the results as expansion of the soul.

CHAPTER 19

THE JUDGEMENT OF HOMOEOPATHS

These pages have ranged from consideration of the fallibility of homoeopaths to the susceptibility of people to be manipulated into sickness by others. By way of antidotes to medicines, damaged tissues, chemical toxicity, dietary errors and more, we have seen how even with the most assiduous of efforts the potential blocks to healing can litter the path to a better quality of life and spoil the work of the indicated remedies. The patient, normally with very little understanding of the processes of healing beyond the need to get rid of whatever is most immediately troublesome, comes gradually to realise that health is hard work. By the same token, often through the frustration of their failures, homoeopaths come to see that there is more to their healing art than the selection of the remedy-energy most like the patient's

At college, homoeopathic students are taught the importance of not being judgemental. They are shown how to take a passive role; to be recorders of the events of a patient's history and documenters of what pathology is developed. The active part of a homoeopath's life is meant to be confined to the selection of the remedy or prescription that is most 'like' the general state of the patient. Yet this necessary teaching is to put aside three things:

1) that not all patients care to be put into an active role
2) that there are times when patients need to be given a lead in order to start them off in a healing direction and
3) that successful homoeopathic treatment is at its best when it is an exchange between two willing participants.

The truth is that homoeopaths have to make judgements about their patients – who need to have trust in their practitioners' ability to make these necessary judgements about them with respect and impartiality. From some of the illustrative cases in these pages you can see that some people have such strange stories or such peculiar characteristics that the gathered information would be confused and even meaningless unless practitioners were able to react at the level of personal understanding gathered from experience.

The study of homoeopathy is almost as therapeutic to a student's constitution and psyche as it is to take a curative sequence of indicated remedies. Most students go through cathartic crises which oblige them to travel down paths they would never have expected to explore. The degree of catharsis is relative to the degree of revolutionary change that is being made to the student's creative and emotional life. What many of them discover is that they must go through a process of 'letting go'; of letting go of such things as imposed parental restrictions (however old they may be), well-rooted prejudices, self-imposed compensatory habits stemming from a lack of self-confidence and old emotional ties that linger as unfinished business in the heart. If this process does not happen then they cannot cope when they begin to meet patients who seek their help; they feel inadequate to deal with what these patients present; they in turn seek help – all to realise that they are, in fact, being asked to deal with something deep in their own bodies of energy.

By academically studying the philosophy of natural healing and by acquiring the essential knowledge about the natural medicines at our disposal, students lay a broad and solid foundation of technique – in much the same way as a footballer does by endless practice or an artist does by copying and sketching incessantly. Then, by beginning to treat others, they start to see how they are required to treat themselves as well. (It is a wise homoeopath who avoids self-prescribing and regularly consults another professional homoeopath.)

The more they recognise of themselves in whatever they are asked to heal, the more they turn the science of homoeopathy into the art of homoeopathy. The more they practise the art, the less they need the rulebook and the more they facilitate the emergence of the intuition. The

intuition, once based on an intellect that is fully conversant with the structure of the natural laws of homoeopathy and the techniques of applying
them, is the most important faculty in its practice. It allows the practitioner
the freedom to make leaps of imagination where the commonplace would
fall short of a patient's deepest needs.

Why should this be? It is because most patients are not very good at
expressing themselves or not good at expressing themselves in the light of
the unvarnished truth and need another to sift through their words and to
observe their characteristic behaviour in order to judge what needs to be
healed *and in what sequence*. Part of the problem is that they have not been
able to express their spirit and emotions well or at all and so they have had
to use their physical bodies to do it for them. It is unlikely that they would
suddenly be able to speak their hearts and minds simply because they have
made an appointment for what they expect to be a medical solution. So the
homoeopath is asked to judge, in his or her opinion, what needs to be
healed. While it may be very straightforward to conclude that someone
won't get better until they have seen a cranial osteopath or have had all the
dental amalgams removed, it often takes more foresight and imagination to
see whether a patient is blocked from moving forward in life because of
emotional or spiritual barriers. Even if a practitioner realises that a patient
cannot get better because he was an adopted child or was in the womb
when the parents were going through a messy divorce or because she was
subjected to emotional blackmail for years by a manipulative mother, the
indicated remedies must be found to spark the healing process of that individual – and they can only be found if the practitioner knows the remedies
'from the inside' and is accurately able to judge just where in each person's
story the healing should begin. Being familiar with remedies is to have intuitive knowledge of them, not just 'book knowledge'. All of which goes to say
that homoeopaths need time to mature. No less do patients: their treatment
is a process of maturation – the release from old habits, resentments and
inadequacies into the fulfilling of their potential.

What makes all this judging more difficult is that no-one can ever tell
in what way a person might react to the well-chosen remedy. While
prescribing for cases of physical pathology, this inability to second-guess
a patient's reaction is less problematic because the major premise is to

establish physical elimination. If that elimination process is set up and it goes according to the laws of nature and proceeds at a safe speed then the healing will be satisfactory. Where emotions and spirit are prescribed for we have to make judgements on the far less predictable reactions of the so-called 'higher bodies'. The elimination (expression) of negative emotional energy can catch us napping if it is shed by means of violence. Can this be right? See for yourself in this case:

Mavis

Mavis was a nurse, married to a doctor. They had one son, now ten, and a lot of debts. Mavis's husband was a reformed alcoholic. She was frigid as a result of undiagnosed post-natal depression and an unconquerable sense (though with no actual evidence) of having been sexually molested by her elder brother when she was younger. She went for counselling and after six months she felt far more energy and self-confidence than she had ever done. What was more, she became aware of increased libido. She even had thoughts of having another child. Her husband, however, felt that he had been traumatised by the years of celibacy and the late-night conversations that they had had during the months of psychotherapy and now that Mavis was physically available to him, he suddenly no longer wanted anything to do with her. Mavis was devastated. She was mortified when she discovered that her husband had been seeing someone else – her best friend.

Mavis decided to *"work things out"*. She did not want to break up the home and felt that they could not separate anyway as she had no financial resources. She asked her husband if they could try reconciliation. He agreed. They went to marriage guidance counselling, but he thought that the counsellor favoured Mavis in every area of dispute and *"anyway, he says that it isn't him that needs the help"*. So a stalemate arose. Mavis and her by now very antagonistic son lived an uneasy existence alongside her increasingly taciturn husband – who began to take up the bottle again. Mavis continued to come for treatment but sporadically as she felt unable to afford it – she felt she was unreasonably indulging herself. She was also seeing a nutritionist who was helping her with her food intolerance.

One day she came to say how utterly defeated she was feeling; how crushed and cowed; how like a doormat. She felt unappreciated and thoroughly unworthy and had no self-esteem left. She said that she felt the same and worse than she had been when she had the post-natal depression. She also said that her menstrual cycle was completely irregular and had begun to be painful. For this state she was given *Folliculinum* 30[1] to be taken once each week.

Eight weeks later she had a further appointment which she phoned to cancel an hour before it was due to start. When told that there would a cancellation fee with such short notice she decided to keep the appointment. She explained that she did not think that there was anything constructive she could say as she had been advised to see her doctor in order to do something about the continued depression. The doctor had urged her to have more counselling (this time paid for by the National Health) and to take antidepressants. She felt guilty that she had so little to report. She apologised for *"messing about with the treatment. I know I've blown the remedies. And now I'm on Prozac."*

Yet, asked how she and her husband were getting on she replied that things were easier even though she had only just started on the antidepressants – they could not have had time to take effect. Then she mentioned how she had felt on taking *"that remedy"*. She became animated for the first time in the interview; it was, she said, as if something had taken charge of her. She felt that she couldn't bear another moment living in the house under the circumstances and she went to find her husband to *"have it out with him"*. So bursting with indignation was she that she told him exactly how she felt and had been feeling for years, she lambasted him for going back to the drink, she told him that their way of life had to change. His replies were apparently non-committal or evasive. Eventually she struck him. Having hit him once she felt the physical power of her emotions and continued until he escaped out of the house. She said that she felt much better for venting her spleen after years of being unable to express herself. Since doing so, she said, her husband was now far more amenable and less truculent. He seemed to respect her more and he certainly paid more attention to their son whose one comment had been, *"Why on earth didn't you do that ages ago, Mum."*

Yet, here she was on an antidepressant, a drug that would only mask the situation and prolong it indefinitely. Though she had felt so much better, she had gone to the doctor because she was so shocked by what she saw as her violence. The remedy had initiated a response in her but she could not trust herself with such new-found confidence. It was not that she wanted to go on hitting her husband; just that she could now see that she was no longer subservient and she was not sure that she could sustain the power of her equality.

Was Mavis's violent action out of character? No, it was an elimination of pent-up emotion, the suppression of which was the result of a stagnant and oppressive relationship. Was it the result of taking the *Folliculinum*? Yes, as that remedy had allowed Mavis to express herself in a way best to release the unbearable tension. Was it right that the homoeopath's choice of remedy had involved two people in the reaction? Yes, as the unhealthy state of Mavis's emotions were inextricably bound up with her husband's – he was part of the equation and was intimately and equally responsible for its being maintained. After Mavis's emotional eruption he became far more reasonable towards Mavis and to their son. She felt that he had begun to listen to her and regard her with a little respect even if their marriage was irreparably damaged.

But would knowing all this cause a homoeopath to avoid such a prescription? One hopes not because it is the practitioner's responsibility to the patient that is paramount. For a homoeopath to avoid the selection of a prescription because he might suspect that the remedy could be dangerous (in an emotional state[2]) is to be guilty of perpetuating a maintaining cause as well as subscribing to the myth that homoeopathic remedies can be harmful. If a remedy sets up a genuine eliminative discharge of emotion (and it could not set up a false one) then that discharge will only involve the patient (however apparently alarming those living in close proximity may feel it to be) and anyone who is contributing, knowingly or not, to their distress.

A brief description of a case from Dr Eizayaga, a respected South American homoeopath, illustrates the point if in a paradoxical way.

> A woman went to the clinic for depression. She lived a life of misery because her wealthy businessman husband so neglected her. She felt that life was bleak and she thought it would be best to end it all. She was given *Aurum*, gold – the most common remedy for this suicidal form of depression. The homoeopath heard nothing for several months but was delighted to see her again at the clinic, this time in the company of her daughter who had brought her children for treatment. The woman greeted him warmly and told him that she needed no further treatment as she felt so very well. Conversationally, he asked her how her husband was. *"He shot himself – soon after I came to see you."*

It is surprisingly common for spouses to take on the pathological energy of their other halves and to become ill with it – even to the point of terminal illness. There are many cases of cancer that are precisely the result of this. When once the sickened spouse is released from this strange position of what might be termed Surrogate Disease Syndrome then the person with the real responsibility for the negative energy is forced to walk their own path with it.

Here is another case that illustrates some of these points:

A Pakistani girl was brought – or chaperoned would be a more correct word – by her older sister and mother to the student clinic. She was nineteen and had been suffering from cluster migraines for over a year. They were extremely debilitating and had begun happening with such frequency and regularity that she was by now quite weak and withdrawn. She found it difficult to articulate her problems well and was obviously relieved that her sister was able to speak for her. Her story was that her father had decided that she was not old enough to go out of the house on her own and that she had to be chaperoned everywhere. He did not trust his daughter; nor did he trust the local social environment. The girl had tried to convince him that she would be alright but he had not listened. In fact, he had been excessively authoritarian about the whole issue and had on one occasion struck his daughter *"for being so insolent"*.

The girl's general health history was good; she had no other physical complaints at all; indeed, her constitution was essentially strong. She plainly suffered from stress, disappointment and humiliation – she was aware that her friends did not have the same sanction put on their lives. She was unable to say what she felt to the person she most wished to express it to – her father. There was no way that her headaches could find an eliminative vocal emotional expression.

When the students came collectively to discuss the case, the general consensus was that the remedy most indicated was *Staphysagria*. This is a remedy we have met before; it is often used for just such a scenario as this where there is disgrace, humiliation, indignation, grief and no means of expression. What is more, it is a remedy that covers patients who are expressing a 'metaphorical' physical symptom picture with an underlying well of unspoken anger.

Staphysagria is also a remedy that often provokes heated and even passionate discussion amongst students who are asked to consider it as a 'like' remedy for a patient; it seems to bring up all those buried emotions that we all have experienced and never found a voice for. In this case, the passion went into the collective sense of indignation that the student group felt for the girl and her situation. It was as if we, the students, were in a position to redress a wrong being perpetrated; by giving this medicine we would be relieving the girl of an intolerable strain. However, student clinics are not medical Star Chambers where justice can be meted out! The supervisor, listening to our discussion and letting us fix ourselves into the conviction that there was only one way of dealing with this girl, quietly and in a disarmingly simple way demolished all that we had been saying. He asked us if we had considered what the consequences of giving *Staphysagria* might be.

It dawned on us that we had almost forgotten that this girl suffered from migraines and that if she did begin to express her anger towards her father, she might well say and do what she might come to regret; that her father might be provoked into saying and doing something that would be irrevocable; that she might, perhaps, say nothing at all but choose the first opportunity to escape from home and be lost to her family which, despite her present circumstances, was of the greatest importance to her and a source of strength. The supervisor expertly guided our thoughts towards a gentler path of healing; one where we would be investing the remedy in the genuine underlying cause.

There is a remedy that covers both fearful headaches and deeply held anger and that has the further aspect that it is often found to be healing by those who have undergone a cultural upheaval such as this family had endured. They had come from Pakistan not so many years before and they had found it disorientating despite the numerous family contacts they had already living in Britain. They felt like exiles. This was lost to the students at first until it was pointed out. It was as if the group's thought process had almost involved punishing the father for his unreasonableness. Much more kindly was the idea that by using the remedy *Proteus* we would be choosing a remedy that would address the background culture shock from which the whole problem had arisen. At the same time we would be addressing the terrible migraines – for *Proteus*[3] covers headaches that arise from suppressed anger.

The results of the prescription speak for themselves. The girl returned in a month. She was accompanied only by her sister and she was quite different. She was able to speak clearly for herself and she did not hang her head but smiled and chatted confidently. She had had no further headaches since the day she took the *Proteus*. What was more, she reported that her father's attitude was completely different. He now said that she was allowed to go out on her own to see her friends. She was back on speaking terms with him; she was clearly very affectionate towards him. She was asked if she had been able to express how she had felt. She looked rather puzzled at the question and simply said, no, nobody had spoken about anything to do with her being confined to the house – to her it was a thing of the past and to be forgotten.

The practitioner's dilemma: intellect or intuition?

Practitioners of any discipline – be it magic, medicine or music – must be alive to the difference between inspiration and technique. We go to college to gather the experience of others and the techniques to imitate our teachers up till the point when we can do the work ourselves. Once we start to do the work ourselves we might notice how we begin to differ in our practice from those who showed us how to do it. What makes this difference happen is our own unique, individual intuitive grasp of every new situation. Skill alone is never enough; acquired techniques cannot prevent any work from eventually becoming 'hack' work. Homoeopathy is just as susceptible to 'a bad day at the office' as any other job. But homoeopathy is not just a job, it is a vocation. It is demanding of rigorous discipline and consistent practice. It exerts a tremendous pressure on its practitioners to excel for as much of the time as possible and any dip below excellence can have the same effects on a homoeopath's creative outlook as a splashy account of Beethoven's Appassionata sonata would have on the pianist.

Homoeopathy is an art form; homoeopaths are forever attempting to 'compose' people back to health. Their purpose in doing so is a service; it is restoring people to their innate creativity, their purposefulness – which touches on our very reason for being. For this they must call on both intellect and intuition – the first being focused on technique, the latter on creativity. Just as the pianist must have respect for the music written on the page but also no fear of doing harm except through negligence and wilful acts of artistic licence, so homoeopaths must have respect and have no fear of causing harm to the patient. Homoeopathic remedies, the practitioner's instruments, can only 'sound' what exists within the patient. The art is to cause the healing vibrations to act together in concert in a sequence and a time frame that is most appropriate to the patient. It is salutary to remember that the artist is – must be – at heart, an improviser, an experimenter who, despite all the training in academic lore, can never guarantee that the next patient will respond to the treatment in an immutably predictable way. No two pieces of music are alike; nor their performances. The same is true of patients!

Towards the most powerful maintaining causes of all

Having examined maintaining causes from the mundane to the bizarre, from the obvious to what any healthy sceptic might find way beyond the bounds of possibility, we arrive at a point where we must cross into territory that only now orthodox science is beginning to explore. So exciting do scientists find this virgin medical geography, so enthralled are they by mapping out every inch of it they can, so vast are the sums of money poured into their research and so sophisticated is their machinery that it comes as a surprise to find that homoeopaths have been familiar with this terrain since Samuel Hahnemann began to hack away the undergrowth – not that scientists would recognise any of it as the same place at all.

The ground we need to cover to complete our survey of maintaining causes is that of hereditary disease patterns – or the genetic inheritance of disease energy. This is highly controversial and is, after all, if we read only medical journalists, the preserve of geneticists. This specialist group of scientists devote their entire working lives to the study of genes and the information carried in DNA. Invested in this work are billions of dollars because it is here that the future of allopathic medicine lies. Without actually telling us that the chemotherapy of allopathy has been a failure, there is an implicit awareness that conventional medical practice has come to an impasse where terminal disease is concerned; ultimately, in the face of the grim, implacable advance of disease, it achieves only as much as a dam spanning a river.

Now there is a universal understanding that chronic disease is influenced by heredity and the hunt is on to find individual genes that betray the origins of diagnosable conditions such as osteoarthritis, cystic fibrosis, multiple sclerosis, Alzheimer's disease, cancer and a host more. Previously, we knew (or were taught to believe) that we lived in a hostile world full of bacteria and viruses all determined to find a suitable host to prey on. Now we are being taught that if the bugs don't get us then there is a bookie's nightmare of a chance that a kink in one of our own genes will. The race is to find ways of manipulating genetic material so that, whatever disease faults an individual might have, there will be a vaccine or some other laboratory-inspired procedure to cope with them. In other words genetic engineering will eventually provide the answer to each and every diagnosable chronic disease state. All chronic disease that is influenced by heredity will be treated at cellular level by the introduction of foreign (if similar though genetically modified) cellular tissue, in the form of vaccines. (One obvious benefit of this theory is that doctors should have far more time to deal with everyday practice.)

Yet homoeopathy already has an alternative map of this jungle and homoeopaths have been more or less familiar with the footpaths that criss-cross it for two hundred years. The map does not look anything like the fantastically elaborate and minutely detailed charts that are being drawn up to show us the intricate biochemical world of genes. Homoeopathic journeys are plotted on a map that is hand-drawn and tea-stained. It has no neat chemical grid references and it is the subject of petty wrangling even among homoeopaths. The topography shown on it can appear to keep changing shape and signposts often point in two or three different directions at once. Things such as grief and spiritual fulfilment, self-destruction and fear of death, atheism and lack of grounding loom up like mountains, and personal relationships, birth trauma, drugs, surgery, lack of forgiveness and dozens of other hazards make the map look thoroughly indecipherable. Nevertheless and paradoxically, like any old-fashioned treasure map, what it lacks in sophistication it makes up for in universal comprehensibility – once the language of homoeopathy no longer causes any difficulty.

Parts I and II of this book have been about that language, the communicable thinking of homoeopathy; its practice and philosophy. Part III is about the hierarchy of inheritable disease influences. It is the natural history of what has become known as the miasms. These are the ultimate maintaining causes. Yet they are also very much more. They are the very breath of human individuality. Though we are talking about disease we are also talking about every individual's journey through life with the handicaps of inherited disease patterns. Our lives are coloured and shaped by what we inherit and it is whatever inherited hazards we manage to overcome in our creative progress through life that mark out our life-achievement – or lack or it.

Untidy and unable to offer any fixed certainties, the homoeopathic map of inheritable disease energy is still the most practical and hope-inspiring guide to healing that practitioners possess. Not only does it show us how disease works on us but it shows why, where, what, when and who as well. It provides a framework for the understanding of homoeopathic and other natural medicines. It explains how disease has influenced art, culture, religion and politics. It also gives us a completely new perspective on evolution. The story of the miasms is also the story of the evolution of disease and how it has paralleled that of humanity. Disease and humanity are inextricably linked because, contrary to the chemistry-based philosophy of allopathy, the one is within the other from the very beginning.

PART III

THE HIERARCHY OF
THE MIASMS

INTRODUCTION

The greatest blocks to cure

One of the challenges to the homoeopath is being able to recognise all the possible reasons why the Vital Force should find itself incapable of throwing off disease. There are many so-called 'maintaining causes' – factors that, until they are removed, will prevent the patient's full recovery; so many, that it seems at times perverse to consider the idea of 'cure'. Chief among these causes for continued ill health and deserving of the closest examination, are the miasms. This rather unfortunate term is given to the collection of chronic, inheritable disease patterns (or disease *taints*) that colour so much of the suffering of humanity.

The term 'miasm' is unfortunate because the original Greek meaning of the word – 'defilement' or 'pollution' – has become altered to cover such lurid descriptions as 'infectious or noxious exhalations from putrescent organic matter' or 'poisonous germs floating in the atmosphere'. Samuel Hahnemann, founder of modern homoeopathy, used the term 'miasm' in relation to malaria in particular, regarding the foul swampy boglands of central Europe as the breeding ground of poisonous gases. It was only later that he used the word 'miasm' when referring to the major chronic inheritable disease patterns. Though there are only six of them, they inform and influence every variety of psychological, emotional and physical condition known to man. Yet, despite the dread that the names of the individual miasms conjure up in our minds, we need also to see and understand that their profound influence is not necessarily all bad. We will come to see that there is almost always something to be gained from the manner in which we individually experience and deal with these perverse, but none the less *natural*, disease influences.

Without the knowledge of these six disease patterns, homoeopathy would be incapable of healing the sick for we would not understand the nature of the patient before us. Our efforts would be limited to dealing with a symptom and not the whole disease as expressed by the whole body. We would be reduced to treating the bunion or the ulcer or the boil, as allopaths are; reduced to the superficial condition without any ability to touch the heart of what makes us susceptible to particular pathologies. With the miasms encoded energetically, we assume, in the patient's gene pool, our success would reach into the system only as far as these inherited disease patterns allowed. These traits may be buried so deeply that they pose no threat while constitutional health remains relatively well balanced. The dragons can remain dormant indefinitely in those whose health and welfare remain in harmony and unchallenged. However, dragons can be awoken by major trauma or minor illnesses and these occur in all of us sooner or later; often awakening one by one. When a miasm blocks the road to recovery there is only one way to remove the obstacle – to treat the energy of the inherited disease pattern with a *similar* but greater energy. The accomplishment of this *always leaves the patient a wholly better person.*

Homoeopaths spend many years becoming acquainted with miasms until they know them inside out, in order to recognise them when they appear. Treating them can be frustrating but in chronic disease it is always necessary. Miasms, fortunately, are subject to the *Law of Similars* ('like cures like') and to heal a person of their influence is nothing short of homoeopathic genetic engineering.

The miasms

There are six major inherited disease miasms. Others are either inheritable traces of epidemic diseases that occasionally seem to inhibit healing in chronic illness (such as malaria or diphtheria) or are influences that cannot be considered as conventional diseases in their own right (such as radioactivity and vaccination). Properly, the six take pride of place.

Before naming the six, it is essential to bear in mind that they are not to be confined to descriptions of diseases found in a pathology textbook.

Though each disease has its own distinctive pattern of process which is described in detail in textbooks, these are only descriptions of their *acute* manifestations. The miasms are in fact terrible *energy forces*. They have *purpose* and *intention* – because *we* have. They are potent forces of human nature – produced by and expressed by *humanity*. As a product of nature in man, we must respect each one in much the same way as we do the intellect and the intuition. Each one is connected to the others; they are not isolated. Each one has many guises. They are all ancient energy patterns – *predating by far the first appearance of the acute diseases that most readily identify the miasms in physical pathological terms*. The earliest descriptions of what we might call miasmatic energy appear in ancient myths; allegorical stories from every culture are imbued with symbology and recount every imaginable negative and positive trait of human psychology.[1] With their origins lying deep within the human psyche, it is only with the passing of aeons that man has found ways of expressing the miasms in physical form with recognisable symptom pictures that have been given diagnostic labels by relatively modern medicine. The six identifiable symptom pictures most readily describe the essential character of the individual miasms.

Everything on the etheric level of the psyche must be expressed, sooner or later, on the physical level as a means of channelling and eliminating. Grief can be expressed as tears or as heart failure; despair can be expressed in loss of hair or vision or in suicide or cancer. Behind these loaded words lie the life stories of individuals, each on their own path with their own set of familial circumstances and with their own inherited weaknesses and strengths. The story of the miasms is the search for understanding why one man should seek his fortune as an adventurer and another as a conniving politician; why one should live unscathed by disease into his nineties and another should suffer years of illness and therapy.

The miasms are progressive and progressively fatal but only because one of their number is subtly dominant. Just as there is a hierarchy of the body, mind and spirit and of disease, so there is of the miasms. Though the most ancient of them is also the greatest, most far-reaching, universal and ultimately incurable, paradoxically it is not that which most bedevils mankind. There is one among the six that can lurk like the jealous Iago in *Othello* and, when ignored or conspired against, inexorably shape our ending.

These six energy states provide a part answer to those burning questions of why and in what way disease changes its shape – why eczema becomes asthma; why tonsillitis can lead to kidney damage; why altering high cholesterol levels indiscriminately might lead to high blood pressure and heart disease; why ulcers can lead to cancer as can the removal of warts and moles; why suppressed acute diseases lead to chronic ill health.

The six are identified as:

Psora
Syphilis
Sycosis (gonorrhoea)
Tuberculosis
Leprosy
Cancer

The most difficult to grasp is psora because it is the matrix of all disease states and *intrinsically exists within every one of the other miasms*. It is protean in its form and all pervasive. The other five miasms are 'children' of psora, and inherit their mother's influence so to speak, while being absolutely identifiable in their own right. Each one of the other five miasms is, before anything else, *a state of being and not just the acute disease that bears its name nor its chronic sequelae.*

Each one of them is defined in whatever guise it might assume by its essential characteristics – *those characteristics remaining ever the same*. They are all clearly identifiable by the way in which their energy works on living organisms and how the affected organisms' energies respond during its presence.

To understand them we will look at each in turn and describe its acute and chronic forms and how the body, mind, emotions and spirit are affected in order to see how this process gives each one its uniquely characteristic picture. Bear in mind that this separating out is only for the convenience of understanding. In reality, there is an inextricable link between them all and they are no more truly separable than the physical body and the spirit are from the emotions in the living form.

CHAPTER 20

PSORA

The word *psora* is from the Greek. It means 'mange' or 'itch'. In the *Oxford Dictionary* its meaning of 1681 is given as 'a contagious skin disease; scabies, the itch'. These are the terms in which Samuel Hahnemann and his successors first understood psora. However, they did not see it just as an acute condition that had a bad record of self-healing, they also came to recognise that susceptibility to the condition could be inherited. Not only was it an identifiable disease which involved a parasitical infestation by the *Sarcoptes scabiei* (a spider mite) but it was also a *state of being* that existed *prior* to exposure to the parasite and that could be passed on from parent to child. What was inheritable was the condition of being *susceptible* to the 'itch' and what became manifest in following generations was likely to *imitate the original disease* in ever more complex forms but always with the accompanying symptom of 'itch'.

In other words, the body that had become susceptible to and supported the parasite, but which had been incapable or prevented (usually through suppressive unguents) from finding its own way to deal with the problem, *would pass on the information within the gene pool that the body had failed to respond with a solution*. Had a cure come from within then it would have been the body's *solution* that was passed on. The important thing here is the concept of inheriting a susceptibility; of inheriting a failing in the Vital Force's resources.

Parasitism and its origins

It is not difficult to grasp the concept of parasitism as being the earliest evidence of disease, not just in man but also in more primitive life forms.

Parasitism – and the susceptibility to being a suitable host for a parasite – is not a long way removed from symbiosis which is 'different life forms living together, each providing the other with support'. Symbiosis was the natural evolutionary progression after commensalism i.e. the harmonious communal living of individual cells that, en masse, form a colony – sponges and corals being the most obvious and primitive examples. By tracing back through history it is possible to see how evolution has influenced the way in which disease originated within the gradual diversification of primitive life forms, firstly bacterial, then vegetable/animal and eventually animal – as symbiosis became perverted into parasitism. As life forms became more sophisticated, so *opportunism* complicated the patterns of disease.

The earliest fossil evidence of ill health appears some 500 million years ago and is no more serious than physical trauma. This was the age of the trilobite and other invertebrates. In the same era there is, for the first time, evidence of bacteria living off decaying material – such bacteria are described as non-pathogenic (not inducing disease). Up until this time bacteria had lived by symbiosis in harmony with other *living* matter. Now they were living and breeding by utilising rotting matter. Bacteria had learnt to adapt to a ready food source – ever-resourceful nature had found a way of cleaning up.

It is with the earliest archaeological signs of air-breathing animals that we have the first primitive parasites. In the Devonian period, some 345 million years ago, when the very first footprints were impressed on land, we find the gradual but ineluctable progress of parasitism, as nematodes (worms) take to wriggling and then later insects take off on the wing. The appearance of myzostomids (sucking parasites) in the Carboniferous era (some 280 million years ago) parallels the advance of the fungi and bacteria – both of which appear to feature so strongly in the development of disease. While the dinosaurs of the Jurassic period (some 150 million years ago) would not have expected anything much worse than accident, attack or poison to affect their health (though there is archaeological evidence of necrosis or tissue death of bone) it is not until the appearance of modern mammals, somewhere in the region of 2-6 million years ago, that potentially threatening conditions such as pus formation are first in evidence.

With the vast timescale of millions of years it is impossible to be precise about the advent of any disease in particular. We have to be content with observing the trends and patterns of behaviour exhibited by those life forms that went on to become *associated* with disease. The physical development of bacteria and fungi may not have advanced much over the aeons but history tells us that their behaviour and purpose has. Bacteria developed first into pyogenic (pus forming) life forms and only later into endemic and epidemic diseases – and then, according to the homoeopathic view, only in response to man's susceptibilities. (It should be remembered that such sophisticated diseases do not occur readily in any but man and his domesticated animals or those that live in close proximity to both.)

The increasing sophistication and specialisation of parasitical animals kept pace with the evolution of other animal life until man appeared and provided a superlative canvas on which to work out their life cycle. Ticks and mites, which had appeared in the Silurian period, 395 million years ago, are related to arachnids (spiders). By 4 million years ago, give or take a few million years, the spider mite was ready to colonise man's first line of defence – his skin. Scabies had arrived, seeming to take (as we shall see) full advantage of man's greatest weakness, his psyche.

Scabies and other parasites

It is more than likely that early man suffered from parasitical worms as well as scabies but, because worms are dependent on a relatively short life cycle and are subject to change in dietary and environmental conditions, he was probably more able to cope with the discomforts of supporting unwelcome tenants in his bowel.

Scabies is the result of being a host to a tiny spider mite that burrows just beneath the surface of the skin. It forms a chamber which becomes filled with a clear body fluid in which it lives and from which it forms runnels to other nest sites where it lays its eggs. Once the procedure has begun, the spread of the condition is speedy. It is very common for it to begin between the fingers but it can originate anywhere on the body. The affected area itches mercilessly but this is part of the reproductive cycle because the scratching breaks open the nest sites, releases the fluid from the vesicles and allows the newly hatched mites to spread to another unsuspecting landlord. The mite is able to survive outside the body of its host for the brief time it takes between the opening of the vesicle and the contact with the new host.

In the case of threadworm infestation, the story is somewhat different. Intestinal worms need an environment where there is mucus production as well as an acid/alkali imbalance in favour of acidity. Worms have the ability to influence their environment to suit themselves and their reproductive cycle. They can alter the host's appetite causing craving for certain food-stuffs and they can release a chemical into the host's system which causes intolerable itching in the nose. When the female worm performs her trick of prickling the anal sphincter of her host (while at the same time laying her eggs) prompting an urgent need to scratch, the chemical that has been released into the system also causes the nose to itch. If the host uses egg-contaminated fingers to scratch his nose, the cycle will begin again.

The life cycle of scabies is continuous and once established in the host needs no further sequence of events. What is more, it can occasionally become fatal (as we shall see) if left untreated. Both worms and scabies are phenomenally successful in evolutionary terms and they have changed little over the millennia. Allopathy may be content to see only the *physical* evidence of these two parasitical states and to ignore the rest of the picture but no-one else should be blind to the effects on the emotions and the psyche that exist in patients suffering from such conditions. To see and understand the *whole* state of the patient suffering from the 'itch' or *the susceptibility to becoming a host,* is to hold a key to understanding how to heal, even the apparently incurable.

Playing the host

A state of being implies not just a physical condition but one in which the physical body, the emotional body and the spirit are all involved. To see why psora should have relevance to the 'whole' we need to be reminded of life on Earth before man. Psora was born in its own imitative version of the 'big bang'. Early, non-pathogenic bacteria discovered that there was mileage to be gained by living off dead or dying matter. In fact, bacteria create their own natural cyclical habitat just as dying vegetable matter creates mulch for the next stage of its natural life cycle. It took a few million years to achieve but it was not such a big evolutionary step to take (despite its enormous consequences) for these now carrion bacteria to begin proliferating on *living* tissue even if the tissue affected was damaged. Fungi followed suit; some primitive arachnids also evolved from being bloodsuckers to skin dwellers.

Parasitism developed as a result of nature's constant efforts to diversify; adaptability is one of the pillars of evolution. However, all parasites seem to have a fatal flaw – when they colonise too successfully the host becomes aware of discomfort due to symptoms arising from the infestation. The result is that the host has to search for relief and the parasite has to develop ways of affecting other hosts. In man's case though, the search is more complicated. The parasites that have most successfully colonised his body are too small and well hidden, either in the skin, the gut or other internal organs, for any 'ferret' to be sent in after them. While a magpie will feast off ticks on the back of a sheep and thus maintain a reasonable and unthreatening level of infestation, man (in common with other furred animals) has no such luxury when it comes to scabies and has to rely on his own wits to discover a solution to what must be his oldest and most intractable chronic health problem. The most sophisticated form of parasitism occurs in man and nature has *apparently* provided no internal, self-healing mechanism to re-establish equilibrium.

What started with single cells diversifying at the expense of another primitive living creature became a search for a solution to an internal disease condition. In furred animals with nothing better than claws or a convenient tree trunk, the search begins and ends with a scratch. With man the search has never stopped because his degree of *awareness* has given him the gift of inventing ever more complicated and radical answers. Paradoxically, it is his very awareness that brings in the first creeping symptoms of incurability, for awareness has caused a rift between intuition and intellect. It is the habit of rationalising everything that has resulted in man investing his deepest anxieties in his health problems – primal psychosoma!

Inherent in the nature of psora is not only the evolutionary search for successful habitation and reproduction on the part of parasites but also the search for a solution to the symptomatic problems suffered by the host. It is a search that leads the host *to look beyond the body* for the answer. If the body finds no *internal* solution to the irrepressible 'itch' then the host must turn to an outside source of relief. Even primitive man needed a 'quick fix'.

The essence of this 'incurability' in the face of evolution and the depredations of a microscopic spider mite are meaningless if we think of man as separate in any way from everything else that happens on the planet. On every level we are an integral part of the continuing evolution of Earth; *we* are part of the evolution of the parasite's world just as they are part of ours and we hold, at a deep and unconscious level, the memory of how we arrived at our present state. This memory includes the path we have taken in our ever-increasing *awareness* with all the specialised mental, emotional and spiritual equipment that has developed with it. Inevitably, any failure to find internal solutions for dealing with disease is buried deep within the memory too. That is the price we pay for our refinement.

We have reminders of our prehistory. For one thing we still have a vital need for symbiosis. Without it our bowels would not function. A variety of different flora colonise the gut and, in a healthy individual, maintain a balance. If the balance in the flora is disturbed then the host suffers not just physically but *emotionally, mentally and in spirit as well*. A preponderance of one bacterium in the bowel over another can lead to constipation or diarrhoea, dehydration or oedema, breathlessness, thrush, weakness, timidity, irritability, impatience, rage, depression and hopelessness. Inherent within us is the certainty, even if we do not recognise it intellectually, that we have to maintain a balance in order to function properly. (The niggling question arises: which came first, the physical and emotional symptoms or the imbalance amongst the natural flora of the gut? As we shall see, the fault does not lie with the natural history of bacteria.)

We can deal effectively with relatively minor imbalances. To put things right, we go off our food or we drink more or we sleep. If it is more drastic then we vomit or brew a fever. These changes continue until the flora is back in balance. However, even in the sympathetic environment of symbiosis there is the threat of suffering if the balance is not maintained.

Our autonomic nervous system provides another reminder of our constant need to maintain balance. It gives us the ability to survive our environment and all its relative dangers. We are provided with an early warning system in the primitive brain – that part of the brain that detects the need for fight or flight, a change of temperature, the urge to eat and so on. The thalamus, hypothalamus and pituitary glands together organise most of our basic needs, according to geography, season, climate, ambience and mood. Our hominid ancestors would have had the same facility and we have retained, at this very basic level, what we need most to survive.

It is when this delicate system is thrown out of sync that we become susceptible to miasms. The experience of discomfort throws us from our regular creative activities of working, sleeping, feeding, mating and child rearing. We take for granted so much of our involuntary and automatic functioning precisely because millions of years of evolution have continued to afford us a supremely balanced system. The more finely tuned our awareness has become however, the easier it has been for that balance to become upset; awareness is an energy of the mind before it is of the physical body. For all the positive genius of mankind, he perceives the negative threat of a hostile environment both within and without.

Parasites, with no finer feelings, spend all their life force on evolving, to keep one step ahead of their hosts. Along with our susceptibility to them, the whole body remembers what it means and feels like to suffer infestation; to be the host of an unwelcome guest – *and the impotence of our inability to rid ourselves of it*. It is here, in the lasting effect on the psyche, that the undermining sense of incurability takes hold. Which is chicken and which is egg? Were the scabies mite and other parasites the original harbingers of angst or was our ancestor riddled with it first, thus rendering himself weak enough to play host?

Before reading the following detailed description of the physical disease of scabies, bear in mind that the meaning of the word 'itch' in the language of the miasms should be broadened to include the metaphorical description of a state of mind; to suffer an emotional 'itch' can be just as life consuming as one on the skin.

Acute scabies - a physical manifestation of psora

In scabies the skin appears reddened and sore and has a dirty appearance. It is very itchy. The vesicles vary in size, colour and geography from patient to patient but are essentially red with scabs and can appear anywhere on the body – the site determined by the point of contact. Dirty, greyish lines radiate out from the eruptions and these are the runnels that the mite burrows. When the surface is broken, the fluid from the vesicles leaks out onto the skin. Sometimes there is bleeding from the inevitable scratching. The itching is usually worse at night in bed when the patient becomes warm. The mite is at its most active when the host is at rest, asleep.

Physical effort tends to cause the patient to flush and sweat – perspiration can cause a temporary amelioration of discomfort. These purely physical symptoms can be made worse if staphylococcal bacteria join the party and create impetigo – a highly infectious complication. With the physical symptoms comes a range of mental and emotional symptoms that affect our whole well-being. There is the sense of contamination and of feeling filthy and we have no immediate means of cleansing it. We have confirmation of this when others steer clear of our contagious state. We feel isolated. Neither we nor anyone else can find a solution to the symptoms. (Remember that here we are speaking historically.)

We have the same sense of feeling punished for something we did not do that we might have felt as a child or a sense of inexplicable guilt – a fear that we have done something wrong but are not sure what. Such symptoms do not appear in the allopathic textbooks on pathology of the skin. It might seem ridiculous to relate one's emotional state to a dermatologist – though greater awareness of stress in relation to skin problems is now gaining acceptance. These mental symptoms are common. They are not recognised as part of the disease because in recent history we have been successful in finding methods of eradicating the *physical* symptoms. From an evolutionary point of view though, mental symptoms are vital because of our ability to pass on negative emotional and mental aspects as well as the physical tendencies of disease.

Scabies can help us see how this can be. It is still with us and it illustrates the traits of psora well. The patient suffering from scabies can become weak from making too much effort and consequently feel apathetic with a disinclination to work; he feels despondent and may lose confidence. He has a sense of unease and anxiety which he finds hard to explain. On waking in the morning he feels oppressed and finds it difficult to raise any enthusiasm for the day ahead. His mood may vary according to the environment or circumstances; he would rather not be alone, even though being in company can make him feel peevish or intolerant. At other times he can become tearful and melancholy but, paradoxically, he can feel oddly elated or cheerful when something quite minor goes well unexpectedly. If the disease is left to progress then the melancholy and despondency – especially about the possibility of cure – will prevail. Fear becomes a major factor. There is an increasing timidity and nervousness. There is fear of the unknown and of the future so extreme that the patient can turn to suicide and for no known cause.

On the way to this appalling state the patient may have passed through anger. This is not surprising when one considers the exquisite degree of irritation to which the itching can take him. The fear and rage are marked by trembling with a resultant weakness and even faintness. There is a tendency for the patient to complain about his condition and to bewail his fate. Needless to say, the patient feels restless and perturbed, withdrawn and without any peace of mind. Scabies is a progressive disease and not all such symptoms are manifest. As every patient is an individual and likely to produce individual variations, the mental and emotional symptoms vary in degree of intensity and dominance. Many of these non-physical symptoms are common to a whole host of well-documented diseases. What is more, any of the mental and emotional symptoms characteristic of scabies can be felt without any physical symptoms being present; if the pysche is so affected, though, the individual is well on the way to being susceptible to developing physical disease.

The treatment of scabies

The treatment for scabies over the millennia has not varied a great deal. *Sulphur* in one form or another has been the common application. When the scabies mite is eradicated from the body and the skin symptoms go away, it is usual for the patient to feel so relieved that a sense of well-being is quickly restored. Yet the body has experienced a potentially devastating condition for which it had apparently no internal healing mechanism. There is no denying the sense of fragility this insidiously imparts into the system.

For the first time, in evolutionary terms, the onset of scabies prompted a sense of incurability or of fatalism. The body was not able to stoke up the liver's fire to burn away the problem. It was not able to vomit the problem away. It was not able to eject it from the bowel or to process it out through the kidneys and bladder. There was no possibility that the problem would be leaked away with a profuse sweat. Nor could the beast be dug out – for early man had no tools fine enough for the job. He might have tried cauterisation but he was probably familiar enough with sepsis not to attempt this too readily. Man surely had methods of killing off the mite and no doubt early patients consulted shamans to have the condition suppressed by concoctions made with *Sulphur* and other minerals or plants, but the cure did not come from within. Each patient whose body registered its inability to deal with the crisis, would have passed on its failure to the next generation.

Scabies and heredity

In slapping on the unguents we still do nothing about the mental and emotional state that gave rise to the susceptibility; it is not just a *physical* susceptibility. Into the genetic melting pot has gone the potential memory of generations of sufferers; as they struggled with the disease, so the lack of success (and thus the *effects* of suppression) was handed down. The psychological effects of the disease are an integral part of the physical presence of the *Sarcoptes scabiei*. It is impossible for man to remain untainted by the mental and emotional aspects – and by extension the spiritual aspects too, more of which will be added later.

The underlying state

There is another parallel and opposite aspect that should be considered. No parasite can gain a hold on its potential host unless there is an intrinsic weakness within the system. It is this weakness that we should try and understand even though it remains conjecture at this time as it is highly unlikely that evidence will be found by either archaeologists or medical scientists.

Modern medicine has a vested interest in asking us to believe the myth that humanity is healthier now than at any time in our history. This depends on one's definition of health and from the holistic point of view it is patently not true; but it serves to convince us that modern medicine has most of the answers and that we can continue to put our faith in it. Ancient man was prodigiously gifted with health. He will have died young, not because he remained unvaccinated or never washed his hands; not because of heart attack, stroke or cancer but because he was at the mercy of the wild animals that he hunted and his fellow man who sought to encroach on his neighbour's patch. Despite an uncorrupted immune system, sepsis would have poisoned the blood of battle-wounded man. Infant mortality was no doubt extremely high, due to ignorance and lack of basic hygiene. He was otherwise likely to succumb to acute epidemics of pestilence – because of his habit of living in close communities where such things breed fast – though there is no particular evidence of this. Early nomadic man was tough enough to migrate to even the most hostile of environments where he learnt to adapt. Nevertheless, he would have been subject to mental and emotional states just as we are. He would have felt the thrills and disappointments of the chase, the terror of the midnight attack, the anguish of grief. He would have known competition and the threat of weather, famine and epidemics. Living 'on the edge' for much of the time expends nervous energy; stress would have lowered his inner resources. It should not surprise us that nomadic man, constantly on the move yet living in close communities, forever looking over his shoulder and wondering whether he would eat again today, should be prey to anxiety and home to the tiny *Sarcoptes scabiei*. Yet despite the high rate of contagion, it is a fact that not everyone who comes in contact with the mite is a suitable host. The same is true of worms or bacteria such as staphylococcus and streptococcus; just as is the case with viruses – some are susceptible and some are not.

The premise here is that while disease may well instigate physical, mental and emotional symptoms, still – even in a case such as scabies – there has to be a predisposing factor for the disease to take hold and one that is *not* from the environment but from *within*. Homoeopathy and the other alternative therapies hold that disease in general is not just a materialistic pathological state that arises out of contact with a threatening environment. The predisposing state for disease can just as easily be the psychological stresses experienced by both primitive man and the whole line of his ancestors. This is not quite the same as saying that every ill is psychosomatic. All and any of the deeply held negative emotions can cause us to become ill. Conversely, any of the different pathologies can bring out inherent negative emotional states. If, as a result, we harbour unresolved mental, emotional or spiritual troubles without giving them a voice then sooner or later nature will find a pathological way to provoke an expression of what lies buried. Disease can rescue us from the festering 'energy wounds' of unexpressed feelings. The relationship between man and disease is a two-way street; it has to be so because the expression and resolution of negative emotional states as the result of eliminative disease are encountered on the road to well-being.

Not everyone is susceptible to parasites

The scabies mite was one of the first– perhaps *the* first – parasite that affected man pathologically and severely enough to be a chronic threat. It was a comparatively sophisticated animal – it had a complete life cycle of its own and it came from *outside* the body. More acute epidemics associated with bacteria and viruses (*inside* the body) caused havoc among populations of early man, leading to death until, with the passing of generations, his physiology evolved to deal with them effectively. The genetic knowlege of *how* to deal with the acute problem would have been passed on by all survivors although the psychological trauma on the collective psyche would also have become a sociological and cultural fear of disease – a maintaining cause of susceptibility in itself. (The bubonic plague which burnt itself out on medieval generations, but is still extant in small corners of the world, is an example of this type of acute infection.) However scabies is the first major disease that man could survive long enough in his own lifetime to be able to pass on his body's inadequate response.

We know that the human ecosystem can be a biochemically hostile place for parasites yet a slight change in conditions can make it ideal for their development. Though it is quite common for one member of a family to pass on worms or lice to the rest, it is by no means a foregone conclusion.

This is not even a question of scrupulous hygiene. Many a watchful mother has been surprised at how one or more of her children never became lousy or worm-ridden in spite of their rolling about on the floor together and never being sure that hands were always washed before meals. Indeed, it is common enough to find lice eggs on the heads of some children that have never gone on to hatch. The fact is that there are many who simply are not ecologically viable to sustain the life cycle of the parasite. If this is true today then it must have been true in Palaeolithic times.

So the origin of man's susceptibility to becoming a host is not clear-cut in historical terms but it is reasonable to consider that the disease state and susceptibility went hand in hand with man's development. As he learnt to suffer and to cope with his environment, so the agents of disease evolved by taking advantage of man's limitations and vulnerabilities. Parasites would never have missed the opportunity of taking hold on someone whose immune processes and self-healing mechanism were weakened by anticipation, anxiety, restlessness, hunger and dread. Illness comes first, bugs follow.

A summary of the relationship between man and mite

Scabies represents the pinnacle of parasitism on man. Though there must have been other diseases (particularly acute ones) that were equally, if not more threatening, scabies was amongst those that had the most long-term, generally chronic effects. Even if scabies is treated with *Sulphur* ointments the body has only rid itself of the *physical* side of the problem. (In fact, it is quite common for patients of suppressed scabies to produce rashes and itches throughout the remainder of their lives – their bodies trying to remind themselves of how it was, in order to find the internal solution.) The state of having been susceptible in the first place is still there with all its potential attendant mental symptoms. While this state persists, the person bearing this burden is likely to pass on to the next generation the propensity for producing 'like diseases' – diseases that mimic or represent what went before and ones that share the same psychological make-up. The following generations produce symptoms *similar* to the original condition in an attempt to find a solution; the purpose of nature here being the eradication of the susceptibility.

What is inherited with psora, from one generation to another, is the state of being unable to deal with the results of an internal imbalance of ecology that has led man to be susceptible as host to life forms that seemingly stepped out of the environment to take possession of part of his life force for its own purposes. As a result man has become generally weakened and he has never found an unaided internal solution – nor will he. If the acute physical condition of scabies is one of the most contagious diseases known to us, the mental state – that emotional 'itch' – that goes with it is even more so. Thoughts in the form of fears, doubts, anger, grief, hilarity or depression are catching and do not require touch to be passed on. Though it might be a controversial issue as far as medicine is concerned, you would find few homoeopaths quarrelling with the idea that such 'thought energies' can be passed on from one person to another; one generation to another. The contention of homoeopathic philosophy is that the gene pool registers energy patterns – it registers states of being as much as facial features, personality traits and patterns of physical pathology. An anxious parent can produce an anxious child; not necessarily one who has been *taught* to be so but one who has inherited the propensity.

Paradoxically, if you were to ask a homoeopath if he had ever been asked to treat a case of scabies, the answer might well be, "*No*". Scabies is not as common as it once was and patients go to the local medical surgery for the fastest possible means of eradication. Yet if a homoeopath were asked to treat it he might well think that his patient was healthier than most! This is because the patient with scabies has produced an elemental acute condition. The practitioner might theoretically be more concerned about a person who was too unhealthy for the scabies mite to be able to colonise his skin. (He might be dubious about his skill to help the patient as his experience would be meagre and scabies often resists the most assiduous of alternative efforts. Even the great Dr Clarke [1] recommends the application of suppressive oils and unguents alongside the internal doses of remedies such as *Sulphur*.)

The legacy of psora

What is the legacy of psora? To find out, we need to match up the acute symptoms of the disease that represents the miasm with the symptom pictures of chronic diseases to see where the similarities are. It is in this way that we know whether a disease belongs in the psoric miasm or not. To learn how to deal with psoric conditions is to hold the promise of how to learn, as patients, to deal with our inadequacies and limitations.

Itching

Firstly there is the itching. The skin is an organ and it is an organ of elimination. Perspiring is one method by which the body throws out unwanted material. The sloughing of skin in flakes or 'dust' is another. Itching can accompany attempts to sweat or it can occur once perspiration begins to dry on the surface. The exfoliation of skin is usually very itchy as well – though by no means always. Internal healing processes often bring on itching as a sign that the condition is coming to a resolution – especially at the resolution of an acute condition. It is common for fevers to end with a mild rash and some itching. Serious acute diseases such as hepatitis also have itching though the skin on its own is simply not adequate for the whole job of elimination in this case. More chronic states have severe itching that can be painful or voluptuous. The patient *must* scratch, even to the point of causing bleeding – and can even derive satisfaction from doing so. After scratching there often remains a burning sensation.

The itching, on the other hand, may be the only evidence of ill health; this might be no more than a 'simple' case of pruritis. However, it can come on with other conditions or at particular times of life – such as the menopause. Older patients can suffer intolerable itching for no apparent reason. The itching may affect only one small area or it may cover a much larger portion of the body; it may appear in first one place and then another. It might affect different patients at different times of day or night. Not all itching is necessarily the result of buried psora; if it is accompanied by other features of the miasm though, it is.

Skin quality

The next symptom to look at is the quality of the skin affected. In scabies it is dry, rough, dirty-looking and often thoroughly unhealthy; it might be accompanied by the itching or not. The patient may have nothing else particularly wrong with him. Psoriasis answers this description well though it has many different ways of manifesting. Not only is there dryness and roughness but there is also soreness and redness. It is characterised by scaliness as the skin cells that surface to replace those sloughed off come up too fast and form thick scales and crusts. Psoriasis, despite the usual textbook description, can be unbearably itchy. It often appears on the hands in just the very place favoured so commonly by scabies. (Or it can be universal and affect every inch of the skin surface.)

Eczema can appear in several forms; the psoric manifestation is, as you might expect, dry, rough, itchy, sore and red. What is more, it has an affinity for the hands and most particularly the fingers and the webs in between – again, just where scabies likes to roost. Eczema (in its psoric form) can leave the skin cracked and weepy or even bloody. If so, the matter that exudes is thin and colourless, just like the contents of the scabies vesicle. When this dries it might leave a granular crustiness that is pale yellow. Just as in the parent disease, eczema is often more itchy and disturbing at night when the patient is warm in bed; some patients feel cold with it, others feel hot. Some have a cold sweat and some a hot sweat – and others have neither.

Dryness

Dryness is an individual symptom worth looking at on its own because it is very characteristic of psora in general. In babies, the first manifestation is often cradle cap, a harmless if sometimes unsightly condition of the scalp which they eventually grow out of. (It is something that parents often try and remove but they do so at the risk of preventing the child from dealing with his psoric past.) The desquamating (peeling) skin can be white, grey, yellow or anything in between; it may come away in flakes or powder or it may cause matting of the hair and tend to 'cake'. (The characteristic unkempt look of psora is unmistakable.)

Other manifestations of dryness are hair that becomes brittle and may even fall out; eyebrows and lashes that are thin and tend to drop out; and nails that are inclined to pit and become crippled. In addition, the orifices tend to become dry and cracked; the lips can peel; ears produce dry and crumbly wax and there may be dry and crusted mucus on the lower eyelids.

Dryness occurs internally as well. In the space between the bones there should be synovial fluid which keeps the joints lubricated. In psora the joints dry out, causing the ends of the bones to rub together. This sets up arthritic changes to the bones as the body's self-healing mechanism heaps calcified deposits at the points of contact as a means of restricting the amount of friction. It is common for those who suffer psoriasis of the elbows, knees or hips to experience drying of these joints.

The dryness of mucous membranes can also involve the gut; psoric patients often have severe constipation. However, in the case of a patient in need of *Sulphur* as a constitutional remedy (to deal with his psoric state), there may well be the opposite – a tendency to have chronically overactive bowels that produce loose motions. Nevertheless, the patient will feel a sense of internal dryness with the bowels losing fluids through overactivity and often the skin sweating profusely - the body is forced to compensate for this constant draining by increased thirst.

Dryness can even be part of the mental picture. The patient might have little or no inspiration or if he does then he will be unable to harness it as his imagination will be locked into routine and drudgery. (Oddly, dry humour – though not outright sarcasm – is part of the positive psoric picture – the ability to see the absurd side of life.)

The vesicle

The scabies vesicle is mirrored in other diseases that have characteristic vesicles. Chickenpox is one and herpes simplex is another. Smallpox was too (though it also had connections with syphilis and sycosis) but it has left the world stage for the time being – it was declared eradicated by the WHO in 1980.

It is probably no accident that herpes in all its forms increased wildly in the last quarter of the twentieth century. Many of those who have suffered from cold sores on the lips or around the mouth will know how itching or tingling precedes the appearance of a blister. This might be filled with clear fluid or it can be various shades of yellow. When the blister breaks, the itching usually begins to ease. Then the crusty scab forms to cover the lesion until the sore is healed. (As we shall see, herpes is a little more complicated than a simple chronically recurrent manifestation of psora. Because there is the involvement of a virus that lies dormant in the spinal column, it has associations with other miasms. However, its uncomplicated surface symptoms are classically psoric in their description.)

It is not difficult to see how chickenpox is related to psora. It is also very similar to a mild form of smallpox. Though chickenpox is an acute disease of childhood, its short-lived appearance is so similar to psora that it has significant implications for both those who had it and those who did not. It is usually produced during the first ten years of life when the body's immune system is at a very active and preparatory stage. The disease actually enhances the immune response and those who do not go through it are the poorer for it. We need chickenpox!

In most cases it is mild – which is one of the reasons why it has been the last to receive attention from the immunologists and their vaccines – but it can be very severe and may affect the lungs, throat, mouth and genitals. Generally speaking, the worse the case is, the more urgently that patient needed to produce the condition – in order to dig deep into the history of the gene pool and express the nearest equivalent to psora which, as we shall see, has been complicated by the superimposition of other miasms.

People who have had chickenpox so severely or inadequately that there are sequelae (follow-on conditions), often go on to suffer shingles (herpes-zoster) which behaves like herpes simplex (in its ability to lie dormant for years within the soft, nerve tissue of the spinal column) but is usually far more severe and debilitating as it affects nerve routes. For those who go through the childhood disease thoroughly and without sequelae, shingles is rare. If mass vaccination against chickenpox is introduced, we can expect shingles to erupt on a massive scale; it will no longer be mainly the preserve of the highly stressed and the geriatric; it will affect children and babies as well – as it has already, in rare cases.

Temperature control

In the acute disease of scabies, temperature can be variable and visit either extreme of the thermometer. At night, as a chronic manifestation of psora, it often rises and is accompanied by sweating or the opposite: a constricting sense of dryness if the skin is inactive. During the day, any slight exertion can produce a raised body temperature and accompanying sweat along with debility; the body is overreacting by producing heat for little reason and causing weakness as well. This condition on its own as a chronic problem is extremely common and is a glaringly obvious manifestation of psora. Seldom though is it seen as a cause for visiting a medical practitioner. (More's the pity! It is a state that can be a precursor to high blood pressure.)

There is also chilliness in acute psora. After scratching in the attack of itching, the patient often becomes chilled as a reaction to both the night-time heat of the bed and the relief from scratching. Many psoric patients manifesting chronic complaints suffer from cold and often complain of being unable to get warm. Psora covers both ends of the scale. To confuse things, in chronic psora we also get frequent swings between the extremes but, instead of these being caused by the mite (as that, of course, is not there), they are due to the reactivity to every little stimulus in the environment on the oversensitive nervous system. In chronic psora the five senses can be acutely sensitive – part of the inherited state of the memory within the very tissues of the body of how it feels to suffer those original symptoms.

So the people who suffer from chronic psoric complaints are representative of every different body type: warm-blooded, the chilly and the thermostatically unstable; the robust; the spare, weak and etiolated; and everything in between. None of this matters to the healthy individual who is able to adjust to every change of environment and circumstance. It is only when the symptoms begin to manifest at an intensity that disturbs the equilibrium, that recognition of psora becomes significant.

There is something else to add. The general lowering of vitality in scabies can bring about impetigo. This is caused by another opportunist: staphylococcus (or sometimes streptococcus). When the body's immunity is compromised, this little cootie causes its characteristic pustular infection.

It is very fast and very infectious. There are itchy eruptions with discoloured lesions, usually around the face but they can appear anywhere on the body. The lesions become crusty, dry and cracked, like psora; they become bloody and weepy, like psora and they can be joined up by 'stains' of infected skin that seem to behave (even if they do not exactly look) like psora. The infected site can and often does produce pus of varying colours – which is an advance on psora.

To summarise: the psoric patient will manifest symptoms similar to any of these states or any combination of them. There are always varying degrees of pattern and severity. Skin, hair and nails will all show the body's state externally with surface lesions mimicking one or other stage of the scabies development. Internally, the nervous system is affected and becomes highly sensitised. Body temperature is affected and can fluctuate out of control. There is dryness not only of the outer skin but also of internal organs or there is an imbalance in the water table of the whole body.

Other characteristic but deeper symptomatology can occur. Because the nervous system is disturbed, there can be vertigo, tinnitus and acute exaggeration of the sense of hearing, photophobia, increased sensitivity or distortion or absence of the senses of smell and taste. The digestion is disordered because the water balance and nervous system are awry; this leads to cravings and revulsion for certain tastes. In constipation (especially of infants) there is a curious craving for indigestible things (such as coal, chalk, dried spaghetti or uncooked potato). Psora is the inherited state of being susceptible not just to external parasitism but also internal infestation; so there is also craving for carbohydrates and sweet things which support the life style of internal parasites. Babies who have worms or nits are doing their psora!

Putting names to psora and its effects

So far there seems not much more than a list of symptoms. It is easier to understand illness if we have a name; we can all understand arthritis and rheumatism, varicose veins and haemorrhoids. With these labels we create a mental picture of what the patient looks like and how they might be suffering. This offers very limited understanding. There is far more to each of these conditions than is apparent, yet we are somehow comforted to know the name of the problem – our reasoning, rational mind is satisfied.

One label that is easy to grasp is psoriasis; arthritis likewise. Yet if we consider Uncle Bill with his flaky scalp or Granny with her stiff knees and gnarled knuckles we are no nearer understanding how they developed their infirmities. We might look in their bathroom cabinets and see coal tar shampoos or analgesics but a moment's thought tells us that these medicaments cure nothing. A second thought might make us wonder why such things do no more than palliate at best and suppress the symptoms at worst.

The history of psora gives us a map of an inherited disease state for which there has so far been no *internal* process of cure but which each of us in our own unique way is mimicking. If we know the salient features of psora and can recognise them in the pathology of the patient we are part way to helping that person change the hereditary pattern of disease. The history of psora is so deep and so ancient that we can never eradicate the tendency completely but we can learn to live with it and to teach our bodies to throw off its surfacing symptom complexes. We can learn to *develop creatively* through it.

Colds

A psoric cold is one where there is sneezing along with chilliness alternating with flushes of heat; the nose becomes sensitive and reddened; there is watery, clear and acrid mucus that tends to burn the top lip; the skin of the face feels dry; the eyes are reddened and sore and they may be very dry or wet from acrid tears. As the cold clears, the nose feels dry and can become crusty; the sinuses feel tight while there is difficulty in blowing anything out; the hair becomes lank and dull; the complexion is pasty and there is a general feeling of being unkempt. Various psoric remedies would be useful. To differentiate between them – because only one of them would be homoeopathic (i.e. similar) enough to deal with any particular cold – other symptoms need to be gathered. Thirst and appetite, quality of energy (nervy and restless or floppy and enervated) and mood would all help to complete the picture.

Joe and Martin have cold symptoms exactly like the ones listed above but one of them is thirsty for long draughts of cold water and the other is thirsty for sips of ice-cold water. One may be disinclined to do anything but read quietly, the other might be restless and preoccupied. One needs *Bryonia* while the other needs *Arsenicum Album* – both are psoric remedies.

Angina

This condition is caused by a reduced blood supply to the muscle of the heart – often because the artery supplying the heart is narrowed due to fatty degeneration. While resting, there is enough blood to keep the heart pumping but it is insufficient during any period of exertion. The patient finds lifting, carrying and walking uphill or upstairs difficult or painful; there is constriction of the chest walls and a variety of pains. The triggers for the condition can be dietary or stress related.

In the uncomplicated psoric angina there is a sense of a tight band around the chest which can become a vice-like squeezing with sharp pains that cause the patient to cry out. There is a sense of weakness and heaviness. The body temperature drops and he feels chilled and asks for covers – though the opposite might happen but this would normally be temporary, during the initial acute phase. The face goes ashen, the hair lank and the skin loses vitality – it wrinkles easily. There are palpitations that are often worse at night on lying down. Digestion often becomes disordered with flatulence and bloating; belching offers temporary relief. An acute episode can be brought on through eating too much or too late in the evening. The blood pressure can range from below normal to very high. The mood is important; the psoric patient will feel and fear he is going to die. At first there is great imaginative activity of mind; there is dread and a sense of impending doom accompanied or followed by restlessness (in the mind if he cannot move) and weepiness. As the condition settles into a pattern there is depression and timidity as well as a resigned negativity.

This description relates to one form of angina but there are others. We only have the 'bones' of the condition. While allopathy would be content to prescribe glycerin trinitrate under the tongue to relieve the acute attack and beta blockers to take care of the chronic state, what should we make of the differences between one patient who has palpitations in the morning as soon as he wakes and another who has palpitations only in the evening? What of the one who has squeezing, stabbing, needle-like pains in the chest while another has crushing pains as if being sat on by a heavyweight? What of the one who is tearful and desperate for attention in contrast to another who becomes implacably angry and unwilling to receive any practical help? Each patient is different and in his own way is expressing psoric heart and circulation troubles. The name of the condition gives us the idea of the territory but gives us very little clue as to the terrain.

The significance of understanding psora becomes apparent when we realise that it gives us not only flesh on the bones of a labelled condition but also that it gives us the blueprint for healing whatever condition it inspires. The *Materia Medica* of the homoeopathic medicines tells us which are capable of dealing with psoric conditions. We can tell the difference between a *Carbo Vegitabilis* (charcoal) patient (exhausted, puffing for breath and bluish around the lips) and a *Cactus* patient (alternately sad, irritable and fearful and inclined to cry out in anguish with the dreadful squeezing, sharp chest pain). Yet all these remedies have core similarities that make them homoeopathic to psora – they share those basic characteristic symptoms of fear and inadequacy, of drying out and breaking down. What makes them different is their individual and sometimes quirky symptoms that are peculiar to themselves.

The third dimension of psora

So why not just use the amyl nitrite spray? It gives instant relief. But then nothing will have been done about the underlying state of the patient, which was not angina, athlete's foot, or any other label you choose to name. The underlying state in psora has always been anxiety, dread, fearfulness, timidity, sensitivity, guilt, low self-esteem and a sense of inadequacy. Nothing in allopathy has ever succeeded in changing this deep seam within our make-up. Nor can it, for chemicals are useless tools in medical archaeology. Homoeopathy cannot cure it either; it can only return to the patient the ability to re-establish balance. To match (even if we cannot cure) the combined energy of inherent inadequacy and the physical memory of psoric symptoms we need similar energies. The *wholeness* of the physical and mental states of psora has to be treated, not just the physical parts of it alone.

In looking at the physical and mental symptoms of psora, have we got a 'whole'? Actually, no. We do not need to introduce this next idea in order to *treat* a patient homoeopathically but we do to *understand* the patient. The physical and mental symptoms of psora are rich enough to match any patient to it, and then define any particular sickness to the point where we can differentiate between the peculiarities displayed by the individual psoric remedies. We already seem to have an adequate map of this great miasm, the mother of all miasms. Yet it is so far incomplete, and for two reasons: the first is that we have not accounted for the innately spiritual side of our nature; the second is that we have not looked for a positive aspect to psora. These two points are very closely linked.

Every culture has myths and legends. In most, these have become so deeply ingrained into the collective psyche that they have become the basis for one belief system or another. Stories and characters were invented to create easily understood metaphors for so many of the inexplicable events and conditions of our world. Social structures can be built round such belief systems. The more socially cohesive a group becomes, the stronger is the whole and the individuals that make up the group all benefit.

As man developed away from other primates he began to show the need to express his awareness of an order higher than his own. Remembering that psora was keeping up with him every step of the way, we can begin to see that his restless nature, searching for answers to the puzzles of the natural world, inevitably invented ever more fanciful and elaborate stories to explain his own inadequacies in the face of the elemental forces around him. Man could no more prevent storm and flood than he could scabies and infestations. He could create shelters and seek high ground but this would not stop the forces of nature. He could cover himself with unguents but the mite kept coming.

As man diverged from other primates he lost the certainty of 'at oneness' with nature that other animals seem to possess – he was on his own. As he adapted and learnt to survive as a nomad and later as an agrarian settler, his physique evolved into that of an upright runner – slighter and less muscular. Though his five senses may have been more acute than ours are, his intellect became gradually more dominant at their expense. His intellect came to dominate his intuition – he saw the material world as his rightful element. As his intellect and materialism gathered pace, so his need to institutionalise his spiritual thinking became stronger – some of the time he felt he was more in competition with nature than part of it. His 'oneness' began to give way to a sense of separation from all other life forms and though it gave him a spurious moral superiority, it caused the agony of self-doubt. It should not surprise us that religions have sprung up to provide not only a social structure but also to explain the presence of a greater hidden force that might at any time cut man off from his most eagerly pursued aspirations. Religions have provided us with a link to God (or the gods) – a link that only man finds necessary and one that has been thoroughly abused from the outset.

Right up until the age of agnosticism and atheism, such belief systems satisfied naïve minds otherwise untrammelled by science and its incontrovertible facts. Even today, for better or worse, spiritual values are part of our make-up even if they are pantheistic, animalistic, monotheistic, 'New Age' or significant by their absence. For most of our history, superstition and servitude have characterised many of the belief structures that have arisen, and in the process societies have gained moral codes and cohesive bonding. When these structures break down, it is as a result of individuals finding them inadequate. What makes the building and breaking down of these structures acceptable is the constant search for, and determination to emulate, goodness. It is in that search that those who have felt the force of spiritual energy feel most 'at one' with either God or Nature – as if they have experienced that unquestioning wholeness with the rest of creation.

This restlessness of spirit, the very essence of psora, is based on the fear of not matching up to the ideals and demands of the 'maker'. 'Feeling inadequate from the sense that we do not control our ultimate destiny' is its central theme. It is not hard to see how this has a bearing on our spiritual inadequacy when life takes adverse turns: 'Our prayers were not answered this time; we were not good enough'. The feeling this engenders takes us further away from the sense of 'oneness with Nature' that we seek so eagerly – if we are principally in a psoric state. No wonder that some writers have equated the story of psora, 'the itch', and the sense of emotional and spiritual inadequacy that goes with it, with the story of the expulsion from the Garden of Eden.

The positive aspect of psora

Every force, question, argument, thought or form has a negative and a positive side – or better, as eastern thought puts it: a yin and a yang (with inherently no idea of right or wrong). Psora manifests not only our susceptibility to being a host, *it is also the knowledge of our limitations.*

The awareness of our place in the scheme of things without the agitating need to venture beyond is the positive aspect of psora. We are all, at heart, psoric. This does not mean that we have to be sick with it – at least, not all the time. It means that we have to maintain a balance not just with the environment but also within ourselves. The balance must be held, though, in all three main bodies: physical, emotional and spiritual (this latter not being limited to any religious sense). While it is held steady, there is no sickness. What is strikingly evident is that of the three bodies it is the spiritual one that most needs to be kept in balance – this is in all aspects of healing and not only in relation to the psoric miasm.

A patient can put up with physical disease if there is no mental or emotional distress. If the cold-infected patient can continue to function as he would wish then there is still a sense of well-being. If the accident victim with a broken leg feels no pressure to heal quickly and get back to work there is no threat to the slower rhythm of life necessary for healing at the body's own rate. If family can accommodate the slower physical speed of an arthritic patient then the pains of the condition will become less threatening and the patient will be able to hold onto their sense of 'oneness' (which is so essential for well-being).

A patient suffering emotional trauma can still learn how to pick up the pieces and re-establish well-being. The feeling of being happy to be alive does not always disappear irrevocably as a result of distress or tragedy. In the psoric state there is usually an awareness that life continues after the death of present hopes or the passing of a relative or friend. If one is hit hard enough by an emotional blow then physical illness usually does follow but often as an end result before a return to the cycle of life. Fainting, diarrhoea or a cold follows a shock or bad news; weakness, poor memory and nervous irritability can all follow on from a death in the family – yet all these can be temporary failings if the patient re-establishes emotional equilibrium. It is as if the physical body is at the service of the emotional and mental bodies, and is allowing the recent distress to manifest in the physical symptoms.

A patient cannot suffer a damaging blow to the spiritual body without inevitable, long-term disturbance to the whole being. It is when the sense of well-being, of being at one with the world, of being purposeful, is upset or profoundly damaged that chronic illness takes hold permanently or until harmony is restored on *all* levels. The physical body is also at the service of the spiritual body but if the latter is disturbed or destroyed then the physical manifestation will be chronic or even terminal. When psora is in balance, acceptance, forgiveness, tolerance, understanding and loving kindness are what can restore spiritual health.

Sometimes it is enough for us to be able to answer truthfully, *"Yes, I feel well"* to the question: *"How do you feel in yourself?"* Yet this answer is often delivered by those who suffer considerable symptomatic distress from some chronic complaint or other. They may well be seeking relief from their existing symptoms, or even a cure, but the integrity of their life force is intact even if it is compromised in its self-healing. In spite of the condition of the physical body and the emotional body, the spiritual body is still intact – *their sense of purpose remains strong.* This is what lies at the heart of well-being; this is what keeps the balance between harmony and discord within the confines of the physical body. When the sense of purpose is destroyed, distorted or perverted then a chronic illness always follows.

The positive aspect of psora gives us limitations with which we can measure and pace ourselves. Psora is a perverse structure of handicaps that we have to overcome in order to achieve whatever we set out to do – and in the process, become stronger and better able to hand on our experiences genetically. If this sounds fanciful then it is helpful to view it from a metaphorical angle. Study of any of the arts reveals often paradoxically simple yet unbelievably complex structures that lie at the heart of any great painting or piece of music. Yet the onlooker or the listener has to work hard to see these internal workings. It takes a trained eye to observe the geometry underlying a Velázquez or a Poussin; it takes an exceptionally keen ear to distinguish the weaving parts of a Bach fugue. Yet it is this very internal strength of structure that makes these masterpieces delight and endure. However, the structure imposes limitations on the artist that hone the creative imagination to a fine degree, to take the work beyond the common-place; the whole becomes greater than the sum of its parts.

This whole premise might be unacceptable if it is *disease* that provides the basis for such a structuring of our lives. Yet it is not really surprising that nature should provide us with a natural process with which to temper our continual development. Disease is a loss of balance; a disturbance that affects our susceptibilities; a state of being where we lose our ability to adapt to circumstances, environment or emotional turmoil – and results in loss, or threatened loss, of purpose. Through our inconsistencies each one of us learns how to maintain essential equilibrium – or not. What makes great artists *great* is not just their extraordinary imagination but also success in the struggle to overcome their limitations in order to produce their creations.

Every patient has a unique story to tell of how they have managed and failed to keep balance – but at the same time, each one has a story of accrued experience. In a patient who is showing essentially psoric tendencies one finds not just characteristic negative traits but also positive ones. These qualities are evident in those who know and understand their limitations and make allowances for them. Some of the positive traits of psora are rather old-fashioned terms that people are now reluctant to use: dignity, steadfastness, stoicism, honour, constancy, humility, generosity of spirit, patience, fidelity and gentility. Other traits include determination, courage, generosity, open-mindedness and clarity of thought. Such qualities have evolved with our state of awareness and each one is an asset in our struggle to maintain the balance essential for good health.

Models of psora

An example of psora personified is J. S. Bach. He was of an equable, cheerful and unpretentious disposition; a man of moral rectitude, God-fearing and possibly somewhat naïve. He was hard-working to the point of being indefatigable – to unselfish ends – and he had an unshakeable sense of purpose. He was open-minded in that he felt no inhibitions in learning his craft from whatever sources were available; he built on the wide-ranging experiences of many other artists from different countries. For most of his life his health was good and he died aged sixty-six from a stroke and possibly pneumonia. However, it is highly likely that his end was hastened by the appalling treatment for his increasing blindness, received at the hands of an English oculist who used repeated surgery and the administration of mercury. How much longer the blind Bach could have survived remains conjecture yet there is no particular evidence that he suffered from other than cataracts – often a psoric manifestation – before being attended by a quack surgeon. (As we shall see mercury was the cause of many a premature death.)

Another example of an essentially psoric person is William Gladstone. He was prodigiously gifted with a capacity for logical thought and hard work. He too was a God-fearing man (though this is not necessary for good health) and one of high principles. His life was remarkable for his dogged determination and single-mindedness of purpose though he was quite capable of holding the reins of several horses at once. His sense of purpose was never selfish or materialistic. If he had a fault by which we can recognise him instantly, it was ponderous and thundering prolixity while standing at the Dispatch box. What made this particularly psoric was that every speech he ever made was thoroughly prepared and exhaustively researched. Unlike Bach, he did suffer bouts of unpleasant illness; he was plagued by erysipelas from time to time. This is a streptococcal infection of an open wound or mucous membrane that is characterised by cellulitis and is often brought on through lowered immunity from anxiety or stress. It is basically psoric in origin as it has a characteristic surface-spreading habit and the central lesion often forms a blister where there is oedema below. However, it can progress to a severe state in which pus, swollen glands and general septicaemia turn it towards a different miasmatic condition. (He died at eighty-nine of old age, cancer of the cheek [2] and painkilling drugs. Common to psoric patients, he was glad in his stoicism to meet his maker even if he found the final journey wearisome and dispiriting.

From literature we can find examples of ordinary folk who show truly characteristic psoric dispositions. Anthony Trollope's Mr Harding (in *The Warden*) is a perfect case in point. He may not be as enviably gifted as Bach or Gladstone but he is similarly endowed with honesty, stoicism, constancy and generosity of spirit. The way he transmutes his anxieties into imaginary 'cello playing' is an eccentricity that exemplifies a psoric's ability to find a way to balance out negative feelings. Charles Dickens' Philip Pirrip and Joe Gargery from *Great Expectations* provide further portraits of the positive aspect of psora. Between them they are possessed of all the virtues mentioned so far and Dickens contrasts them with characters that have long since lost their psoric way and passed into deeper and uglier miasmatic territory. Miss Haversham, the ancient, jilted bride, seeks to enjoy vicariously the emotional torture of whoever will love her protégée, Estella, a frigid girl with a heart of stone.

John Milton, in his blindness, showed psoric stoicism when he wrote of his predicament: 'They also serve who only stand and wait.' Rudyard Kipling, too, understood the psoric state in its positive aspect and, in his magisterial poem 'If', he clearly recognises how best to maintain one's focus and equilibrium even if implicitly he knows just how hard it is. These two poets' productive natures may have been irrevocably influenced by their heartbreaking experiences but their creations reflect their success in channelling the energy of their suffering for the benefit of humanity.

Purpose in psora

In mentioning creativity and productivity it is necessary to consider the underlying qualities in the psoric state. Inspiration and its translation from thought to material form or end product tends to be slow. Psorics need long apprenticeships. Their nature is to be methodical and thorough; speed makes them anxious. Though they are clear-sighted and often quick-thinking, they take time to make decisions for fear of missing details. They rely on experience and often learn best by making mistakes – even though this costs them lost energy due to nursing regret and damaged self-esteem. Their progress is usually marked by patience and perseverance; 'dogged does it'.

The essence of psoric productivity is service. This must surely derive from deep in the psyche of ancient man who saw that it was by common effort that survival was best ensured. Though this service is for the good of others, it carries the reward of self-satisfaction (in its purest sense). In all the other miasms the spirit of humanitarian service is compromised and tarnished by negative and egotistical influences. Psorics have a sense of inadequacy – if only through a certainty that nothing one might do could ever be perfect – and an innate sense that there is a source of higher power and wisdom. Well-balanced psoric people lead useful and fulfilling lives that follow a steady and relatively uninterrupted flow, coloured by self-respect and respect for others, morality, solid grounding and faith in the sense of purpose – though this last may be entirely unconscious.

The rarity of uncomplicated psora

This all begins to sound nauseatingly pious – or thoroughly boring. Yet we are trying to view the history of psora alone, through the filter of the twenty-first century. There is so very little pure psora left amongst mankind. Some peasant cultures, untainted by the influence of the western world still exist but these are dwindling. Among them are psoric people who lead slow and steady lives rhythmically punctuated by daily, monthly, seasonal and annual routines. In modern Europe such patients are found only in communities that resist fast changing times. In third-world countries that are still miraculously untouched by too much commercialism, missionary zeal, rampant politics and vaccination, psoric people are found in greater numbers. Occasionally, one comes across a patient whose life history is so free of threateningly chronic ill health and who is so well in every other way (except the relatively superficial complaint that they have brought for treatment), that one can only stand back admiringly and dispense only the barest minimum to effect as thorough healing as possible. Here is a delightful example:

> A woman aged seventy-six came for treatment some good few years past. She had suffered psoriasis on the back of her neck for most of her adult life. She said that it did not bother her much but thought that as

homoeopathic treatment was now so readily available that she would like to try and get rid of it. There was nothing else wrong with her at all though she mentioned that twelve years before she had experienced a bout of troublesome constipation which she had dealt with by taking up yoga. (The constipation, which had started some two years before the yoga sessions, was relieved within two days.)

The psoriasis was rough and reddened across the nape of her neck; it looked sore but she said it was only so when she caught her comb on it. The skin flaked off in pearly white scabs but left no raw patch beneath. The only itching she experienced was on her back while lying in bed at night. She did not get uncomfortably hot in bed but did admit to sticking her leg out from under the cover to keep it cool. (Her husband complained that she had to have the bedroom window wide open *"so that it's always blowing a gale"*.) In temperament she was quiet and unassuming. She enjoyed gardening and loathed cooking – though she was good at it. She adored being a grandmother and said not a word of criticism about her alarmingly eccentric daughter-in-law. She was quite unable to remember any incident in her past that might have caused her any grief except *"the usual upset everyone must feel when a parent departs"*. She could not recall what had been happening in her life at the time that the psoriasis first developed – *"though I do believe it was around then that I got married!"* Remarkably, she had not a grey hair on her head.

She was given *Sulphur* 1M and on her return in a month she was able to say that not only was the psoriasis some 50 per cent improved but also her energy was better – though she had not reported any difficulty with this before. She was asked to wait before anything further was prescribed but after some six weeks she reported that she felt that the psoriasis was returning. She was given *Sulphur* 50M and this time she returned after two months with an almost clear neck. *"I can wear all my dark clothes now without the embarrassment of white flakes all over my collar!"* Some six months later she mentioned that there was again a slight return of the skin condition. This time she was given *Psorinum* 50M. She has remained free of psoriasis since then. (It has to be admitted that not all cases of psoriasis are so amenable to treatment.)

Psorinum: the energy of psora in remedy form

Does such a case constitute proof of anything very much? Not in itself but if we look within it at the remedies that effected the healing and the reasons for their administration then we can find something more deserving of critical appraisal. We have already drawn the parallels between the psoric miasm and the suppressed energy of the scabies mite and have noted the susceptibility to being a host to it and to other parasites. We should turn next to the remedy made from the body product caused by scabies itself – the serous fluid taken from the vesicle formed by the burrowing mite. However repulsive this may seem, *Psorinum* has been a remedy since Hahnemann's day and has proved its worth for two centuries. It was proved in the way laid down by Hahnemann; the symptom picture it evoked in the healthy people who took it in order to prove it stands testimony to the patients suffering similar symptom complexes who need it to recover. Moreover, although Hahnemann was known not to have used it very much (except in fairly hopeless cases), clinical evidence has since been able to establish an even wider area of symptomatology that it will heal.

Dr Clarke, in his *Dictionary of Practical Materia Medica*, written almost a century after Hahnemann's work, gives us a clear portrait of this nosode. With the benefit of the collected clinical experience of many of Hahnemann's successors as well as his own, he set out a detailed analysis of the types of patient who would need and benefit from the serous remedy: the way it works; the results that one might expect from its administration; the physical, mental and emotional symptoms it is capable of both engendering and healing. The following is an edited account of it.

Psorinum is suited generally to psoric constitutions particularly when there is a lack of reaction to other remedies (i.e. the patient simply does not get better in spite of an accurate assessment of the case and the administration of well-indicated remedies). A dose of *Psorinum* will galvanise the patient's self-healing mechanism and in so doing will allow the previously given remedies to work. This is often the case in patients who have suffered a long-term chronic complaint. (When Hahnemann gave this remedy to hopeless cases there was an apparent extension of life.)

Psorinum is suited to patients who suffer from psoric complaints (particularly of the skin, the glands, the bowels and the orifices) in which one of the salient features is a foul and filthy smell best described as the odour of stale excrement. No amount of washing entirely removes this smell. Such people have little sense of cleanliness or personal hygiene. (This is markedly less common as a symptom state these days but not because the psoric miasm has gone away; not only has society a less tolerant attitude to a lack of personal hygiene but a patient's psora has been so overlaid by the other miasms that it is not able to surface so obviously. Homoeopaths are faced with treating a hydra of miasms, one of which – in its symptom picture – covers scrupulous cleanliness even to the point of insanity.)

Psorinum is suited to pale, sickly individuals – especially children – who do not develop well and are, in consequence, delicate, weak and antisocial. (This is common enough but not as usual as a similar state that is the inheritance of the tubercular miasm – this looks the same but for the latter's unique tendency to foster attractive, bright, restless, emotionally oversensitive people who nevertheless need lots of social stimulus.)

Psorinum is suited to patients who are subject to producing conditions (particularly of the skin and the glands) which are frequently suppressed. This is true most significantly of those who have skin eruptions eradicated by ointments or internal drugs. The process of suppression itself tends to encourage the waking of this miasm – as long as one of the other miasms is not already predominant. It is also indicated in patients who do not have the energy to produce external expressions of disease; the skin is unable to react by producing eruptions. (This is an important failing as the end product of so many acute diseases is just such a skin reaction.)

Psorinum is suited to those whose central nervous system is hypersensitive. They are easily startled; they misinterpret sensations due to distortion of one or more of the five senses – misperception of: taste (things may taste burnt or bitter or coppery); smell (things may smell foul or not smell at all); touch (there may be numbness, pins and needles or smooth things feel rough); sight (there are sparks, dimmed or blurred vision or objects seem to tremble); hearing (there is tinnitus and distortion of voices and other sounds). This degree of sensitivity of the nervous system is just as much pathology as the rest of the range of symptoms, not least because it causes the patient to feel more acutely his state of physical inadequacy. *A defective nervous system exaggerates the perceived hostility of the outside environment.*

Seldom would a patient present himself at the homoeopath's clinic suffering in every particular. The image of psora can sometimes be pared down to a few keynotes. This is helpful to the practitioner when the patient does not at once appear to fit into any of the above descriptions. These keynotes include:

i) lack of vital reaction, not just to other well-indicated remedies but to any form of treatment whatsoever – including allopathic sometimes;

ii) lack of recuperative powers, especially after an acute disease (and when other psoric remedies have failed to ignite the Vital Force into self-healing);

iii) hopelessness and despair of ever recovering – this is the mental/emotional parallel to (and fatalistic acceptance of) the lack of reaction;

iv) emaciation (loss of weight) – especially after acute diseases;

v) foul body odours;

vi) hypochondriasis with peevishness – a psoric ailment is often marked by fear of the effects on the system of what might become dangerous symptoms (there is a fear of inflammation; of fever; of constipation).

Whenever one or more of these keynotes is a salient feature of a case then *Psorinum* must be considered as an agent of healing. The effects it creates in proving and in healing sickness show acute scabies, with its physical, mental and emotional and spiritual picture, to be a good representative of the chronic state of initial unwellness in which the body, mind and spirit becomes susceptible to drying out, cracking up and breaking down; accompanied by anxiety about security, health, the future and inadequacy.

Sulphur

Confusingly, much of what has been said about *Psorinum* so far could be applied to another remedy – *Sulphur*. This is another of Hahnemann's legacies. He discovered that *Sulphur* is the greatest of all anti-psoric remedies – it is capable of being the healing agent for so many of the depredations of psora on the whole body. Not only is it a remedy, when shown to be 'like', that has the power to initiate the body's self-healing of scabies (or any form of 'the itch') but it is also able to relieve the system of the tendency to produce psoric disease states generally. (He stopped short of claiming that it would cure psora altogether – indeed, he stated that psora was incurable.)

In homoeopathic literature *Sulphur* is often mentioned in the same breath as psora in discussions on the miasms. *Sulphur* crops up in more symptom rubrics (lists of curative remedies) than any other medicine. It has a reputation for being required sooner or later in any long-term treatment of chronic disease. Hahnemann often felt it expedient to begin to unravel a case with an initial dose of *Sulphur*, whether or not it was specifically indicated, simply because of the universality of psora and its influence.

Sulphur is made from a volcanic, crystalline substance and is one of the earliest (if not the earliest) known medicinal substances. It is still the basis of some drugs manufactured by pharmaceutical companies. It has been recognised and used indiscriminately (in its material form) for its uniquely suppressive powers. In homoeopathy it has become (in its dynamic energy form) the agent of the opposite effect; it is the most commonly used remedy for promoting the expulsion of toxicity from the body. (Not surprising when you consider that it comes from a volcano that is a point of eruption and elimination on the Earth's crust – its skin.)

Sulphur and *Psorinum* share many features but they are distinguished relatively easily by just a few factors. (It is not difficult to tell when one is indicated in a case and not the other.) *Psorinum* is suited to those who become predominantly chilly. The body's thermostat no longer maintains body heat; the chronically ill patient may need to wrap up well even at the height of summer; he might feel uncomfortable without a hat the whole time; there is likely to be a dread of the winter and cold weather. *Sulphur*, on the other hand, is likely to suit those who are overheated – if not all the time then at particular times of the day; at night when the patient must throw the covers off or stick a leg out of bed; on the least exertion when his face becomes suffused with red and he pours sweat; while sitting idle in the evening.

Psorinum tends to have strange appetites. There is ravenous hunger but food is crammed in without relish; there might otherwise be ravening hunger which disappears as soon as eating starts. *Sulphur* is characteristically hungry at 11 a.m. and will raid the fridge. *Sulphur*'s appetite is decidedly in favour of the rich and spicy which *Psorinum* would find

412

unappealing. When well, a *Sulphur* patient (i.e. one who is likely to produce *Sulphur* symptoms when ill) is usually quite energetic even if he or she dissipates the energy unnecessarily on idle activities. When ill, then energy is at a premium and he goes into a floppy state. *Sulphur*-hungry patients tend to drape themselves over furniture – if they care what people think (which is not so likely) – or they slump in an untidy heap. *Psorinum* patients have as little energy as *Sulphur* patients but they are more restless and anxious, chilly and sensitive.

Frustratingly, these are generalisations that can be contradicted. *Psorinum* patients can be overheated and indolent while *Sulphur* patients can feel extremely chilly and preoccupied. However, these are exceptions to the rule. More often than not *Sulphur* is well followed by *Psorinum* anyway in relatively straightforward cases. The delightful woman with psoriasis quoted earlier is a case in point; the *Psorinum* was needed because the *Sulphur* was not sufficient on its own to hold the cure. (This is an example of a nosode being given to 'underpin' the achievement of a major remedy that would not otherwise hold – even where the 'picture' of that nosode is not strictly speaking fully evident. It is given more for the general *theme* of the pathology.)

In the mental, emotional and spiritual spheres both remedies are applicable to many shared symptoms. Both types of patient are subject to deep melancholia – to the point of suicide. This relates to the patient's sense of worthlessness and hopeless despair. There is irritability and confusion. They cannot stop thinking of their condition; it becomes obsessive. There is weakness of memory and a tendency to make mistakes in speaking, answering, understanding and visual perception. (This brings to mind Oliver Sacks' case of the man who mistook his wife for a hat. For such an apparently healthy man to make such extraordinary mistakes with his vision would probably lead a homoeopath to administer *Sulphur* in a high potency.)

Both remedy states include a sense of having done something terribly wrong; the patient may have a guilt complex yet often cannot identify its cause. In each case this can spill over into spiritual territory as patients might feel that they have been judged unworthy for salvation. This sounds as if it comes straight out of the eighteenth and nineteenth centuries and is increasingly uncommon in our time. Or so it would seem – except for the number of people who confess to being unable to make headway with their spiritual development; they feel inadequate and sometimes lament that this aspect of life is more difficult nowadays, not least because the Church is no longer as powerful a focus of our lives. For a patient to express their sense of a need to be more spiritually aware suggests that the psoric miasm is beginning to surface – especially if there is a sense of inadequacy with it. Once such patients have had a dose of *Sulphur* or *Psorinum* or both, they seldom mention such worries and even go on to describe how well they do with their chosen mode of spiritual expression. (It must be added that other remedies also cover this rarely considered area.)

Psora – and *Psorinum*'s and *Sulphur*'s influence over it – is only part of our evolutionary condition and is no more than an influence over our perception of ourselves and therefore how we perceive ourselves in spiritual terms. The remedies, in influencing the whole system, allow us the energy to change whatever is oppressively and therefore potentially pathologically threatening to our peace of mind. As everyone (apart from the died-in-the-wool syphilitic) derives some if not all of their sense of peace from a state of 'oneness' with God or Nature or their own expression of purpose, it becomes evident that remedies can have a profound spiritual effect. (It goes without saying that remedies cannot influence the mode of spiritual expression. Remedies effect benefit on Buddhist and Baptist alike.)

Sulphur is a 'constitutional' remedy. This word is open to debate but it is meant here in the sense that, in general terms, the whole-body life force can be encompassed by the description of its energy. Not everyone is of the same 'whole body' type and all the great constitutional remedies have the capacity to answer the description of more than one. *Sulphur* covers several.

Take the tall, stooping academic with unruly hair, long and far-from-clean fingernails with a wrongly buttoned cardigan, who tramps the corridors of learning with an absent-minded expression; or the expatriate policeman, pin-neat and leather-tanned, who likes nothing better than a hot curry and a siesta; or the weekend pub-crawler who can down a gallon of beer in no time to fill his pot belly while cracking risqué jokes, in order to relax from a week of hard labour; or the spotty youth lost in his exam work and found again on the football field, who spends any other spare time slumped in front of the television, oblivious to everything else going on in the house, or chomping his way through boxes of takeaway junk food. They all need *Sulphur*.

Consider the businesswoman whose disconcerting confidence alarms all who do not know her well and whose idea of relaxation is to dash off to France for the weekend and sit with shoes off, sipping wine, plotting her boardroom moves. What about the dumpy granny who misses her bus stop because she is dreaming up knitting patterns or lost in thoughts that she would not be able to remember if you asked her? They all need *Sulphur* in spite of being well. They need *Sulphur* to *keep* them well.

Those described above are all inclined to abuse their health disgracefully and *Sulphur* can be administered prophylactically to help maintain their superlative constitutions. If any of these people were to produce a medical complaint it would be likely to be a psoric one – a skin eruption; a bout of chronic but uncomplicated diarrhoea; stress headaches with visual disturbances; piles; high blood pressure; memory loss. Whatever it might be, it would be of slow onset but gradual and inexorable; it would impinge on the person's lifestyle, eventually to the point of troubling the patient enough to force them to seek help – only, with the psoric miasm, it can take a very long time to reach this moment of crisis. The underlying threat though would be the same; the symptoms would threaten the person's sense of adequacy on one or more levels.

The initial trigger for the condition that distresses the person enough to ask for treatment may be mechanical, bacterial, functional, emotional or mental; if the condition is similar to psora and to *Sulphur* then *Sulphur* will heal – and if it cannot achieve this on its own then *Psorinum* will often complete the job. It would be fatuous to prescribe on the core symptom of 'a sense of inadequacy'. To recognise when a patient needs *Sulphur* constitutionally and to confirm the choice we have a 'map'. Provings and clinical experiences have given us a vast canvas to work with yet often all we need is a knowledge of the essentials of the remedy.

Sulphur's great keynote characteristics are:

i)   uneven distribution of circulation causing flushes of
        heat in various parts of the body resulting in red face

or lips, hot feet at night, heat and sweating of the
chest etc.

ii)   a dislike of, and feeling worse for, excessive heat; the sun, a
      heater or the warmth of the bed all aggravate.

iii) a sensation of weakness and emptiness that makes the person
      want to rest even after the slightest exertion and most of all after
      having to stand for any length of time.

iv)   a tendency to suffer from fast-acting bowels; chronic diarrhoea
      or the propensity for loose motions is typical of the remedy.

v)   a marked tendency to skin complaints in the form of rashes,
      pimples, blotches, boils, acne, eczema, psoriasis or simply
      chronic itching with no other symptom.

Other characteristics of *Sulphur* include:

vi)   either forgetfulness of or a marked aversion to washing – a
      distinct lack of cleanliness at any rate.

vii) sensations of burning; many of the pains of a *Sulphur* patient are
      best described as fiery or burning.

viii) a tendency to enjoy alcohol too much; *Sulphur* is one of the
      most common remedies for alcoholism (though this condition
      has syphilitic connotations).

ix)   a tendency to cramp.

There are typical mental aspects worth noting too: daydreaming to the
point of being absent-minded; the curious perception that things of little
worth are of great value (many a collector is a *Sulphur* patient); sudden
flashes of hot temper that burn themselves out as quickly as they erupted;
childish lapses of temperament in adults; egotism and pride to the point of
self-delusion; melancholy and despair that one can never live up to personal
expectations. On a more positive note, *Sulphur* types are given to flashes of
extraordinary inspiration that come out of the propensity for daydreaming.

These attributes might well exist in people who are not even contemplating making an appointment to see the doctor but they are all capable
of tipping the balance into a pathological condition. As they are characteristic of the energy of *Sulphur* it can be seen why the remedy is of such

consequence and how it can be used to dispel ill health before it manifests threateningly – if at all.

Calcium: a variation on the psoric theme

There are other psoric remedies that deserve just as much room in a ho-moeopath's drawer. It would be impossible to allow space for them all here; there are too many. Nevertheless, it is worth taking a look at just one other great psoric remedy; the one that stands opposite and complementary to *Sulphur* – *Calcium Carbonate*.

Calcium is another legacy of Hahnemann. He made the remedy from the middle layer of oyster shells. (Others have used carbonate of lime precipitated from a solution of chalk in hydrochloric acid.) Through proving it he discovered a remedy only rivalled by *Sulphur* in its importance in the treatment of psora. It would be impossible to practice homoeopathy satisfactorily without these two remedies; their energies are similar to those of the healthy constitutions of a majority of mankind. (*Phosphorus* and *Silica* complete the square of psoric remedies on which constitutions are based and homoeopathic practice would be inconceivable without these as well. This last concept of having just four basic constitutional types would no doubt be debated furiously by the many proponents of the different philosophies of homoeopathy!)

How is *Calcium* psoric as a remedy? Naturally, at its heart is the sense of inadequacy; the feeling that something dreadful will happen and that one will be unable to cope. A range of feelings from anxiety to anguish are experienced in response to even quite trifling things; this can lead to despair, extending even to a fear of insanity. It is easy to be discouraged in activities and projects; memory and the five senses can be weak or lead to the misinterpretation of the environment or communication which leads to impatience or intolerance and anger, varying from the desire to 'opt out' to the desperate need to be with those who can offer security.

People needing *Calcium* can be easily frightened or they take umbrage quickly and lack the will to see the cause from any other perspective. When agitated they lose their sense of direction and thought processes become uncoordinated. Distress brings on physical symptoms quickly – racing heartbeat, flushing of the face, cold sweats, gastric disturbances and a general sinking feeling. Those showing a need for *Calcium* are often worried about their health even to the point of obsession.

On the positive side, *Calcium* types (forgive the categorisation!) are hard-working in a methodical and determined way. They leave no stone unturned and become impatient with those who would settle for less. If *Sulphur* is capable of inspired flashes of genius, then *Calcium* is noted on occasion for its insight and intuition. When well, they can cope with any amount of work as long as they are not made to feel that they are too slow or inaccurate – though they can take constructive criticism as long as it helps them to complete the task satisfactorily. They are content (unlike the typical *Sulphur* patient) to work at mundane things; they derive satisfaction from setting everything in order. (This is why they enjoy puzzles and jigsaws; they tend to doodle on telephone pads or exercise books.) They prefer to be early or punctual because to be late would mean having less time to think and might prevent them from completing an allotted task. All this can lead to their becoming bogged down in the minutiae of a job; this slows them down further, makes them late and, consequently, agitated.

While a *Sulphur* type explodes with anger and then forgets it, the *Calcium* patient builds up resentment slowly before declaring anger but then holds on to the negative feelings. It takes a long time and much patience to placate a *Calcium*. A *Sulphur*, infuriatingly, often forgets that there was ever a cross word uttered. (No surprise that *Calcium* is a little more common in northern climes while *Sulphur* characteristics are seen to predominate in Latin countries.)

Though both cover despair and anguish, *Sulphur* people have a greater awareness of things on a global scale and any sense of personal defeat is often due to the world's inability to recognise their talents. *Calcium* people, with hardly a glance up to see anything beyond their immediate environment, lament when things go wrong that the world is an unsafe and hostile place to be in. This is not to suggest that *Calcium* types are small-minded or inferior in intellect; nor that *Sulphur* characters are all fire and no substance. *Calcium* is not always slow and cautious and *Sulphur* is not always quick-witted and intemperate. However, within the confines of the psoric miasm,[3] these tendencies are often prevalent. With them go their counterpart characteristics: when *Calcium* shows brilliance and speed there is often a loss of stamina and the will to follow through which is succeeded by anxiety, frustration and tears; when *Sulphur* erupts into activity the result can be lethargy, indifference and a lack of grounding. (It will become clear that when the picture is clouded by one or more of the other miasms reactions to initial activity can be radically different.)

In a psoric state, the *Calcium* physical type is often described rather more specifically than the *Sulphur* physical type. This is unfortunate for students as it limits the perception of the range of this remedy. The typical *Calcium* person is supposed to be pale, flabby, chilly and costive. *Calcium* babies are said to have a chalky or translucent complexion, large, chubby features, round heads and sweaty necks. They are all supposed to be fair. Such children are given to having night terrors. These details are true and different from the typical *Sulphur* subject. Nevertheless, it is not the whole picture. *Calcium* people can be sturdy and well built. They do not have to be fat; they can be lean or well padded with musculature. However, they have to work harder to keep their weight down; they have to exercise more consistently to build up muscle. Because their metabolism works at a generally slower rate and as they are distinctly chillier mortals than *Sulphur* types, they have a tendency to lay down fat easily. *Sulphur* characters, too, can run contrary to type and be obese and sluggish, chilly and constipated – but this is more likely to be through downright abuse of the body's health. (What is more, this would be a case of a *Sulphur* personality influenced by one of the other miasms - sycosis.)

In the range of physical symptoms, *Calcium* contrasts well with *Sulphur*. Apart from the difference in body heat and metabolism, *Calcium* tends to be more associated with skin eruptions that weep clear fluid rather than bleed; there is more glandular activity than in the case of *Sulphur*, which erupts onto the surface with blood and heat. There is slow growth rate with delayed teething in *Calcium*; there is a tendency for excitement to disrupt the body clock so that routines are interrupted. There is an oversensitivity of the senses causing alarm and despondency. Weather changes affect the system far more readily and with greater variety than in a *Sulphur* patient whose average response is to collapse into a chair or rush to the lavatory.

419

The appetites of *Calcium* are quite different from *Sulphur*. Children who attempt to eat things that are indigestible such as coal, chalk, uncooked spaghetti or potato peelings quite commonly need *Calcium* (while this may be to do with teething, it is not always so). Sand is a great favourite with them and there are recorded cases where it has actually helped move the bowels.

Such descriptions and comparisons can be instructive in illuminating a couple of principles:

i) Minerals (and plants, animal products and anything else with electrodynamic force) really do have specific energies and energy traits that are similar to those of people – both when well and in sickness.

ii) Knowledge of the differences between such energies provides us with the wherewithal to treat the sick – for it is the peculiarities of a patient's sick energy that betray with what medicinal energy he or she heal themselves.

In the new millennium, unfortunately, it is uncommon to find patients who are intrinsically so well as to answer the description of just one remedy, so our knowledge of relationships between remedies is essential. It is worth noting that the healthier the constitution (however serious the condition it is supporting), the nearer it is to needing mineral remedies. Minerals are older and often have simpler mental/emotional energies than the plant and animal remedies (though that is not to say they are less deep or distressing).

From the comparison of *Sulphur* and *Calcium* above, the relationship that both have to psora and to *Psorinum* is apparent. *Psorinum* is not as commonly given as a remedy but it is essential to clear as many obstinate traces of the miasm as possible from the system. Both minerals share symptoms with both the miasmatic state and the disease product yet all three remain distinct energies in their own right. It is the common threads that make them psoric, but their peculiarities that make them individual remedial agents. People can be psoric and still express their individuality.

However, nature is thoroughly perverse; neither *Sulphur* nor *Calcium* are so simple as to be confined in their healing properties to one miasmatic state. These remedies are so prodigiously endowed with interweaving energies that they are of inestimable value in treating diseases characteristic of all the miasms – though they and all other major remedies appear quite differently when influenced by the other miasms; something that is not apparent from the *Materia Medica* but only revealed by long hours of practice.

Role models for psoric remedies

J. S. Bach's method and industry might well put him into the *Calcium* camp and a convincing case[4] has been made for Mozart to be considered for a place there too. Sir Walter Scott must undoubtedly take a seat at the top table; his prodigious flow of words with its painstaking descriptive passages is typical of this mineral's energy. Henry James, equally verbose, was more likely to have needed *Sulphur* – he was quite capable of muscular writing that rambled purposefully across the hill and dale of a sentence leaving the reader to fend for himself. John Betjeman, with his quiet humour and sly digging insight would add some sparkling levity. Alfred, Lord Tennyson, with his fairy-tale wizard's beard and stooping appearance would have had a seat next to James.

Queen Victoria was born a *Calcium* type. Her short dumpy figure and rounded features are so typical of the mineral. (Her relationship with and her grief over Albert, led her constitution to be overlaid with a layer of *Pulsatilla* though, for she had that remedy's particular tendency to cling and to weep with a feeling of being abandoned.)

Henry VIII was born a *Sulphur* personality. His square jowl, sturdy frame and rubicund face all attest to that. However, something happened which caused him to change from the comparatively simple psoric into a tyrannical brute. The same something – though with very different results – befell the gentle Franz Schubert. Born an ugly, cherubic *Calcium* personality, he became a deeply haunted man driven to write the darkest but loveliest music of the soul. Van Gogh, born a *Sulphur* persona – he probably died a *Sulphur* persona – suffered likewise. We might remember his cornfields and sunflowers but cannot forget the black crows, lowering self-portraits and lopped-off ear. Then there is another composer, Frederick

Delius, a restless, outdoor *Sulphur* whose final years we remember almost as much for his blindness, paralysis and irascibility as for his musical portrayals of windswept seascapes and drifting, ethereal songs. In the same guise, destiny stalked the great storyteller, Isak Dinesen (Karen Blixen). Starting out more as a passionate *Sulphur* than anything else she quickly progressed through a whole gamut of remedy states that encompassed unendurable symptoms until she reached her emaciated, withered, old age.

What did these sickened people encounter that served them so ill? What was it that caused them to leave the relative calm of psora for the unmitigated horror of their terminal condition – and let most of them suffer for such an interminable time? This disease force is very old; it was described at least 5,000 years ago but had its roots further back in prehistory. It is absolutely incurable by any conventional methods of treatment. Allopathy claims that it can be eradicated but only because it bases its wisdom on the disappearance of *physical* symptoms. It has an acute form, a chronic form, is hereditary in its effects and seemingly indiscriminate in its choice of hosts. Its name is syphilis.

CHAPTER 21

SYPHILIS

The world of syphilis is dark and complex; to be understood it needs to be examined first from its roots. The story of this extraordinary disease does not begin with the conquistadors nor even with the latest evidence of bone, over one million years old, with unmistakable signs of the characteristic necrotic effects of endemic syphilis. We have to look further back than this, even though we lose sense of the timescale involved.

The origins of syphilis lie in the matrix of all disease – psora. We need to return to psora in order to understand how the deepest sense of inadequacy, with its inherent imbalance, developed beyond the point which caused the susceptibility of being a host; how it evolved into a sense of feeling isolated, rejected and threatened; where intellect became detached from intuition and man lost contact with his sense of spirituality; where purpose took on exclusively worldly connotations and the promise of peace of mind through fulfilment became notable for its absence, replaced by a craving for temporal power and self-justification. This is a place where the ego is all consuming and self-referential. It is in the psyche that we find the first threads of the initial steps away from psora into subtly obscure and treacherous territory. An exploration of chickenpox, odd as it may seem, can help our understanding of the evolutionary steps that man and disease took in the inexorable advance inwards and its effects on the three vital bodies.

Chickenpox and shingles

Chickenpox is there before we see it and has more than one guise. It begins to manifest as an infection that looks more like a cold with a mild fever than anything else. This leads, in an uncomplicated case, to a general malaise, fever, sometimes a headache and then a rash that develops from successive crops of macules (spots) into papules (pimples) and then vesicles containing fluid. The spots itch and scratching breaks open the eruptions. In a more complicated case, the rash stage may take much longer to manifest than the fourteen-day incubation period that is generally allowed. Instead there is a persistent racking and mucousy cough with general weakness. This can persist for many days before the first surface symptoms come out. They are frequently accompanied by feverish cold symptoms that in a simpler case would have been despatched sooner. Such a severe case suggests a lowered immune system; too weak to put the pocks onto the surface.These cases almost always show signs of having the eruptions internally first; not just in the mucous membranes of the mouth but also in the larynx and even in the lungs, vagina and the anus where scarring can occur.

Not everyone suffers chickenpox to the same degree or with the same symptoms. Many get away with no more than a few isolated spots while others are covered from head to foot. Those in between show that the disease has a certain affinity for certain areas of the body: the trunk, the armpits, the scalp and the genital region. In addition to spots, the condition can also be marked by the swelling of glands in the back of the neck and sometimes under the arms. Some patients have a marked fever while others have no temperature at all. Some become photophobic with reddened, sore eyes while others suffer a loss of appetite and thirst. But we need to emphasise again that *it is not the disease that dictates the symptom picture – it is the patient and his individual expression of the disease.*

Chickenpox is the result of infection by the varicella-zoster virus. It is the same that causes shingles (herpes zoster). Shingles is an *acute* disease only nominally; it has *chronic* implications. It is a complication of chickenpox that manifests years after the initial infection[1] because the varicella virus went underground. It is not, in all cases, expunged by the body's immune system. Many cases of chickenpox do not resolve properly since the virus finds a home in part of the spinal column – the posterior root sensory ganglia – where it is safe from the immune response mechanism. Here it lies dormant until activated by psychological or environmental stress of some sort but it might also be the result of certain types of allopathic drug.

Once it is activated, the virus reveals itself to have a different personality from its original, childhood one; it has matured into something far less obliging. It has a different modus operandi, to start with. The first signs are of tiredness with burning and irritation on the skin. This occurs in a confined area and traces the course that the virus takes along particular branches of the nerves as it emerges. Favourite places include the abdomen, the ribs, the forehead and scalp – sometimes involving the eyes. It often manifests on one side only. Having travelled along the nerve pathway it breaks out on the surface at the ends of the nerves in an eruption that superficially resembles chickenpox. The vesicles are usually larger and far more painful. There is also a greater variety of colours – some are pink, others are either red, purple or even black. Some are dry while others are pus-filled.

As the irritation and rash develop, there is also a mild fever and general malaise. What bothers the patient most is the burning sensation on the skin where the dermatomes (areas of skin supplied by a single nerve root) are affected. It can take anything from three days to a week or more for the eruptions to break out. They take a further few days to form scabs which eventually peel away. Sometimes the area of skin affected is left without sensation because the process has caused nerve cells to die. If the trigeminal nerve is affected the condition can cause eye problems. The virus can come out in vesicles on the cornea having travelled along the optic nerve. This may lead to visual defects due to scarring and residual neuralgia. A further complication is the result of the opportunist staphylococcus invading the surface skin where it has been rubbed or scratched and causing its usual septic trouble.

Shingles is officially described as a disease that only strikes once. Some unfortunate patients go on to experience shingles more than once – sometimes it is an annual or biennial event for a while and sometimes it is intermittent and the result of further bouts of insupportable stress. When the eruptions (or 'shingles') are healed, that should be and often is the end of the episode. However, many cases continue to suffer neuralgia and this is particularly evident in the elderly and in those patients who have had eruptions on the scalp or over the kidney region. Sometimes the pains are unendurable and lead to severe depression and even suicide.

Psoric chickenpox thus shows its relation to shingles – both are from the same source and have superficially similar eruptions. For the latter to happen, the body has played unwitting host to a virus that lives almost at the very core of the body's mechanism – the spinal column. The varicella virus found a way of eluding the immune system to create a survival scheme that would result in a sophisticated method of reproduction in the future – it is possible to be infected and develop chickenpox from someone who has shingles. (It is not possible to develop shingles from a chickenpox patient because it is the period of dormancy and maturation in the spinal column that creates the secondary disease.) Bearing in mind that the childhood diseases are nature's way of improving the immune system and that chickenpox is related to the psoric state, it is hypothetically likely that chickenpox (and therefore shingles) is a very ancient disease indeed.

The putative link between chickenpox and syphilis

Evolution of man, beast and disease is marked by patterns of behaviour and described by changes in and variants of those patterns. Living beings intent on survival must invent new structural forms or behaviour or both, in order to adapt to changes in the environment. This is just as true of viruses and bacteria as it is of the infinitely more sophisticated creatures that act as their hosts. We can spot evolutionary sequences in disease too; *not through physical attributes but through the patterns of behaviour and reaction demonstrated by the living hosts.* Thus it is that we can trace a connection between the viral shingles (and chickenpox) and syphilis which is bacterial.

It may seem far-fetched that viruses have links with bacteria – it is not possible that there is any generic connection. (Or maybe it is!) What we are looking for are the *similarities of symptomatic expression as a reaction to the presence in the body of the disease energy with which a virus or bacterium is associated.* We are looking for the way in which diseases appear, through the body's mode of expression, to mimic each other. Just as 'like cures like' so 'like follows like'. Specifically we are looking for the way syphilis, the acute disease, might be similar in its bodily expression to chickenpox or shingles. In order to make this connection absolutely clear, we need to go back to the earliest form of syphilis to see how the body expresses it – then we can see how 'like' its behaviour is in comparison with varicella.

Endemic syphilis

Syphilis did not spring fully armed into the world. Endemic syphilis or yaws, as it is more often called, is a more primitive form. It is also known as frambosia because of the raspberry-like skin lesions that develop. It is associated with a spirochete – a spiral-shaped bacterium that is suited to burrowing – called *Treponema pertenue* and it causes destructive symptoms of the skin, bone and other internal tissues. It affects the populations of tropical and subtropical regions who are poorly nourished. Children are mostly affected by the initial attack but there is a chronic state that comes out at the time of puberty with necrosis of bone and destruction of mucosa. The method of infection is through contagion. After the initial contact there is a three to four-week period before sores appear on the skin where the spirochete first made entry. This is known as the 'mother yaw'; it is extremely itchy and highly infectious. It spreads easily as soon as the patient begins to scratch – so more growths appear anywhere on the body. There is fever; the bones and their joints ache. The lesion eventually opens up to form an ulcer. Typically, the new growths appear on the hands, feet and genitals. The ulcerated lesions often appear to have a caseated (cheesy) crust.

Yaws lesions will eventually heal over, even without treatment which is normally a large dose of penicillin. Left to its own devices however, the affected body will take up to six months or more to finish with the spirochete – but not before other people inevitably have been infected. Before it departs, the bacteria is likely to have caused deformity or destruction of the nose, the palate, the upper jaw and tissues of the legs. It can leave the victim crippled. Archaeological evidence of its existence reaches back to some one and a half million years ago. It is probably considerably older than that.

Syphilis – the acute disease

Bearing in mind the way in which many living things learn how to mimic others for their patterns of behaviour and survival, we now come to syphilis in its acute form. Many of its symptoms have already been seen in the other diseases described above. That is, despite its unique definition, syphilis will cause the body to react in ways similar to those of other disease agents.

Treponema pallidum is the name of the syphilis spirochete. It is admirably suited to swimming and burrowing which is exactly what it does through lymph and tissue. Initial infection is mostly through sexual contact. An infected person with an open ulcer (or chancre) passes on the spirochetes to their partner. At the point of contact the spirochete burrows into the skin, forming an ulcer that has a raised red rim, a base that is grey and lardy, while the whole is usually painless. The spirochete quickly multiplies while a scab forms over the ulcer. The ulcer heals over even without treatment and will only be present for two to six weeks. The scar may disappear or remain for some time after; in some cases it can linger for years. Once the chancre has appeared, the lymph nodes nearest the ulcer swell. Indeed, if the chancre (or chancres) is small enough, this swelling may be the first sign that the patient is aware of. If the condition is not treated at once then the patient will go on to experience the secondary stage of the disease.

Some time after the chancre heals – a week to six months or so – a pale red or pinkish rash appears, sometimes over the whole body (though it has a marked affinity for the palms and soles); it is accompanied by a fever, a sore throat, a headache, joint or bone pain and loss of weight and energy. (It is no coincidence that measles bears a strong relation to this condition.) Hair may fall out, not just from the head but also other parts of the body. The eyes become sore and can be reddened and photophobic. Moist and highly infectious sores form around the genitals and anus and can take on the appearance of pox. Libido can be increased with the result that the patient ensures the reproduction of the disease. This stage can last from three to six months or more. If left untreated, the patient will progress to the latent stage.

There may be no physical symptoms during the latent stage though patients would always test positive as the spirochetes will have become established in lymph glands, bone marrow, vital organs and in the central nervous system and the brain – they have a predilection for the soft tissue of the most sensitive and important parts of the body where they can lie dormant for years. It is thought by allopathic medicine that between 50 and 75 per cent of sufferers spend the rest of their lives with no further trouble and it is unlikely that there is any further infectivity. (This statistic is based on tests that are unreliable due to the frequency of 'false negative' and 'false positive' results.)

The final stage is what gives syphilis its terrible reputation. It has not been called 'the Great Masquerader' for nothing. After the disappearance of the secondary stage symptoms, the spirochetes disappear into deep tissue of the body and go quiet. They can remain in this dormant, apparently asymptomatic state for years. Then usually after a trauma, an accident or an acute illness, the tertiary stage of the disease starts its destructive, terminal last act. Wherever there is a concentration of spirochetes, gummae (rubbery tumours) appear. The tissue beneath is gradually eaten away. These gummae can appear on any part of the body, externally or internally, therefore any system of the body can be affected including the brain and central nervous system. It can cause myocardial infarction, aortic aneurysm and other coronary disease; blood disease; neuropathic conditions such as paralysis and ataxia; meningitis and epilepsy; mental derangement and insanity. If the spine is particularly affected (causing the condition tabes dorsalis) then problems in the digestive tract will arise as well with emaciation and the gradual breakdown of neural responses. Spontaneous bruising, recurrent skin lesions including copper spots and symmetrical eruptions, persistent susceptibility to opportunist infections, blindness and loss of other sensory functions are all among the symptoms of this inexorable disease.

The similarities with yaws cannot be missed, the two main differences being that yaws is not necessarily sexually transmitted and, in itself, is not fatal (though it can be the cause of death if the lesions prevent the ability to eat and drink). Syphilis is not confined to the tropics, nor does it *primarily* affect children, though mothers will pass on the condition to their babies. (It is in this aspect that syphilis is regarded as hereditary by allopathic medicine but not in the same way we are taught that heart disease, arthritis, rheumatism or osteoporosis are – though in truth it is the reverse as syphilis can be responsible for all the latter.)

Nevertheless, both yaws and syphilis are caused by a burrowing spirochete; both develop acute symptoms of fever, malaise, joint and bone pain and lesions. In both, after a period of dormancy, new sites of infection form and both soft and hard tissues are destroyed in the long term (although the timescale differs). It would appear that syphilis is the more sophisticated of the two. It is as if the *Treponema pallidum* is an aggressive mutation of the *Treponema pertenue* and that, by becoming a sexually transmitted disease, it ensured far wider distribution in the world. Yaws is successful by any standard but because it must rely on contagion it is possible to avoid it through awareness of the risks. Not always so with syphilis; initially the sores are often too small to notice. Furthermore, with the heightened libido, reason often does not come into consideration till too late. Whether or not yaws is the parent disease, must remain speculation but in the miasmatic scheme of things it is more than possible especially when history and geography are both conducive to the idea.

The next step is to look back at the way the body behaves in the presence of varicella/herpes zoster compared with *Treponema pallidum*. The chickenpox virus invades the system producing fever, malaise and a rash which develops tiny ulcer-shaped lesions which are fluid filled; there is a sore throat and joints ache; the lymph nodes enlarge in the neck (and elsewhere when it is a severe attack). In those who are susceptible, the virus then goes into a *latent* stage and buries itself in the soft tissue of the spinal column where it lies dormant. Once activated, zoster causes disease of the nerves (pain and sensitivity) and the skin (infectious lesions with scabs)[2]. It is mostly a condition of the elderly. It is as if psoric chickenpox manifests later in life as syphilitic shingles. This suggests that the psoric state can transform into the syphilitic state with the deepening of disease. Psoric chickenpox, with its surface lesions, can manifest – in those susceptible to harbouring the virus – as something deeper, more insidious, more painful, less easily self-healed and more threatening when it appears as shingles[3].

Syphilism or the state of being syphilitic

The moment that the word 'syphilitic' is employed, another dimension is implied: that syphilis is – before being an acute, infectious disease an all-pervasive state of being that is capable of influencing the health of a person who may never even have had the acute manifestation. Clearly, not everyone who suffers shingles has had acute syphilis. However, everyone who has shingles with burning, black or bloody eruptions, restlessness, sleeplessness, bone pains and acute exacerbation of symptoms during the night is manifesting the syphilitic miasm. The behaviour of the body in manifesting the acute disease that we call chickenpox and its later expression, shingles, is mimicry of deep hereditary susceptibility. *It is not the acute disease called syphilis that is inherited genetically from one generation to another. It is the state of susceptibility to syphilitic conditions that is.*

What is inherited is the propensity for the individual to produce symptoms similar to those that would be manifested in syphilis – 'syphilism', to coin a word. This state is so ancient that it predates the accepted, but necessarily provisional, date (the 1490s) for the first appearance in Europe of the disease we now know as syphilis. Our brief survey of chickenpox, shingles and yaws shows that more than one disease is capable of eliciting similar syphilitic body reactions. Nevertheless, where a forebear has actually suffered from the acute ravages of *Treponema pallidum*, it is far more likely that any progeny will carry the hereditary incubus of this susceptibility – the syphilitic miasm.

Syphilis in history

Since the furious epidemics of syphilis that swept over Europe in the early sixteenth century the universality of the syphilitic miasm has been assured. The finger of rationalist history points to Columbus's first imported cargo from the New World as the tinderbox that ignited the fire of syphilis. The initial waves of epidemics at first seemed as potentially devastating as the Black Death but, with time, these lessened in intensity to become immediately fatal only in exceptional cases. Eventually, the majority of cases (allopathy's 50 to 75 per cent) seemed able to overcome the acute symptoms without any apparent chronic sequelae. However, the use of the various *suppressive* treatments for the acute disease – which have included, most famously, mercury and latterly antibiotics – has meant that the miasm has been well and truly grafted onto the family trees of a large majority of the world's population.

The allopathic belief has always been that once the mercury (now, mercifully, abandoned) or antibiotics have killed off the multiplying spirochetes (which they can only do in the first and second stages), the disease is finished. This is hardly supported by statistics that tell us that syphilis has shown no consistent fall in occurrence since the introduction of penicillin,[4] the most successful allopathic treatment yet. (Indeed, there have continued to be 'waves' of syphilis, as natural a phenomenon as the weather, in spite of aggressive programmes of suppression.) What is also overlooked is that there is an energy that drives the spirochete and *it is an energy of purpose* that has a response in the host that ensures its successful regeneration. *It is the negative potential within the host that has created the environment for the disease; not the other way round.*[5]

Antibiotics may kill off the physical body of the bacterium *but they do not destroy the dynamic energy* – any more than they do in the case of, say, a streptococcal infection or a so-called viral fever. (Remember how mucus and catarrh, diarrhoea or constipation, headaches and rashes can all be the results of suppressing such an acute condition – and not just as the body's reaction to the drug but as continued evidence of general disease within. Witness too the *Belladonna* case where suppression led to a personality change in the patient – see Part 1, p 36.

Why syphilis should be capable of sustaining its own form of 'life after death', across so many generations, is a question whose answer lies both in the human psyche and in the way that that psyche has allowed the *Treponema pallidum* to evolve from its origins. At least since the sixteenth century (if this is when the modern form made its entrance) the *dynamic energy* of acute syphilis, whether the physical bacterium has been destroyed or not, has been establishing itself in the gene pool. The importance of individual reaction is as strong in syphilis as in any other disease and not everyone suffers the same intensity of symptoms or the same inevitable fate – though the statistics put out by scientists are both suspiciously reassuring and highly debatable.

This should not surprise us. Firstly, syphilis is a covert disease; far more people suffer it than is ever recorded. (It is possible to contract the disease and be absolutely unaware of any infection and this is particularly true of women who may develop the painless chancre only deep within the vaginal tract.) Secondly, many people who have had syphilis early on in their lives fail to report the fact when discussing with their physicians some other seemingly unrelated condition. They either assume that the problem of acute syphilis was cured years ago or are unaware of ever having had it. So the connection goes unregistered. (This is particularly so with young people who report their VD early on, have it suppressed while their immune system is otherwise in good shape and then carry on with life.) Even if a patient were to suspect that his previous condition of syphilis were in some way responsible for his present ailment, the allopathic physician listening to him would not know what to make of the information. Almost nothing in his training would tell him what he could do about it – beyond referring the patient for tests to show up the presence of antibodies in the system. He is forced to treat the symptoms in front of him, not realising that these may show all the hallmarks of a syphilitic condition.

Although it is common knowledge that, say, coronary disease and deep ulceration (to name just two) are often symptoms of tertiary syphilis, it is largely assumed that these conditions can and do manifest in people without the least connection to anything worse than old age and/or because an immediate ancestor suffered the same condition. (A patient with an aneurysm – dangerous ballooning of an artery wall – might well be asked if his father or mother had heart disease; no-one would think to ask if one of the patient's parents or grandparents had syphilis.)

To summarise so far:

i) We have suggested that there is a link between psora and syphilis that is demonstrated in part by the similarities of expression of varicella-zoster and syphilis and in part by the fact that the patient is still a host.

ii) We have described the 'textbook' version of yaws and syphilis which is strictly limited to the *physical* manifestations of each disease.

iii) We have described the similarities between the tropical disease yaws and syphilis with the suggestion that the latter is the more sophisticated version.

iv) We also mentioned without elaboration that man's psyche makes it possible for such an evolutionary process to happen.

v) We have suggested that allopathic medicine, while successfully treating and eliminating the *physical* expression of syphilis (i.e. the spirochete), has not only been unable to halt the disease but has been entirely unaware, and in denial, of most of the psychical and hereditary aspects of syphilis.

A fuller picture of syphilis

The textbook description of syphilis only examines the physical characteristics and takes little or no account of the mental and emotional symptoms, let alone the spiritual. Nor does it tell us that, once the secondary, infectious stage of the disease is passed, the state of mind, emotion and spirit of the patient is still subject to the illness in its chronic third stage. These omissions leave us with a false picture that must be remedied in order to understand the role that syphilis plays for both good and evil in man's destiny.

This is closely related to another issue; that syphilis is a disease that evolved with man over a great many generations until it found a spectacularly efficient method of reproduction. That it was able to do this tells us more about the nature of man than it does about the spirochete. To understand this we have to go in search of an evolutionary purpose in man's relationship with syphilis and syphilism.

The psyche of syphilism in history

Syphilis is not just a physical disease. As with scabies, there is a characteristic symptom picture of the mind that is always present to some degree. In the initial stages these mental and emotional symptoms may be less marked than in the later stages though they can be present even before infection occurs – as part of the general susceptibility. We have a clue to the diversity of these symptoms from knowing the plight of such famous syphilitics as Henry VIII, Franz Schubert, Robert Schumann, Nietzsche and a host of others.

We know Henry VIII to have been ill-tempered, irascible and given to irrational outbursts of violence that led him on more than one occasion to regret his actions. He suffered from indecisiveness at times as well as despondency. He was suspicious and yet easily persuaded by his intemperance, rather than logic and prudence. In spite of this he was capable of great insight and shrewdness. Early in his life he had shown little sign of the mood swings that syphilis can engender, apart from his inability to remain faithful to his first wife even while he loved her. By the time he met and married Anne Boleyn, though clearly infatuated, the driving force had become his desperation to sire a male heir.

Schubert was altogether different. He showed all the attributes of the melancholic. He was known to his friends as someone who had two sides to his nature – light and dark. One was the jovial drinking companion, the other a mysteriously inward-looking man who seemed to be racked by shame and guilt. In his final years he suffered from the characteristic skin rashes of syphilis as well as the ignominy of losing enough hair to warrant investing in a wig. There was little of Henry VIII's foul temper; Schubert was essentially the mildest and gentlest of men with a disarming and wholly genuine humility. Yet there are suspicions that he was not far from being alcoholic and his acute bouts of melancholia were marked by searing self-doubts. He was able to channel the expression of this profoundly dark side into some of the most poignantly intimate music ever penned. Though some historians are quick to point out that he did not die of syphilis the fact remains that syphilis made him acutely susceptible to his final illness, typhoid, and that it guaranteed the outcome by reducing his immune system to nothing.

Robert Schumann, too, died of syphilis but in quite different circumstances. In his case, the syphilis attacked his central nervous system and sent him mad. He believed that he had probably contracted the acute disease in his youth and it is entirely feasible to assume that it was responsible for bringing out his famous character split (he rationally called his two selves Florestan and Eusebius, the light and the dark, the passionate and the melancholic) at first evidenced in his diaries and then in his writings as a music critic. While he was able to sustain the fabulous wealth of musical invention, he was able to balance his two opposing but complementary sides. The inevitable progress of the disease, however, gradually made this precarious feat impossible – he became possessed of multiple phobias, was unable to concentrate, his memory failed him, he was subject to alternating bouts of extreme elation and blackest despair; he suffered seizures, bone pains and disorders of the five senses; he attempted suicide. He died, peace-fully it is said, in a lunatic asylum even though he had episodes during his final two years of violent behaviour that necessitated the use of a strait-jacket.[6]

From just these three examples it can be seen how diverse the effects of syphilis are, even if the common threads of ultimately terminal mental, physical or spiritual *destructiveness* are always present. Not everyone who contracts the disease will suffer in such ways. This is evident from an experi-ment carried out in America by the US Public Health Service to determine the effects of untreated syphilis; it lasted from 1932 until 1970 and was based on the cases of 399 black men, all of whom had been positively diag-nosed. Effective allopathic treatment – penicillin – was deliberately withheld from these patients and they were duped into believing that they were receiving health care and therapy. As part of the study, blood tests and lumbar punctures were routine, the latter being responsible for some of the symptoms that were subsequently registered. The experiment was closed down in 1970 due to media pressure. Millions of dollars in compensation were awarded to the surviving families, a good proportion of whom were known to have contracted the disease. One of the most obvious results of this dubious medical research is that it showed that some people survive with latent syphilis for longer than others. While some of the men died within a few years of first contracting the disease, others survived into their nineties. No explanation of this disparity has yet been forthcoming. To get anywhere near a reason we need to return to Schumann briefly.

Schumann was, it is widely accepted, a manic-depressive. We do not need to dredge through the archives looking for evidence that he con-tracted syphilis in his teens – there is a lot of evidence to suggest it, beyond the records of the asylum he died in. We should look instead to Schumann's family. His father was a hypochondriac and a depressive who died suddenly aged fifty-three. Within one year, his sister committed suicide by jumping from a window when she was only nineteen. These two deaths occurred when Robert was fifteen. What is important here is that suicide by leaping from a height and sudden death in depressive illness are both, by nature and in terms of homoeopathic philosophy, syphilitic events. This is not to imply that either Schumann *père* or his daughter had syphilis but that the family was significantly tainted by it in the gene pool. Robert Schumann already had the propensity for suffering from syphilitic mental conditions – and this would have fostered the susceptibility to becoming infected physically. To show how this is possible it is necessary to set out the extent of the potential mental/emotional symptoms of the syphilitic nature.

Syphilis in the mind

The earliest signs of acute mental and emotional aberration due to the presence of *Treponema pallidum* are dullness and oppression; a sense of impending misfortune. There is depression and sulkiness with a distinct aversion to contact with other people. The patient tends to have morbid thoughts and to harbour suspicions, though he or she might be sufficiently aware of their lack of foundation to dismiss them straight away. The dullness leads to slowness of reactions and to developing fixed ideas about things. The patient may complain of not being able to collect his thoughts; of feeling heavy and unmotivated. These symptoms do not necessarily follow parallel with the physical symptoms – there is no strict programme to syphilis.

There is a creeping restlessness and a sense of dissatisfaction. Night-time brings aggravations of these symptoms and many syphilitics feel relief to see the first light of day. They are most likely to feel despair as the dusk draws into night. The mental unease is often enough to drive them out of bed. While some become irritable others become self-recriminatory. All this mental and emotional distortion may take months to develop and even years – but when the symptoms do manifest they are absolutely typical of the body's reaction to the treponema. Patients can become obsessed with phobias – such as a germ phobia which causes compulsive washing of the hands; there is a desperate need to feel safe from infection or anything that might threaten security. If allopathic treatment has been administered much of the acuteness of the picture is removed because the *intellect* is now lulled into feeling 'cleansed'. Antibiotic treatment removes the immediate threat of the physical evidence. There are no more rashes or swollen glands; hair stops falling out; bone pains subside and body functions normalise. At least this is what happens in the vast majority of those treated allopathically.

Nevertheless, the whole nature of the patient is tainted and characteristic symptoms can emerge at a later date. The picture of an old syphilitic (though this does not necessarily imply geriatric patients) might be any combination of the following symptoms: susceptible to mood swings between furious and violent anger and mild, amenable humour; prone to fits of despair with suicidal thoughts; bouts of memory loss that increasingly look like senile dementia – inability to remember faces or things that have just been said, yet perfect memory for events long past; tendency to weep and complain but with an aversion to being consoled; perversity of will. There is a fear and conviction of never becoming well again and this can alternate with a total lack of interest in the future. There is cynicism with which the patient attempts to cast gloom on all around. There can also be a dread of not becoming successful; the patient becomes single-minded and hellbent on making a name for himself or pots of money, or both! There is an extension to this; the patient, like Henry VIII, becomes obsessed with carrying on the family line.

If there are episodes of 'over the top' euphoria it is on these occasions that the patient is at his most lethal in his sexual relations. Not only can the syphilis be passed on (physically in the first and second stages but energetically in the tertiary phase) but also the sexual act can be violent. Sexual abuse is not uncommon. Fits of black depression can follow sexual release.

In latent syphilis, as in its inheritable miasm, depression is common. As syphilitics brood and do not give much away, others may be unaware that anything is amiss, beyond the fact that the patient has become a bit more introverted. Such people are capable of suicide and there is a tendency to do it without the least warning, even though considerable planning might have been required. These are the people who suddenly open the window of the ninth floor and jump out. What is remarkable is that so often they leave behind a sense of devastation in those who knew them, almost out of proportion.[7] Imagine the effects on a family when a teenage son, without warning, is found hanged after failing to meet their own expectations in examinations. Distressingly often these people, having led apparently exemplary lives as loving parents, suddenly go berserk and massacre their family.

Latent syphilitics might be verging on the senile or they may seem to be excessively sharp-witted. In those who become possessed of extraordinary will power to succeed, their minds become obsessively focused on what they are setting out to achieve. This blinkers them and often leaves them with dulled imagination – though they may be cunning – or suppressed emotions so that they are unable to give and receive affection or love. If their ambitions are thwarted then they become either violent or utterly depressed – even to the point of suicide or murder; remember the 60 or more financiers who are reported to have jumped out of their office windows as soon as the Wall Street Crash happened in the 1920s. (Even if it is not true, it is exactly the kind of anecdote that illustrates syphilism.) Money and gold play a vital role in the natural history of syphilis. They are tangible evidence of worldly success which, in someone who has lost touch with their spirituality, becomes imperative as a *raison d'être*.

The spirit of syphilism

Despair in a syphilitic goes into the realms of the spirit, for there is a creeping realisation that there is probably no God at all. The general feeling of paralysis of purpose, especially if materialism proves to be an empty vessel, is accompanied by a sense that life has 'let him down'. There is no God because the infinitely forgiving God we are all taught about from Sunday school onwards 'would never allow this to happen'. In the absence of any spiritual guiding force the syphilitic can become more concerned than ever with the material world – either through accumulating the trappings of success or by despising and fearing everything around him. Sometimes this is all apparently reversed; the syphilitic becomes ever more overtly religious and spends a lot of energy in communion with God. Often such a mental state involves plea-bargaining with God – "*I will promise to be obedient to You and do Your bidding if only You will grant me what I seek most…*"

The combination of genius with syphilis results in warped states of mind that can lead to the acquisition of enormous power. Howard Hughes, the American millionaire who died a senile recluse, was a good example of a wealthy, obsessed syphilitic. Al Capone, the vicious gangland boss of the 1920s and 1930s, died in retreat from a stroke, with the mental age of a child of less than twelve, having once been the undisputed head of

Chicago's massive bootlegging empire. It is not too great a step to seeing how the interaction between man and syphilism can lead to criminality and inhuman behaviour. The abuse of power and the manipulation of wealth inevitably involve vice and corruption, the more readily in a world where the protagonists have lost their spiritual base. Even where lip service is paid to the Almighty, hunger for power can remain the driving force. The Spanish Inquisition was an instrument of domination and destruction for three centuries in the name of God but actually in the pursuit of power. (If we are to believe the history books, syphilis was introduced in the 1490s, ten years *after* the Inquisition was established. The first *epidemic* of syphilis was recorded in the 1494-5 Franco-Italian wars when Spanish troops were involved. As might have been gathered by now, the dynamic *nature* of syphilism was abroad in the world long before the gold-trafficking Spaniards came home.)

Ultimately, the physical symptomatology of syphilis matches that of the mental/emotional side; both tend to *self-destruction*. The insidious eating away of body tissue is paralleled by the creeping corruption of the mind. At the same time the spirit is, at first, ignored and then denied. The three parts of the whole are riven; yet the outcome is not all gloomy and gruesome. Schubert and Schumann may have ended their lives with corrupt physical bodies but their heroic struggle with life, channelled through their art, is there for us to emulate – if not in fact, then in spirit. The world would be a far poorer place without the musical glories of Hugo Wolf, Delius, Smetana and Mozart, not to mention all the other composers who did *not* have the acute disease itself but certainly demonstrated a syphilitic nature in their lifestyles; Tchaikovsky (a depressive with suicidal tendencies) and Mussorgsky (an alcoholic) being just two of them. It would be poorer, too, without Goya, Van Gogh and El Greco; the theatre would be unthinkable without Oscar Wilde (who died of syphilitic meningitis) – or Henrik Ibsen (a psoric) who understood the syphilitic nature so completely and whose plays are among the most powerful and precise testaments to the all-consuming nature of syphilism.

Tolstoy's Anna Karenina and Flaubert's Madame Bovary both went to their self-destructive ends unable to resolve the strata of emotional upheaval that they had experienced in their short lives. Anna was impulsively pulled to her messy suicide beneath the wheels of a train by an overwhelming mixture of grief and vengeance[8]; Emma Bovary drawn to her agonising poisoning by hopeless despair for which she could hold no-one to account but herself[9]. Both women were passionate, unconventional spirits determined to explore the limits of their sensitivities; they were restless explorers of the boundaries of human experience, particularly those that involve the excitation of the five senses and sexuality – as we shall see, this is tuberculism to a T.

If syphilis, the acute disease, is no more than the *physical representation* of a pre-existing state of spirit and mind, what is the nature of the miasm or energy that predates the advent of the physical disease? What is it that makes us *susceptible* to syphilitic conditions? Some of the great myths and legends of the world seek to answer the same question. It is inherent in the stories of the Greek gods on Olympus. What takes place in the Garden of Eden is the story of psora. The expulsion from Eden is the story of syphilis.

Whatever causes a sense of isolation can turn the mind to hopelessness, despair, even suicide; to hate, revulsion and aggression or, paradoxically but positively, a return to psora, that is Eden; witness the story of Job.

Syphilism is the spiritual wilderness where either victims or their abusers are found. It is an earthbound place where there are few and ephemeral material comforts. It is the legacy of violence committed against the soul – perhaps first perpetrated by one nomad against another whose temporary acre was greener than his own. It is no accident that *Treponema pallidum* swept across Europe at the beginning of the Renaissance – that moment in history when reason began to break down the parochial fence and open the floodgates of exploration for material gain.

Because accessibility to God (or spirituality, at least) is so indescribably difficult to achieve while wandering the wilderness, the search for power is a common pursuit. The destruction of most of the empires of the world has been based on the envy and greed of those who stood outside the capital walls – but it is the corruption within that has always hastened the inevitable end. Nazi Germany, one of the most spectacular national examples of collective syphilitic behaviour, was partly the result of bitterness, hatred and a sense of isolation felt after the Treaty of Versailles. Hitler was a good example of one who showed classic syphilitic characteristics; paranoid and subject to rages alternating with moods of calmness and gentleness; delusions of grandeur; an absolute sense of his own rightness with a determination to impose his will on all within his sphere of influence. He was also typically syphilitic in destroying himself and those nearest to him at the moment of his reckoning. His Russian counterpart, Joseph Stalin, was similarly afflicted. With all the power of a rational genius for evil, he conducted his regime of violent insanity for 30 years and was responsible for more deaths than anyone else in history. Restless, suspicious, cunning, vicious and ruthless, he nevertheless could be mawkishly sentimental. Not only that but he understood to perfection how to manipulate the evil in those lesser men who were attracted to his power.

It is this dark side of man, the abyss or wilderness, that is the negative *essence* of the syphilitic miasm. It is in all of us, to some degree or other. It may manifest in any one or all of the three bodies: physical, mental/emotional or spiritual. Sooner or later we all need to face it, even if it is only at the end of a very long life.[10] A study of the most hideous moments of history shows how terrible it can be: Genghis Khan's campaigns, the Crusades, the terror of the French Revolution, the Bolshevik uprising, the Holocaust, the Valentine's Day Massacre and September 11th.

It would be quite wrong to see the miasm as all black and negative. It would be a mistake to compare syphilism with the other miasms and see it as 'worse'. Syphilism is not a one-way street to despair and destruction; it is a challenge to our creative purpose in being here. Though it can feel like the abyss, the 'black hole', it is, nevertheless, the place where a person has the choice to surface and recover or remain forever in the dark and face defeat. Syphilism is not unsusceptible to the will to change for the better; it is not unsusceptible to treatment. For this to happen, one must throw off the need to feel powerful over others and the compulsion to accrue material possessions to bolster one's lack of faith in the abundance of life.

Syphilism can bring out the very best: here we might list all the works of the great composers who had syphilis or manifested all the signs of the syphilitic miasm; we might mention all the paintings and poems of similarly afflicted artists. These would be representative of creativity that, in showing the influence of the syphilitic side of the human psyche, offers us a mirror in which to view ourselves so that, seeing, hearing or feeling the creative energy of another, we can witness how we might cast off the shadow of the miasm – even for a short moment. Mozart gave us *Don Giovanni* to exemplify the hellraising disaster of choosing the easy and attractive options of temporal power and dominion over others through ruthless ambition and rampant sexuality; then he gave us *The Magic Flute* to show us the balance – this is a work about similar choices but this time the protagonists win through their baptism of fire by electing love and service.

Could something have been done to heal these historical or literary people? They would certainly have been given antibiotics today – a very material solution – and long before they entered the final stages of the disease[11]. Yet, so successful is the teamwork between man and this disease that allopathic treatment has failed to deliver us from the scourge of syphilis in spite of its apparent success in treating the physical symptoms.

Treatment of syphilis, ancient and modern

Antibiotics were only discovered in the 1920s; before then, physicians who were versed in herbalism rather than chemistry relied on methods of treatment that have been buried beneath the success of penicillin. There are a number of plants that had a reputation as cures for syphilis[12]. They have long since disappeared from any reputable allopathic pharmacopoeia but still appear in the *Materia Medicas* of herbalism and homoeopathy. One of these plants, *Stillingia sylvatica*, (a member of the order of *Euphorbiaceae*), was popularly used in the southern states of the USA as the only cure necessary. Dr Clarke, in his *Dictionary of Materia Medica*, reports that not only does the plant tincture cause symptoms in the provers similar to those manifest in syphilis but also that there are records of cures:

> '...a case of secondary syphilis treated by Preston, one of the (original) provers. The patient, a man, suffered extreme torture from bone pains. After receiving Stillingia he slept well. The immense nodes disappeared from head and legs; and from the most deplorable, down-hearted (sometimes almost raving from derangement), miserable, thin-looking object, he changed into a buoyant, joking, rotund-looking fellow.'

Clarke also writes that the '*proving shows an action closely parallel with that of syphilis, attacking the genito-urinary organs, throat (pharynx, larynx and trachea), mouth, head and bones.*' He further reports that *Stillingia* '*has removed nodes on the forehead, tibia and elsewhere and arrested caries of the nasal bones.*' Such healing action was noted after the patients had either chewed the root or taken the tincture – so the results were nothing to do with homoeopathic *potencies*. Clarke[13] himself prescribed this remedy in syphilitic cases and had success with the removal of chronic symptoms.

Corydalis, (*Dicentra canadensis*), is another plant known for its power to heal patients with syphilis; records[14] of clinical experience show its affinity for symptoms of secondary syphilis including chancres, ulceration of the scalp, falling hair and enlarged glandular nodes.

A tree, *Calotropis gigantea* (from India), has been proved but not fully. The juice, root and bark were used in the East '*for their emetic, sudorific, alterative and purgative qualities*'. A certain Dr Gramm, (writing in the *Minnesota Homoeopathic* Magazine of August, 1897) was able to report that he had used the tincture '*with great success in cases of syphilis when mercury can no longer be given; in anaemia of syphilis; secondary syphilis.*' This introduces the most famous of all drugs that have been used extensively for the destruction of the syphilitic infection: mercury – though its effects are far different from the benevolent effects of plants.

Mercury, a metal and a medicine

Mercury was to the physician of the eighteenth and nineteenth centuries what antibiotics and steroid drugs have become to those of the twenty-first. It was prescribed most prominently for syphilis and gonorrhoea, and used in different forms; either as corrosive mercurial salts or as calomel, a sub-chloride of mercury. The latter was an early example of a 'slow release' drug as its action was deemed somewhat gentler and slower than its vicious parent.

One of the intentions behind the administration of mercury was to bring on salivation as a means of exciting the body to relieve itself of toxicity. The effect was devastating for the symptom of salivation was no more than a toxic effect and one that was minor in comparison with other side effects:

ulceration, pustules, falling teeth and hair, caries of bone, gastric disorders and neuropathy; not to mention the psychological symptoms. The patient would, however, be freed of the symptoms of syphilis because the energy of the material dosage of the metal was superior to the beleaguered spirochete and to the body that was attempting to produce *natural* reactions. The body, invaded by the metal, could not support the lifestyle of the bacteria. This is the result that the physician wanted because he would have considered the suffering due to the poison preferable to the disease. What he and all his colleagues did not consider was that mercury is *homoeopathic* in every way to syphilis; it is *the* natural counterpart to the body's symptomatic response to treponema. (It is not the only remedy for syphilis by a long measure but it is the substance that possesses the *most similar energy* to it by far.)

It was because physicians gave the mercury in *material* dosages that it was so devastating. Had they taken the step that Hahnemann took – of diluting and succussing the crude, material dose until there was only the electrodynamic energy present – they would have become homoeopaths by default. *Mercurius Solubulis*, to give the medicine its full name, was one of Hahnemann's discoveries. (He prepared it by precipitating mercury from a solution of nitric acid by means of caustic ammonia.) Mercury in homoeopathic potency has the potential to alter the body's energy to the degree that it will, without toxic effects, eliminate the depredations of the spirochete – unless too much physical damage has been done already. As it was, the material mercury suppressed the physical pathology of the disease but replaced it with a reaction that was equally pernicious leaving the dynamism of the syphilitic state buried deeper still in the psyche.[15]

Although mercury was abandoned as a drug to treat syphilis early in the twentieth century, it was used for a little while longer as a treatment for septic throats. Someone with quinsy might have had their throat 'painted' with the mercury; this would result in the suppression of the pus exuded by the ulcerated membranes but also cause the disease itself to change its shape. That shape, because of mercury's similarity to syphilis, would take a syphilitic turn and the patient would then suffer chronic syphilitic symptoms – such as bone pains and night sweats. It was the advent of penicillin that put paid to mercury as a marketable treatment – and not before time. (Though as we have seen mercury still finds a place in modern medicine; dentists still using it. It is also indefensibly in childhood vaccines, certain laxatives, nasal sprays, antiseptic creams and some contact lens solutions.)

And yet, *Mercurius* is an absolutely indispensable homoeopathic medicine. It is to the syphilitic miasm what *Sulphur* is to the psoric state. It is of invaluable use in the treatment of so many who might suffer the consequences of the syphilitic miasm becoming uppermost in their state of health. There are other metals, as well as plants and even animal remedies that will treat someone suffering from either syphilis or its hereditary influence, but few challenge the supremacy of *Mercurius*. To illustrate this we should look at what this remedy could cause a healthy prover to produce in the way of symptoms.

To list all the details of mercury would require several pages of very small type. However, some of the essential details show how common a picture it presents:

Mental/Emotional:
   i)   Constant anguish and restlessness with tormenting thoughts[16]; moving from place to place, unable to settle.
   ii) Fear of going mad, of being unable to think, of being unable to make a decision; dread of having done something wrong or even criminal; desire to escape or run away.
   iii) Angry and even full of rage; tends to pick quarrels; morose, truculent and suspicious; avoids conversation; tells lies.
   iv) Makes mistakes in speech, writing and all forms of communicating (it is a remedy for homoeopaths to consider when treating children with learning difficulties); either very slow and confused or very hurried in speaking.
   v)   Poor memory.
   vi) Easily swayed by others and tends not to trust his own thinking processes.
   vii) Dejection, apathy and lethargy; disgust for work and for life itself.
   viii) In children there is also a tendency to be mischievous, cheeky and insolent.

ix) Very quick changes of mood from happy and cheerful to miserable and irritable.

x) There is also a tendency to become alcoholic.

General symptoms:

i) Inflammations of any tissue but particularly along the alimentary canal.[17]

ii) Ulceration of any tissue. Pustules, boils and local infections that contain pus and blood.

iii) Rheumatic pains that dart and shoot; cutting pains, cramps and contractions.

iv) Bones – especially long bones, shoulders and shins – affected either by softening or becoming easily fractured.

v) Weakness and lethargy in the limbs with restlessness.

Modalities:

Pains and other symptoms all:

i) Worse for or aggravated: at night, from heat, from sweating, changes of weather, draughts.

ii) Improved with: even temperature, rest.

Skin:

i) Tendency to itch and fester; useful in festering eczema.

ii) Sweat is watery or greasy but usually causes the patient to feel worse rather than relieved.

iii) Ulcers contain blood and pus and have a tendency to suppurate; ulcers burn and spread.

iv) Skin tends to peel away and exude clear fluid and blood which is worse for itching.

v) Eruptions tend to focus on the face, extremities and genitals.

Keynotes:

i) Salivation with thirst especially for (ice) cold drinks.

ii) Fœtid breath which smells rotten, sour or 'catarrhal'.

iii) Metallic taste in the mouth.

iv) Very quick switching from one temperature to another.

v)   Night sweats which come on with every change of temperature from chilled to warm.

vi)   Swollen glands especially of the throat.

vii)   Right-sided – many symptoms manifest primarily on the right side of the body.

There are also symptoms of the genital region that are very significant when comparing the effects of mercury with syphilis:

i)   There is both the increase and then the absence of all sexual desire with libido becoming insufferably urgent or so absent that the male organ and the uterus can become withered.

ii)   There are pains that match syphilis; burning in the urethra; dragging or tearing as well.

iii)   The whole area becomes damp with sweat that smells rank.

iv)   The inguinal glands swell.

v)   The skin becomes eczematous and sloughs off; there is intolerable itching, to the point of being 'voluptuous'.

vi)   In women, there is a vaginal discharge that is white and corrosive, causing itching, redness and soreness; this can spread round to the anal region.

vii)   The ovaries and uterus can swell and become oedematous and the menstrual cycle can become either shorter or longer and painful.

viii)   There can be uterine haemorrhage with the period.

The effect on the digestive tract is no less terrible in those who are susceptible:

i)   There is burning and ulceration; heartburn and peptic ulcers are within its sphere.

ii)   Food allergies are frequently a concomitant symptom.

iii)   Jaundice comes in its range as mercury is a liver remedy too.

iv)   There is a lot of mucus secretion, much of it in the throat, chest and mouth; it is always foul, being thick and purulent.

These are some of the symptoms reported by provers of the remedy and by physicians using the remedy on patients who were relieved of the symptoms under its influence. *Mercurius* is veritably protean as a remedy in its homoeopathic dilution. Not all who proved it (or those who need it) suffered from all these symptoms at the same time. A patient may need *Mercurius* for nothing more than a few cold symptoms. (A typical *Mercurius* cold is characterised by sneezing fits with alternation of heat and chills, sweats, especially at night and increased thirst for cold water. It is frequently described as a rising cold; one that starts in the throat and goes up into the nose and sinuses.) Or the patient may be well in almost every way but have some problem that pops up from time to time, especially when there is stress, causing sufficient distress to interfere with normal routines.

A man came claiming to feel well except that he was bothered by irregular bouts of genital herpes. He would get small blister-like eruptions on the right side of his penis that itched furiously. This was at its worst when he became warm in bed and he was quite unable to desist from scratching. The blisters would burst and become small red pimply ulcers. He would become sweaty in the crotch area and he was aware that the odour was unpleasant. Sheepishly, he added that he was almost constantly aroused while the itching was there. He was suffering from the herpes at the moment. He was given *Merc. Sol.* 30 to be taken at the rate of one tablet every four hours until the eruptions had cleared.

He has relied on *Merc. Sol.* to clear himself of the herpes ever since. He has the outbreaks less frequently and this has been all the treatment he felt he needed. (Much could be done to eliminate the problem but a lack of insight into one's condition is a syphilitic symptom.)

Here is another case, quite distinct:

A girl aged twenty came for treatment of her chronic iritis. She had inflammation of the right eye which was red, sore and burning. The lids were red and puffy and the lower lid was sore from the acrid tears that flowed permanently from the duct. There was a mass of capillaries to be seen in the cornea and the eye drooped. She was depressed and had no energy. She said that she could not have cared less about her university course which she felt was unusual for her. The condition had begun very soon after her adoptive father – of whom she was both afraid and in awe

– died suddenly of a stroke. She added that she was surprised at her own reaction as she had always felt that she would be relieved when he died.

Mercurius is, besides all that has been listed, a remedy for emotional shock. She was given *Merc. Sol.* 200, one dose to be taken each day for three days. Within seven days the eye was clear of all symptoms. Her mother reported that her daughter had "*a horrendous cold, an absolute streamer*" and that she had also had a cathartic explosion of anger and tears in which she had accused her parents of all sorts of things – some of which the mother refuted as being without any foundation. In spite of this, both the mother and the girl felt that there had been an overall lifting of spirits and energy as well as the elimination of the iritis.

Iritis is a common second stage condition of syphilis, so *Mercurius* is no surprise here – though there was no question of her having had the acute disease. However, in this case the *connection* was confirmed. The symptoms returned some three months later. She was given a dose of *Syphilinum* 100, since which she has remained entirely free of all the symptoms of iritis. (Just as it is quite common to use *Psorinum* to consolidate or support the action of psoric remedies, so it is with *Syphilinum* in relation to syphilitic ones.)

These two cases have an obvious connection to syphilis (both the miasm and the disease) – even though neither patient had contracted the disease – because the physical symptoms of both genital herpes and iritis are similar to symptom patterns found in their acute forebear. Furthermore, had the man come back for more long-term treatment to address his underlying tendency to produce the herpes, he would have, sooner or later, needed a dose of *Syphilinum*. As he did not return we can only speculate as to how he would have responded to *Syphilinum*. Experience in countless other cases, though, suggests that, with time, he might well have been relieved of the herpes.

It is also well known that *Mercurius* and *Syphilinum* have a strong affinity. It is very usual to see a prescription sheet on which *Merc. Sol.* is followed by *Syphilinum*, but the two are *not* interchangeable. It is unlikely that a patient showing all the keynote symptoms of one would improve if he were given a dose of the other instead. If the case shows a distinct similarity to *Mercurius* symptoms then nothing else is likely to suit. However, if it is seen to fail where it is clearly indicated, then a dose of *Syphilinum* will more than likely be the remedy to cause the patient to improve – the nosode kick-starts the system to respond to the indicated remedy.

This can be a very confusing area as *Syphilinum* shares so many of mercury's symptoms: the profuse salivation, the night sweats, the ulcers, the bone pains, the skin eruptions and so on. Yet it is a different remedy. Like all the nosodes, it has two functions: it is used to liberate the patient from the underlying grip of the miasm however much the case calls for another remedy (as in the above case of iritis); and it is a remedy in its own right which can be given to any patient who exhibits a similarly dark, forbidding energy which might occur in any or all of the three bodies.

The bleakest side of syphilis

This 'dark, forbidding energy' can be almost palpable because of all the perverse, tortured passion that lurks beneath. If you are familiar with Edvard Munch's famous picture *The Scream* then you have seen the artistic expression of one who knows syphilism from the inside – even the strange, black, spermatozoan squiggles that border the painting seem to point incriminatingly to the spirochete.

Charles Manson, the Death Valley murderer, stands as a real-life example. He suffered from syphilitic insanity complicated by drug addiction. Looking at a photograph of him one first sees a demonic force of evil rather than anything human. Many photographs of other murderers and criminals show similar brooding or maniacal energy as if the subject were possessed of some malign force. Francisco de Goya, Spain's great painter who probably suffered from syphilis, knew all about this black, abysmal power. His fourteen so-called 'Black paintings' attest to his having been witness to the dreadful terror of the darkest, least fathomable depths of human energy.

On a more commonplace level, some syphilitic patients appear with lowering, shifty looks, dark circles beneath their eyes, lank hair and little to say for themselves. Sufferers of anorexia nervosa, heroin addicts, alcoholics and AIDS patients can appear like this. Such people are often tormented within themselves but quite unable to express in what way. Sooner or later they would need either *Syphilinum* or a syphilitic remedy like *Aurum*,

Mercurius, *Kali Iodatum* (potassium iodide), *Nitric Acid* or *Fluoric Acid* in order to lift this grim energy.

Like the spirochete, the miasm can remain dormant for years. It might, once awakened, still be very difficult to spot. Not all pathologies are obviously syphilitic. The spirochete hides and so does the miasm; it is as if it does not want to be tracked down and 'outed'. The patient becomes elusive – does not tell the truth; does not turn up to appointments; makes excuses for not taking the remedies; subtly manipulates family relationships (and the practitioner); avoids responsibilities. All practitioners, allopathic or alternative, would agree that there are just some patients who obstinately refuse to get better. In spite of their apparent willingness to cooperate, they actually do not comply with instructions properly and become watchful and suspicious. They play mind games and, because there are no rules, those on the receiving end can never win. They obfuscate and confuse while appearing to be rational. The practitioner is left wondering whether he or she has either misinterpreted what was said or somehow 'missed a trick'. Such malignant energy is fed by those who would – often unwittingly – collude with it. It seeks to provoke; tears and anger in those being manipulated stoke the embers. Starved of reaction from its victims, syphilism weakens.

It is distressingly common for a miasmatically syphilitic patient to get to a point in treatment, where all seems to be progressing satisfactorily, and then leave. The syphilitic miasm can become a way of life, albeit a dark, self-destructive one. It can be more than life is worth to make the effort to throw off the shackles of self-destructiveness. The pain and anguish can seem like loaded dice; some can fall into so dark a space, that there is no light at the end of the tunnel.

There are two sides of this coin: some are aggressors, abusers, manipulators; others are victims, passive-aggressive and thoroughly abject. In Scottish history the Stuart dynasty gives us the repellent Lord Darnley, riddled with pox, weak but weasley, determined to manipulate people and events to his own ends. The way that his life and that of his wife, Mary, Queen of Scots, were enmeshed with the evil machinations of Scottish politics is the very stuff of the syphilitic miasm. A world away, look at the paintings of Modigliani; his later portraits of his etiolated mistress lack the least spark of life in the eyes. Modigliani was an absinthe drinker and drug addict who died tragically young and utterly corrupted. Within hours his 'victim' mistress, heavily pregnant, threw herself from her bedroom window. Neither was in any way malign, simply unable to climb out of the pit of negativity. Yet, perversely, many (but by no means all) seem to prefer to remain in their syphilitic state and for a number of reasons.

A woman, who worked as a secretary for an enterprising boss who was 'into' alternative therapy, came for treatment because the appointment had been made (and paid for) on her behalf. She had suffered from multiple sclerosis for a number of years and the symptoms were beginning to affect her ability to work. She had darting pains in her arms which also tended to ache. She had less sensation in her left hand than normal and felt a creeping numbness in her left side generally. This came and went depending on how stressed she felt. In addition, she had visual problems. These were very characteristic; when she looked fixedly at anything such as the television or what she was typing, she would gradually lose the colour in her sight and the central vision would blur leaving clarity only on the periphery. Not only did she have so-called 'polo-mint vision' (central scotoma) but she saw things as if she were looking at a film negative – without colour, everything she saw was in varying shades of grey.

This 'picture' of the physical symptoms – and they are not necessarily common to all MS sufferers – was characteristic of just one homoeopathic remedy: *Carboneum Sulphuricum* – a close chemical relative of lampblack! She was given the remedy in the sixth potency; to be taken once every day. The result was far better than anticipated. When the patient returned she reported that the visual symptoms had all disappeared. (Curiously, in relating this she showed no emotion whatever. Where most would be relieved or elated, she simply reported the facts.) Furthermore, the pains in her left side had almost completely disappeared and she felt that her left arm was recovering its strength – though the right one had "*some way to go*". When she was asked what differences these changes were making to her life, she simply replied that she was now able to do all the work given to her. She was asked to continue taking the *Carboneum Sulphuricum* 6 on a daily basis and to return in six weeks time. She was also told that, if she felt that progress slowed down or went backwards before the next appointment, she could call the clinic.

She never appeared for the next appointment. No word was heard from her even when the clinic receptionist phoned to find out if she had been unwell. The practitioner, exceeding his brief, called the woman's boss and asked him whether he knew what had occurred. He promised to find out and reported that his secretary had forgotten the date and had then decided not to bother about any further treatment. The boss had asked if she were quite well now to which she had replied that she was much better in spite of the pains in her arms which were now getting worse again. Her boss persuaded her to return for another interview, paid for the missed meeting and the new one and gave her a whole day off to go to the clinic.

This consultation was the last one. She explained that she had got married to her partner of several years and that, in all the celebrations, she had neglected to take any more tablets. Gradually the pains had returned though her vision remained good. At the moment she was suffering from aching and numbness as well as "*a creeping tiredness*" that she associated with the MS becoming active again. The physical symptoms she related were all still similar to the *Carboneum Sulphuricum* – which, she agreed, had made her symptoms diminish. She was given a bottle of it and asked to return in four weeks. She never did. When her boss was contacted he said that his secretary had left and he no longer knew where she was as she had left no contact number.

But this story has no flesh on the bones; you only know a fraction of it so far. The physical symptoms are not enough to base any judgement of the case on at all. Although the practitioner was left with frustration – what a fantastic effect the *Carboneum* 6 was having! – he was privy to a whole range of detail about the woman's life that only a few others knew about. The woman was the victim of parental abuse. As a child she had been whipped, beaten and shut away in a room. She remembered her mother applying make-up to her face before she was sent to school so that the bruises would be less apparent. She grew up in an atmosphere of distrust, fear and hatred. Eventually her parents split up and the beatings ceased but then she became the subject of her step-uncle's libidinous attentions when her mother remarried. At seventeen she had married to get away from home and found that her new husband was not so very different from her father. He was violent and abusive as soon as he had too much to drink. "*He slapped me around, mostly at weekends. I will say he did work hard in the week but I was the one who had to pay for it.*"

She had two children before she was twenty-one and when her husband became abusive towards the children – "*because they cost too much to feed and clothe, he was that mean*" – and she also discovered that he was having an affair she decided she had to seek a divorce. After a lengthy legal procedure – further drawn out because her husband at first claimed that she was incompetent to have custody of the children and then that he was unable to afford any maintenance – she found herself living on her own with her children. *"It was such a blessed relief but even then I'd wonder who it was coming in through the door. Every time I heard the cat flap go I'd jump in case it was my dad or Mick. It was ages before I could sit in an armchair…it just felt too unsafe to settle; the only safe place was my bed. I didn't have to think any more once I was there. It was then, when I began to settle in myself, that I got the first symptoms."*

Some years later she met the man who became her partner. *"He's such a gentle man. At first I did wonder if he was a bit pansy but he isn't at all. He can't do enough for me. He's always making me things and fetching me tea in bed. He has his odd ways but he makes me smile, I can't help myself."* This is what she had said about her partner during the first consultation. At the second, the story was somewhat different.

"I'm not sure I've done the right thing at all. It was lovely up until the day I married him. From then on he's been a different man. He can't stop swearing and cursing. He's got so mean, just like Mick. He's so rude to the children and they're full of backchat. Then the other day he seemed OK so I suggested we go for a walk. We got into a silly argument and suddenly he just pushed me so that I fell down the bank. Some other people were there and I fell over a bike. I was hurt but he just took no notice and stalked off home. I couldn't believe he'd do a thing like that in public – and then just leave me there."

There were no tears as she related her history. Everything was delivered in a deadpan voice and the only expression was the odd wispy smile. When asked if she were inclined to weep when alone, she said she did not cry any longer. *"No tears come. I wish they would."*

When asked if she ever felt anger towards her aggressors she replied, *"If I started to feel angry I'm afraid of what I might do. It's very dark in there and I'm fearful of what I could dig up. My brother suggested psychotherapy once but I said no thanks; it's no good raking over all that stuff – that's only more trouble."*

There are many such patients who find that getting better involves too much effort. The condition they suffer is preferable to the journey through the emotional minefield that has to be made in order to achieve health. There is nothing that anyone else can do however much we might see what needs to be done and how it could be done – the patient must always have the choice; it is his or her inalienable right for good or ill. *The negative choice, though, is part of the syphilitic miasm.*

Those suffering a destructive illness are seldom ostensibly alone; even if the family and friends have deserted the patient, there are still those concerned and charitable people who are often willing to come to the rescue even if they are sometimes roundly abused for their pains. It is often the case, too, that those suffering from syphilitic conditions have very few true friends; in their hearts there is usually loneliness, silence and separation. If such a patient maintains the sympathy, love of partners or children then there is almost always in them a sense of toil and sacrifice that seems to be a heavy emotional burden. The patient seems to be able to play on their sympathy and to manipulate to their own advantage the sacrifice of care and time that is made for them. It is common for the carer to be oblivious of this abuse, or if they are aware of it then they accept it. Where this is not so then the patient becomes the victim and is sometimes mercilessly manipulated or abused, physically and emotionally, by those who are apparently in a position to be of most help. This would apply to the woman in the previous case study.

Either one of these scenarios is relevant in MS as it is a deeply syphilitic condition. MS bears the hallmarks of one aspect of the last stage of syphilis: nerve damage, paralysis, loss of some or all of the senses, a sense of inevitability about the outcome, for they almost always believe they are incurable. So marked is this symptom in MS and other so-called incurable conditions, that it is often part of a homoeopath's strategy never to suggest that the patient is 'getting better'. Such patients do more for themselves if they are allowed to continue in their belief that the homoeopathy is only palliative. This is particularly true of cases where irreversible neurological damage has taken place, but in those cases where the patient is 'caught' early on then it is possible for the patient's system to remove all trace of physical symptoms – though such positive changes would only occur if the *psyche* received healing as well as the physical body. One such case that illustrates the effect of the syphilitic energy on the mind is as follows:

A woman who had had MS for eight years came for treatment. She said that she realised her condition was incurable but had heard that homoeopathy could help with sleeplessness. She maintained her treatment well and experienced, somewhat to her surprise, considerable relief from all her symptoms. Only when she felt under any stress did she become aware that her symptoms were returning; she would get numbness and tingling back in her arms and she would experience fleeting sensations like mild electric shocks through her body. One day her husband, who had been suffering from persistent heartburn and gastric discomfort for several months, read an article on stomach ulcers, their cause and the threatening results of leaving them untreated. He conceived the idea that he had cancer of the stomach and became inconsolable – yet he would not go to the doctor. He knew that he was going to die. At this point, his wife began to wonder what on earth would happen to their business and the children if or when her husband died. From that moment on she had no symptoms of the MS. "*They vanished!*" This improvement lasted until her husband plucked up the courage to go to the doctor and then the specialist, both of whom assured him that he did not have cancer at all. Up to then his wife, free of her usual inhibiting symptoms, was more purposeful, more energetic and less depressive and anxious. As her husband returned to normality, with a diet and some antacid jollop, so her symptoms crept back.

Certain remedies have manifestly demonstrated that the physical symptoms of MS[18] and other syphilitic, degenerative diseases can be positively affected. Nevertheless, it remains a fact that the true incurability of any one patient (barring the physical trauma that has caused permanent physical damage) lies within the psyche – and how that psyche is affected by the syphilitic miasm. It is occasionally enough that the chosen remedy for the physical symptoms also matches those of the emotions (which is the ideal homoeopathy); the patient does well and achieves what is generally considered 'remission' of symptoms. More often than not, however, it will be necessary to complement the chosen remedy that most similarly covers the physical picture with other remedies that cover certain aspects of the long-sickened psyche. In *all* cases of heavy-duty physical pathology the stricken psyche is of longer standing than the manifestation of physical symptoms.

Among these complementing remedies will be ones known for their affinity for the relief of long-held grief or deeply buried anger, frustration or emotional mortification. There will also be occasions when *Syphilinum* is called for as a support to the main indicated remedy. It is not uncommon for a syphilitic patient to react to an indicated remedy (such as *Mercurius*) by producing a severe acute disease such as a sore throat with swollen glands. It only becomes apparent that the body is crying out for *Syphilinum* when the acute persists beyond endurance and fails to respond wholly to the remedy chosen. The treatment of such an aggravation is an ideal moment to prescribe *Syphilinum* as it relieves the acute symptoms and wakes up the system to the inner ability to quell the general state of syphilism.

There will also be emotional crises during the long-term treatment. If the patient is prepared to go through with healing their history of psychic trauma, they will need remedies that are chosen for their specific ability to deal with the particular quality of the crisis and which complement the main remedy. Acute crises of grief are common when dealing with long-term cases (though, in truth, they are never really acute except in timing) and they respond well to remedies like *Aurum*, *Natrum Muriaticum*, *Ignatia*, *Lachesis*, *Oak*, *Amethyst*, *Emerald* and *Staphysagria* (the delphinium).

Our knowledge of syphilism, the miasm (not the acute disease), gives us a map by which we can read people and their susceptibilities. We can use this because we have not only the *physical* picture of the disease but the *psychology* as well. Syphilis, the infectious disease, shows us the inherent third dimension that is so often hidden – *a state of being that underlies the surface appearance*. This is vital to successful treatment because so often the syphilitic miasm is only manifest in just one or other aspect and only rarely in any unmistakable appearance. Remember that treponema's effects are those of a master of disguise. We need to illustrate the miasm further by relating other cases so that its true colours can be witnessed. This will also afford us an insight into methods of treatment and the different remedies for treating both raw syphilis and its hereditary/genetic effects.

Cases to illustrate the miasm

A seven-year-old boy was brought for treatment. He had been coughing for some time and his mother feared that it was chronic and had even wondered if her son had had whooping cough and his present state was the result. All the symptoms that he displayed indicated the need for

Phosphorus; he had a dry cough with a burning sensation in the chest; his voice was thin and cracked; he was unable to speak for long without a paroxysm of coughing; he was extremely thirsty for cold water; coughing exhausted him; he had moments when he would suddenly seem to recover, being bright and cheerful, but these did not last and he would collapse in front of the television. *Phosphorus* 200 was prescribed and within two days the cough that had lasted six weeks, disappeared.

Within two weeks his mother phoned to say that since taking the *Phosphorus* her son had been having accidents in which he hit his head. On one occasion she had taken him to casualty because she thought he had suffered concussion. She rang because she had suddenly thought that perhaps the remedy had something to do with this. The boy had also just bashed his head on the kitchen cupboard for the third time that day.

The boy was prescribed *Arnica* 1M for the effects of bruising and physical trauma. The mother reported that he was pain-free by the following morning and the bruises disappeared within two further days. Soon afterwards she rang again to say that the coughing had started up again. The symptoms were all the same as before so *Phosphorus* 1M was prescribed. No sooner had the cough cleared for the second time than the mother was on the phone to say that her son was having more accidents involving his head. She was seriously worried, not least as she had seen the relationship between giving the *Phosphorus* and the proneness to accidents. Though the symptoms of bruising and pain were the same as before, *Arnica* was not given. This time another remedy and one that covered that curious symptom of 'accident-proneness', was prescribed. The boy had *Syphilinum* 100.

The effect of this remedy was immediate. The mother reported that the pains in the head disappeared, the bruising subsided within 48 hours and no further accidents occurred. Furthermore, he had no return of the cough. In addition, she reported that the boy had a growing spurt and became far more amenable and cheerful.

Accident proneness and resulting bruising are miasmatically syphilitic conditions. *Arnica* and *Phosphorus* are both syphilitic remedies – meaning that both remedies cover symptom pictures that look like aspects (albeit different ones) of syphilis. When syphilitic remedies only partially heal a condition then *Syphilinum* will very often effect the cure. *Phosphorus* and *Arnica* may well be indicated by their symptom pictures but if these do not complete their action then there is an underlying state that needs to be addressed. If *Syphilinum* does that job of clearing the hidden root of a condition then it is of syphilitic origin.

> A little girl of two and a half was brought for treatment by a very harassed mother. She had two children, the older of which was asthmatic. The girl was constitutionally well but given to throwing monumental rages. Her mother said she was, for most of the time, a thoughtful, serious child; she often had a frown on her brow, either from effort in doing something or from thoughtfulness – though she almost never showed any other emotion. At least, not until she began having the tantrums.
>
> *She is utterly without reason and she's so ruthless. She absolutely must have her own way and she will keep up the shouting and screaming for so long that I give in, in the end, because I feel she will do herself some damage. She doesn't seem to care where she is or who is watching – she becomes oblivious to her surroundings. She is just hellbent on getting what she wants. And her face…it goes dark! There's real hate!"* (At this point the mother wept.)
>
> The child herself was present. She made no sign that she was aware of what was going on and the mother spoke in a low tone trusting that her daughter was fully occupied with the doll she was dressing. Nevertheless, when the girl brought the doll over for an inspection, she sank her teeth into her mother's leg. She was given *Syphilinum* 200. The mother waited for a full month before reporting that, from the moment that her daughter had been given the remedy, there had been no further tantrums in the house; she had lost that frown and permanent seriousness and was now more likely to be found playing with her brother, instead of alone as she used to. She was also no longer getting sweaty at night which was a symptom that the mother had forgotten to mention.

Some syphilitic remedies

Essentially, a syphilitic remedy is one that would hypothetically treat someone manifesting the particular symptoms of the acute disease in a manner as 'like' to the reactions in a healthy person who had proved that individual remedy. *Mercurius* is the most obvious example but there are many. In fact, there are 48 listed in the repertory of symptoms compiled by James Tyler Kent, the American homoeopath who practised at the end of the nineteenth and beginning of the twentieth century. In more recent repertories over 150 are listed. Some of these remedies have come to be seen as archetypally syphilitic: in addition to mercury and its close relatives, *Mercurius Iodatus Flavus* (green iodide of mercury) and *Mercurius Iodatum Ruber* (red iodide of mercury) some of the others are *Arsenicum Album*, *Aurum*, *Kali Iodatum* (potassium iodide), *Nitric Acid*, *Phosphorus*, *Silica*, our old friend *Sulphur* and *Thuja Occidentalis*.

If a remedy has the capacity to heal someone of syphilis then it will also heal others who suffer from syphilitic problems. It has already been shown how *Mercurius* has the appearance of syphilis in any part of its life cycle, how it can heal someone who suffers from a condition that is related to syphilis even when that disease *is not* and *has not* actually been present. The same goes for all other syphilitic remedies. We can illustrate this point by taking one of those remedies listed above and comparing it with syphilis, the disease, and *Mercurius*, the remedy.

Nitric acid

Nitric acid is a formidable poison. Like mercury, it was used by allopaths in the nineteenth century to treat all sorts of conditions including syphilis. It was used in a mild dose to cure excessive thirst in those with chronic fever symptoms; it was also used to suppress the profuse secretions of the mucous membranes in those with lung disease. It was applied topically to warts in an effort to burn them off. It was used to seal chancres (syphilitic ulcers). It also established a reputation among homoeopaths as a remedy that was much needed in the treatment of patients with disease suppressed by mercury (allopathically prescribed) . The homoeopathic preparation was found to be of inestimable value in antidoting the effects of mercury poisoning. Its credentials as a syphilitic remedy are established beyond doubt by its proving.

Nitric acid shows that it has an affinity for certain parts of the body as most poisons do. Arsenic affects the stomach, guts and blood; hemlock, known to homoeopathy as *Conium*, affects the nerves and causes ascending paralysis; the poison from the bushmaster snake, Lachesis, causes coagulation of the blood, especially around the throat, and results in death, virtually from strangulation. Nitric acid can be just as vicious as these but is chiefly known for its affinity for the muco-cutaneous surfaces that make up the orifices of the body: the mouth, the urethra and the anus. In its material form it can affect the body both through its fumes – which cause suffocative attacks, spasms of the throat and severe inflammation of the lungs – and in its fluid form – which acts as an irritant that burns the surfaces it touches; it has a cauterising effect.

Where nitric acid is in contact with the skin it causes ulceration of the upper layers of tissue, turning them yellow. It can cause the skin to appear blistered and the wounds bleed easily especially on being touched. These facts all become keynotes in the *Materia Medica* of the homoeopathic remedy. In acute syphilis, *Nitric Acid* (the homoeopathic preparation) will heal small blistered-looking chancres that bleed easily. These eruptions can appear around male or female genitals, on the prepuce under the foreskin or on the labia. They can also crop up around the anus or around the mouth. The appearance of the lesions is very similar to herpes and indeed the remedy has a spectacular reputation for treating this condition.

Already we have a differentiation between *Mercury* and *Nitric Acid*: one has larger ulcers that have a pustular or cheesy base and that spread with red, raised edges while the other has smaller, contained spots that bleed easily especially on being touched. The blisters of *Nitric Acid* can burst and encourage the eruption of further ulcers leaving a general surface area with a scurfy, sloughing appearance. The eruptions of *Mercurius* tend to itch and burn while those of *Nitric Acid* have a pain that cannot be mistaken: there is a sensation of pricking as if a pin were being jabbed into the skin. There are, as with syphilis (and mercury), bone pains, weakness, lethargy and an aggravation of all symptoms as soon as the sun goes down which continues through the night until the sun rises again. There is swelling of glands; at first in the groin and lower abdomen. With this come shooting and drawing pains. The throat can be affected; the glands swell and the pricking of pins happens at every swallow. The right eye is another particular site of trouble; there can be sensations of sand or grit with haemorrhaging into the cornea. (*Nitric Acid* is another major remedy for iritis, a common symptom of secondary and tertiary syphilis.) Both *Mercurius* and *Nitric Acid* tend to sweat around the crotch causing soreness and redness but only *Nitric Acid* has urine that is listed in the *Materia Medica* as being like horse's urine.

Mercurius is capable of healing ulceration around the anus too but not to such a marked degree; the ulcers and fissures of *Nitric Acid* are true torture. Every passing of a stool, however small, causes cutting and stabbing pain which leaves the area sensitive and bleeding for some considerable time.

The mental picture of *Nitric Acid* is unmistakable. There is none of *Mercury's* changeability of temperament; it is all gloom and doom. So miserable is its reputation that, on one occasion, a homoeopath who sought treatment for her menstrual problems and who was not permitted to know the name of the remedy she was given, burst into floods of tears on her return appointment when she was then told what had effected the satisfactory result. She explained that she was embarrassed to think that she must have been so terrible to live with that she had needed *Nitric Acid*.

The patient is nervous, irritable, melancholy, quarrelsome, easily startled and thoroughly difficult. He never stops 'nit-picking'; nagging and disparagement are hallmarks. There is restlessness and anxiety and facial expressions are limited to one – frowning. *Nitric Acid* is the master of the acid-drop comment; malicious sarcasm is its stock in trade. The patient is excessively sensitive to all sorts of external stimuli – from irritating noises to thunderclaps. He or she can be driven to distraction by having to listen to people talking too much. This sensitivity causes more weakness and enervation. Some patients fear insanity almost as much as they fear for their general state of health. Such a mental/emotional picture is extreme and not uncommon in secondary syphilis. However, it is also common enough, though perhaps not to quite the same intensity, in some who have never had syphilis at all. Take the example of the wretched homoeopath who was unable to diagnose her own symptom picture.[19] Her case was of the utmost simplicity:

> She was feeling unkind and unhelpful towards her husband. She blamed him for causing the irritating, painful and debilitating leucorrhoea[20] that she had been suffering for nine months. She declared that she was absolutely fed up with it and if the treatment did not clear it up she would go to the doctor instead. She "*half suspected*" her husband of a one-night stand and had grown to believe that he was lying when he dismissed the suggestion. She had stopped all love-making and was now blaming him for looking at other women. She had aphthae on the tongue

which, she said, plagued her. These are little blistery ulcers. She was given *Nitric Acid* 10M and the condition gradually cleared up over the following five weeks.

It is easy to discern the suspicion, the mean spirits, the quarrelsome nature of the syphilitic here. It is also an illustration of how a person who might have been expected to recognise these things was quite unable to do so when she was in the state herself. It is entirely characteristic that she sought to blame her husband. It is not surprising that so many of the remedies for syphilis and the syphilitic miasm are, by nature, extremely unpleasant; nor is it strange that being in the sway of an energy that is similar to any of them should cause the sufferer to be blind to what is needed to effect a cure – not least as they almost always look for blame outside themselves. The syphilitic state is always reluctant to release the host from its coils.

It is not always so easy for the practitioner to see what needs to be done. There are some cases where the syphilitic *Nitric Acid* state is not presented in the classic picture described above. Take the woman in her late fifties who came for treatment for her arthritis and her high blood pressure:

She was a pleasant person who only seemed concerned about the frequency of her headaches (in the back of her head) and the pain in her hip which made her lame. She had not a cross word to say about anyone. She did have shooting, stitching pains in her hip (but then, this symptom is covered by countless others). It was remarkable just how patient she was; she returned so often for treatment that was apparently not really helping her. At first, the practitioner was inclined to believe that the allopathic medication for the control of her blood pressure was in some way interfering with the remedies – but this is an easy trap to fall into. Finally, the homoeopath changed tack altogether. Having concentrated almost exclusively on the arthritis and the headaches – because the patient seemed to be so unaffected by any emotional concerns – he asked how she got on with her father; he was not sure why he asked this but he was glad that he did.

"*That old bastard! He's more trouble than he's bloody well worth. I can't see why he's hanging on for so long. He's just a misery guts. Every time I turn round he's there asking me some darn thing or another. He's forever giving me the jumps – he creeps about the house in carpet slippers so I never know he's there. I'm pleased to get to work in the morning, though I never know what I'll find when I get back. He's a liability. And, of course, I'm the muggins who has to look after him, aren't I. I can't go away on holiday and they never come down and give me a break."*

Her normal passive expression was transformed to one of scowling distemper. She was given *Nitric Acid* 30 to take once a day. The headaches were relieved almost at once and the hip pain was improved by 50 per cent. She continued to take the remedy because she lived with the cause of her illness: her relationship with her father. Their feud had been ongoing for many moons and she admitted that the only thing that would change her attitude and feelings was his death. She was very pleased that homoeopathy had given her the means with which to survive, with greater comfort and equanimity, her continuing struggle with her father.

So, though *Nitric Acid* is not exclusively a syphilitic remedy, it possesses all the criteria for belonging to the list of remedies that contribute to the healing of this terrible disease and its miasm. It has the ulceration, the destruction of tissue, the bone pains, the aggravation of symptoms at night-time, the pathological activity of the glands, the nervous disorders, the blood dyscrasia and the mental/emotional upheaval. Anyone who manifests symptoms that mimic this condition and who has characteristic *Nitric Acid* hallmarks falls into the category *syphilitic*. This is true when any of the other remedies mentioned are presented as characteristic energies of a patient's pathology. Not all syphilitics need either *Nitric Acid* or *Mercurius*; the variety of syphilis and its miasm is bewildering but if you can retain the essential details common to all syphilitic remedies and to the disease itself it becomes apparent when a patient has succumbed to his inherent 'syphilism'. It is the characteristic idiosyncrasies of the individual remedies that determine which one is required. As has been intimated, this can be either imperceptible in its mildness or it can be an implacable, incurable enemy.

Polychrests

Some syphilitic remedies are polychrests; *Mercurius, Arsenicum, Silica, Phosphorus, Sulphur* – all belong in this group. They are frequently needed for all sorts of conditions; they do not always carry syphilitic connotations; most are also tubercular or sycotic. They even appear in first-aid kits available from homoeopathic pharmacies. At the thinnest end of the syphilitic wedge these remedies are curative of quite negligible problems – the common cold, sore and watery eyes, diarrhoea and vomiting, mild skin rashes due to too much exposure to the sun or from contact with an irritant; all problems that would clear up on their own given time. In this capacity, they seem to have nothing to do with syphilis or its miasm. These remedies are simply demonstrating their enormous capacity for adaptation.

Many of us need the remedies for minor complaints on a routine basis. Nevertheless, if anyone requires *frequent* doses of a potentially syphilitic remedy then the underlying miasm is nearer the surface than we would suspect from the minor nature of the complaints. Someone who needed intermittent but repeated doses of, say, *Mercurius* for throat troubles would sooner or later need *Syphilinum*. The more severe or chronic the ailment, the sooner is the nosode likely to be needed.

In the case of the major polychrests, there may be no apparent pathology at all. These remedies all have starkly identifiable personalities of their own. Agatha Christie's Hercule Poirot is a classic portrayal of *Arsenicum* 'in health'. The dapper detective is pin-neat; he is fastidious to a fault; he has a keen and scientifically orientated intellect. Nothing escapes his sharp eye and he makes use of what he discovers. He is the very opposite of his friend, Captain Hastings, who is the epitome of a psoric *Sulphur* – the perfect foil for an *Arsenicum*. Poirot is a 'doer'; Hastings is a romantic dreamer. (Though '*Sulphur*' people can be doers too.) Even Poirot's acute health problems are *Arsenicum* type colds – the sneezing, the need for a tisane and a clean *mouchoir* and removal to bed upon the instant of any worsening of the condition.

But Poirot is obsessive. He is passionately involved with his moustachios to the point of being absurd. His cleanliness is bordering on the ridiculous. We see these details as eccentricities but they are very minor examples of insanity. What prevents him from tipping over into anything more threatening is his genius and his resolute will to create order for a good purpose. Sure enough, in his last case Poirot not only deals with what he describes as the worst form of criminal (a conniving, reclusive manipulator of other people's weaknesses) but he himself dies of a syphilitic condition after having engineered the death of his villainous victim. While

Poirot can be dismissed as a character of fiction, another *Arsenicum* personality cannot. Robespierre, who led the Reign of Terror during the French Revolution, was as pin-neat, obsessive, suspicious and fanatical as Poirot but with rather different results.

Giving either Poirot or anyone else *Arsenicum* when they are 'in health' will not change the personality – and certainly it would have been too late to save Robespierre from the guillotine as Hahnemann was only just beginning his life's work in the 1790s. But it can protect them from tipping into the negative syphilitic state; a miasmatic prophylaxis, so to speak. It is not exclusive to treating the syphilitic miasm though; such work is carried out all the time with all the other miasms, as you shall see.

What about the whole question of heredity? Who are homoeopaths to make any claim about the genetic encoding of syphilis[21] (or any other of the great miasmatic diseases)? Homoeopaths are observers of patterns of behaviour that manifest both in patients and their diseases. Furthermore, those patterns are observable as skeins of negative energy running through families.

Family history

None of the cases cited would be so intrinsically interesting if it were not for the investigation of family history. Homoeopaths will always ask about the health of forebears. They will ask what parents, uncles, aunts and grandparents died from or what they might suffer chronically now. Such details often give a further clue to the identity of the miasms at play. (Though with psora there is less need to be so precise as homoeopaths accept that it is to be found sooner or later in every patient.) In the case of the accident-prone boy who needed *Phosphorus* and *Arnica* (p. 458), there were grandparents who had had heart attacks – which might have reflected psora except they suffered them in their forties and fifties, and that is more syphilitic. In addition, there was an alcoholic uncle and cancer in both sides of the family. In the case of the small girl with the tantrums (p. 460) there was a history of depression, a suicide in the mother's family and the father had asthma and bronchiectasis (in which the tissues of the lungs are damaged leaving holes in which purulent matter can collect). The mother herself had suffered several miscarriages with severe haemorrhaging which can often be characteristic of the tubercular/syphilitic state. So it was not surprising that these children produced the conditions that were resolved through the use of *Syphilinum*. A hereditary thread is always there in syphilitic cases even if it is significant by the complete *absence* of any information – many patients are quite unable to find out anything whatever on the health of their fore-bears. To illustrate this thread of family history, as well as taking a closer look at the thicker end of the syphilitic wedge where tragedy waits, we can describe the case of an alcoholic.

Helen came for treatment for her son. He had warts and 'abdominal migraines' (another way of describing tummy aches with a psychosomatic cause). When his mother saw how well the child progressed, she booked herself an appointment. She suffered from insomnia and high blood pressure even though she was only in her early thirties. She had experienced blood pressure problems during her pregnancy but they had disappeared after the birth of her son (who was now seven) and only returned when she discovered that her husband was gambling. She had learned of this by accident while talking to her GP who inadvertently referred to "*Gary's vice*" as if she knew all about it.

"*When he realised I did not know what he was talking about, he clammed up. But he'd said enough for me to want to find out more. I was devastated. I spent a week not knowing if it were all true or not.*" It had been three years since Helen had confronted her husband with the evidence. He, at first, denied everything but quickly changed his tack and became dismissive saying "*what did it matter, there was plenty more money where that had come from*". He became, from then on, very surly for most of the time though there were moments when he would be almost euphoric.

"*He can almost be his old charming self again but I can't trust it. I'm always wary – especially if he's been drinking. He has taken to doing some very odd things. He hides things away so that I can't find them. My rings and other jewellery; he'll swear he hasn't seen them but then I find them in his sock drawer. He hoards things in odd places…but then can't find where he's put anything. He hides his empties in the boot of his car and thinks I don't know when he slips off to the bottle bank at 10 o'clock at night. He denies knowing anything about it when I ask. I've caught him out lying on several occasions. We can't communicate any more; I've got to the point where I've almost given up trying.*"

She went on to explain that though he was very good with their son, taking him out to the cinema and out for rambling walks, he almost never volunteered any conversation with her anymore. He would say that there was nothing to talk about. If she initiated any conversation, it would end in a slanging match which he would terminate by telling her that it was all her fault because she was "*so damn insensitive to his needs*".

"*I feel that this all has to be causing me the sleeplessness and preventing my blood pressure from coming down. There is so much tension in the house. I blame it on his mother…partly. He's exactly like her and he is a martyr to her every whim. She can't bear me because I always stand my ground with her but he always rushes to her defence, which infuriates me – not that I ever say much these days. She's rather pathetic now, crippled with arthritis, but I have to say she's been a blight on his life and pretty poisonous to me. She didn't like the age difference to start with – he's 22 years older than me.*"

Helen had recently consulted a new, very sympathetic GP who had told her that, in her opinion, her husband was a depressive personality and probably "*on the borders of being alcoholic*"; she had recommended that he should seek help.

"*I was absolutely devastated but then I just felt relief, so much relief. I realised that I was not just making it all up; that he couldn't blame me for everything. I felt such a fool – and it all makes sense, really. It's come just when I needed to make sense of so many things. His latest thing is that he's got in a firm of security experts and he's getting them to turn the house into a fortress. For heaven's sake, we live right off the beaten track and there's not much of value anyway! And we can't really afford it anyway.*"

Gary, the husband, came for treatment. It was not immediately clear what it was that had inspired him to come. He spoke elliptically, seeming to jump from one thing to another. A gaunt man with cadaverous cheeks and a hunted look, he found it difficult to meet the practitioner's eyes. During the usual questions about his daily routines he was reminded that his doctor had told him that he was probably a depressive.

"*I suppose he knows what he's talking about. Helen says her doctor said the same thing. They both think I'm alcoholic. They're like a couple of witches stirring the pot, talking about the way I am. It's quite unnerving. None of my friends have said they've noticed any difference in me and they're the sort of blokes that would…say if they had, I mean. It's true that I have been under tremendous pressure recently. Now I've got this filthy cold and I have to be absolutely on the ball this week. You'll have to give me something to get it out of my system.*"

At the end of the interview he declared that he did not have the same faith in alternative medicine as his wife had and that he would just as soon go to the doctor's for antibiotics for his cold and if it did not clear up in 24 hours he would do just that. Though the cold did clear up on a dose of *Pulsatilla* 200, apparently he also went to the doctor – but for another reason. He developed a severe pain in his chest with violent palpitations. He began to get hard pains in his head which came on with waves of heat. He also began to tremble and shake uncontrollably.

"*It felt as if my face and head were suffused with blood,*" he later reported. "*I couldn't think straight. Everything went blank and I had real trouble with knowing what I was supposed to be doing. I was dead scared. My blood pressure was sky high apparently! But it came down after a couple of days. Nevertheless…*" But he didn't finish his sentence.

The doctor had sent him to a private clinic from which he discharged himself after ten days – he could not bear the claustrophobic atmosphere and he believed that the drugs he had been given there had made him feel worse. He had not been given a clear diagnosis.

Over the following months he continued to come for treatment. He was given *Aurum* in a daily dose. Not only is *Aurum* a remedy that covers just those acute symptoms that he had complained of but it also has despair, anger, paranoia (the feeling that all the world was against him), intolerance, suspicion and a tendency to weep uncontrollably – all of which he manifested. (Some of this information was given by Helen.) It also covers the syphilitic night sweats that he had begun to produce as well as the trembling and extreme sensitivity of the five senses that he now admitted to having felt for the last few months. It was more than possible that he had experienced an attack of delirium tremens.

"*I'm a mess and I know that I have to do something about it. I've probably lost my wife and I don't want to screw up my job. I don't mind admitting that I am shit-scared. Every time my pulse races I wonder if I'm going to have a heart attack.*"

He also had the syphilitic's (and *Aurum*'s) fear of heart disease. In his consultations he spoke about things other than himself. He mentioned the children (he had two by a previous marriage), his parents, his wife, his colleagues and his best friend. He spoke of them as if he were an observer of their movements and not as if they had connections with him. He was critical of his wife and colleagues yet he was terrified of losing the support of either. He was nostalgic about his parents even though they had made his early life "*a misery*", according to his wife. (They had lived abroad and had sent him home to boarding school. They made flying visits to see him and the aunt he stayed with at Christmas.)

The one person he mentioned with genuine affection was the aunt who had stood guardian to him. She had never married and was not talked about in the family. She was much older than his mother and only a 'half' aunt as she was the child of his grandfather's first marriage. Talk of these family members led to a discussion of how healthy they had been.

"*They all had excellent health. My mother is still alive and she's well though she does have arthritis. Both my grandmothers lived into their late eighties. I never knew my mother's father as he was so much older anyway.*"

Yet later, Helen revealed that his father had had high blood pressure and angina for years; his mother was diabetic (late onset); his paternal aunt had died in her fifties of bone cancer; his paternal grandfather had had TB in his late teens and died of emphysema in his sixties. Most revealing of all – and this information came from him – was that he had been born one of a pair of twins but his twin brother had died some two weeks before delivery.

"*My mother can't be drawn on the subject. She simply refuses to talk about it. I only found out because of something my father once said in an unguarded moment.*"

Such a family history is distressingly commonplace. One day he came for treatment and was apparently in turmoil. His erstwhile guardian aunt had died and he had been to the funeral. He was shaky and tearful. Helen had once said that he took less interest in the aunt than he professed but at this moment he was clearly affected. He began to explain that he had met an old Roman Catholic priest at the funeral who had told him "*more of the old girl's history than was quite good for me to know*".

"*This man had been an old friend of Eleanor's and he told me why she had always been* persona non grata *with the family. She was their skeleton, I s'pose. Apparently, during her childhood, she had lived with her alcoholic mother and her 'lodger' and he consistently raped her up to the age of about fourteen. He would beat her mother up. One day he broke her neck. My aunt apparently found her in the kitchen. She was taken to hospital and lay in a coma for ages. She never recovered. My aunt then went to live with her father, my grandfather, but he had recently married again and his new wife – my grandmother – resented Eleanor so much that she shut her up in the attic for long spells. She attempted suicide twice – she jumped out of the window but only broke some bones and she took her stepmother's sleeping pills; she took too many and made herself sick instead. Somehow she managed to pull herself together but she more or less lived quietly and alone after that.*"

By the end of this story he was sweating profusely and shaking uncontrollably. Tears ran down his face which he wiped brusquely away. He went straight into a peroration about his wife's lack of sympathy, her callous treatment of his family at the funeral and her lack of respect for anyone's feelings but her own. He had thought of hiring a private eye because he had begun to have suspicions – he did not say of what.

What he cannot have known is that he was in the deepest syphilitic thicket. His family was riddled with the miasm (alcoholism, physical and sexual abuse, buried secrets, broken families, violence, threatened and attempted suicide, silence in the face of emotional devastation) and now it was his turn to attempt to deal with what had started so long ago. When the miasm takes such a firm hold it is extremely difficult to shift. It is as if the miasm has taken possession of the person; it hides from attention but spreads out to wreak havoc on those close by. Just as syphilis, the acute disease, causes its victims to be libidinous in order to take part in the reproductive spree, so the miasm seems to reach out and infect as many around as possible.

Money, being a worldly crutch, is something of an agent for the miasm to work with. Alcohol is just such another. Secretiveness and deviousness are, almost, methods of its employment. There is a sense of doom with an inability to extricate oneself from the abyss. Indeed, there is a perverse inclination to draw others into the pit. In the darkest hours, love and kindness are not embraced with relief but are twisted and manipulated. For those, like Helen, who see the threat to their stability that a deeply syphilitic person can be, the only safe course of action is to create a distance. Emotional involvement with such a person will only lead to irreparable damage and grief. Yet, so often, these tragic souls have a terrible attractiveness.

When they first married, Helen had no conscious inkling that her new husband would be the source of so much turmoil in her life. She had not started out with, nor developed now, any reforming zeal to work on an afflicted soul who needed rescuing. (Though this is often the beginning of a syphilitic disaster.) She had had a 'rosy picture of domestic bliss'. Yet here he was, thinking of employing surreptitious tactics – to find out what his wife was thinking and doing; he was smoking to excess and had started to drink again, more than he could cope with. "*I need to smoke and drink just now. The need to relax is more important than trying to give them up.*"

He was resenting his wife's freedom from his problems; feeling that she had completely given up on him. He genuinely wanted his wife to stay with him but he was puzzled that he could not please her by doing everything that she told him he ought to do. (Instead, of course, of taking responsibility for himself.) He felt confused and found it difficult to remember words or appointments that he ought to keep. He confessed to having thoughts of suicide – these began after he had heard of his aunt's terrible history.

"*I can't even pray for all this to go away! I've never believed in anything much beyond success.*" There speaks a syphilitic. The prognosis of his case was not good. In fact, he continued to prevaricate. Rather than looking to himself for the release of his disturbance, he sought ways of incriminating his wife for all his problems. He complained of trivial incidents to the homoeopath and the psychotherapist, the acupuncturist, the masseuse and the cranial/sacral therapist to whom he went in turn. So plausible and convincing was he that it was sometimes difficult not to wonder if, in fact, all was not exactly as he said it was. Though he continued to take the homoeopathic remedies they seemed only to work on a partial basis. The headaches and the chest pains did not return; the acute side effects of the drugs had been eliminated; greater clarity of mind was achieved. Whether or not it was the smoking and drinking that compromised the efficacy of the remedies, his response to treatment did not include any sign of seeing how his way of life undermined his future chances of health. He failed to see that the tragic family history was something he had to face and deal with – though not because any of it was his fault. He did not grasp that he had to make the changes that would effect a curative resolution and help his damaged family. For by coming to an acceptance and understanding of his own life's predicament – the circumstances of his birth, his abandonment by his parents when they left him in a boarding school, his addictions – he would have been showing those in his family who cared enough to see how they too could have come to terms with their grief. He would also have been showing his son, despite his young age and lack of anything but emotional understanding, how he set about self-healing. He did manage to find tears for himself which would well up unbidden. "*I'd cry at a Disney cartoon!*"

But this was only the surface. The original dose of *Pulsatilla* had done more than deal with the cold. *Pulsatilla*, on its deepest level, is famous for its feeling of abandonment and loss. After taking it, Gary began to experience all the serious symptoms of acute high blood pressure. The symptoms that his system expressed were those that answered to *Aurum*, most often used in chronic, syphilitic conditions where there is a background of despair, grief and deeply held anger. *Pulsatilla*, the humble pasque flower, (one of the closest complementary remedies to

Aurum) had brought to the surface what Gary had been suppressing for years.

The *Aurum* did relieve the physical symptoms; it did help him to see the importance of holding his family together even though he could not resist the temptation of sniping at his wife from time to time. He did control his gambling. Yet, when it came to his emotional turmoil he was unable to drop his guard in spite of his desperate wish to keep his family together. His desperation was genuine but he had the syphilitic's need for the control that is necessary for the continuation of fertile soil for the miasm itself. This is a curious paradox; he seemed to abdicate responsibility for change to his wife and practitioners, but he held tight reins on his deepest emotions. He was not in control of the drink or the smoking beyond the refusal to attempt to give them up. He claimed that, at fifty-six, he was too old to dig into the past and upset anyone else in the family.

"My mother is an old woman. I can't ask her about my twin brother. I don't see the point…it's all gone, in the past. She knows all about my aunt but I know she'd never talk to me about it. There was bad blood but let things alone I say."

Helen moved out when her son began cutting up her clothes with a pair of scissors and carving lines into her favourite jazz records.

The old cliché says it all - 'the sins of the fathers…' What shapes do these sins take on in past generations and where can we find the syphilitic miasm in our forebears. The answer is always the same – in whatever is *actively self-destructive*. MS, motor neuron disease and some forms of heart disease have been cited already. There is a mass of others: addiction to certain drugs, alcoholism, Alzheimer's, aneurysm, anorexia nervosa, almost all autoimmune disease, bronchiectasis, celiac disease[22], certain congenital malformations, Cushing's syndrome, emphysema, Friedreich's ataxia and so on through the alphabet with some in capitals: leukaemia, lymph cancers, manic depression, schizophrenia, suicide.

Syphilis, in its last stages, is universally acknowledged as the master of disguise and can erupt into life as almost any terminal pathology. The miasm is only showing the same propensity when patients produce any of these conditions. After all, the miasm has been with us far longer than acute syphilis which is only the climactic physical expression of the state of being that is syphilism. AIDS is just such another expression, a nadir of evolutionary development in man's capacity to find ways of expressing his deepest, darkest angst.

It is rare and suspicious in these times and in western Europe to come across a patient whose family history is innocent of anything more than relations who die in their nineties. Even the most disarmingly simple cases can harbour hidden depths of rank miasm. See for yourself in this case:

A woman aged sixty-three came having been referred by her osteopath who could not deal with the patient's sinus problems without auxiliary help. This sinus condition was chronic and had been troubling her for some ten years. When she spoke her voice was coloured by the obstruction in the nasal cavities. Her throat was always congested and she complained of a continuous post-nasal drip. These factors, she insisted, contributed to her having a perpetual cold which sometimes led to a severe chest infection for which she had always felt obliged to contact her doctor who inevitably gave her antibiotics. *"It's not that I'm ungrateful for them because they do get rid of the infection...but they make me feel so wretched."*

She was asked about the quality of the mucus that she manufactured. It was green and thick. *"Quite disgusting, I'm afraid. How horrid for you to have to ask about such things."* And she play-acted a delicate little shudder. She was a precise and charming person who presented herself immaculately. She did not like talking about her health at all; it was *"such a nuisance"* and there were *"so many more people in the world worse off than me."* She led a happily married life and was comfortably off; she and her husband took two annual holidays and in the remainder of the year she did 'good works' – she was also a staunch member of the Women's Institute. She had two children both of whom were successful and firmly married to the right people (*"...at least, I'm very pleased."*). They both lived abroad in exotic places and she loved going to them so that she could enjoy the grandchildren. *"They are absolutely delightful but quite a handful so I'm glad I don't have them on top of us all the year round. It's nice to go out there and do my bit, though."*

She was given remedies that were well indicated.[23] They made some difference and she felt as if *"things are shifting but slowly"*. She was aware of having more energy, though it did not last. She thought that her chest felt clearer and that she could breathe more deeply. Further than that there was little change. This woman's appearance should have betrayed the underlying problem. Although she dressed neatly and gave the impression of being a scrupulously clean and tidy person, her complexion was as dark and earthy as Boris Karloff's. She had the look of someone who did not eat very healthily – not the greasy, spotty complexion of those who live on fast foods – but the anaemic, shrivelled look of the prematurely aged whose faces are corrugated with tiny lines. In spite of her bright little button eyes and her clipped and energetic talk, she gave the impression of being tired and worn out but with enough energy left to keep up a pretence of vigour.[24] Because her appearance suggested a darker side to her story, she was asked to look back in her past and see if she could remember anything that could have been a sufficiently strong trauma to have disturbed her system profoundly enough to prevent remedies from working.

She thought for a few seconds and said that there was only one thing that might have done this. She described how her sister had been murdered while they were on holiday in Jamaica. She had insisted on going out in the evening on her own; had too much to drink and would not listen to reason.

"The last time we saw her was not a good way to remember her. She demanded that my husband should give her some money and then shouted abuse at him when he refused. We stayed up for a while and were just going to call the police when she rang through to say that she wanted to come back but had no money for a taxi. She was crying down the phone, snivelling really...like alcoholics do...and then said she was, well, 'bloody well going to walk back if you'll excuse my French' if no-one would come and fetch her. She slammed the phone down before we could ask her where she was. Of course we would have picked her up. We'd had to do it before, for heaven's sake! My husband rang the police and told them what had happened but they didn't seem interested – it was a busy night. So he went out to look for her. He came back at 2 a.m. saying that he just couldn't carry on. We couldn't sleep though. In the morning the police phoned to tell us that she had been found. They wouldn't say how she was, just that we should come to the hospital as soon as possible. It was a nightmare of a journey – we didn't know what to expect. When we got there we were asked all sorts of questions that didn't seem relevant at all and they wouldn't tell us where she was! I was almost hysterical. Eventually an officer came in who told us that she had been gang-raped and left, apparently for dead. A taxi driver had found her and brought her to the hospital and then called the police. The doctors did all they could but she had multiple injuries which caused internal bleeding and then she had choked on her own vomit.

"I do look back at that time and wonder sometimes. It was almost surreal and yet in a funny sort of way it didn't – and doesn't – surprise me. It was always on the cards that something like that would happen to her. She was always the black sheep. She married an alcoholic who ran off with all her

money. She was in and out of clinics either to dry out or for depression. She found herself in all the wrong places at the wrong times. She must have broken every bone in her body before she was 25 – she was potentially a brilliant skier but she ruined any chances she might have had by having several car accidents that left her in fairly constant pain. She couldn't get into the driving seat without streaking off at 100 miles per hour. She was exhausting. So it wasn't a shock. It was strange to think that death had put a stop to all the difficulties of being her closest family – it touched me as well."

The patient stopped and seemed to go into a reverie for a few moments. She had just been describing the syphilitic nature of her sister's life. Based on no more than this association with her sister and the curiously withered, sallow complexion, she was given *Syphilinum* 100. She reported a significant improvement when she returned in eight weeks but she felt that she had reached a plateau. She was given *Syphilinum* 200 and this "*did the trick*". She was told that she should keep the appointment that she had already made for some ten weeks later as the progress had to be carefully monitored. This was more for the practitioner's benefit as he wished to be certain that the remedy would hold and that the patient would not trip up at the 'last hurdle'. At this next consultation the patient claimed to be feeling good still but that some of the physical symptoms were returning. As there was no hint of the miasm at all but every indication that *Pulsatilla* would match the picture, it was given in the 1M potency. This remedy now worked much better than it had done, several months before. The prescription sheet suggests that her treatment progressed more thoroughly and swiftly after she was given the *Syphilinum*.

Other signals that betray syphilism

This prompts the question: are there any other telltale, physiological signs that betray the syphilitic miasm? Complexion is often a good guide to judging a person's acute health but it can also be indicative of a chronic state or miasmatic condition that underlies and threatens to undermine even the most robust constitution. Syphilism can be apparent when there is a sallow, gaunt look. Eyes can give away much or little; a syphilitic often has a straight glare with a dark expression or, when something less than the truth is being said, there is a veiled quality or an elusiveness. Dark rings round the eyes often suggest that a person's kidneys are weak but when the shadows are permanent it is likely that syphilism is lurking.

Stunted growth with an anaemic appearance is a common enough sign in children. Disproportionately small, scoop-shaped noses are another; very occasionally one meets someone born without supporting cartilage though this is a condition now corrected early with surgery. (It is also a potential sign of the related leprosy miasm.) Teeth that are peg-shaped or have serrated edges are also signs. Syphilitic children are not likely to be well proportioned. They have large heads and puny physiques; they are often weak and have bones that break easily. They have a drawn look and the eyes are often rather sunken even if they are sharp and piercing in their gaze. In both young and old, rapid emaciation is a sure sign of syphilism at work.

There are indications on the skin: eruptions that appear on the body symmetrically; eruptions that have a coppery colour; spreading and deepening eruptions or ulcers that begin to give off a fœtid odour; ulcers that will not heal. Skin lesions that turn gangrenous or that readily ulcerate can be added to the list. Moles that threaten to turn black and then malignant are an indication. It would probably be syphilism at work in any young person who has such bad acne that the skin bleeds easily, is pitted and scarred.

It is usually, however, the typical behavioural patterns that homoeopaths come across in practice. Wherever the threads of *self-destructiveness* are evident then syphilism is at work. Depression, despair, envy and manipulative power play, calculated wickedness, cold rage or well-disguised passive aggression with the victim state writ large – these are all well-documented traits. We may be touched by it in the least of ways – baby teeth that come through rotten; crippled toenails; a temporary obsession with the fear of disease; very poor hair growth. Or we may be affected by becoming the unwitting accomplices of a family member who seems to need all the help they can get but who in reality is surreptitiously leeching on everyone's energy. We might know someone who is struggling to deal with their syphilism by being dangerously anorexic or drinking themselves into oblivion or – and this is often hard to spot – orchestrating disharmony within a family through acid drops of gossip that play one member off against another. Shakespeare knew a thing or two about syphilitic evil: Othello only throttles his wife because he is the unwitting victim of Iago's unbridled, furtive syphilism.

Most of us begin with relatively good health and it is only through our negative physical, mental or emotional experiences, to which we fail to adjust, that anything like the syphilitic miasm might stir within to cause 'dis-ease'. Nevertheless, the stronger the miasm is within the family, the more susceptible to chronic illness the person will be; the more they will suffer from suppression (through drugs and vaccines) and the sooner it will arise to be dealt with in the next generation. The less satisfactorily it is dealt with by each succeeding generation, the more urgent and deadly it becomes. Yet none of this happens without purpose; the expurgation of negativity; little short of the phoenix moment.

There is a curious aspect to all this that should be mentioned as it is surprisingly common. It is usual for families in which there is a strong but hidden syphilitic strain, to throw up just one member of the pedigree who seems to embody all the attributes of the syphilitic miasm so powerfully that it is as if their life's mission is to take the whole burden of the miasm so that others in the family might restore some semblance of 'normality'. A further example will illustrate the potential for this extraordinary situation.

Where the buck stops with syphilism

Two large and local families – farmers, blacksmiths, market gardeners and tilers among them – had been, twenty years since, united in the marriage of two of their children. The families were rivals and riven with antagonism. Many of the older generation were long lived but either spinsters, bachelors or gaga. The remainder were in their late sixties and seventies and suffered retirement in poor grace with conditions ranging from anal abscesses and suppurating ulcers that threatened gangrene to psoriasis and MS. There was alcoholism, violence and incest – most of which lay buried in a wall of suspicion and recrimination which was pointed and repointed by years of sniping and gossip.

The pair who had married were apparently untouched by any of this malignancy. Both were strong of constitution and hard-working. They were seen as the ideal couple and were the focus of hope for some who might have seen the need to develop a healthier strain in the families. These two were in their forties and had two boys and a girl. The mother was cheerful, industrious and mother-hennish. The father was gaunt, deeply tanned and taciturn. Both were very worried.

The younger of their two sons, who was sixteen, was depressed and given to fits of 'blacking out'. He was subject to bouts of either unimaginable rage or inexplicable self-loathing and recrimination. He would flip from one to the other without warning. He would blame his parents for all manner of things – they were the cause of his failure in exams; his inability to make friends; his frail health. He would accuse them, one at a time – for he seldom attacked them together, choosing to play one off against the other – of undermining his confidence; of preventing his friends from coming to the house; of misleading him about what other members of the family were up to; of spoiling his brother and sister and leaving him out. At other times he would weep or remain silent for days, shut away in his bedroom, reading or simply staring into space. He would apologise to his parents and say how he realised that he was so unreasonable and how difficult he must be to live with; he would ask for forgiveness and declare dramatically that he knew that he did not really deserve it and that he would be better off dead; that he was no more than a burden on the rest of the family.

The parents confided in no-one except a close friend who had been a witness to some of the paranoia. They did not believe in doctors and had not sought professional help. They had been advised by the friend, however, to consult a homoeopath about the frequently recurring headaches that Brian was now suffering. These could be so intense that he would be unable to lift his head from the pillow without screaming, they would cause loss of vision and tonic[25] spasms of the lower extremities and the abdominal muscles. It was this symptom picture that the homoeopath was, at first, asked to treat. So severe had the condition become that he was virtually bedridden with 'cluster migraines'.

Over the next few years a host of different conditions arose which always seemed to respond to remedies. So marked was this that the parents, who were clearly an introverted couple wanting no outside influence to alter the routines of their household, came to trust in the efficacy of homoeopathy. It was clear that not only the distress of the original headaches and other physical ailments were relieved but that some of the mental and emotional picture was apparently resolved. This latter aspect of the case was only gradually allowed to be seen. While the mother was down-to-earth, practical and more able to speak of emotional issues, the father was not, giving the impression of wanting to remain closed. While she spoke of the trauma of living with the difficult behaviour, he only made the odd, cryptic comment. What was also clear was that every time the practitioner was able to give a remedy for the underlying mental/emotional state – because the latest physical problem had been resolved – the boy would throw up another acute condition that would seem to cut across the action of the last remedy.

This situation is a common phenomenon in any practice – though not to such a degree. The boy often suffered sore (streptococcal) throats, mouth ulcers, boils (staphylococcal infections), abdominal pains, testicular pains, violent cramps, trigeminal neuralgia and rheumatic pains in all the joints. If none of these were present, then it was likely that he would be in a state of rage or of self-loathing. As this mental state was the psychosomatic background to his general condition, it was always the state which needed the most attention and deepest treatment. So often, though, the acute ailment that followed a major, constitutional remedy (i.e. one based on the 'whole' picture) would seem to set him back mentally and emotionally once the physical symptoms were better. He would be 'washed out'; he had no vitality with which to overcome the attack on his immune system and nervous system.

After some time, both parents began to ask, individually, for treatment. It was through this that it became apparent that their son's condition was not a curious aberration in an uninterrupted stream of normality. For one thing, the parents distrusted each other profoundly. They suspected each other's motives particularly in relation to the children. Each felt that the other was a disappointment; neither respected the other. There was a deep well of enmity that had, it transpired, been there since early on in the marriage. She resented and grew to loathe his family whom she saw to be a threat to her independence through their influence on her husband. He could not cope with his wife's mood swings which were due to her difficult menstrual cycle. She complained that he would never talk to her; that he was not prepared to look at emotional issues. He grumbled that she undermined him all the time. She felt deeply offended that he would spend so much of his time with his parents, even his mealtimes, while he felt she was headstrong, immovable, implacable and determined to have her own way. There was no middle ground. Both found respite in their work. Civil communication was at a premium.[26] While they were responsive, like their son, to treatment, there was little evidence of any shift in the family dynamics. They remained obstinately grim until the family crisis some six years after that first remedy was given for the 'cluster migraines'.

Suddenly the headaches began again. This time they were dull and oppressive. They caused dimness of vision. There was unconquerable sleepiness and torpor after waking. Over the following few weeks, double vision came and went; there was nausea and vomiting; episodes of memory lapse. He became unable to complete any school work and spent days at home. He complained of pains in the back of the neck and head which were more or less continuous and had cramps in the legs at night. His appetite diminished alarmingly over days at a time but then was restored for a short while when he would eat substantially – only for this to be followed by headache, nausea and vomiting. Coughing aggravated the headaches.

Quite soon after the initial symptoms of this phase began the parents finally agreed to call in their local GP for a referral to the hospital. Tests were duly carried out and included X-rays and brain scans. The results showed brain tumours that were inoperable. The question of radiotherapy was mooted but rejected on the grounds of the advanced state of the condition. The boy was given not much more than a month to live. Because of the speed of proceedings the parents found themselves carried along on the tide of orthodox advice. They later said that they did not know or understand what was happening except that the doctors had needed to keep their son in for observation.

The boy was given antiemetics, painkillers and diuretics (to reduce oedema in the cranium). While in hospital, he developed a sore throat for which he was prescribed antibiotics. This caused thrush and a bladder infection for which a different antibiotic was given. A skin rash with itching then appeared all over his trunk for which he was given nothing (but which was swiftly resolved with *Sulphur* 200). Eventually the parents were told that there was nothing further that could be done for their son and that he should be allowed home; they would be put in touch with someone who would explain about specialist nursing care. The boy came home and was settled in his bedroom. He showed no signs of the original behavioural troubles; he was calm and pleasant in his manner. He asked to be put back on the homoeopathic remedies that he had been using for the pains, nausea and vomiting before going into hospital. He said that they were more effective and meant that he had no bowel or bladder trouble.

"*I know they don't stop the pain but they make it softer; they do help me not to be sick and I can keep my food down better. One of the drugs gives me a real ache here (he pointed to his liver) and it makes me feel tired.*" He showed a remarkable stoicism and courage. His mother reported that he had asked her if she realised that he was going to die. "*He said it so gently, when I wasn't expecting it. He told me not to cry but then he went on to mention all the things he was going to do when he got up.*"

Yet as this tragedy was unfolding there was no let-up of the enmity between the parents; if anything it became worse. The mother reported that her husband would accuse her of causing the disease that was killing their son.

"He knows I could never do enough for him; I feel so isolated – all his father's family are behind him and I know they are full of accusations. They don't live the day-to-day routine and can't see how strong my boy is – emotionally I mean. He's so changed. I'd never have believed that he could be so strong with all that he has to put up with. I don't know how much longer we've got though it is miraculous that he's gone on for well over a month longer than they told us. None of his father's family come to see him – well, they haven't since the beginning, not really; that hurts him so much. He wants them to visit; he said he felt they needed to as much as he wanted them to. It was as if he feels he could do something for them but they won't come. They don't want to risk seeing me – but I wouldn't have them in the house. They could come when I'm not there; I'd go out specially if they really wanted to come."

Against all expectations the boy lived for two more months than had been predicted. He died peacefully in his bed while his mother was out of the room. *"I couldn't have done any more for him, could I?"* she said. *"His father insisted that he was going out to work as usual and I only nipped down to the kitchen to turn the oven off."*

At the funeral both families were well represented and many friends and acquaintances filled the pews. It was generally agreed that the service did justice to the boy and his life and death. Afterwards, the parents came individually for treatment. Both expressed their grief; the mother openly and with dignity, the father with fortitude and a candour that had been hard for him to muster before. It was only after they had spoken of their unmitigated sadness that each began tentatively to intimate that they had harboured thoughts of separation. The father admitted that he probably would never have stayed with his wife if there had been no children. She now felt that her life had to be devoted to getting on with living and with her work – she made curtains and covers. The two older children were now in their twenties and able to fend for themselves although finding it hard to come to terms with what had happened. The father spoke of his disappointment at never having fulfilled his ambition to go to Africa. She speculated on the freedom she would now enjoy – suggesting that now she was able to let go of the burden she had shared with her husband of the caring for their sick son. They both talked of feeling the unbearable pressures of living the last twenty odd years together and though still united by their common grief, the first cracks of light were creeping into their lives.

Both these people had shown the depth of their feelings for their son in their loving, caring attentiveness. It was only after his death that they had understood how deeply they were mutually incompatible. Furthermore, the mother was sure that it was not just herself and her husband but the terrible enmity of their families that somehow coloured their boy's death. It was the twisted attitudes and antagonisms that had always been there. Neither she nor her husband was able to suppress entirely the well of recrimination that fed their attitudes towards each other. Yet they began to conceive the idea that life apart would be less destructive – only after they had buried their son. For the mother this came with the desperate thought that it might have been their antagonism that had been the root of their loss.

What neither parent could have known was that their son had been battling with his own version of the syphilitic miasm. He had frequently been prescribed syphilitic remedies such as *Mercurius* and *Arsenicum*, *Aurum* and *Nitric Acid*. *Mercurius* had dealt with the streptococcal throats, the night sweats, the burning thirst, the metallic taste and profuse salivation; *Arsenicum* had dealt with cold sores, chills, headaches and nausea; *Aurum* had greatly alleviated the barren moments of despair, the almost suicidal self-loathing; *Nitric Acid* had lifted the moods of grim hatefulness and vindictiveness, the quarrelsome nature and the despondence felt after hurling abuse at his parents. *Baryta Carbonicum* had succeeded in dealing with retreat from communication and a sense of dullness of the brain which had, at one stage, meant that the boy had been violently opposed to going into school at all and had refused to see any of his friends. He had also had *Syphilinum* in various potencies over the years of treatment and almost always with positive results, the main one being the increasingly fewer bouts of the behavioural, mental/emotional symptom picture. *Syphilinum* was able to support the action of the other remedies.

As homoeopathy always seeks to heal the deeper pathology of the spirit, mind and emotions before expecting the physical symptoms to be eradicated, it was reasonable to see the boy's case as one of general, albeit extremely slow, progress. That is, until the final illness. The suddenness, finality and dramatic sweep of this condition was the very essence of the syphilitic miasm in its extreme. A family group, clustered around the bed of a terminally sick patient, gripped in despair and grief were yet at loggerheads. Friends and relations all crocheted a blanket of gossip that made the boy's mother feel negligible in the world's eyes. A pall of doom hung over the home. The truth lay in the fact that the parents were never able to resolve the malignant conflict between them which was inherent in the families. The years of bitter hate seemed to culminate in the plight of this one boy. His condition appeared to draw a response of gradual change from relatives close enough to observe the events – though it came too late. Out of the ashes could have come opportunity as both mother and father admitted their inner thoughts of mutual hostility. They had the seed of renewal in the recognition that twenty years of marriage had not been a happy success. The appalling lesson of the syphilitic miasm had offered them a chance to break a mould that had been established generations before. Despite her overwhelming sense of loss, the mother was more than prepared to pick up the threads and start afresh. The father, quite unprepared by circumstance or upbringing – *"We're a family that never talk. There's no need for all that."* – remained obdurate in his silence; he even refused to help choose the headstone or visit the grave. Silence is yet another ploy of syphilism.

Truly, it is not fanciful to see disease in this light – of teacher. The terrible history of this case is by no means an isolated example. It is one of many that could be selected to illustrate the way in which disease throws up opportunities for us to seize in order to create change that is beneficial. The price can be far beyond what we would willingly offer, but the greater the cost the more urgent the need to grow away from negativity. Of all the states of being that beg for healing, the syphilitic miasm can be the darkest, the most negative, the most desperate, the most intractable and the most unremitting. To the seasoned practitioner, it can seem to elude the most assiduous efforts to remove it; it can require the utmost patience and even cunning to deal with it. Yet it is still capable of allowing a person the chance to grow if they are willing to participate in the healing process.

The practitioner does not decide when to treat the syphilitic miasm; he must follow what the patient throws up to be healed. At no time does a homoeopath have 'power of choice' over what the patient should have treated; his obligation and responsibility is to *observe* and set out to heal that which is presented by the patient. In the syphilitic state there is much to obfuscate and confuse – but this is part of the very picture of the acute disease which is but the pinnacle of man's *material manifestation* of an ancient state of mind and spirit.

To speak in these terms is to suggest that we are susceptible to being possessed by a malign energy – and that is exactly how it appears. We should not be fooled by our tendency to believe that everything bad for our health is bound to come from outside. That is the approach of the rationalists and the biochemists – who would have us believe that germs are 'out there', aggressive and hungry for life. We alone are responsible for the syphilitic nature and have created the opportunity for treponema to establish itself within us as part of its life cycle.

There *is* a physical aspect of the syphilitic state to address – either in the acute when treponema is present, or miasmatically, when we see symptoms *similar in appearance* to any arising in acute syphilis. To concentrate on the physical aspect exclusively is not just potentially fatal to the patient, it is negligent of the *whole* and that includes all that the patient may pass on to their children. This is a medical crime beyond measure as the lives of the succeeding generations are either compromised or forfeit.

In Ireland during the 1920s a man of forty was married to a woman, much younger than himself, who had led a sheltered life as the only daughter of elderly parents. The man was devoutly Roman Catholic having been brought back to the faith after years as a rake. His priest had mentioned there was a young woman in his congregation who needed to be 'brought out of herself'. This man had wooed and married the girl who, history relates, had accepted his proposal in the belief that it was the wish of both her mother and the priest. Within a few months the wife became pregnant; six months into the pregnancy her husband was dead of tertiary syphilis that he had contracted in his late twenties or early thirties. A daughter, Ninette, was born and she was fit and well. The mother and daughter moved to London, where there were relatives, and led a quiet life until the start of World War II. During the war Ninette met a young man who had been invalided out of the navy – he had been involved in an accident in which his sight had been severely impaired. The young man was determined to become a university professor and to marry this young Irish girl. He succeeded in both aims.

This couple went on to have eight children; six daughters and two sons. Two of these children died in infancy. The surviving children were relatively healthy and the family prospered. Ninette coped well but she was a nervous and exacting person who fretted for much of the time. She was also unhappy in her marriage; she looked down on her husband, finding him boorish and ill-mannered. She nagged him mercilessly. He responded by retreating to his study and working harder than ever. She was forever complaining that she would die before she saw any of her children settled satisfactorily; she felt that her husband never supported her ambitions for their offspring. Neither did she appreciate that he hoarded money when she would dearly have liked to own their own house – they lived, still, in the cramped, rented accommodation that they had acquired after their third child had been born.

Ninette developed breast cancer when she was forty-seven. Both breasts were removed and she was told that, if she survived the next two years, the outlook was good. She did survive – but then developed liver cancer, five years after the breast operation. The youngest daughter – who provided the facts of this case history – living at home, as yet unmarried, witnessed her mother 'wasting away'. Of Ninette's children only this youngest daughter remained apparently unscathed by ill health though she had suffered severe acute conditions as a child. She had had pyelonephritis (a dangerous condition of the kidneys), quinsy (several times) and rheumatic fever (which had left her susceptible to arthritic symptoms in damp weather).

The oldest child, Maude, had had her spleen removed. She had also contracted hepatitis and peritonitis; the latter was carelessly treated and resulted in septicaemia. This daughter went on to have three children of her own, one of whom was a manic depressive and another who produced two little girls who suffered multiple allergies and asthma. Ninette's other children fared little better. The third surviving child, Diana, developed breast cancer at exactly the same age as her mother. It was not surprising, relatives commented, as this daughter was so like Ninette. Diana was no stranger to illness as a thyroid condition had been diagnosed some five years before and she was obliged to take drugs for the rest of her life. She too was very unhappy, having married into a wealthy family that had a history of alcoholism.

Ninette's surviving boy was healthy; he never suffered from any disease whatever. He appeared robust and fit but he had a tendency to drink too much – though he would not have been labelled alcoholic. He was also a gambler. He never married but had plenty of girl friends. He made money somewhere in the city and no-one ever dreamed of asking him anything about it. He was a closed book.

The sister who followed him was unable to have children; she was born with no uterus but they did not discover this for some time and only after much frustration and emotional agony. In the end, she and her husband adopted a son and settled into a contented parenthood that worked extremely well.

The last but one daughter was the fittest of all the children. She had an exemplary childhood, suffering the childhood illnesses mildly and having nothing further to trouble her. She was of a sunny disposition if somewhat bossy. She was also the most attractive child with her long blond hair, large eyes and insouciant manner – all of which roused her siblings' enmity. This daughter, Henrietta, married a man ten years her senior and she adored him. He was tall, dark and handsome and a wastrel. He was an inveterate gambler, he drove fast sports cars recklessly, he drank uninhibitedly and either ate nothing or dined on rich and spiced foods that fed his duodenal ulcer. He died, drunk, at the wheel of his sports car.

The youngest daughter, having struggled with those illnesses early on in her life, was comparatively healthy. She had four children but her daughter was born with a congenital heart defect; the main artery to the lungs was narrowed which meant that she was prone to breathlessness, fainting, raised pulse rate and enervation. She did not grow well as a baby and had no stamina. She was a very unhappy little girl, very demanding and inclined to throw tantrums. All her strength appeared in the form of absolute ruthlessness in her demands for attention – her parents were entirely in the grip of her will; she knew exactly how to manipulate them. It took them some years before they realised that the fainting fits, though genuine, were also produced to order and did not constitute a threat.

This family history suggests potential material for some television saga – until the miasmatic threads are picked up and traced back to the reformed rake who began the story in the 1920s. Every one of his descendants showed signs of being syphilitic even though none had actually contracted syphilis. Ninette, the daughter, showed every sign of needing *Arsenicum Album* for her constitutional state: she was thin, chilly and precise. She was punctilious and demanding and had standards that it was hard for others to achieve. She was a 'doer' and she did. She was a worrier and it wore her down. She had three miscarriages, a stillbirth and suffered the death of an infant through meningitis, a condition that can have a syphilitic connection. She herself died of metastasised cancer after a radical double-mastectomy – an operation that bears the destructive stamp of the syphilitic miasm, however necessary it might be.

Ninette's eldest daughter suffered complications that resulted in the loss of a vital organ. She had skirmishes with death on the operating table and as the result of bungled treatment – her reaction to which included heavy blood loss requiring transfusions. The syphilitic element here may seem tenuous until you realise just how many people who are close to the miasm suffer these inexplicable incidents; as if they attract them.

The next surviving daughter who is on thyroxin permanently, for Hashimoto's disease, and has had breast cancer, also demonstrates her legacy; Hashimoto's is the result of an autoimmune condition which is generally syphilitic in origin. (The body turns on itself and sets up self-destructive activity within the system.) Behaviourally, too, she showed her syphilitic nature by marrying – and staying with! – an abusive alcoholic to the detriment of their two children both of whom became emotional cripples.

The 'black sheep' son would appear to defy the trend of the miasm – yet this is not so. Some syphilitics appear to enjoy superb health. They can abuse their system with impunity. Here indeed is the origin of *The Picture of Dorian Grey*; Oscar Wilde was an accurate observer of the syphilitic state. Small wonder that he died of syphilitic meningitis. Ninette's son is just such a one to die without warning; one might predict a massive heart attack, a stroke or galloping cancer, perhaps of the kidney – or even a messy end in his Porsche. He is too emotionally shut down and too careless of his physical body not to have to pay for his legacy dearly. (It should be remembered that, were he a patient of homoeopathy, his practitioner would need to be able to consider such things in order to create a strategy of treatment that would take such self-destructive behaviour into account.)

Julia, born without a womb, shows us more physically what the miasm is capable of. Syphilis, the disease, is capable of tissue destruction. If the gene pool can carry the memory of tissue destruction then it is capable of reproducing it in the pursuing generations. To be born with defective or absent tissues is essentially syphilitic. (Cleft palates, perforated septums and spina bifida fall within this category.) Julia, however, successfully overcame her infertility; she learnt to accept her fate and leads a happy and fulfilled life.

Henrietta, healthy and vibrant, seems to buck the trend of the miasm but, unlike her brother, she too has found success and happiness. After her first husband died a syphilitic death she married again. This man was not the dashing socialite; he was slow, steady and seemingly dull – though actually, and much to her surprise, he has turned out to be "*a*

489

most endearing and charming person who adores his wife and their two children". Her brush with 'syphilism' came in the form of being ineluctably drawn towards someone who was fatally branded with its mark. Her grief at her first husband's death threatened to destabilise her almost to the point of being suicidal…but not quite. She chose the more psoric option of survival and acceptance. She may not have spent her life with the man who was capable of stoking her deepest passions but she had the common sense to realise that was no reason to waste what else life had to offer her.

The youngest daughter 'did' all her syphilitic miasm when she was a child. The last childhood illness that she had was measles. From the time she recovered from it she has enjoyed excellent health. Measles is the childhood disease that is associated with the hereditary miasm of syphilis; it looks like the second stage of syphilis. In childhood, measles is vital to enhance the immune system and to prepare the body against the depredations of the syphilitic miasm. It is to syphilism what chickenpox is to psora. Not surprisingly, therefore, one of the results of mass immunisation against measles is repeated outbreaks of meningitis. The latter being one of the potential acute results of tertiary syphilis as well as a well-known complication of measles. If the body is not able to put out a skin rash then it will have to do the disease in another way. (One of the best reasons for young people receiving regular homoeopathic treatment is that any miasmatic history in their make-up can be worked on before they become parents; the risk of serious complications in their children from a disease such as measles is then minimised or eradicated.)

Ninette's granddaughter, who has the pulmonary artery defect, did not escape her great-grandfather's poisonous will either. She was the first one of his descendants to take homoeopathic remedies consistently from an early age. She was given *Aurum* for her moods, her lack of growth, her physical weakness and her syphilitic inheritance. The result was spectacular. She grew steadily; her hair, no longer matted and split, bushed out; her complexion, once dark and bloodless, blossomed; her fainting spells reduced in both frequency and intensity; she developed a sense of humour and a most infectious laugh – where before she would cry if anyone had found something to laugh about.

This transformation did not happen overnight. She was given other remedies as they became indicated for both acute infections (to which she was once very prone) and for stages of development. She had *Baryta Carbonicum* when school work seemed to demand too much of her compromised stamina. She went into a state of dull torpor which this remedy eradicated within a very short time. She needed *Sepia* at the approach of puberty. Her first periods left her exhausted and with an irritable bladder but these episodes were dispelled with this remedy. Not surprisingly, she also had *Syphilinum* on a number of occasions when her old, infant black moods surfaced again – but each time they did, they were weaker and more easily expunged. Today, although she still has the narrowing of the pulmonary artery, she is well and able to cope with whatever she wants to do. She compensates for her problem by sleeping. She does not feel her condition curtails her way of life at all.

One of the incidents in life that this girl will never forget is the time she had chickenpox. This is where we began this chapter and it will not surprise you to know that this bout of chickenpox was spectacular. Her entire body was covered with it; not only that but she had it in her mouth, her vagina and her anus. Her scalp was so eruptive that her hair, what little there was of it, stood up on end. She screamed when she had to pass a stool or water. She scratched her arms and legs till they were raw. It was four weeks before she recovered and it was months before the last evidence of the spots was gone. Though she had not had any homoeopathic treatment at this time (she was twenty months old) the parents were strongly of the opinion that her recovery was something of a turning point. They still had to put up with the moods and tantrums; there was still the fainting and enervation. Yet they felt that the urgency and emergency in their daughter's life was somewhat lessened. They still became panic-struck every time they spoke to the doctors who monitored her progress every six months, but left to their own devices and at home they felt that some of the heat had gone out of the situation. Once the homoeopathy began to take effect and show results, they became far more relaxed and even blasé. (They even issued their daughter, when she was old enough, with a packet of *Ignatia* 200 for those moments when she felt she needed a fainting spell.)

Summarising syphilism

To sum up – syphilis is an acute, infectious disease that:

i)   Has been established, certainly in the western world, since the Renaissance – and probably, in a milder form for longer than that.

ii) Has no known cure within allopathy beyond the physical manifestation of its symptoms.

iii) Is only fatal once it has reached its secondary or tertiary stages which are no longer considered acute but are chronic by definition.

iv) Is potentially lethal to the children of the host, whether the physical presence of treponema has been eradicated or not, because the consequences of being affected by the dynamic energy of the spirochete become hereditary – this being a sophisticated method of ensuring the continued reproduction of the original disease *energy*.

v) Can become, once established in successive generations, a 'collective force'; an energy entity that is capable of manipulating the psyche of the host (or hosts) to draw others into its web – with the express intention of gathering more power.

vi) Is the ultimate and physical expression of a negative and destructive force within man, in the same way that man, himself, is one of the ultimate expressions of Earth's evolutionary forces; both are a fantastically sophisticated 'crystallisation' of basic and primitive natural elements.

If we ignore the syphilitic side of our nature, begun so long ago, then we do not pick up the baton of responsibility for the renewal of the human race through constant purposeful change and positive development. The miasm insists that either we accept its depredations and suffer the destructive consequences or we acknowledge its presence and choose a more creative, expansive and positive path. This is no less true of a patient seeking treatment for headaches and hair loss than it is for someone who is terminally ill with AIDS. The positive aspect of syphilism is the chance to recognise and resolve all that is terminally negative. It is the very reason for the myth of the phoenix and the fire of renewal. Science, in attempting to eradicate disease only on the physical level, demonstrates that it is unaware of the reality that disease is constantly reinventing itself. This is not because disease is an independent driving force of nature such as the weather or the sea. It is because humanity has a purpose for disease and that the more disease symptoms are suppressed, the more *humanity* is suppressed. It is this that is not yet understood by allopathy.

It will come as no surprise, either, that there are 'new' acute diseases cropping up in the world that are so similar to syphilis that the only way of distinguishing between them is to do laboratory tests to see what sort of bacteria is 'causing' the mischief (in reality being only associated with it). Chancroid, for example, is a rare disease associated with a strain of the *Haemophilus* bacteria – normally linked with lung conditions or meningitis – which is beginning to gather pace in the East and in the tropics. As its name implies, the body creates ulceration; it also has most of the other features of syphilis. Furthermore, it is often – but not always – present in the body at the same time as herpes, chlamydia and treponema itself. It is interesting to note that though it has been more evident during wartime, there have been recent outbreaks in the USA and even in Europe during periods of political stability.

But it is not only the sexually transmitted diseases that we should be watching. There is a rare but probably increasingly common disease called Kawasaki syndrome that is suffered by children which bears the stamp of the syphilitic miasm. This condition comes by stealth, looking like a childhood fever, and can leave the patient with a defective heart and arterial system. With the high fever come swollen neck glands, a red rash, red eyes, inflamed throat, cracked lips, stiff neck and characteristic purple blotching on the palms and feet. These symptoms might be mistaken for measles – our old syphilitic friend! – and, indeed, Kawasaki syndrome has been known to follow on or be confluent with it. Yet we do not need the association with childhood's measles to confirm the syphilitic nature of Kawasaki; it is enough to know that it causes similar acute symptoms and the chronic results of inflamed heart muscle, pericarditis, damaged veins and arteries, the formation of clots and even heart attack – in infants! There is 'no known cause' of this appalling condition but hospitalisation and treatment has to be swift. (Though obvious homoeopathic treatment such as *Belladonna*, *Apis* and *Pulsatilla* may well be needed, it is essential that such a case should have prompt and thorough monitoring in hospital.)

So syphilis is not simply the natural history of treponema. Nor is it all that has to be told of chronic illness.

CHAPTER 22

SYCOSIS – THE STORY OF GONORRHOEA

Syphilis is only one half of the equation

It is not nature's way to allow any life force to exist without a balancing counterpart. Syphilis is no exception. If syphilis is single-mindedly aggressive and destructive, gonorrhoea is exuberant in its profusion and profligacy. Syphilis is yang to gonorrhoea's yin. These two diseases are complementary and closely related through their common root of psora, both still being in essence susceptible to playing the host (though playing host to very different unwelcome guests). As infectious diseases they appear to be entirely different and, when studied as physical conditions, they should be studied separately. (Little distinction, if any, was made between the two, right up until Hahnemann's day.)

However, neither syphilis, as we have seen, nor gonorrhoea are simply *physical* diseases. They have a natural history that includes a life cycle (the present), a miasm (the past) and a prognosis (the future); the latter being dependent on the two former. Gonorrhoea (like syphilis) has a mental/emotional aspect that is sufficiently consistent in its basic elements to be regarded as symptomatic of both the acute disease, despite inevitable variations among individuals and, in part, of the inheritable miasmatic influence. Furthermore, gonorrhoea is an *energy* and one that is both distinct from and equal in its potential to syphilis – though curiously, as we shall see, it is often at the service of syphilis for the latter's own nefarious purposes. As you have seen with syphilis, so it is with the energy of gonorrhoea – it only reaches its full potential when it manifests physically, emotionally and spiritually in man as a chronic disease state when it is

494

known as sycosis. (It is interesting to note that domesticated animals, like horses and dogs, with relatively high brain capacity, also manifest syphilism and sycosis. Perhaps it is due to the close relationship between man and his animals.)

If eradication of the physical presence of the disease were all that was required then there would be no further need to write more on a subject that has been exhaustively documented for many generations. But it is not. Gonorrhoea has accompanied man for many hundreds (perhaps thousands) of generations; it is one of the most 'successful' infectious diseases in the world and, despite the worldwide availability of penicillin and its derivatives, is still one of the most common. Indeed, through the aggressive suppression of both diseases, all that has been achieved is their diversification. Instead of just treating syphilis, now we are also dealing with AIDS and the massive proliferation of viral diseases; instead of treating just gonorrhoea, now we face a cohort of differently named, usually bacterial conditions and their complications that still bear all the hallmarks of their mother disease. (These include nongonococcal urethritis, nonspecific urethritis, post-gonococcal urethritis and non- specific genital infection.)

Seeing bacteria and viruses in a different light

"Yes," shouts the chorus, "but syphilis is a bacterial disease and AIDS is viral; gonorrhoea is caused by a diplococcus while urethritis is caused by chlamydia. How can the gonococcus be parent to the chlamydia and how can treponema be parent to a virus?" The 'parent' analogy does not work if you see disease exclusively in the light of disease agents invading the body. *See it in the light of the body responding in similar ways while in different disease states.* Then the gonorrhoeal reaction becomes common to *whatever* 'causes' the symptoms of gonorrhoea whether it is a gonococcus or chlamydia; the syphilitic reaction becomes common to whatever 'causes' the symptoms of syphilis, be it a spirochete or a virus. So, just as AIDS is syphilitic because the body mimics its reaction to syphilis in the presence of the virus, so nongonococcal urethritis is gonorrhoeal because the body reacts similarly when chlamydia and *Neisseria gonorrhoeae* are around. It matters not one jot that the organism that has found a home is a virus or a bacterium or a fungus – unless you are searching for a drug to remove it.

What has always mattered most, is the quality and method of the body's reaction once the Vital Force has been sufficiently weakened to allow such a tenancy to become established. That alone will illustrate the history and dictate the healing. If the Vital Force has been weakened in a syphilitic way then it will demonstrate syphilism, whatever the associated agent; if in a gonorrhoeal way then it will demonstrate sycosis, whatever the associated agent. (If the Vital Force is not weakened at all then it will sort the problem out by itself!)

What does 'sycosis' mean?

Before setting out to explore the curious world of gonorrhoea we need to explain the word 'sycosis'. Hahnemann is widely credited with coining this term for gonorrhoea and its miasm but its first appearance in medical literature goes back to 1580 when it was used to describe various types of ulceration or 'morbid growths' on the skin that had the appearance of figs. It was this that led Hahnemann to speak of the 'fig wart disease'.[1]

Warts are part of gonorrhoea, either as a result of allowing the acute condition to run or as a result of suppressing it. They are frequently present or commonly arise during the treatment of the acute disease, its chronic sequelae and the miasmatic tendencies. Such warts are usually raised and relatively soft with the appearance of a cauliflower or a coxcomb (if they stand more proud and with raised roughness or even spikes). The most common areas affected are the hands and genital region. They can appear on the mucous membranes just inside the body as well but this is often directly associated with the suppression of gonorrhoea or its miasm.

In allopathy, gonorrhoea is regarded as a bacterial disease yet, confusingly, warts are considered as viral in origin – there are some 60 related human papilloma viruses that are implicated. The most contagious are genital warts: condylomata. Verruccae are 'viral epidermal tumours' on the feet and are still regarded as contagious by many allopaths; molluscum contagiosum[2] is also described as a contagious viral skin disease – the raised pink papules appear on the trunk, in the armpits and in the groin, mostly on children. Yet both are usually associated with the sycotic miasm. In homoeopathy these two kinds of wart are not seen as infectious or contagious in the conventional sense; the infectivity is more to do with *the energy of the sycotic miasm becoming active in one person and waking the same dormant miasm in another*. When a child is manifesting sycosis strongly enough to put the typical symptoms onto the surface of the skin – that is, he or she is attempting to eliminate the miasmatic tendency, then the necessary force of eliminative energy can be enough to trigger the same healing force in others who have a similar purpose – *the removal of the susceptibility to sycosis*. This is illustrated by the fact that when one among fifteen children in a playgroup develops molluscum, several but not necessarily all will produce the same – and not because the affected ones all touch each other. *It is energy that is catching* whether it is conveyed by a bug or due to individuals interacting.

Warts are only the most obvious physical attribute of the gonorrhoeal miasm. Sycosis is universal and is no less part of humanity than syphilism – it has good reason to be there. So, to describe someone as being in the sycotic state is to say that he or she is manifesting signs and symptoms that are 'like' the signs and symptoms commonly associated with acute gonorrhoea – not just the physical attributes. When they are doing this, the Vital Force has a healing purpose even if it is unable, without help, to complete the process of elimination.

Some statistical information about gonorrhoea

A significant statistic is worth mentioning at the outset: 60–80 per cent of women who have sexual contact with an infected man will develop gonorrhoea while only 20–30 per cent of men contract the disease. This suggests that the *penetrating* partner is less likely to be infected than the *penetrated* partner, which is interesting in the light of the mental/emotional picture of gonorrhoea because the inevitable analogy of 'victim' and 'aggressor' arises. (This tendency has also been noted in the infection rates of HIV.) It would be well to remember this detail as it colours many aspects of the psyche of sycosis – *it is the particular condition of the psyche that predisposes anyone to sycosis* – and its relationship to the syphilitic and tubercular miasms.

STD and the law

Gonorrhoea and syphilis are covered by the Venereal Disease Act of 1916 which means that they are notifiable diseases that must be treated by allopathic medicine. This has meant that many cases that might have been treated naturally by alternative means have not been. Alternative practitioners are obliged by law to report cases or to refer them to the appropriate clinics at once. However, there are many cases of gonorrhoea and syphilis that are never reported, let alone treated. There are others, more commonly gonorrhoea than syphilis, which are satisfactorily treated through homoeopathy and usually because the patient, having heard the practitioner's advice, still decides to accept the alternative route and avoid the suppressive treatment. In other cases, the patient, having been already unsuccessfully treated by antibiotics, has decided that allopathy's failure to eradicate the acute symptoms is a good excuse to try out homoeopathy.

The acute form of gonorrhoea

Officially, gonorrhoea is caused by *Neisseria gonorrhoeae*. This particular bacterium is a diplococcus – a spherical bacterium that occurs in a paired or double formation as a result of incomplete separation after cell division. This, too, is an important factor; it is as if the bacterium is caught at *the moment of separation* – which, as we shall see, is a core symptom of the sycotic psyche. The gonococcus is deposited on the mucous membranes of the genital tract, rectum, throat or eyes either during sexual contact or in childbirth. It takes anything from two to fourteen days to incubate, after which the characteristic symptom picture will arise.

If the infection is restricted to the urinogenital tract then the symptoms can include painful urination and a pustular urethral discharge which might be white, cream, beige, yellow, green or khaki and may not have an odour (which is often either rotten or fishy). There is a frequent urge to pass water but the flow is often restricted causing a split or sprayed stream or dribbling. This is because the membranes of the urethra are swollen, causing restriction of the tube. There may well be pains with either the urging or the passing of urine. These can range from an ache in the bladder and urethra to sharp pains that are often described as trying to 'pass broken glass'. There can be itching that ranges from the mild to the insufferable.

If these symptoms are ignored or unsuccessfully treated then complications can occur quite soon. Men develop an ache in the testes and these may swell with epididymitis (swelling of the tubules connected to the testes). Prostatitis is another common symptom. There will be tenderness around the pubic area and it can have an effect on bowel function as a swollen prostate gland can cause pain during the passing of stools.

For women there can be acute inflammation of the pelvic organs which threatens fertility. This is accompanied by pains that might be extremely severe and debilitating; from deep aching and cramping with the sense that the internal organs are all dropping out, to a feeling that the abdominal cavity would explode from pressure with sore, burning pains that spread from side to side. The variety is considerable and this is reflected in the number of different homoeopathic remedies there are for such conditions.

Sometimes in the later stages of the acute disease, the patient might produce genital warts of any size between that of a pinhead to something the size of a thumb – though these do take some time to mature. If there is a large crop the patient often has an accompanying sweat problem which has a characteristic, sickly sweet odour. They can be painful and sore or they might have no sensation at all. Warts can appear not just on the genitals but also on the perineum, on and around the anus or between the legs. They can also appear in the mouth, on the gums or tongue.

Apart from these specific symptoms there are generalised ones. There is fever, headache and malaise with muscle aches and pains. This can feel like 'flu and, if the urethral discharge is limited or absent, this ''flu' may be the initial diagnosis. There then can follow a rash of red blotches over the skin which develops into pustules filled with yellow, foul-smelling pus. The patient becomes very susceptible to staphylococcal infection so it is not uncommon in advanced cases to find a tendency to boils.

If the infection is rectal there is usually trouble with defecating. There is a sense of urging to pass a stool but on going to the lavatory there is nothing. This is proctitis or swelling of the rectal membranes and can be very painful. Straining to pass motions can lead to piles. If the infection is in the throat there is swelling and pustular, catarrhal secretions of foul yellow or green mucus. The same infection in the eyes is mostly restricted to infection passed from mother to baby as it is born. This is characterised by inflammation of the conjunctiva, redness of the cornea, swelling of the eyelids and a thick purulent discharge of yellow or green pustular mucus. Wherever the infection is focused, the general symptoms of malaise, fever and muscle pain often accompany. (Babies can display this symptom picture even if the mother is apparently free from infection. It makes no difference to the homoeopathic diagnosis; the newborn infant is suffering from sycosis and the cause will be the latent sycosis in the parents.)

Confusingly, no *acute* symptoms of gonorrhoea might be present at all. Women, particularly, may become infected but show no outward sign of symptoms – yet be capable of infecting a new partner (or a newborn baby). Such cases are discovered only through assiduous back-up services at VD clinics. The treatment is the same for these asymptomatic people as for those who are producing the full panoply of symptoms – antibiotics. (Antibiotics are often useless in asymptomatic cases as there may be no bug to kill off; only the energy of the disease that is not susceptible to allopathic treatment.)

The administration of an appropriate drug is intended to remove the gonococcus from the system. Because it is a diplococcus that inhabits mucous membranes, it is far more susceptible to drug therapy for longer than syphilis which can hide deep in the body's tissues and is out of reach once it has crossed the blood-brain barrier. Gonococcus is restricted to multiplying *in situ*. However, it is prodigiously exuberant in its growth and, in those who are susceptible, it can invade a considerable area quickly.

Gonorrhoea, history and the pox

There is no certainty of when it first developed and because, unlike syphilis, it causes few obvious changes to bones (in its acute form at least), it is unlikely that archaeology will be able to help us reconstruct its prehistory. Though the chronic effects of gonorrhoea include deformity of joints through rheumatoid arthritic changes, gonorrhoea is not credited with having been their cause. As with syphilis, it is not really of particular moment to hunt for the advent of the gonococcus. It is more important to find the origins of the sycotic *miasm* which, in fact, have to be searched for amongst the history of other diseases that produce 'like effects' on the human body.

You will remember in the description of chickenpox that there are similar symptoms not just to syphilis but also to acute gonorrhoea. Setting aside the urinogenital picture, the fever, malaise and rash are common. In many cases of chickenpox the rash develops pocks filled with psoric, watery fluid but in others these can go on to become pustular and easily infected by staphylococcus – both symptoms can occur in gonorrhoea. In many cases of chickenpox, the rash and pustules are gathered around the pelvic and genital region. A common picture would be of the child who is restless and achy with sore muscles, feverish and irritable with itching and swollen cervical glands. The eyes might be sore, stiff and swollen and produce sticky, purulent matter. Just such a picture might be seen in gonorrhoea. A homoeopath would recognise sycotic chickenpox. Acute psora can go either way – into syphilism or into sycosis.

There is another disease that has similar characteristics, not just to chickenpox and gonorrhoea but to syphilis as well. This is a disease that science has been chuckling to itself about since 1980 when the WHO declared it had been eradicated entirely – in spite of a frozen stock of it in both America and Russia. Smallpox cast a blight on the world in a series of major and minor epidemics until, the official story goes, vaccination starved it of its livelihood. It may seem unnecessary to describe it here, nevertheless it is quite intriguing to note its place in the hierarchy of disease. The initial signs of smallpox were headache, high fever, nausea, backache and malaise with bodily fatigue. This was then followed, as the fever abated, by a rash that concentrated on the face and periphery of the limbs. This rash developed into flattish red spots that formed blisters containing thick, foul, yellow pus and which were covered by thick scabs. The eyes were often affected. When the pustules dried up, the scabs fell away to leave pock marks. So far we have similarities to chickenpox and to gonorrhoea.

It is also interesting that the variola virus which 'caused' the smallpox was of a curiously similar shape to the gonococcal bacterium It was an ovoid sphere with a biconcave core that appeared to be in the process of dividing. Though little is known about how the virus conducted its business once it had manifested within a host, the effect was clear – it proliferated by

501

growing massively and then exploding to release more of itself into its new environment. The parallel with gonorrhoea's activity is obvious. If we go a little further we find something more sinister.

A certain form of smallpox was a killer and it had a peculiarly nasty method of despatching its hosts. The virus could affect the internal organs: the throat, the liver, lungs, spleen, intestines and heart. If the patient's immunity was already severely impaired, the pustules that developed on the internal mucous membranes became confluent and the damage to this soft tissue was such that internal haemorrhaging could lead to death. The internal flesh was eaten away by the depredations of the virus. What is interesting here is just how syphilitic this is – and how similar to the way that the body behaves in the presence of new 'flash' viruses such as Ebola, the flesh-eating horror from Africa that appeared in the 1980s.

From this it is possible to see smallpox as both sycotic – because of the effusion of pus – and syphilitic – because of its tissue-destroying nature. This is not all; smallpox had different guises. In another form, it appeared as haemorrhagic-type smallpox in which bleeding into the skin preceded the characteristic lesions. It should not be ignored that AIDS can be characterised by very similar symptoms. Could it be a coincidence that in the year that the WHO declared smallpox had finally been eradicated, entirely due to vaccination, AIDS made its dramatic appearance on the world stage? Was smallpox eradicated or did we find another way of expressing it – so that it looked as if it had changed its spots?

This anarchic and frightening idea might seem to be nothing more than the musings of the alternative fringe but, before dismissing it, we should look at the putative origins of this appalling disease. Smallpox was first described by a physician of Baghdad, Rhazes, who wrote of his method of diagnosing it in 900 AD. The Romans, in 189 AD, already knew as much about it as they cared to find out; they suffered a ferocious epidemic then and lost up to 2,000 citizens daily. Yet it is suspected by some that smallpox first appeared in the East over 2,000 years ago and by others to have originated no less than 10,000 years ago in North Africa, from whence it was conveyed to the rest of the civilised world by Egyptian traders. The Pharaoh, Ramses V, is reported to have died of smallpox in 1157 BC and the disease had certainly reached most of Europe by the 700s AD. Hernando

Cortés, the conquistador, is reputed to have introduced it to the Aztecs who were decimated in an epidemic that lasted some two years and cost 3.5 million lives. In the eighteenth century it is said that 60 million people died in a series of epidemics across Europe. By the time the British were waging war on the Americans in the 1790s, they were largely immune to the epidemic that raged through the colonial ranks and that they themselves had deliberately started.[3]

The relationship between smallpox and cowpox is well known with the latter, a disease mostly manifest on the udders of bovine animals but transmissible to humans, being seen as far milder. It has been suggested that man's relationship with cows prompted the mutation of cowpox into smallpox. The variola virus made an evolutionary leap by finding man to be a suitable host. The prevalence of the syphilitic and sycotic nature of man could have made this possible. Yet, the survivors of smallpox, in spite of appalling scarring and even blindness, could be assured that they would never suffer anything like it again – the disease conferred immunity on its victims and increased resistance in their progeny. The same had been true of the Black Death though. In the case of this disease, there was no subsequent programme of mass vaccination so it was allowed to run its destructive course until it burnt itself out. (Outbreaks do occur even today but they are short-lived and relatively easily contained confirming the efficacy of allowing man to run the gauntlet of an epidemic disease in order to confer on himself immunity.)

Smallpox is no longer with us in any obvious form. It is the only disease in the history of mankind that science might legitimately lay claim to having eradicated. Yet if we look back at gonorrhoea and syphilis we can see that this may be a hollow victory. The lesson we keep having to learn about disease is that the *agents* of disease keep evolving and 'eradication' often means 'enforced evolution'. But there is something else to take into consideration as well: *it appears that the dynamic energy that gives a disease its driving force and purpose, makes use of another 'vector' if its original agent is compromised.* Man, author of his own disease states, will still produce similar maladies whatever the bug associated with the symptomatic results.

So syphilis (the energy), subject to as great a drug onslaught as any transmissible acute disease, can be evident by its activity in chancroid, AIDS or lymphogranuloma venereum – even if spirochetes never show up on a slide. Sycosis (the energy) may not have so reliable a steed in *Neisseria gonorrhoeae* (because of its relative susceptibility to antibiotic treatment) but it has found other mounts to run its course in the body. For this to be possible, we must accept that the disease is not bug-induced but body-inspired.

There were people who didn't 'catch' smallpox, in spite of epidemics; there were people who, though bitten by vector fleas, never produced symptoms of the plague; there are people who have not developed AIDS despite what the blood tests show. *Evolutionarily acquired immunity is nature's answer to susceptibility.*

What smallpox shows us, with its similarities to syphilitic and sycotic traits, is that disease energy is protean in its capacity for assuming different guises. We may not know where the starting post for gonorrhoea (or syphilis) is but we can see how tendencies towards its inception developed relatively early on in man's evolution. The tendencies are demonstrated by the types of disease reaction of the bodies playing host.

Medorrhinum: the essence of gonorrhoea

The most direct way of showing these symptomatic tendencies is by describing *Medorrhinum*. This is the nosode of gonorrhoea – the medicine made from the pus discharge of someone suffering from the disease. This energy medicine, the potentised remedy of the toxic product, epitomises the range of effects that the body can express in response to the *Neisseria* bacterium as well as standing as representative of the vast swamp of mental and emotional symptoms that belong to the miasm.

Medorrhinum is no different from any other remedy in that it can be proved; indeed, it has been and, once again, we can turn to Dr Clarke's dictionary for the full exposition of its potential symptom picture. (The following is culled and summarised from his essay and the report he wrote on the provings from which he worked, as well as containing additional material from a wide source of *Materia Medica*.)

Medorrhinum has effects on all three of the bodies, physical, mental/emotional and spiritual. It affects the psyche, the nervous system, the mucous membranes, the lymphatics, the endocrine system, the musculoskeletal system and the skin. It can thus be considered a 'constitutional' medicine. It has profound implications in terms of heredity for it will treat children of stunted or dwarfish growth – which is a frequent result of inherited sycosis or syphilis or both. (Dwarfism in sycosis is usually characterised by heavy, broad features with wide-set eyes, a fleshy but flattened nose and 'thickened' skin – which can have the texture of chamois leather; sometimes it is referred to as orange-peel skin – though this is not exclusive to dwarfism. Dwarfism in syphilism is characterised by small and sometimes distorted features and bone structure with little musculature, dark complexion with somewhat translucent skin.)

It will treat those who produce symptoms similar to those found in acute gonorrhoea but out of a constitution compromised by the inheritance of sycosis; chronic pelvic inflammatory diseases in both men and women are subject to the curative influence of its energy. It is useful in the treatment of rheumatism and arthritis where there is inflammation, swelling and weakness in the affected joints and limbs. It is used in the treatment of nervous disorders where the patient experiences numbness, tingling, weakness and trembling. It is called for in hypersensitive people who suffer from intense nervousness and exhaustion; this sensitivity of the five senses can be so extreme as to be almost extrasensory – the patient might be negatively affected by the presence of others who are 'not on the same wavelength'. It is a vital medicine in the treatment of those who suffer from long-term chronic sycosis that has led to the formation of tumours and cancers.

Medorrhinum, being the nosode of acute sycosis, is one of the most common remedies in the treatment of warts especially genital ones. Related to this is its action on the removal of polyps (which have a close connection with warts) both external and internal. (The production of warts and polyps is often a positive sign that the body is working potential malignancy out of its system; a reason not to be too quick with acid or the knife.)

When it comes to the lymph system, this medicine has influence over swollen glands especially when there is an accompaniment of oedema, soreness and heat within the body. The endocrine glands are profoundly affected as well; the pituitary gland, which controls the activity of all the other ductless, hormone-producing glands of the body, governs water balance, hormone cycles and sexual development and activity – all of which can be perverted in one way or another by the influence of sycosis. Hence *Medorrhinum*'s value in restoring its balance. (The remedy is often most useful at moments of natural development when hormones are at their most active such as the baby/toddler stage, puberty and the menopause.) As for the skin, *Medorrhinum* is of service to those who have a tendency to staphylococcal infections which involve the manufacture of pus.

These are the so-called 'generalities' of *Medorrhinum* – the general areas of activity on which the energy of the remedy (and the disease) will play. We get a little nearer to clear identification when we look closer at specific symptoms. For example, there is a tendency to headaches in the back of the head and precisely in the area of the cerebellum; these bring on or exacerbate the tendency to vertigo and even fainting. The nervous sensibility of the patient can also increase the likelihood of dizziness. Headaches are induced by the slightest brain fatigue. (Take a pause before you condemn a colleague for overdramatising a dull head. Skiving work with minor ailments might be a sign of far deeper water than you suspected.)

The special senses are all affected.

i)   Sight becomes blurred or hazy with the feeling that one can see images that are not there. (This is matched by the delusional symptom of being convinced that one has seen something out of the corner of the eye and which causes anxiety. There is double vision as well.

ii) Hearing can be so affected as to cause deafness yet, paradoxically, induce extreme sensitivity to sounds at the same time.

iii) The sense of smell can be entirely lost; this is particularly true of patients who suffer from chronic rhinitis or nasal polyps.

iv) Taste is often putrid or 'coppery' or metallic. Mucus production in the back of the nose and in the throat will contribute to this.

v)   The sense of touch can be acute or entirely absent. If touch is perversely sensitive it might go hand in hand with that extrasensory feeling that one is in the presence of something antipathetic. The patient might often say or feel something like "*Someone has just walked over my grave*" and shudder. He or she might complain that they feel "*really spooked*" by a particular place or person; as they express this they will often make gestures as if they have been contaminated.

Medorrhinum has quite specific cravings – one of which is considered 'a gift' by homoeopaths: a passion for oranges and orange juice. (One small boy, who had such a craving for oranges that he ate the peel of all the other boys' fruit at the school dinner table, had hands that were covered with warts, some the size of peanuts.) There is a craving for alcohol; in young people not accustomed to heavy drinking, there is a thirst for shandy. Coca-Cola is another craving though this is covered by other remedies as well. The increased desire for all things salt, sweet and sour (and the combination of all three) that has become widespread since the 1960s is very much a sycotic phenomenon and is part of the picture of *Medorrhinum*. (Fast food and the desire for it is a sycotic phenomenon of our ultramaterialistic society.)

The stomach, abdominal and digestive symptoms of *Medorrhinum* are many and varied but of no especial interest in trying to identify the uniqueness of the energy. We need to move on to the urinogenital tract to find greater differentiation. Here are the characteristics of all sycotics: dull pains in the kidneys, ureters (the tubes from the kidneys to the bladder), the bladder or the urethra. These pains which can be so severe that they cannot be ignored, can extend to or begin in the ovaries or the testes. Often when these pains are of sycotic origin, they are accompanied by a foetid or fishy smelling sweat in the same region as well as a general feeling of malaise or 'flu-iness' with weakness and light-headedness. There is congestion of all the pelvic organs with a sense of constriction during discharge – there may be cramping pains during menstrual bleed or slow, dribbling or sprayed urination. The pelvic organs can be suffused with excessive quantities of blood which has pooled due to portal stasis – a condition usually caused by an overloaded liver too busy to accept more return blood from the lower half of the body. There is water retention in the abdominal cavity and in the lower extremities. At times of crisis – periods, the menopause, excessive stress – both sexes can experience an intensification of sexual desire. (*Medorrhinum* has been known to cure young children of prepubescent masturbation.) Itching of the external genitalia can cause considerable distress.

Medorrhinum is one of the most common remedies to be found on the prescription sheet of any asthmatic – it is often vital as a support to other remedies which would not otherwise work well or at all. It will often do nothing for 'dry' asthma; it is indicated in the 'wet' asthma of sycotics where the lungs fill up with volumes of thick and purulent catarrh. (Dry asthma is more a tendency of the tubercular/syphilitic constitution. What makes *Medorrhinum* so associated with 'wet' asthma is the quantities of purulent catarrh that can be produced. This is similar to the general tendency of sycosis for producing pus and mucus loaded with bacteria.)

Another 'gift' of a symptom is very peculiar indeed – the patient finds breathing and coughing easier when they turn on their front, bury their head in the pillow and have their knees up under the chest so that the bottom is in the air. This is known as the knee/chest position and, though *Medorrhinum* is not the only remedy that is called for in patients who display this symptom, it is a strong indication in asthmatics for its use. The position has a purpose to cause the thoracic diaphragm to be stretched and pulled downwards creating more air space in the lungs, parts of which may be filled with mucus. (Many a parent has noticed that their toddler has adopted this position in which to go to sleep. Sometimes this one symptom is enough to confirm that the remedy is needed for wilful behaviour or inability to go to sleep before the parents go to bed.)

Medorrhinum affects the heart. It has been found of great value in cases of high blood pressure, palpitations after even the slightest exertion, burning sensations in the chest that seem to be radiating from the heart, sharp pains in the chest that would suggest angina and heart problems that accompany or follow on from gout.

Sycotics suffer their symptoms more during the daytime while syphilitics suffer them more during the night even though there are exceptions. This daytime aggravation has a lot to do with the fact that a sycotic's body clock is often out of sync. (In a syphilitic the body clock may also be adversely affected but there will often be a state of anxiety or fearfulness associated with the night.) A true sycotic patient will often give himself away by saying that he is much more awake at night and that he could go on working (or, more likely carousing) into the small hours. *"How do you feel when you wake up in the morning?"* is very often answered by a grimace and one word: "*Lousy!*" This should not surprise us because the sycotic is into abusing his liver with junk food laced with salt, sugar and spices well into the late evening when the body's metabolism would rather be quietly going into absorption than digestion. By 7 o'clock the next morning the liver has not had a chance to finish doing what it has to during sleep before the system is flooded with coffee or tea which the patient needs in order to stimulate the body into gear for the working day. (Not surprising, that addiction to coffee and tea is sycotic!) *Medorrhinum* will not be the only remedy needed to deal with such a situation but it will be on the prescription list.

We do not yet have a unique picture of this remedy that would encapsulate the essence of the sycotic miasm or mark it in a case that would show it to be the most similar, indicated medicine. We might have those 'strange, rare and peculiar' symptoms to do with oranges and odd posture but if they are absent from the patient's case history we need something more. It is in the mind and emotions that we find that definition of *Medorrhinum*. So particular is it that it cannot be missed – for one of the chief mental symptoms of this energy is obfuscation; so confused and muddled can the patient be that the elicitation of mental/emotional symptoms becomes a problem in itself. This patient, either wittingly or unwittingly, is not going to tell the whole truth. Sycotics live a life of avoidance of issues and hard facts; the sharp clarity of everyday life is just too hard to grasp. Sycosis engenders not just confusion in the patient but a will to confuse others.

The physical discharge of catarrh and pus is matched by the emotional discharge of cloudy, befuddled thinking and speaking. This can be very mild so that any listener might only find himself bemused by the sudden jumps in subject matter. It can occasionally be so glaringly obvious as to appear that the speaker is bordering on the deranged. More often there is nothing more than a confusion of words. Spoonerisms are a typically sycotic trick of the mind. Common terms for ordinary things can escape the speaker; he can be 'lost for words'. Even before he opens his mouth, a sycotic patient might feel 'far off' and not 'with it'. There is a distortion of time as it passes so that events of yesterday can seem to have belonged to last week. A lack of confidence in the ability to express oneself with words in turn leads to hesitancy in speaking or clumsy attempts to start or continue a conversation. There is an inability to finish what one wants to say so sentences lose their momentum; this might often be punctuated by frustrated foot-stamping in a child or giggling in an adult. (Often this remedy is indicated in children with learning difficulties.)

Medorrhinum/sycotic patients have a real difficulty in concentrating. They may start off well but there is no staying power. Here is the person who reads a newspaper article several times before getting the gist even of the first paragraph. Many such sycotics give up reading books because of this inability to focus on the written word for long. They end up reading magazines. This poor power of concentration is linked to a sense of anticipation that can become so strong as to be described as dread. The patient will express this in fear of the future, of examinations, of what someone might tell them, of what others might be saying about them, of illness, of being out of control, of being overemotional. They often complain that everything seems to be unreal. This gives them a sense of insecurity that can lead them to feel unsure of their own sensory equipment. However, there is often remarkable accuracy about the prognostications that come out of their anticipation. These people can be extraordinarily sensitive to things that have not yet happened and be startlingly right. Unfortunately there is a downside to this ability. Many sycotic people have this extrasensory capacity which, once they realise it commands attention from others, they play on for all that it is worth. Here we find mediums and sensitives. So often they do have a striking gift for 'seeing' but it is not unalloyed. They get 'carried away' by their own words, let inaccuracies creep in and say more than is necessary or right; they go into areas of their clients' lives where they have no business to go.

There are genuinely gifted people who do have the ability to 'see', the gift of the 'third eye', but if they are not sycotic they will never speak without being asked and they would not accept payment for their services. Genuine extrasensory perception is psoric for it is only in psora that intuition is sufficiently finely balanced with pure heart, intuition and intellect. Those who talk about being 'in touch' with their 'higher selves' are often showing up a sycotic internal rift between body and soul; a spiritual wishful thinking.

The energy of *Medorrhinum* is associated with delusions: that someone is behind, following – and the patient will admit to wanting to turn his head to look; that faces are lurking and eyes are watching; that he can hear whispering – which is often about him; that there are people out to harm him or do him down. There are terrible fears: of the dark; of saying the wrong thing, especially in public; of going insane. Children often have irrational fears of the dark even when they do not have nightmares. When they do and it is accompanied by sleeplessness, *Medorrhinum* is often called for – a symptom picture that has to be differentiated carefully from the state into which syphilitics can go. Many children who suffer from terrible nightmares are actually showing signs of having their minds 'infected' by television programmes. They are sycotic children in that they have a fascination for and a horror of these programmes; they are addicted to them quickly because the speed of image change and excitation through colour and content on the screen produces higher levels of adrenalin than they can cope with; they become hyperactive as a result or they appear 'out of it'.

The symptoms related above might lead you to suppose that there is too much anxiety and insecurity to produce enough energy to exhibit a bad temper. This would be quite wrong. *Medorrhinum* has one of the most foul moods imaginable. It is especially apparent in children because adults tend to be afraid of losing their temper in case they lose control. A child in a sycotic strop would seriously explode. There is screaming, crying, biting, striking, stamping, throwing things, tearing at clothes (their own as well as other people's) and *a capacity for changing the reason for the original bad mood that is quite bewildering*. They can be described as being thoroughly unreasonable, uncontrollable and inconsolable. They are 'beside themselves' with fury. In adults, if they do 'lose it', there is a lack of control that can be alarming and even dangerous. In a syphilitic there is usually sufficient calculation for any outcome of fury to be part of the desired result; in sycosis the actions carried out in fury, are uncontrolled and the person perpetrating them is not fully aware. A sycotic will scream obscenities, will spout lies, will threaten dire consequences but that will lead to exhaustion, weakness, frailty and distress. A syphilitic will choose his moment to express his wrath. It will be launched with venom and deadly accuracy. He will wait, sometimes years, and the wait will be in order to achieve the optimum effect so that vengeance in one form or another will be fully exacted – just read Dumas' *The Count of Monte Cristo* (the ability to nurture evil is peculiarly syphilitic.) If the fury of a syphilitic is not directed towards a person but

511

is due to a situation then the temper will be turned in upon himself and will result in deep depression. A sycotic will be depressed about the lack of control and what that can bring about. A syphilitic will be depressed about his worthlessness if he has realised that there is only himself to blame for his predicament.

Strangely, there are some apparently syphilitic traits that *Medorrhinum* has a reputation for healing. One is self-mutilation.

> A girl was brought for treatment, aged eleven and well developed; she wore make-up and nail varnish and already needed a bra. Her problem was not immediately apparent for she wore a long-sleeved blouse. She complained of painful periods and went into considerable and unnecessarily gory detail. The impression she gave was that she was avoiding an issue that needed to be aired but enjoying the attention and the chance to express herself uninhibitedly. Eventually, the girl was asked about her arms – the practitioner having been primed by the mother. At this she lifted the sleeves and showed deep scars and cuts along the forearms. She explained that she used a broken compact-mirror to cut herself when she felt bad. She did not know why she felt bad but she just found herself cutting into her arms. She had been doing this for some eighteen months, superficially to start with but with more determination lately. What made this sycotic rather than syphilitic was that she had no intention of seriously hurting herself; she avoided the main arteries and veins. She was doing it to gain some form of attention – her mother had married again and was seriously depressed herself. The cuts, the inappropriately adult demeanour, the precocious development all suggested *Medorrhinum*. She was given the 200 potency and from that day on she stopped cutting herself, stopped using make-up, no longer had period pains and made a good relationship with her stepfather. (Next time you spot a youth with a safety pin through his nose or a stud in their navel think of this remedy! If one of your children wants to have designs tattooed on their body you will know what is being illustrated.)

Medorrhinum can 'flesh out' the picture of a person whose 'bodies' are separated and, thus, not grounded. Balance seems to be almost completely gone and the subject is at the mercy of mood swings, confusion and an inability to stay centred. The image of the diplococcus bacteria caught, as it were, in the process of separating, is mirrored by the sycotic person appearing as if not fully 'in the body'; he or she is unfocused and distant. Sycotics tend to be artistic by nature because the 'right-brained' activity of artistic endeavour can be a form of productive escapism – the imagination can run riot.

Syphilitics are so determined to keep control that focusing every effort on one thing (and making a success out of it) tends to cause them to be 'left-brained' in their activities. Their focus and intention are geared to calculating results. Children with syphilitic tendencies are thus more gifted in maths and sciences; sycotic children turn out to be artistic or gifted in English and history. Either might suffer from learning difficulties but the syphilitic will have few problems with numbers and the sycotic will have a marked facility at drawing. In a nutshell, syphilism is cold, hard, sharp and focused; sycosis is diffuse, unfocused, ungrounded and escapist.

That *Medorrhinum* has the ability to evoke this composite and multilayered picture and to prove its worth by healing those with a similarity of symptoms, shows that the energy of gonorrhoea/sycosis should be given its due respect. It also shows the futility of trying to contain it through suppressive drugs.

Aftermath of the 1960s

The swinging sixties marked the first years of the contraceptive pill and this meant that casual sex was perceived to be less hazardous in terms of unwanted pregnancies and more fun as there was no longer the need for 'protected' intercourse. This was also the decade when recreational drugs – particularly cannabis – first came openly onto the scene. (Opium, cocaine and morphine addiction were well and truly with us already but were far more covert.) The combination of the Pill and cannabis (which initially enhances libido as well as loosening inhibitions), coming together in the postwar generation, was bound to have negative consequences. These went unnoticed at the time because those years were so superficially carefree and they went unremarked for many years after because the myth about their own youth was perpetuated by that generation.

In truly sycotic fashion it was a period of unreality, lack of grounding and loss of focus. Sexual liberation and an apparent explosion of pop-culture creativity went hand in hand.[4] The revolutionised attitude to sex degenerated into sex for sex's sake – a sensationalist, masturbatory process. Joe Public was no longer satisfied with watching the bedroom door shut at the end of a film. Bodies became an essential part of the drama. Famous bodies became very public icons of desirability. The imagination was no longer sufficient.

It was galloping promiscuity that led to an explosion of venereal disease. It also led to the hectic and ultimately frustrating race to discover more antibiotics to deal with the increase of sexually transmitted diseases. It did not take the bugs very long to become resistant to the drugs or to change into what orthodox medicine saw as other guises to cause similar disease characteristics. To avoid confusion – which is, of course, a prominent mental state of sycosis – we should look at the *energy* of the sycotic miasm (within man) in relation to the different bugs it has been able to influence in association with the acute disease.

Gonorrhoea and its diversity

There are two types of reaction to the gonorrhoea bacterial energy. There are those who develop the disease, produce a pustular discharge, a fever, swollen lymph nodes, one or two other symptoms and then get better. Once they have had the disease and eradicated it by the efforts of their own immune system, they are immune to the gonococcus for life. (This is increasingly rare.) There are others who develop the disease and do not get better. They are not able to throw it off because of a weakened immune system, a hereditary susceptibility or because they have sought allopathic help *before the symptoms have run their course* – or all three.

Since the 1960s allopathy has been forced to deal with the new agents of gonorrhoeal-type disease. The best-known is nonspecific urethritis (NSU); inflammation of the urethra characterised by aching and possible itching in the genitals with a clear, white, cream or yellow discharge. It is nonspecific because tests often show up no identifiable bacteria on the slides. This condition can be severe enough to cause symptoms in the prostate gland or uterine and Fallopian tubes. It is often the same as nongonococcal urethritis (NGU). This is more or less the same set of symptoms but the disease agent is usually chlamydia which is a curious, coccoid bug that causes phagocytosis (bacterial cell destruction or bug munching) so that it can live and multiply among the debris – an intriguing mix of syphilitic and sycotic traits. Trichomonas is another cootie – it uses its hairs as if they were oars to move about; this is normally a microbe that is associated with the gut but it can cause vaginal itching and discharge and is found in men as well. Candida (a fungal infection) is often present in the patient when either of these two bacteria is about but is unnoticed or ignored. It is as if the yeast and sugar-hungry candida contributes to the predisposition to a sycotic infection. (Certainly candida lowers the immune system and affects the Vital Force.)

Then there is post-gonococcal urethritis. This is baffling to both patient and practitioner as it is a condition where the gonococcus has been eradicated by drugs but the patient is displaying all the symptoms of still harbouring the germ. Sometimes, if another swab or urine sample is taken, the test shows up, perhaps chlamydia – which had not been there before, so another round of treatment is begun. It is a myth to suppose that once the bacteria are gone, so will all the symptoms be. The energy of the disease remains in spite of the physical suppression.

Allopaths are of the opinion that it is better to have NSU than gonorrhoea because there are fewer sequelae. This is more apparent than true. Chlamydia is relatively young and has not had time to show its mettle. It is easier to suppress the early symptoms (cystitis) that arise with its presence than it is with *Neisseria* but it is another mistake to believe that chlamydia, though it causes a less severe *acute* condition, can be so easily dismissed. It is sycosis that we are dealing with – *the energy that allows the manifestation of the bacteria in a ready host.* The results of suppressing any of these conditions are potentially the same and the complications from suppressed gonorrhoea or NSU are unpleasant and can, indirectly but ultimately, be lethal.

Treating acute gonorrhoeal infection

> A young man came for treatment for *"an embarrassing situation"*. He had been on a business trip with two older men. They had persuaded him to 'go out on the town' with them. Though he had been reluctant, he went

and had regretted it ever since. He was now suffering from "*some sort of infection down below*". He described this as violent itching on the head of the penis which woke him up every morning; there was, at times, a thick yellow-green discharge; there was discomfort from a thick sweat in the groin area. He had itching of the scrotum and the anal region. He was particularly disturbed because he realised that he should not have sex with his fiancée while these symptoms continued but he was aware that his libido was unusually urgent and he was running out of excuses and will power to avoid contact with her. He was asked if he was aware of any other changes.

"*I'm not getting much sleep because I keep having to get up to pee but then when I do there's not much to pass. The urine is quite dark and I did wonder if there was any blood in it but it looks more like brick dust. It can really hurt too; but the pain is not in my bladder, it's more in the top of my legs.*"

He looked 'pasty' and unwell.

"*I've got no self-confidence. It's not like me! I keep getting these moods of feeling really down, like a sort of sadness but I have nothing to be sad about. I feel snappy and I keep arguing with Kathy – though that could be the effort I'm making to avoid the dreaded subject. I feel so negative – and this weather is really getting me down. (It had been very wet and cold.) I feel I'm not here half the time; I can't concentrate.*"

The specific physical symptoms were typical of the remedy, *Natrum Sulphuricum* (sodium sulphate). He was given it in the 200th potency. He reported back within 48 hours to say he had spent all the previous day "*trotting to the loo*" and had passed enormous quantities of urine, the discharge was now almost clear and far less profuse; the itching was minimal and there was no sweating. He was able to pass water without any discomfort and he was sleeping normally. He was much happier in himself and felt that all his self-confidence was back. However, he was disturbed because he had pains in his head like the headaches he used to suffer after he had been in a skiing accident in his early teens. He had fallen, turned over and hit the back of his head on a fallen tree trunk. He had headaches until he went to a chiropractor who had "*fixed my head back on my spine.*"

This was a return of old symptoms and not surprising; *Natrum Sulphuricum*, apart from being a remedy for gonorrhoea, is a major remedy for injuries to the back of the head. It was the remedy this man would have needed at the time of the accident. By fortuitous circumstance he suffered a bout of gonorrhoea that called for the same healing energy underlying his head injury. Though he may have had no physical signs of the injury – the mechanics having been dealt with – he suffered ever since from a lowered immune system evidenced by his frequent, catarrhal colds (again a symptom of *Natrum Sulph.*) and it was this that caused him to be more susceptible to the gonorrhoea. (Such apparent coincidences are very common in homoeopathy.)

The pains in his head were entirely gone within three days, as were the last symptoms of the gonorrhoea. He was then left with a lower-back ache – sometimes a symptom that follows on from the successful treatment of a head injury – which was removed with a dose of *Sulphur* 30. He was very grateful but felt very guilty that he no longer needed to be entirely honest with his fiancée about his recent health trouble.

Another, older man came for treatment with a similar condition.

"I've been to the clap clinic," he blurted out, *"but that was a bloody waste of time. They took samples, told me I had NSU, told me what I should and shouldn't do – as if I didn't know! – and gave me a prescription for antibiotics. They haven't done anything at all. I'm fed up with the whole thing. If this can't be cleared up with homoeopathy I shall have to go back to the quacks and get something caustic to shove up my willy. This itching is driving me nuts."*

The other symptoms he had were an aching in the left testicle which was worse when he was sitting; sweating in the groin and anal region which had a peculiar, sickly smell; a yellowish discharge which came and went. He also felt depressed and *"woozy in the head."*

"I can't think straight. I keep losing the thread; I can't think of the simplest words. I find myself reading something and when I get to the end of it I haven't the faintest idea what it was all about. But what really bothers me is this infernal itching."

He was asked about his urinary symptoms. *"I keep wanting to go but then there's not much there. In the morning I find I can pass enough but it takes ages to come through the plumbing. It dribbles and splutters, it's a damn nuisance."*

The urine was not strongly odorous or coloured but it tended to burn as he passed it. He had noticed what he described as granulated crystals collected at the end of the urethra. He was given *Thuja Occidentalis* 200 and he felt *"horrendously worse"* for 3 days. He said that he had 'flu-like symptoms and had had to go to bed. He *"ached from head to foot"*. He felt that he had been through a fever but he was now better. The urinary symptoms, the discharge, the pain in the testicle and itching in the penis were all gone. He had *"another gripe, though."* He mentioned that the warts

517

that he had once had under the foreskin were resurfacing; there were two and they were itchy. He was asked, perhaps rather late in the day, if he had ever had gonorrhoea to which he agreed that he had, some ten years before. He also confirmed that the symptoms then had been similar to those of his recent chlamydia infection. That acute bout had been suppressed with antibiotics after which the penile warts had appeared. These had been lasered away.

Though the patient was pleased that the acute infection was gone, he still complained of poor energy and irritability. *"Which is not so different from how I usually feel, I s'pose."*

He found it hard to get to sleep and then was difficult to rouse in the morning. His joints were stiff and achy and his muscles felt sore much of the time. This is a simple picture of suppressed gonorrhoea which had been reawoken by the *Thuja* sent in to treat the chlamydia infection. When the *Thuja* had completed its cure of all the acute symptoms of the NSU, he was given a dose of *Medorrhinum* 100.

The result of this prescription was that the warts both increased in size very rapidly and took on a 'cauliflower' appearance. They began to 'break up' after some four weeks and by six weeks after the remedy they were not much more than granular roughness on the surface skin. While these warts had been changing the patient had experienced other changes. He had an attack of gout in his right large toe, he had headaches which he described as 'liverish' and he had two 'colds' during which he coughed up quantities of thick, foul, yellow-green mucus. *"If I'd known what those beastly little pills were going to put me through I'd have probably not gone through with it."*

However, two months after his initial appointment he was clear of his acute NSU, free from the chronic symptoms of suppressed gonorrhoea and he was now far more energetic and felt better in himself. *"I can read a newspaper now and I know what I've read. I don't have to go back to see what it's all been about. And I'm not making all those little mistakes with words any more."* For a busy executive who spent much of his time reading reports, this was a considerable relief.

These two cases demonstrate three things.

i) Gonorrhoea is gonorrhoea whatever label you give it and whichever bug turns up on the slide. It is not the bug that calls the tune; the bug is the result of disease and not the cause.

ii) Gonorrhoea may have characteristic symptoms but it does not always present in the same way. Like syphilis, there are subtle differences in the acute gonorrhoeal picture between one patient and another. It is these differences that determine which homoeopathic remedy is curative. So *Natrum Sulph.* would not have been curative in the second case any more than *Thuja* would have been in the first. (*Nat. Sulph.* does not cover the granulation that *Thuja* will produce; *Thuja* does not cause pains in the tops of the legs like its colleague.)

iii) The treatment of gonorrhoea or its relations (NSU) is often not just a case of healing the body of the acute. Frequently, other health problems that have been lurking come up as a result of ridding the body of the acute. This means that the remedies become the tools for 'medical archaeology'. Both cases show how, once the healing process has been initiated, the body will not necessarily stop at dealing with the presenting problem; it will continue to bring to the surface whatever is underlying. The 'holistic process' becomes an *evolution of cure*.

These cases also show that gonorrhoea is curable without antibiotics. It always was, even before Hahnemann's day. There are plants that have a reputation for dealing with the condition: *Cannabis sativa, Caulophyllum* (blue cohosh), *Equisetum* (scouring rush), *Tussilago petasites* (butterbur), *Petroselinum* (common parsley). Each of these has a distinct symptomatology in gonorrhoea and would have the potential for cure. It is unlikely, today, that any patient suffering from acute gonorrhoea who presented themselves to a herbalist or homoeopath would have a picture of such good general health that the *herbal tincture* of one of these plants (i.e. the material dose) on its own, could inspire the body to eradicate the disease. Almost all of us have immune systems that are too compromised to be able to rely on the energy of the raw material substance alone to cure such a powerful source of susceptibility-cum-infection.

As in the case of syphilis, before the advent of antibiotics, allopaths – ignoring or having lost the art of herbalism – had to rely on mercury and nitric acid to suppress the symptoms. This is ironic when you consider how close (and yet how far from) they were to the truth – that *Mercurius* and *Nitric Acid* are both capable of curing gonorrhoea, without suppression, when given in nuclear energetic dosage and when the symptoms are individually appropriate. Both remedies have their syphilitic reputation as well. It also shows how easy it is to confuse syphilis and gonorrhoea without an obvious physical differential diagnosis. Unless the physical symptoms of the acute infection make it clear that one or the other is the immediate, presenting problem, then the practitioner is thrown back on his knowledge of both the chronic effects of suppressed gonorrhoea and syphilis and the hereditary effects of the two miasms/diseases. Having looked at the physical aspect of acute gonorrhoea, it is time to see what happens if, instead of cure, there is suppression.

What occurs after suppression of gonorrhoea

A man aged forty was, he explained, suffering from the beginning of arthritis and, as his father had had it before him, he was anxious to "*nip it in the bud*". He had stiff knees and aching hips; his right hand sometimes felt weak and the wrist felt as if it were swollen. He was asked if there were any environmental conditions that seemed to make these symptoms worse or better. "*I have noticed that I don't get the pains when it's hot. I've been craving the sun and I certainly felt great when we went to Spain; I feel as if it absorbs something out of me, I can't explain it any better than that.*"

Other useful details included the fact that there was some inflammation of the left knee; that, on rising in the morning, his joints all cracked and he felt rather unstable on his ankles until he had been moving about for a while; that he loathed the winter with the cold and damp; that a hot bath and massage both made him feel better for a little while. He also mentioned other details that were not apparently so germane to the situation.

"*I feel muzzy in the head a lot of the time. I do find it very difficult to concentrate and that's getting worse. It feels as if I'm a little bit removed from what is going on. I catch myself looking on at what's going on around me as if I wasn't all there and suddenly I come to and find I'm watching myself. I have to make a conscious effort to collect myself together. My wife has commented a lot recently how far off I seem to be. I dismissed this at first but it is getting to be a habit. I'm a bit worried in case it affects my work. I can't afford to make a mistake.*" (He was an accountant.)

In the course of routine questioning certain other, apparently quite trivial things came to light. Yes, he did find it more difficult to fall straight off to sleep at night in spite of a hard day's work; yes, he did have to get up to pass water in the night and yes, it was difficult to wake up in the morning feeling refreshed – "*I have to have at least one cup of tea before I feel human*"; yes, when he passed water, it did often come out in a split stream rather than a single one: "*How on earth did you know that? Does that really have anything to do with the arthritis?*"

"*Did you at any time in the past have any urinary tract infection that was treated with drugs?*" "*Yes, in my twenties I had to go to the doctor for something like that. He referred me to the VD clinic and I was given antibiotics. It was all a bit of a surprise really.*"

He was given *Thuja* 1M in a 'split dose' – three pills to be taken at the rate of one every two hours. He was asked to return for a follow-up appointment in six weeks. When he returned he reported that he felt very much better in himself; all the muzzy-headed feelings were entirely cleared and he found that he could concentrate for long stretches of time. He felt "*far more with it*" and he no longer had a sense of foreboding that he had forgotten to mention at the first interview. "*I realise I had been unaccountably anxious a lot of the time. But that has all gone now. What I've got now is what my neighbour – she's a nurse – tells me is gout! My right big toe is killing me.*"

The ball joint of the right big toe was inflamed and reddened and he said that he had sharp, hot pains in it. These were excruciating when he walked and better when he rested and put his leg up on a chair. He no longer had any stiffness in the hips or the knees and a much clearer head in the morning. He was now getting up with the light which he had not done for years. "*And I've no longer got split pee!*"

He was asked to steer clear of any alcohol, red meat or rich, spicy foods and to avoid acid-forming foods such as tomatoes and oranges. He was given *Medorrhinum* 200 (three doses; one every two hours) and *Sulphur* 30 to be taken daily for two weeks at bedtime. He was asked to return again in six weeks. This he did and reported that the gout pains had got very much worse on the night of his last appointment. He found that the pain was unendurable and had taken paracetamol. However, by the next morning the pains had diminished considerably. There was now no inflammation. One other detail almost escaped his memory; on the day after he had taken the *Medorrhinum* he passed quantities of urine that, at first, was very dark and foul-smelling but which eventually became more and more pale and watery. "*I must have peed about four pints that morning!*"

521

His wife came for her regular appointment some four weeks later. She was very grateful because her husband was so much nicer to live with now. He was not so short- tempered and not so prone to mood swings. He was less inclined to drink and he no longer ate junk food before he came home in the evening so now he could enjoy his supper.

This is absolutely typical of rheumatism as the result of suppressed gonorrhoea. It has many hallmarks of sycosis, bar the warts – which are not always necessarily evident in a case. It is also typical of suppressed gonorrhoea in someone who is relatively healthy. It had taken twenty years for the chronic symptoms of suppression to manifest in a fashion that was so disturbing to the health of the patient that he felt the urgent need of treatment. It can take much less time or even more…but out it must come.

Had the patient not had the condition treated homoeopathically he could have expected the same fate as his father: gradually more crippled by the rheumatism with increasingly strong drugs to relieve the pain; other heart drugs as angina and then atheroma (plaque built up in the arterial walls) and ischaemia (reduced blood supply to the heart muscle) develop – these latter being the direct result of suppressing the miasmatically influenced rheumatism. In an otherwise healthy individual it might have taken another twenty years to get to this point and, at 60+, no-one would equate the heart symptoms and crippled body with the dual suppression of gonorrhoea and rheumatism. (In rheumatism where there has been *no* previous urinary tract infection, the same process nevertheless pertains. The inherited miasmatic taint of sycosis is cause enough to lead the patient along the same path to a pathology that will eventually mimic, in one form or another, the disease whether it was acquired or inherited.)

From this case we gather that suppressed gonorrhoea affects joints and muscles by causing inflammation, heat and pains. For this to happen, the liver must be involved. The liver processes toxic waste from the blood, amongst many other functions; it should then deliver this waste to the bowels and kidneys for elimination. The suppression of gonorrhoea (or the inheritance of the miasmatic tendencies) disturbs this function and prevents the thorough excretion of toxins. Rather than allowing a build-up of potentially harmful waste in vital organs, the liver does the next best thing – it delivers the waste to the least threatening places in the body for storage, the spaces between the joints. If it can, it will send the rubbish (in the form of crystals) to the joints at the periphery. This explains why gout, a sycotic disease, should often be in the toes – as far away from vital organs as possible.

After suppression of the acute disease, the body is no longer attempting to eliminate the gonococcus by producing volumes of pus and mucus, but is *still suffering from the presence of the* energy *that encourages the growth of the bacteria*. It attempts to continue its eliminative work without being able to focus on a physical representative of the infection. The result is the body *starts to copy the effects of the original disease out of its own tissues.* Unlike syphilis, which mostly sets the pattern of self-destructive processes, gonorrhoea, when suppressed, sets up increased growth of epithelium (the cellular covering of internal and external body surfaces), so that warts, nodules and tumours are formed, or crystallisation occurs in which the body manufactures calculus (renal and gall stones; uric acid crystals). It will also continue to produce mucus, catarrh and pus but in areas other than just the urinogenital tract; the lungs, throat and sinuses become involved and produce phlegm ranging from 'white of egg' to thick, green and purulent.

In general, overproduction of catarrh by the mucous membranes, causing congestion, secondary infection and lymphatic stagnation is very sycotic. (Syphilis might create abundant mucus but it would be of secondary importance to the destructive nature of the condition and there would also be a degree of paradoxical dryness, weakness and wasting and blood would usually mix with the exudate.) This is a rule that can even be applied to a cold that leaves the patient with severe sinusitis; the frontal and maxillary sinuses might produce thick, foul, yellow or green catarrh continuously while there could be a post-nasal drip that clogs up the throat. Even the eyes and ears can be involved, both producing the characteristic discharges.

Rather more chronic and serious is the case quoted by Dr Clarke, in his dictionary:

Miss X, twenty-three, had suffered chronic blepharitis (inflammation of the eyelids and a well-known complication of acute gonorrhoea) since the age of eleven. She was extremely light sensitive, to the point where *"this prevented her going into society"*; she found reading difficult and by the morning she had agglutinated lids that were painful to prise apart due to the dried and crusty pus that had collected. She had been given homoeopathic treatment already but to no avail. The man she now consulted happened to have treated the woman's father for gonorrhoea many years before, prior to his marriage, and this caused him to consider that the intractable eye condition had a relation to this. She was given *Medorrhinum* in high potency in repeated doses, each one causing an amelioration of the eye symptoms until cure was established. History does not relate whether the physician had suppressed the father's gonorrhoea or only treated the man sufficiently to alleviate the symptoms but had left the underlying energy of the infection. As the *Medorrhinum* was successful and it is highly unlikely that the child had had acute gonorrhoea, we are left to suppose that the miasm had still been handed down.

In this case, it was the energy of the patient's Vital Force, tainted with sycosis, that dictated in what way the disease state should be expressed; there had never been a bacteria to suppress in the first place. Here is a similar case:

A mother brought her son of three months old. Since the day after his birth he had produced yellow pus from his left eye which had to be bathed with warm water and bicarbonate of soda. Sometimes the right eye began to do the same thing but it never became as bad. The child was developing normally and, because there were no other signs of particular stress, the mother had rejected the idea of antibiotics or eye drops.

"*The only problem otherwise is that he can be really whingy and whiny. He won't let me put him down when he gets like that and as it's usually in the evening when I have to get the supper ready for everybody, it's a bit of a nuisance.*" This picture – of a clingy child with a pus discharge from the left eye – is typical of the remedy *Pulsatilla*, another medicine with a reputation for dealing with acute gonorrhoea. The little boy was given *Pulsatilla* 1M, a single dose. Within two days there was no further trouble from the eye and his mood changed dramatically. He became cross and awkward and he refused to feed from the breast; this lasted for 24 hours. Then he settled down and went back to his usual placid self but without the clinginess.

However, within a fortnight the mother phoned to say that the eye condition had flared again though his mood was still good. She was afraid that he would revert to his former distress. This time he was given

Medorrhinum 200 after which there was no return of the blepharitis. A later inquiry of the parents revealed that there had been no urinary tract infections in either. Nevertheless, there had been sycotic pathology in the grandparents – gout and rheumatoid arthritis.

Conditions with a sycotic soil

So-called 'wet asthma' is another condition that has its roots in sycosis (see the description of *Medorrhinum* on p. 504). The lungs produce such quantities of thick mucus that breathing is restricted. The gluey catarrh can remain stuck in the bronchus and bronchioles encouraging opportunist infection by pneumococcus, haemophilus or pseudomonas bacteria. Patients with this type of asthma are much more prone to attacks during cold, damp or humid weather and far less likely to suffer in hot, dry conditions. They are also susceptible to acute attacks during the daytime and find a certain amount of respite in the hours of darkness. Syphilitic asthma, on the other hand, is more likely to cause trouble during hot, dry weather, at night-time and with less emphasis on mucus production than on restricted breathing from tightening up of the tissues of the walls of the tubes in the lungs.

These details give us differentiating keynotes. Sycosis generally is more trouble in the daytime with amelioration at night while syphilitic conditions show the opposite. Sycosis suffers from the damp, either when it is cold or hot and humid while syphilism is the opposite (though it can cause terrible suffering during winter weather). These differences may be present in anything from gout and valvular heart disease to behavioural difficulties in toddlers.

There are other keynotes that help us to differentiate between the two miasms – some quite specific and peculiar. The sweat of the sycotic patient is more greasy and appearing on the face, especially on the forehead and in the middle panel of nose and chin, gives the patient an almost waxy appearance. Body sweat can smell sickly sweet and foetid. Facial skin can take on the texture of chamois leather (orange-peel skin) but only in someone with a deep history of sycosis. Young people with severe acne that leaves craters in the skin show not only sycotic tendencies but also a syphilitic one and the whole is a reminder of the connection with smallpox.

The digestive system of the sycotic patient is often a battlefield. There is a susceptibility to liver and gall bladder trouble and to pancreatic and spleen problems. (The pancreas is vital in the digestive processes of fats and sugars; the spleen is involved in the immune system process and the break-down of old blood cells and the forming of new ones.) As most forms of hypertrophy (enlargement) and inflammation are of sycotic origin, any of these organs can be affected. It is common to find a history of overindulgence with both food and drink; many sycotic people are, at heart, self-indulgent hedonists. Fast-food stores cater for sycotics. It is no wonder that the liver, stomach, spleen and pancreas, the organs of the solar plexus, suffer. So, too, does the gut. It has to work overtime to process excessive amounts and then excrete all the waste. With the junk food, snacks, sweets and alcohol, the liver and gut have their work cut out to discriminate and eliminate efficiently – made all the worse by added sugars and salt which are potentially aggravating burdens on the digestion. Addictive behaviour is part and parcel of sycosis.

It is not surprising that so many patients who come with pathology of the pelvic organs are sycotic, given the nature and origins of gonorrhoea. Any of the organs of the sacral plexus (bladder, prostate, testes and penis; the ovaries, Fallopian tubes, uterus and, by extension, the female breasts) are liable to inflammation, congestion, hypertrophy and overstimulation from hormone imbalances. Ailments of any of these organs can, when influenced by sycosis, be triggered by natural stages of development such as puberty or the menopause. (They can also be triggered by the indiscriminate use of hormone altering drugs such as the Pill and hormone replacement therapy.) So, prostatitis, orchitis (swelling of the testes), balanitis (inflammation of the glans), ovaritis, polycystic conditions, cystitis, salpingitis (inflammation of the Fallopian tubes), fibroids, PID (pelvic inflammatory disease), endometritis (inflammation of the lining of the womb), endometriosis (abnormal development of womb lining outside the uterus) and mastitis all share sycosis as a common thread.

It is the character of the common symptoms that illustrates this. Sycotic pains are aching, burning and sore and they are accompanied by swelling and inflammation. There is often oedema (water retention) and swelling of the lymphatics. At the same time there is stiffness and weakness of the musculature, either local or general. In addition, the sycotic patient is prone to pressure headaches with pains that are centred in the occiput and that can come through to the front of the head; there is a sense of a tight band and the head feels heavy. Vertigo and light-headedness are never far away.

Judging sycosis

So much for the physical and general symptoms of the sycotic miasm, many of which, you will have noticed, are features of *Medorrhinum*. Amongst the individual remedies for sycosis there will be a wide variety of expressions of these characteristics. Some are remedies that have an affinity for particular parts of the body – even though they do affect the whole.

i) *Nitric Acid* has a strong affinity for the orifices of the body and the adjacent mucous membranes.
ii) *Argentum Nitricum*, (silver nitrate), has more of an affinity for the abdominal cavity with its extraordinarily disabling flatulence and diarrhoea.
iii) *Natrum Sulphuricum*, already mentioned in relation to asthma, has a strong association with the liver and the lungs.
iv) *Sepia*, the ink of the cuttlefish, is universally associated with the pelvic organs.

Each one of the sycotic remedies has an individual mind picture as well and, though there may be characteristic sycotic symptoms such as confusion, ungroundedness, loss of control, anxiety and anticipation in every one of them, there is always something uniquely characteristic to identify each one. Any homoeopath has to be able to make these differentiations in order to understand not only the case in hand but also to be able to judge whether or not it is sycosis, syphilis or some other miasm that needs to be addressed. Here follows a 'failure', to demonstrate the subtle differences that ask to be taken into account.

An anxious woman brought her four-year-old son to the clinic. He was asthmatic and had been since he was three or four months old. He was taking steroids and inhalers and she was deeply concerned that his condition was hampering his physical and mental development. During the interview it was noticed and commented on that the boy's hands were covered in warts. The mother's reaction was instant – she put her own hands over her son's in order to cover them up. "*Yes, we've got an appointment tomorrow at the surgery. They're going to freeze them off. He really is so embarrassed by them.*"

The little boy looked quizzically at his mother and withdrew his hands. He was quite happy to show his warts to the practitioner and even counted them to make sure that all of them had equal attention. The homoeopath then asked the mother not to have the warts removed as this would be detrimental to the body's healing process. He said that the warts were just as much an expression of the child's health state as the asthma and that the two conditions were actually distantly related. "*How can warts and asthma be related? One is a breathing problem and the other is just a skin thing.*"

It was then explained that the asthma and the warts had a common origin and that, after the whole story of the boy's health had been heard, some time would be spent in describing how this was possible. The mother seemed to go along with this though she appeared to be sceptical. She answered all the questions factually and a typical picture of sycotic asthma was gradually revealed. The boy's birth had been relatively easy but, soon after he had been born, he developed "*conjunctivitis*" which was treated with antibiotics. After several treatments, the discharge and inflammation of the eyes had cleared but he then developed wheezy breathing. The symptoms had changed little since that first developed; he had 'wet' asthma with wheezing and bubbling in the chest which, the doctors told her, was worse on the left side of the chest. He was always worse in the winter but he was never really 100 per cent well except in the warmest of the summer weather. Apart from these symptoms and the warts, the boy had no problems. He was, said the mother, a very calm boy. He was completely placid and never showed any temper at all.

"*Actually, he is a little far away most of the time in a world of his own. He's a bit young to be described as a daydreamer but that is how it seems. If you put him in front of a television he'll be content for hours – and you can't get any sense out of him as if he's right inside the screen. I'm not sure if it's good for him.*"

While his mother was speaking, her son was sitting on the floor, absorbed in arranging plastic bricks. In contrast, she was sitting forward in the armchair with her hands clenched into fists, agitatedly rubbing her knuckles together. Her expression was intense and anxious. In answer to the question about the family history of ill health, not very much of interest came up. Most of the relatives were long-lived.

The practitioner then asked whether either the mother or the boy's father had ever had any kind of urinary tract infection. The effect of this question was instantaneous and dramatic. *"How do you know? What makes you ask such a question? How can that be relevant? I don't understand."* She was sitting bolt upright in the chair and looking almost aggressive. The practitioner said nothing, expecting her to continue once she had become used to the new dynamic of the interview. After a few seconds and a number of different facial expressions, she continued, gabbling.

"Well, yes, I did…but it was long before he was born. I don't know how long. It was all such a confusing time. I didn't really know what I was doing or what was happening to me. There were no symptoms; none that I was aware of. I'd always had a discharge, ever since my periods began – and they started very early. I was only ten. Then my husband – we weren't married at the time – told me that I had to go to the clinic to be checked out. They put me on antibiotics. Then I had to have the warts lasered. That was a bit later; I don't know how much later. Oh, God! Can this really have anything to do with the asthma? What can I do about it? It's all so sordid. It's so degrading. I'm so ashamed!"

She began to weep quietly. The little boy took no notice whatever though he had stolen a furtive look at his mother as soon as the atmosphere had changed in the room. She said nothing more and hardly acknowledged what the practitioner explained about the remedies. She agreed to return in four weeks for a follow-up appointment and nodded when she was told that she could ring at any time if she became worried about her son's condition. She took the prescription away with her; she was so distracted that she left the consultation without any of the usual formalities. On the following day the mother rang and left a message on the answering machine: *"Would you cancel my appointment on the 4th of November. I shan't be following through with the treatment."*

This case highlights several things about sycosis that are very common. The boy and his mother showed different aspects of the miasm. To take the mother first; she was anxious, nervous and on her guard. Anyone might be during any kind of medical interview; what was particular about this person was the intensity with which she expressed herself and the loaded, brooding atmosphere which filled the room. Her emotional state extended beyond herself to affect her surroundings; it was palpable.

She felt guilt and remorse that part of her history had touched her son's life with a negative influence. Even before she came she 'knew', she had been able to identify – though without any full understanding – what the source of the problem might be. Telling her of the connection between the boy's wart-covered hands and the history of suppressed gonorrhoea only served to confirm something that she seemed innately to have suspected. Yet her primary reaction was to be protective of the secret of her shame. It cost her much effort to confess that she had been infected with gonorrhoea. (The expression on her face as she thought of it suggested that she was becoming aware of more of the ramifications.) Though she now saw with clarity the hereditary nature of her son's asthma she felt confused and distracted. At the end of the interview, she appeared to be 'beside herself'.

Her son presented quite a different picture. Though he seemed to be suffering only from the physical aspect of asthma, he still betrayed sycosis through his manner. He was 'far away' and a 'daydreamer'; he had difficulty in concentrating. These are typical descriptions of the sycotic miasm. Yet he was not so far away that he was not aware of his mother's emotional turmoil. He was a child who seemed to have learnt to observe and absorb while revealing very little on the surface. This is not uncommon in true asthma; it is as if the disease is the only form of expression that can be permitted. It is hardly surprising that so many people – and children in particular – who are treated for asthma such as this, begin to show emotional reactions that were never manifest before, as their physical symptoms recede.

Perhaps it was this that persuaded the mother to abandon homoeopathy before it began. She had been advised that her son might well begin to exhibit emotional symptoms that he had never shown before. This, too, is sycotic; strong emotions erupting in others are, to a sycotic patient, too much. They feel overwhelmed by them and as they are already overflowing with their own emotional maelstrom, the last thing they want to deal with is another person's emotional baggage. This is true even when the relationship between the people concerned is as close as that of mother and son.

Another possible reason for the mother's decision was that she might have realised that she too needed treatment. Not only that, she could have thought that her husband also needed to address his history. Having come to see whether homoeopathy could treat the asthma – she did not ask for 'cure'; she asked for 'help' – she left with the realisation that her whole way of thinking about health and her past history would have had to change radically. It is unlikely that she was prepared to cope with that.[5]

In both mother and child there was a 'split'. The mother's focus was divided; on one hand she wanted to do the best for her son and on the other she was inhibited by the knowledge and shame of the background. She had thought enough about the boy's condition to realise that she did not want to continue with the suppressive treatment without something to reduce the side effects she had been made aware of over the past three years. (She knew that he was being held steady by the drugs but that it was a precarious balance.) She also felt the onerous burden of having to accept responsibility for her boy's condition and all that that entailed – including the obvious need to receive treatment for herself. As so often, confusion resulted. Many would have gone on, not because they had made a conscious decision that homoeopathy was the best course of action but because they could not make any clear-cut decision at all. In this case, the woman, possibly having discussed everything with her husband, saw that she had only one choice – to go the whole way with all the family or not to do it at all. Quite conceivably her husband strongly objected to the whole idea of homoeopathic interference.

The 'split' in the boy occurred between his psyche and his emotions. He was aware of a lot more than he was going to allow others to see. His system had settled into a pattern of using the disease to 'do' his emotions. It is unusual for a child not to be angry when frustrated. One of the most frustrating things is being unable to do something because there is not enough breath in the lungs. Asthma or no, it is unusual for any child not to show symptoms of emotional distress or irritability. He simply compensated for his compromised breathing by remaining fairly inactive.

But all this is hypothesis. These ideas about sycosis are hanging on no more than suppositions. The main reason for relating this episode is to introduce you to an atmosphere, a colouring. Both the intensity of anxiety and confusion and the 'distance and far away-ness' described are only two parts of the picture of sycosis but they are both very common and important. They are engendered by the 'split' between the intellect and the intuition that is at the heart of sycosis.

Where does the balance lie in sycosis?

In psora there is always a relative balance between intellect and intuition; the latter being able to hold sway, in good health. Instinct and intuition are of more value to *survival* than their younger brother – intellect. In syphilis and syphilism, intellect gains the upper hand for an obvious reason. To be in the grip of negative emotions such as fear, hate, suspicion and avarice, the intellect is needed to maintain the advantages over others that a syphilitic feels most successful with. In the case of a yin syphilitic (a victim state), the intellect is needed to convince the self that all the negative self-destructive habits that maintain the miasmatic thrall are perfectly acceptable.

In sycosis it is as if intuition and intellect, something akin to two etheric organs of awareness, are unable to communicate between each other especially when the person is under pressure. Things are 'black or white', overwhelming or insufficient; there is either confusion or abstraction, conflict or withdrawal. In spite of a high degree of sensitivity, shades of grey are hard to discern. The mother and son showed the two ends of this same polarity.

Though this split is of the mind, it is epitomised in gonorrhoea by the structure of the gonococcus, with its semi-divided nucleus. Not only is the bacterium split but its reproduction by subdivision is a continuous process of the same. This physical aspect, as we noted earlier, is mirrored by the mind and emotions; no less is it true of the spirit, too, as we shall see.

The brain, housing the mind, is itself divided naturally into two halves. The left and right sides cover different functions but all the myriad connections between them serve to maintain balance and coordination – physical and mental. The left side is often regarded as principally being associated with robotic, calculating, organising activity. The right side is more associated with the sensitive, feeling, artistic aspects. In syphilism, it is as if the left side takes control while in sycosis it is the reverse. The syphilitic will seize control through rules, orders and rigid discipline. The sycotic is far more likely to worry that there is *no* control; life is chaotic and there is often a desperate struggle to maintain control but the aesthetic sensitivity is greatly enhanced. In the syphilitic, the intellect is put to the task of maintaining order – and by whatever means; in the sycotic, there is such a profusion of ideas, worries, burdens and mental clutter that the intellect has a struggle to keep a grip, leaving the person to rely on faith, hope and the charitable patience of others – sycotics often assume that charity is one of life's perks.

You have to bear in mind that such a stark contrast, between the syphilitic and sycotic activity in the mind, is very limiting. In simple, healthy terms there is the scientist, with his left-brain activity, who maintains balance by enjoying the arts (and even being a fine exponent as well). Then there are artists with flighty imaginations who are clever at their own business management; both show a balance of left and right brain activity. Does this mean that all scientists are syphilitic and all artists are sycotic? No, it doesn't. Healthy people maintain a balance between left and right brain activity even if there is a bias to one side or another and they do not need to express any miasmatic symptomatology to demonstrate how far away they might be straying from contentment.

Before sycosis makes trouble

We have seen how the syphilitic miasm can be manifest in health, even if relatively harmlessly. (Remember Hercule Poirot: the *Arsenicum* type who himself commits murder in his final case.) Sycosis can also influence health without necessarily being pathological. Picture a plump cheerful woman with a broad grin framed by full lips. Too much eye shadow and tinted hair draw attention to themselves. She has a gravelly, chuckling laugh and an ample bosom. Her dress is full but cut low on the chest. You expect to see her knee-deep in children and washing-up. When you greet her, she embraces you fondly with a slapping kiss, stops whatever she is doing and sits down to enjoy your news or a thoroughly titillating gossip. She plies you with quantities of strong tea and tells you to keep helping yourself to the biscuits. This is a picture of comfort and warmth that is welcoming and irresistible. Such is sycosis before the scales are tipped into a negative picture. Generosity of spirit, when influenced by sycosis, can be debased to a grosser vibration and become generosity of the flesh, the Nell Gwynne syndrome.

Sexual generosity is a theme of sycosis. Consider the janitor's daughter, sixteen, who lived in a block of flats where a lad of fifteen, the natural son of the maid of a wealthy family, lived. She was quiet and smiling with a gentle sense of humour; he was a silent, lonely person who was only permitted to be in the maid's room or outside in the mews. These two struck up a friendship. She was extremely pretty; he was gaunt and immature. She was open and gregarious; he was anxious and lacked self-confidence. Though she had several boyfriends, she nevertheless made time for her quiet neighbour. She saw no conflict in making love to him while forming potential relationships with other boys – one of whom she eventually settled down with. Her generosity served its purpose well, for the young man gained confidence and worldliness through their tender friendship. Such can be the nature of sycosis even if it is living close to the edge. These two understood and read each other well and were in control of the distance that their relationship could run without falling foul of emotional complications. But in any other situation, where one or other might not have been aware of the limitations, there could have resulted pain – emotional or physical.

Finding sycosis among the famous

It is easy to be judgemental and disapproving of anyone who is cheerful in their abandonment because we know how near to the edge they walk – medically as well as morally. It is, after all, not such a big step between indulgence and overindulgence; profligacy and promiscuity. Many have become famous for their orgiastic appetites and while some have managed their lives well in spite of them, others have not fared so well.

Queen bee of the silk-sheet club must be Mae West. Bedizened in diamonds and decked out from her all-white wardrobe, she was notorious for her outrageous behaviour and her deliciously wicked bon mots. Knowing her own worth and maintaining a keen sense of creativity all her life, she died aged eighty-seven, far older than most other famous hedonists who were less able to control their appetites and destinies. It could be argued that she fulfilled (but to excess) a sociological role: she epitomised the spirit of freedom that stripped off the Victorian straitjacket. Such a social service was, nevertheless, bound to be seized on as permission for greater licentiousness and this is what stamps her career with the label 'sycotic' for such effulgent sexuality can only encourage libidinous activity that is bound to lead to more sexually transmitted diseases.

Perhaps the secret of Mae West's success and her longevity is in the fact that she knew exactly what she wanted, how to get it, how to enjoy it and when to stop. She knew her limitations – something that most sycotics have great trouble with – and she understood that stepping beyond them was the road to grief. She never married so she steered a steady if very steamy course. She played a sophisticated game with men all her life and won hands down every time.

Queen Elizabeth I seems to have played a similar game but only in her mind and much to the frustration of her suitors and political advisors. She loved to be surrounded by elegant, dashing and intelligent men who added lustre to her court. However, unlike the sycotic Anne Boleyn, her mother, whose rages were quite possibly influenced by unbalanced hormones, Elizabeth's fickle mood swings always had an element of stage management. She remained in control. Perhaps tragically or perhaps conveniently for her, she was always aware of her responsibility to keep the balance of European power. She avoided marriage with any eligible suitor and contented herself with liaisons that have fuelled speculation ever since.[6]

If Miss West and Queen Bess both managed to keep a balance between their practical and emotional needs, Marilyn Monroe was a disaster. This beautiful sycotic, whose pouting lips mesmerised a generation of men and caused a revolution in women's cosmetics (an area of commercialism that is distinctly driven by sycosis), never knew the meaning of balance and order. As Hollywood's major gift to the media she was quite unable to control her own destiny. In becoming an icon of kittenish sexuality, living in the imagination of her fans, her own identity was subsumed until she fell victim to booze, sleeping pills and the Kennedy brothers. This was the ultimate public-image 'split' of sycosis; the fiction of the screen obliterated the reality of a gifted and intelligent woman.

How nearly similar is the story of another queen, Caroline of Brunswick, the Prince Regent's wife. Gifted with more wits than her reputation allows, Caroline was rejected by the prince[7] because of her appearance, manners, body odour and his own continued liaison with another woman. She was of a sycotic nature and build; her head was out of proportion to her body and her neck was too short; she had a rounded face and form with a tendency to put on weight and her eyes were slightly tilted towards her temples.

Caroline was dogged by scandal for the rest of her life but, through her wild indiscretions, she did nothing to stop the opprobrium that was heaped on her. Being a woman of considerable appetite, she died an appropriately sycotic death. She developed an inflammatory condition of the bowel caused by an obstruction which did not respond to the usual purgatives or antacids. The doctors plied her body with mercury, castor oil and jalap,[8] and still with no immediate result. She died in agony and delirium after putrefaction of her body had already set in. It is quite likely that she had some form of tumour in the colon which, after her trial and a wild celebration of her acquittal, suddenly took on fatal proportions. Added to which would have been the appalling prescription of suppressive medicines – it is typical of the 'advanced' sycotic to have a cupboardful of drugs.

The split between what she was suited to be and what she was forced to be, inflamed the sycotic miasm within her psyche so that she lived a chaotic existence. Her personality, however, remained intact for she was a kind and generous woman who sought to do good and the best she could.

Addiction: how sycosis can lead to syphilism

It is not difficult to see how sycosis is responsible for the addictive personality. The sycotic is often the victim of his or her own compulsion to overeat, to drink excessively, to smoke, to be promiscuous and to spend inordinate amounts of time at parties. Most of these activities and especially the addiction to recreational drugs, cause a fundamental split between gratification and fulfilling the demands of 'purpose'. The sycotic wastes much time in conviviality, the pleasures superseding or even becoming the purpose. Usually addiction sets in due to an innate sense that true purpose or creativity has been diverted or lost or is just too difficult or too dull by comparison. Under these circumstances sycosis begins to meld with the syphilitic as despair sets in. Syphilism and sycosis are but two sides of the same coin. No-one exemplifies this more acutely than J. F. Kennedy.

To understand the shambolic and sycotic nature of JFK's life, one needs to look at his forebears first. His father, Joseph, was one of the most repulsively corrupt men ever to hold high office in any American administration. He was an egocentric materialist without scruples of any kind. He was a serial womaniser who had no compunction about ditching his lovers when he had done with them. He was, to all intents and purposes, an absentee father. His nine children all suffered as a result. His wife, Rose, turned into a rigid disciplinarian; a stickler for social correctness who nevertheless found it impossible to keep all her children from straying. The loveless home she ruled over was a breeding ground for tragedy.

JFK grew up to be sickly and rebellious. He suffered mystery illnesses that baffled the doctors. Frequent spells in hospital as a teenager, undergoing humiliating tests, served merely to exercise his libidinous eye. As he progressed through school and university his list of sexual conquests grew ever longer. His anxiety about contracting syphilis was real though his concern over gonorrhoea was, perhaps, less acute. He suffered from satyriasis – a pathological or exaggerated sexual desire. It is often a complaint that has its roots in heredity (a mix of the sycotic and the syphilitic) and in an unhappy upbringing; it is also a precursor to sexually transmitted diseases.

He was quite unable to give any heartfelt emotional commitment in any of his relationships; he used women. Though he may have been a charismatic, charming companion who was steadfastly loyal to his family and close friends, he was also at the mercy of his rampant sexuality. Beyond the purely physiological, his head, heart and genitals did not connect in any way. Here was another aspect of the fundamental split that lies so often at the heart of the sycotic miasm. The central themes of sycosis, the divided mind, the addictive tendency, the pursuit of excess and the lack of control, all reached their apogee during JFK's presidency.

We now know that Kennedy suffered from venereal infections for the whole of his adult life. Though his White House doctors treated him with massive doses of penicillin for his chlamydia infections, it is more than possible that JFK had become infected with gonorrhoea much earlier and had it suppressed. (It is common enough, as we noted earlier, to have gonorrhoea suppressed only for the patient to become susceptible to chlamydia. It is equally common for chlamydia to hitch a ride and be present alongside the gonococcus but to remain after the latter has been eradicated by drug treatment.)

However, a much more immediately threatening condition underlay his chronic genital infection – Addison's disease. This is a condition that is potentially fatal and must be treated with steroids. The adrenal glands begin to atrophy causing a deficiency of two essential hormones, aldosterone and cortisol. This leads to a severe imbalance of certain minerals which are essential in maintaining the correct water tables in the body. The symptoms of Addison's include dehydration, nausea, vomiting, anorexia, loss of weight, fatigue and an irregular heartbeat. Hypoglycaemia (low blood sugar) is a complication and, if bad enough, leads to confusion and coma. In addition there is a deficiency in sex hormones and the skin becomes pigmented. In Kennedy's case the disease was an autoimmune process and one that laid him open to infections of any sort. Quite when it had started is a mystery though its causation can often be psychosomatic; he certainly suffered a good deal from stomach problems and loss of weight with distressing regularity from his teens – before he contracted any STD.

These teenage symptoms had no label but he was variously described as having colitis, a duodenal ulcer and malaria. JFK's lifestyle was hardly that of someone suffering from Addison's; not only was he a sexual athlete but, once into politics, he was a campaign workaholic as well. Yet, by the time he reached Congress he was a chronically sick man with partially destroyed adrenal glands; a sycotic/syphilitic state if ever there was one. There can be no doubt that his frequent suppressive treatment for the venereal infections increased the threat of the autoimmune Addison's. So this is the man who was the icon of the free world. Even after the truth has emerged, the myth is almost impossible to dispel completely. His tragic death was curiously fitting. If he had not succumbed to the sniper's bullets, he would have died soon enough; it would have been carefully diagnosed as natural causes but, in truth, would have been the results of heredity, venality, addiction and medical intervention. In any case, the sycotic came to a tragic, sticky syphilitic end.

It is entirely characteristic of sycotic-tainted man to enshrine such sickness in a miasma of heroic myth. It is something that the media, always at the service of sycosis, is peculiarly qualified to do. Being unable to judge the difference between fact and fiction, then, is a core symptom of the sycotic state. In politics the sycotic wants to believe the best and the most. Thus political 'spin' is the skilful manipulation of the sycotic tendency with its fears and anxieties, its sensibilities and lack of real grounding. (The syphilitic wants to believe the worst and the fewest, so often listens to the skilful prophets of doom who, at the same time, can promise to deliver what will be of most – usually financial – advantage to himself.)[9]

An example of sycosis channelled to good advantage

As an antidote to the depravity of sycosis, it is worth while to cast about for an example of an inspiring and positive biography that has emerged from this miasm with credit. The life of pianist and composer, Franz Liszt, illustrates positive sycosis well. He was born in 1811 to a devout but ambitious official at the court of Prince Nikolaus Esterhazy, a feudal nest of prodigious music making. Liszt was a sickly child who suffered much from acute infections with high fevers and convulsions. (No doubt, had he had the advantage of homoeopathy he would have been prescribed *Belladonna* quite frequently.) Nevertheless, he quickly demonstrated his phenomenal gift for playing the piano and by the age of eight he was not only able to read music as proficiently as the rest of us read words, he was able to improvise freely. By the age of twelve he had already become something of a celebrity for his sheer technical virtuosity, and begun his composing career by producing numerous piano pieces and an opera. In fact, the spate of notes increased to a ceaseless torrent by his teens. His influence on the history of music generally is acknowledged by most of the composers who have followed him. It was the staggering quantity of his music that first suggests the influence of sycosis.

He was a divided soul. Growing up in a family of devout faith, he had a lifelong devotion to the church that was the source of some conflict for him. Liszt's career as a child prodigy gave him fame and fortune. As his celebrity ratings soared, so did the temptations – he never married but had a series of wealthy and aristocratic mistresses. Liszt found the public image of lionised virtuoso hard to balance with his spiritual sensibility. His musical gifts gave him worldly experience in abundance but it also gave him the means to express his faith; within his art he was able to live out the two sides of his nature. He 'retired' from the concert platform more than once. He took minor orders in the Roman Catholic Church and was known as 'the abbé Liszt' yet he continued with concert tours till late in his life.

Liszt's struggle with his inner dæmon was about the need to overcome the base materialism of the world in order to find fulfilment in the more esoteric realms of religious experience. He never fully achieved this. Yet, in his last years he was a lonely man in spite of being so sought-after as a teacher.

By the end, his health was not good though he had been far less ill during most of his 74 years than many other artists of his stature. He suffered from various maladies including osteoarthritis, cataracts and congestive heart failure. It is likely that he died from a heart attack which came on during a final bout of bronchopneumonia. (He was attended by a doctor in the final hours who injected camphor directly into the heart which may well have been the immediate cause of death though it is inconceivable that he would have survived very much longer anyway.)

So what evidence is there beyond the putative 'split' in his psyche that Liszt was a sycotic person? His appearance is a give-away. His face was covered in wart-like moles. This is a common sign of sycosis in someone who has inherited the taint rather than had any acute sycotic disease such as gonorrhoea; it is a following generation's solution to bearing the sycotic trait and manifesting it harmlessly. Then there are Liszt's illnesses. It is highly likely that his chronic congestive heart failure was in part due to his lifelong addiction to smoking. Smoking is a sycotic addiction because introducing nicotine into the blood stimulates the central nervous system so that fine motor control is enhanced and, at the same time, it induces greater alertness – both enabling the person to accomplish more than they would normally be able to do. Smoking encourages an excess of potential energy. It also can lead to failure of the right side of the heart.

One of the concomitant symptoms of chronic congestive heart failure is oedema, the retention of water that 'pools' in parts of the body. In Liszt's case he suffered from oedematous feet and ankles, and ascites or dropsical swelling of the abdomen. This condition often brings on liver trouble which would have made Liszt's drinking habits more of a hazard. It would not have been surprising if his liver were involved in his terminal state as he had suffered jaundice earlier in his career, probably as the result of contracting hepatitis, a condition that can severely weaken this organ. He also had, in his final months, the typical 'barrel chest' of someone with pulmonary oedema which is consequent on failure of the left side of the heart. Oedema and the swelling it causes is recognised in homoeopathy as being primarily sycotic. In addition, he had chronic blepharoconjunctivitis which is a swelling of both the eyelids and the conjunctiva with a sticky, pustular discharge – very sycotic. He may also have had gout; one contemporary observer noted that he had swollen fingertips but this could equally have been due to the osteoarthritis.

The consequences of the smallpox vaccination

Something else which had a bearing on Liszt's health occurred when he was quite young. At the age of six he was vaccinated against smallpox and reacted very badly; he became extremely ill. This event happened in 1817, twenty-one years after Jenner first began his investigation and practice of immunisation, first with cowpox and then with vaccinia, a hybrid vaccine that seems to have been introduced, somewhat mysteriously, to replace the original cowpox serum. This is relevant because smallpox vaccination is one of the reasons for latent sycosis becoming manifest in a patient. That Liszt recovered from the side effects and went on to become a healthy adult does not detract from the fact that smallpox vaccine, once introduced, leaves its indelible mark on the whole system. The acute side effects would have been the body's immediate reaction to the *material substance* of the disease matter but the *energy of the toxin* and its effects on the body's Vital Force would not have been removed so easily. It could lie dormant for many years, unable to create malignant changes to an otherwise balanced system but it would eventually manifest in some pathological condition.

Depending on the individual and his susceptibilities, the pathological effects might become anything from chronic headaches with high blood pressure to severe and even crippling rheumatism. Countless patients who have suffered from respiratory disorders that complicated heart pathology or from the growth of tumours, probably owe the triggering of their condition to having been vaccinated. So strongly is the link forged between what the great homoeopath, Dr James Compton-Burnett, called vaccinosis (the systemic poisoning through the introduction directly into the blood stream of smallpox toxins) and sycosis, which Hahnemann had been at such pains to describe just less than a century before, that it becomes imperative to understand how the smallpox vaccine has complicated our lives.

There are several sources of evidence for this premise over and above the clinical evidence of patients who reported their adverse reactions to being vaccinated. None have been investigated by anyone other than homoeopaths because the evidence is circumstantial and clinic-based. (It is hardly likely that science would subject artificial immunisation, one of the most hallowed tenets of contemporary allopathic medical philosophy, to critical examination in the light of hearsay evidence.) Nevertheless, the information cannot be ignored as it tells us so much about the health state of most of the population of the world – even so many years after vaccination was abandoned. The evidence comes from the knowledge of:

i) the remedy made from smallpox itself, *Variolinum*,
ii) the remedy made from the vaccine that Jenner and his colleagues developed, vaccinia, and
iii) the remedy made from *Thuja occidentalis*, a conifer tree that has proved of inestimable value in its ability to reduce the acute and chronic side effects of vaccinosis.

Of these three, only *Thuja* has received a full and exhaustive proving; with the others we are reliant on reports of cases cured by their administration in homoeopathic potencies.

Variolinum,[10] the smallpox nosode, is chiefly thought of as one of the remedies for clearing up the last symptoms of shingles – the nerve pains, the scars and discoloration of the eruptions. It is also useful in herpes cases with similar, recalcitrant symptoms. That it should be able to do this suggests yet another link between syphilism and sycosis as well as confirming the connection between smallpox, herpes and varicella-zoster. The deeper link with psora is not missing either. *Variolinum* will cause the healing of psoric skin conditions such as clusters of dry, red, raised pimples which itch like fury. It is in the mind that *Variolinum* shows its affinity with sycosis; there is confusion even to the point of feeling that one will go crazy.

Vaccininum, made from vaccine material, has many similar features including a very characteristic symptom of smallpox – a chronic backache with pains in the lumbar region that make the patient feel the back is breaking. Its most obvious connection with sycosis is in the skin symptoms it is capable of initiating: 'Eruption of pustules with a dark red base…filled with pus of a greenish yellow colour…' though the mind symptoms are close to sycosis too: 'Crying. Ill humour with restless sleep. Nervous, impatient, irritable; disposition to be troubled by things.' (Even its headache is sycotic in that it feels as if the head is split right down the middle.)

Thuja occidentalis

It is with *Thuja occidentalis* that we come to the very heart of sycosis. Nature has provided a living energy, in tree form, of this miasm. When *Thuja* is made into a remedy it is capable of treating a vast range of states though, as always in homoeopathic remedies, there is a unique unvarying core of characteristics by which it can be recognised. Why it should be that a rather unassuming tree from the swamps of Pennsylvania is indispensable to the healing of so many varied ills, is a mystery. Yet its physical attributes and life history mirror so many of the aspects of sycosis:

i)   sycotic patients feel worse in damp and chilly places while *Thuja* loves cold swamps;

ii) sycotics tend to be 'water retentive' and so does *Thuja*;

iii) the cones of *Thuja* resemble a mass of green warts and sycotic patients may produce crops of warts and, though they are not green, often the urethral discharge that might be an accompanying symptom is.

We owe its discovery as a remedy to Hahnemann who came across it in a rather particular way. He was consulted by a young noviciate in some distress and embarrassment. He complained of a urethral discharge which was pale green and thick in consistency. Before Hahnemann could ask any questions that might have called the young man's morals into doubt, the monk emphatically denied that he had ever had any relations with a woman as he was strictly celibate. Hahnemann, taking his patient at his word, questioned him on every aspect of his health but he was unable to discover any reason for the condition. Hahnemann invited himself round to the monastery to spend a day with the patient so that he could observe at first hand the novice's daily life. Nothing of any note occurred until the young man took his usual postprandial stroll around the monastery gardens. Then Hahnemann noticed that his patient, on passing a thuja tree, plucked off a bit of foliage and began to chew it. This was enough for Hahnemann. He told the patient to desist from chewing; the young man's problem was cured completely. Hahnemann then made a remedy of the tree and he set up a proving of it which is the basis of one of the cornerstones of homoeopathic prescribing. Not only did Hahnemann discover that *Thuja* is the epitome of sycosis but he realised that it is also an invaluable remedy in all the other miasms as well.

Having been given the clue to its use in gonorrhoea and suppressed (chronic) gonorrhoea by the noviciate's urethral discharge, Hahnemann went on to show that *Thuja* is capable of stimulating a system into healing both the acute and the chronic symptoms of the disease. Not only will the characteristic discharge be removed but also the fishy smelling sweat, the cauliflower or coxcomb warts which can tend to bleed easily, the glandular swelling, the headaches, the anxiety, the nervousness and the impoverished memory and intellect will all be healed by *Thuja*.

That is not all. Hahnemann's acolytes and others after them realised the enormous importance of using *Thuja* to heal the side effects of the continued practice of vaccination. This may have started with the successful use of *Thuja* during a smallpox epidemic by a German homoeopath called Boenninghausen. Others followed his example, confirming *Thuja*'s curative power over this terrible disease. Then Dr James Compton-Burnett made the discovery that vaccinations did not need to 'take' (i.e. to show a marked skin reaction) for vaccinosis to be established. He wrote that 'not a few persons date their ill health from a so-called unsuccessful vaccination'. To us this means very little as the practice is now abandoned but, at the time, it was considered better that a patient should show a skin reaction at the site of the vaccination and, if there were none, it was seen as a sign that the patient had not been effectively immunised.

What is incontrovertible is that vaccination was the practice of introducing toxic disease material directly into the bloodstream by placing the infected serum onto a surface scratch on the skin. Homoeopaths quickly discovered that *Thuja* had the effect of eradicating the side effects of this action; not only were skin reactions – which included pustular swellings – swiftly dealt with but also internal symptoms as well. These internal symptoms were many and varied. They included – and we quote Dr Clarke – 'neuralgias (of which [Dr] Burnett gives many examples), morbid skin disorders, indigestion and constipation; warts and new growths of many kinds.' Burnett described his use of *Thuja* for many cases of vaccination poisoning and the symptoms that resulted: paralysis of the left side of the body, with hypertrophy of the spleen; breast lumps; angina; lipoma (fatty tumours); rheumatism. In one case Burnett was called on to treat a ten-week-old baby whom he found to be 'ghastly white and in collapse'. The infant had been breastfed by a wet nurse who, just the day before, had been revaccinated at the Marylebone Workhouse; her arm was painful, swollen and had a pustular eruption at the site of the vaccination. Burnett concluded that the boy was sucking in the vaccinal poisoning with the nurse's milk. He had no proof, of course, as this was the 1890s and there were no lab tests to confirm such a theory. It was just as well for the patient that Burnett prescribed on his hunch, as *Thuja* 6, given to nurse and baby, swiftly cured them both.

In homoeopathy it is universally accepted that the introduction of smallpox disease material into the bloodstream was extremely detrimental to the health. It set up chronic disease that was related both to the symptom picture of smallpox as well as to other, less well-defined states that did not appear in any descriptive medical text but were recognisably connected to the sycotic miasm. *Thuja* is one of the most commonly used remedies and is fundamental to any practitioner's work; the fact that it still occupies that place in the homoeopathic pharmacopoeia suggests that vaccination, even so long after it became obsolete, still casts its shadow down the generations.

Though it is not an official statistic, it is worth mentioning that many patients whose parents spent time abroad and were often given multiple vaccinations, come with complaints that require *Thuja* as a first prescription – or, if that is not given initially, it is often needed before any pathology will yield to treatment – to clear the vaccine dyscrasia. This suggests that vaccination has a hereditary effect. This should not surprise us as to have a disease imparts natural immunity not just to the sufferer but to the following generations; we learn the evolutionary art of becoming immune. Vaccination against smallpox was an *unnatural* method of acquiring a disease – as it was introduced directly into the bloodstream – and the shock to the system that this created would have been enough to be registered by the gene pool. Vaccination became a secondary miasm, a hereditary disease taint and one that complicated and set off the major one of sycosis.

More than a few people who were vaccinated died as a result. It is well documented that many had side effects that ranged from the minor to the severe and survived – but with impaired health. It is also known from reported cases that others, who had a *natural* immunity to smallpox after being given homoeopathic immunisation (*Variolinum* or *Vaccininum*), threw off the *material* dose vaccination at once or, if not, were relieved of the side effects by either *Thuja, Vaccininum* or *Variolinum*. What needs to be understood is that, even though patients might have recovered from the side effects of the vaccine *material*, their physical and mental bodies did *not* throw off the *disease energy of the vaccine* – which, after all, was a form of smallpox – unless they were given homoeopathic remedies. Remember the habit of dormancy displayed by diseases related to smallpox.

Vaccine damage (the symptomatic result of vaccination) was only the initial set of symptoms – and it was always unique to the individual, with some producing skin reactions and others not, but all eventually producing internal ones; the *chronic* effects followed later when the system was weakened by the excesses of the sycotic miasm. So, the energy of the vaccine toxin is kept from causing any observable chronic disease effects by an otherwise healthy constitution; it would have to wait till time and the awakened sycotic miasm began to tell on the system. Though Liszt, who was so *acutely* ill as a result of vaccination, was an inveterate smoker, it remains a moot point whether he might have enjoyed a longer old age had he been given *Thuja* to relieve his system of the vaccine dyscrasia early on in his life. What is certain is that many of his disease symptoms were characteristic of sycosis complicated by the smallpox vaccine. What is equally sure is that *Thuja* is among the indispensable remedies in dealing with the effects of artificial immunisation right up to today.

Thuja, however, is about more than correcting the imbalance created by vaccination and much more than its ability to galvanise the body into throwing out gonorrhoea and its noxious, degenerate disease relations. *Thuja* is, possibly, the first remedy that homoeopaths come across that can be prescribed for nonmedical conditions; this is as paradoxical as the energy of the medicine itself and needs a careful explanation.

Thuja's role in discouraging developmental stagnation

We are brought up to believe that medicines exist solely to heal the symptoms of the sick. With this premise goes the negative reaction of expecting that the need for medicines implies that something is pathologically wrong with the body or the mind – or both. This leaves medical practitioners, orthodox or alternative, facing patients who expect their problems to be taken away. If they are more enlightened, the patients know they have to take responsibility for their own health but nevertheless feel that their symptoms have to be shed as if they were an unwelcome impediment. Yet, so often, *symptoms reflect a state of being that is indicative of a patient's growth and development.* They can come and go according to the ability of the patient to deal with life – and only become pathology when there is stagnation. This stagnation might be due to many causes – such as parental control, lack of confidence, not wanting to grow up, even a mechanical trauma – but the effect is to hold the patient in circumstances that prevent the steady growth of creative potential. Whatever the cause of the stagnation, the result will be a sense of unease that has to do with the person sensing – probably without being able to articulate it – that he or she is 'on the wrong path'. This unease need not be *dis-ease* – though that would follow if no change were initiated. So this point of not moving forward can be a precursor to illness but it is treatable before illness occurs.

Thuja is often prescribed for just that condition where a person is at an impasse and unable to create sufficient change in life to spark off the creative or developmental fire. Such a person might come with a range of *mental and emotional attitudes* rather than *symptoms* per se. As often as not, one of the first things that they say is, "*I'm a bit of a fraud really as there's nothing actually wrong with me.*" They might add, "*I should be seeing a counsellor rather than a homoeopath!*" Whatever they may say, they are asking for help to make changes that will be self-motivated and potentially creative.

In the course of an interview with such a patient it is common to find that they have been feeling out of harmony with themselves – "*I've not been myself lately.*" It is not unheard of for this simple sentence to be the sole reason for prescribing *Thuja* – if there are no other indications. Though many remedies, especially sycotic ones, also cover this feeling, it is *Thuja* that has it in spades and that is so often needed when not much else of a symptom picture is available. A good confirming – if leading – question is, "*Do you feel as though you are at a crossroads and the signposts have been removed?*" The answer, when *Thuja* is needed, is so often, "*Yes, that's exactly it!*"

The sense of unease that *Thuja's* energy can unlock in a person is only the earliest of warning signs. *Thuja's* capacity for creating and curing symptoms that only start here but go on to far more worrying conditions, is prodigious. One step on from unease is feeling ungrounded and lacking in direction. Then there is lack of concentration with easy distraction – because the mind is elsewhere with either anxieties or daydreams. There is an inability to make decisions and a consequent feeling of inadequacy. This leads to a feeling that one's livelihood is threatened as one cannot keep up with the pressure of having to make important decisions everyday.

This is frequently followed by *Thuja's* darker side – the need to cover one's tracks. Where any shortcomings are evident a *Thuja* will seek to hide them and often by subterfuge. This is especially common within relationships. The person is unable to face the consequences – as they see them – of telling the truth whenever a difficulty arises. So they fib or evade. Scott's wry lines: 'O, what a tangled web we weave, When first we practise to deceive!' so often aptly describe a *Thuja* patient's dilemma. Indeed, it is common enough for a *Thuja* patient to attempt to conceal – even unwittingly – all sorts of information from the practitioner which leaves the latter with the feeling that there is no core or top and tail to the case. It is not unknown for homoeopaths to prescribe *Thuja* intuitively on this nebulous sense that the patient has eluded being identified by their remedy energy state.

If a homoeopath were to see fifteen new patients who were not suffering any particular pathology, it is quite likely that at least three, perhaps even four of them would need *Thuja* as a first prescription. They would come with a sense of anxiety and inner unrest; they might find eye contact quite difficult; there would be a difficulty in expressing exactly what they wanted to say and even a doubt as to what they actually meant. There might be a feeling that they were out of touch with what they regarded as their normal context; with this would go a hesitancy and a loss of confidence. They might trip up over words or forget an everyday word or expression. They might start a sentence and not know how to follow through with the ideas they wanted to express and then end up with *"Well, you know what I mean."* The mental confusion would be hard to disguise.

Confusion is as central to *Thuja's* energy as it is to *Medorrhinum's*. One of the ways that this is manifest in terms of mental symptoms is 'fixed ideas'. A *Thuja* patient will often have attitudes or opinions that are unchangeable. They are often based in routine or tradition. Thought processes are thus dictated by habit. The reason for this is that habit creates stability amidst confusion. It is not unusual for a *Thuja* businessman to be very capable in the office – the habit of being efficient does not fail him – but once outside the office he becomes very uncertain about what he is really doing.

Many a spouse has complained that their partner obstinately continued to believe that black was white – because to change would mean that the edifice of the past would begin to crumble. A countersymptom to this is vagueness. *"Oh, do you think so? I'm sure I don't know." This is a favourite answer of the Thuja* patient as to give a definite answer might lead to making decisions or holding definite opinions they would have to defend. *Thuja* always wants time to become certain – a condition that obstinately eludes it.

Having a 'bee in one's bonnet' is also part of the 'fixed ideas' syndrome. A favourite theme is that those in authority have 'a thing' against one. Imagined criticism and slights can assume enormous proportions with inhibiting results. This is a very simple version of the frankly psychotic. One step further on, *Thuja* is known for dealing with such curiosities as:

i) 'as if a strange person were at his side'
ii) 'as if the body, especially the limbs, were made of glass and would break easily'[11]
iii) 'as if an animal were living in the abdomen'
iv) 'as if the whole body would be dissolved'[12]

It is not uncommon for patients to express their strange feeling that they are watching themselves. *"It's as if I'm not really doing what I'm doing, I'm sort of observing me going through the motions."* Some people have a curious sensation when looking in the mirror; they see themselves, from outside, looking at themselves – a three-way mirror, in effect.

It is not surprising that *Thuja* should be so important in the treatment of dyslexia and dyspraxia (the inability to coordinate well), conditions that are not, strictly speaking, medical; they are not diseases. These disorders, which so inhibit conventional learning, engender the most profound confusion. Dyslexics and dyspraxics find that the world is not as they experience it and they are unable to make the same sense of it as their peers and they can see that they are different when they compare themselves with others. This is ample reason for these children (and adults) to remain in confusion; they are separated from whom they feel they really are. As a result, many of them attempt – and often very successfully – to compensate for their 'mistakes' by covering up, avoiding what they can't achieve and concentrating on what they know they *can* do. The strain of maintaining these compromises is a limitation on the resources of the Vital Force. So, many such people go through a catalogue of acute childhood conditions involving ears, throat, tonsils and bladder; headaches and bowel problems are not uncommon either. What the mind and emotions cannot deal with must be expressed by the physical body and with *Thuja* the immune system is put under considerable strain.

The emotional picture of *Thuja* is not easily expressed unless there is an acute crisis, major or minor. The subject can be overexcitable and easily stimulated to the point of agitation yet will not reveal this unless anger or despair is reached. Every little thing is the occasion for worry and anxiety. Thujas are great planners for disasters even to the point of making provision for the failure of contingency plans. The subject of such effort might be making sure that someone will be around to pay the window cleaner but, at the other end of the spectrum, can be exemplified by those who would instal a nuclear shelter in their gardens in case of a catastrophe.

There is anything from both moroseness and whining ill temper – *Thuja* children are forever saying things are 'unfair' – to sadness and suicidal despair. There is a distinct unwillingness to become involved in intellectual activity; it costs too much energy. The mind wanders off too much to be able to sustain any threads of thought unless they are the subject of anxiety.

Thoughtlessness and forgetfulness mean that many parents say their children are selfish and unwilling to help out with even the simplest household activities. They do not make their beds or offer to help wash up. They do not clear away their plates or brush their shoes. All this may well be good, old-fashioned sloth but, if so, it belongs in the house where there is little parental discipline. If *Thuja* is needed then it does not make any difference how much discipline there is. No amount of threatening to cut off pocket money or leave the ice cream in the freezer will change the pattern. The patient is unaware of *how* to change. In fact, there can be genuine distress that they cannot find a way of complying with the rules of the house. There is parental disbelief that any effort is being made at all; this is a pity as it shows a lack of realisation that there is a genuine problem. This leads to frustration and misunderstanding on both sides and provides fuel for bitter feelings for years to come. The truth is that *Thuja* patients often have a real difficulty in being able to *reflect*. They may well understand things perfectly clearly with hindsight; it is too late to change what has happened. This is not so far from the learning and reading problems of the dyslexic; understanding with hindsight is somewhat similar to reading backwards.[13]

Thuja patients may become adept at covering their tracks but they make a habit of tripping themselves up. Take as an example the mildly dyslexic boy who cannot finish his homework in time if he works from his own notes; he copies what another boy has done not realising that he is copying the same spelling mistakes that are characteristic of his friend. When the teacher faces him with it, the boy denies what he so obviously has done – thus making matters worse by stoking the teacher's irritation as well as disappointment. "*It wasn't me, miss*" is another phrase that hovers about the lips of *Thuja* patients. What they suffer, though, is self-mortification because they did not really want to be blatantly dishonest – not least because they now see how quickly they have been found out – and they no longer have the chance to put it right. They find it difficult to project into the future and predict what the good consequences would be of their making a full confession and a genuine apology – often for things they did without any prior understanding of wrongdoing. Like the dyslexic's reading ability, they can see backwards but not so easily forwards at how they can create positive change for good.

Thuja people, of another hue, can project their confusion onto others. Being able to disguise their own problems with a facade of congeniality or seriousness, spurious confidence or downright officiousness, they are able to convince other people of their own 'rightness'. Politicians often labour under the *Thuja* yoke – either it encourages them to go into politics, or political intrigue influences their energies so that they go in a *Thuja* direction. Politics beyond the hustings and the Houses of Parliament is also *Thuja* territory; its energy is manifest wherever there is manipulation and devious persuasion – in the office, the boardroom and the bedroom. Other remedy states have similarly malign energy but none so adept at attempting to fix things to the manipulators' best advantage – the purpose always being *to secure the ground on which they stand*. The primary purpose of all those in need of *Thuja* is to be fixed and steady. This is because, whether the patient is a 'victim' type or otherwise, *Thuja* is a state of being stuck, of being unable to progress while in a false position that was either handed on to them by parental or scholastic influence or imposed by familial tradition. It is a place of doubt and doubting. It is a state of being caught between two (or more) conditions or influences that may be either intrinsic or of external origin.

This point is neatly illustrated by the physical aspect. *Thuja* is the primary indicated remedy in those who suffer from the alternation between asthma and eczema. First one condition will arise and, when it is either better or suppressed, the other will come up. A prescription of *Thuja* will often limit this alternation and lead to a state where the practitioner can deal with the underlying causative miasm of both diseases – which will be either tuberculism, sycosis or psora (or, quite likely these days, all three).[14]

In psychosis, *Thuja* is a frequently needed remedy. This is just as true for severe cases, where there are mental aberrations, as it is for milder forms such as depression that might be temporary. One very common situation is postnatal depression. Another is the menopause. However, any change might tip a person into needing *Thuja* if that change makes them aware of their insecurities, their fragility and their lack of perspective.

Moving house, changing jobs or grieving can all bring out the *Thuja* in us – though it is only those events that have negative connotations that might dull our powers of reflection and cause us to feel 'out of place' or distanced from our norms. With the sense of doubt, the frailty, the lack of grounding goes the sense of *separation* from normality, routine and the familiar.

Antidepressants and sleeping pills create a need of *Thuja* for they separate the patient from the normality of their unwellness. The drugs suppress the symptoms that, however distressing, are the patient's *reality in disease*. Many patients who are keen to come off their psychotic drugs are fearful they will return to their original complaint and suffer their own symptoms again. They go into a state of confusion and distress that is often greatly eased by *Thuja* – even while they are still on the offending drug. It is as if the drug has removed them to a curious limbo of partial 'nonfeeling' and the initial response to the administration of *Thuja* gives some integrity back to the nervous system so the split from reality is partially healed. If the patient is weaned off their drug it is likely that the original psychotic symptoms will, at some stage, return. Then it is a matter of prescribing for that original symptom picture and its cause; this is often a critical time and not all who attempt to go through with it succeed. Those who go back on their antidepressants prefer drug-induced stagnation to the struggle with the inner dæmon.

If this were not a controversial area then the next might be. *Thuja* is quite probably the most significant remedy in the treatment of those who are troubled by sexual ambiguity. It is, perhaps, unfortunate that homosexuality is listed in homoeopathic books as a symptom yet this should not suggest that the condition is a disease – though such a point has been debated seriously on more than one occasion. The point is that homosexual feelings can be the *cause* of symptoms that create distress in soul and psyche. The obvious and understandable feelings of guilt and shame are enough to bring out the *Thuja* state. Even in our enlightened times of tolerance, being drawn to the same sex both physically and mentally can still be a source of bewilderment, and feelings of separation. This is equally true, if not more so, of bisexuality. It is not being homosexual or bisexual that is the problem; it is the hesitancy, the indecision, the 'outsider' mentality and, even now, the fear of revelation that make *Thuja* such an indispensable energy medicine for those in so fragile a space. *Thuja*-ness is symptomatically expressed by those who are disturbed by the confusion created by their sexual orientation; as a remedy it encourages wholeheartedness. In some cases, when abuse has created profound confusion in someone who might otherwise have grown up with no hang-ups, *Thuja* has been of inestimable value in bringing the person to feeling 'at one' with him or herself.

Another area in which *Thuja* is greatly needed is in heavy pathology where the patient is threatened with either a severe change of lifestyle or the thought of death if the illness is terminal or potentially so. Morbidity is a preoccupation of part of the *Thuja* mind. There are persistent thoughts of death or of dead people (though this symptom is not exclusive to those who are seriously ill); this impinges on the dream state as well. The same theme of anxiety over security is there but it is now turned towards the state of physical health itself. *Thuja* is one of the remedies that has a mortal dread of cancer or heart disease – so strong can this be that it is a mental symptom that may have to be taken into consideration when prescribing.

The knowledge of one's own mortality does different things to different people. Other remedies have a fear of death:

i)   *Arsenicum Album* which fears the pain and indignity and the loss of control of bodily functions;

ii) *Aconite* which has an almost 'spooked' terror of meeting what is on the other side;

iii) *Phosphorus* which has a fear of being dead and left alone in a total void.

Thuja's fear is of separation between mind, body and soul and of the agency that can bring that about. Through administration of the remedy, when indicated, this symptom state can be relieved. The patient may be eased either into a more positive frame of mind which will enhance the chances of recovery or into the final passage.

Some cases to illustrate the range of *Thuja*

This description of *Thuja* has thrown up some controversial ideas which are best illustrated through case studies. You will notice in these that *Thuja* is not used to the exclusion of other remedies. This is because *Thuja* is almost never the only remedy indicated in any patient's case; *Thuja* is always a station on the way from somewhere to somewhere else. It is rightly called a constitutional remedy because it is a polychrest that treats the whole being but it is a remedy state that is transitional – the 'crossroads' remedy – whatever the condition. It is a remedy that encourages personal development, even 'soul growth', if you will.

> A boy of five was brought by his mother for his asthma and behavioural difficulties. He was taking conventional medicine for the asthma; two puffs of a steroid inhaler each day. He had a history of croup, frequent colds and bronchiolitis (inflammation of the narrow air passages in the lungs). He had been in hospital on two occasions when he had been put onto a nebuliser to restore his breathing. He had no obvious signs of distressed breathing but, on listening to his chest it was obvious that his upper airways were congested. His mother said that he could not run far without wheezing and that every morning he brought up lots of yellow mucus with his daily coughing fit. She mentioned that he seemed to be coming down with another cold. His mother was more concerned, however, about his behaviour as she felt that the steroids were helping to maintain his physical well-being. She described him as being very whiny and tearful with obsessive fears and anxieties; his thinking processes seemed to be way beyond his age.
> *"I don't think it's quite right that he should be going into such a worried fret every time he watches something not very pleasant on the television. If he sees a report on a famine somewhere or refugees then he looks so anxious and he wants to know what we're going to do about it all. He imagines all sorts of scenarios of how he'll ring up hospitals to get them to send doctors out to some far-flung place he's never heard of. He will go on about it till bedtime and then the next morning he's forgotten about it! Then it all happens again unless we switch off the television in time. He can even get like this over something on a*

*cartoon programme. He tries to persuade my husband to ring up to get help
organised. Once he's off there's no stopping the questions; he'll go into every
detail trying to get a more and more vivid picture of all the horrors and all the
whys and wherefores of how it happened. Is it just me or is this really normal?"*

As the boy was hot and bothered with the cold as well as clingy and
whingey he was given *Pulsatilla*. This caused an exacerbation of his cold
and brought on an asthma attack which was successfully treated with
Arsenicum and *Sulphur*. When he returned for the first follow-up
appointment, six weeks later, the mother reported that his breathing had
generally been much better; she had noticed that the slight wheeze she
had always been used to was no longer there. She had maintained the
steroids to be on the safe side. She returned to the behavioural difficulties.
He had become quieter and less urgent in his anxiety but he now wore a
worried expression on his face most of the time.

*"He seems to be more introverted than he was. He might have been worried
a lot but it came in bursts; the rest of the time he was OK. He was able to laugh
and fool around with his brother. Now he seems so serious all the time."*

When asked if she had noticed whether he had any coordination
problems or had shown any sign of regressive behaviour patterns she said
she had noticed that he did not seem to be speaking very clearly.

*"He's quite indistinct sometimes and there's almost a stammer. His teacher
said that she had noted that and that he doesn't seem to be paying attention as
much; he's in a dreamworld of his own is how she described it."*

A final question, that was perhaps not strictly necessary, elicited the
expected reply. *"Does Steven prefer to play with children of his own age or
with younger ones or does he, even, prefer to be in adult company?"*

*"He does prefer to play with his much older brother or to be with adults.
He's awkward with children of his own age. We thought that was to do with his
being above average in his learning ability – he can't write properly, he's all
over the place with that but he's been reading since he was three."*

Steven was given a bottle of *Thuja* LM1, potentised *Thuja* drops,
which his mother was asked to give him each day. This she did until their
return visit six weeks later. He had had no colds or croup. He had no sign
of congestion on the lungs. He was far calmer, less whiny, less anxious
and had not worried about any of the disasters on the television. He had
not watched much of any kind of programme at all. His mother declared
he was a different boy. He had grown so that she had had to buy new
shoes and she was about to get him new trousers – things she had begun
to worry about as he had remained the same size for six months.

She had noticed two things that she wanted to ask about. Steven now had a verruca on his left foot and his feet sweated profusely. She was assured that both of these things were not uncommon as a result of *Thuja* and that they were simply an expression of the body's discharging mechanism. She was asked not to put anything suppressive on the verruca; it would fall out when the time was right but if it caused any pain, she should phone the clinic for advice.[15]

Six months later Steven's mother was able to say that he was now very happy to play with friends of his own age and that he was concentrating well in class and that, although he still found writing and drawing hard, he was making progress in that too. She was now ready to start weaning him off the steroids as she felt he no longer needed them.

A girl of eight, very plump and forward, was brought to the clinic suffering, her mother said, from premenstrual tension.

"*My God! Anybody would think she was eighteen! She's quite the little madam. You never know what mood she's going to be in. She'll come down to breakfast all bright and breezy and wham! she's biting your head off. Something is definitely not right here. She flounces about the house and she's ever such a flirt – even the milkman gets it! As for the paper boy, well, she just moons out of the window till he's passed. I can see we're going to have to be careful with this one or we'll all be in trouble, won't we?*"

Further questions revealed some other pertinent facts. Natalie had been developing breasts for the last few months and they were tender. She felt her joints were painful but the pains shifted from one to another. She had a vaginal discharge that was green and foul smelling – with a fishy odour. She also felt that there was something wrong in her tummy though she had not mentioned it before; she had a sensation as if there was something 'squiggling around' in there now and again. She was deeply embarrassed by these symptoms and felt that they caused her problems with her friends; she was afraid they would be aware of the fishy smell so she had begun to avoid close contact. This had made her friends think that she was being stand-offish so they had begun to make snide comments about her. She felt that she was left out.

She was not sleeping so well and was having 'nasty' dreams. She would dream that she was flying but then would fall out of control and instead of hitting the bottom she would wake up with a jump. Neither did she know why she could be so horrid to her mother and sister. They irritated her so much. She could not control herself when she swore and screamed at them; when she did that, she felt so exhausted afterwards.

She wanted to cry a lot too, she confessed, and some of it was to do with worry over her Dad who was away from home so much with his work. She felt relieved when he got home. Sometimes she had gone out to look at his car to see if it had any sign of an accident on it. She did feel something awful might happen to him. He was such a fast driver.

This was a very sycotic case. Though Natalie was only eight she seemed to have a physical condition that was very similar to gonorrhoea; one might say, mimicked it. She had advanced pubescent symptoms that are typical of sycosis in small girls – the hormones go 'over the top' long before they should. "*She's got a full crop of hair…down there,*" said her mother, making graphic gestures that left the girl squirming in embarrassment.

She was given *Thuja* LM1, one drop to be taken each day and *Medorrhinum* 100, once each week for four weeks. The result of this was reasonably satisfactory to begin with. The breasts were less tender, the discharge became intermittent and the abdominal movements[16] disappeared altogether. However, by the follow-up appointment the breast tenderness and the discharge were getting worse again. It was six months before the symptoms finally succumbed to ever increasing potencies of the *Thuja* and the *Medorrhinum* That it was the remedies that made the difference was shown by the process of improvement; the discharge became gradually less odorous and paler, turning from green to yellow and then to a clear viscous fluid before finishing. The breasts stopped growing and lost their tenderness. Then Natalie produced two warts on her hand which eventually grew and diminished till they disappeared. Her moods began to be less volatile. She re-established her friendships and she even stopped gawping at the paper boy.

It is highly unlikely that Natalie's symptoms would have yielded to either *Thuja* or *Medorrhinum* on their own. The vitality of the condition was so strong that only a sustained assault with both remedies could restore Natalie's own Vital Force to take full charge of her body. The *Medorrhinum* was used to support the *Thuja* because sycosis was so obviously the underlying miasmatic influence at work. Such cases are not uncommon and they usually need great discretion and patience. It was an enormous advantage that the family was a close and loving one.

These cases show that *Thuja* was needed in conditions that had both physical and psychological aspects. The following case is of a boy who seemed to have no physical pathology at all. He had not been taken to see the family GP or a specialist as the parents never considered that he had a health problem as such. His mother was concerned about her son's learning difficulties.

George was seven and bright. He never stopped asking questions and had a prodigious memory. *"He's exhausting,"* his mother whispered so that he would not hear, *"there is no let-up. He has to know everything. He reads all the time or watches programmes like 'Tomorrow's World' and he seems to soak it all in. His vocabulary is extraordinary; it's almost worrying because he doesn't sound like a seven-year-old at all, more like a rather pompous teenager. I've written a few notes down about things as they are better not said aloud,"* her voice tapered off into silence as she mouthed the last few words.

'George is very solitery [sic]. Doesn't seem to want to make friends. Can look quite lost and far away – in a world of his own.
Still sucks his thumb. Bites his nails.
Seems to have two left feet. Very clumsy. He used to fall over a lot but this is better now.
May be dyslexic. Often writes letters backwards. Can't do sums – even simpel [sic] addition. Easily distracted; teacher has mentioned his concentration lapses in class but she's not too worried as he always seems to know the answers. She is concerned that his written work is so behind and has suggested we get him tested'

George roamed about the room, picked up toys and put them down, came back to his mother and rubbed his face on her shoulder and then on her lap, sat down on the floor with a book and shifted to a pile of cushions on which he lay down, put his thumb in his mouth and began to hum tunelessly. He may have had a cherubic face but his expression was rather serious. The practitioner asked George what his birth date was. He straightaway looked at his mother with a frown as if asking for reassurance.

"I think," he began ponderously and paused, *"I think…it's in July, yes!"*
"Would you mind writing down your name and address for me, George?"
He reluctantly put down the book and came over to the desk, not because he wanted to but because his mother snapped her fingers at him and made urgent beckoning movements. He seemed to know the impossibility of ignoring the pursed lips and set expression. He took up the pencil awkwardly in his left hand and wrapped two tensed fingers over the top of it, two beneath it and left his thumb sticking straight out away from his rigid fist. The pencil was gripped in place by the base of his

thumb. As he wrote, the top joint of his thumb waggled with every movement he made. George's tongue was stuck out of his mouth and moved in sympathy with his hand. The effect was almost tortured.

When he had finished, he left the sheet on the desk and moved back to the cushions and the book; he took no further interest in what he had done. The writing was compact but it did not sit on the lines exactly. The capitals were almost comically elaborate while the other letters were set at different angles to each other with no uniformity. Some letters were very faint while the majority were written with heavy enough pressure to cause the back of the paper to be embossed.

"*Do you remember your telephone number?*"

"*No.*"

"*Oh, George, really!*" said his exasperated mother. "*He doesn't like pressure; he hates being shown up. He knows it perfectly well but he does sometimes get the numbers mixed up.*"

A direct question was asked of his mother; "*Does he ever show any signs of concern or worry about anything outside his familiar surroundings?*"

She thought a moment and then said that he was always concerned about the world, about pollution and the plight of animals and the sea – she had noticed that he was almost obsessed about what she could only describe as the health of the planet. "*Don't you think that is rather strange for someone of his age?*" She was back to mouthing.

George was given *Thuja* 1M. This he took in three doses at two-hour intervals. He was asked if he minded coming back in eight weeks time to which he said that he did not. When he returned in just over two months, the first thing his mother said was that George had gone into regression.

"*He's been making the most extraordinary baby noises; he has his thumb in his mouth all the time; he has tantrums like a two-year-old. I nearly rang you up to ask what on earth the remedy should be doing but I resisted. Just tell me that this was expected!*"

It was explained that a remedy can encourage children to go through development stages that they had, for some reason, missed. George had always been a very placid child and had "*never caused us any bother*"; he had never been through any 'terrible twos', he had never crawled but had instead shuffled his way round the floor either on his bottom or on his pot.

"*He was always so bright and quick that we perhaps didn't notice that he wasn't doing things in the right order. It's true, we did seem to miss out on the toddler stage as if he went straight from infant to baby-teenager.*"

George no longer plied his parents with questions; he no longer watched the television; he did not look serious all the time. His mother reported that he slept better, he read *Asterix* comics instead of books; he had asked for a friend to come over to his house to play (though it had not been very successful); he had stopped weeding the cat's grave in the garden (something she had forgotten to mention on the first visit).

"It's not all good news though. He's had a bad cold and he's all stuffed up. He continually snorts and refuses to blow his nose. He always used to be able to do that without any difficulty so I don't know why he says he can't now. He has also become very clingy to me recently, since the cold really. He winds round me all the time. And the slightest thing I say can make him quite tearful. This isn't really like George at all."

He was given *Pulsatilla* 100 in order to deal with the lingering symptoms of the acute cold as well as the present mood that he was in. *Pulsatilla* is complementary to *Thuja* so would not have interfered with any more development changes already set in train and still to come. The next visit confirmed this as George was quite different. He was happy. He sat in a chair beside his mother, occasionally swinging his legs. There was a cheeriness and clarity about him that had not been there before. He had received a very good school report and the teacher had noted progress though he still had to struggle with his writing. He no longer avoided doing written homework but did ask his father to help him with it. His mother said that it was as if he now accepted that he had difficulties and was prepared to face them. There was only one thing that his mother wanted to clear up: he still had the remains of the cold. The mucus was much better but he had developed a nasty hacking cough. She had taken him to the doctor who had given him a short course of antibiotics but they had not touched it.

There was a history in the family of TB. One of George's grandfathers had TB during World War II. George was given *Bacillinum* 200 for his cough and it disappeared entirely within three days. *Bacillinum* is one of the TB nosodes made from the sputum of a tuberculous patient. It is a very common remedy in the treatment of chronic coughs that are persistent, dry and hacking and that disturb the patient at night and on waking in the morning. Furthermore *Bacillinum* is complementary to *Thuja*; it is not at all uncommon for a *Thuja* patient to need a tubercular remedy soon after initial treatment as *Thuja* so often brings up other, underlying miasmatic influences apart from sycosis – though, as you will see in the following chapter, TB is often a sycotic disease.

561

One of the reasons that homoeopaths can find *Thuja* so difficult to grasp and to see frankly indicated in a patient, is that it is a remedy that is associated with (and needed in the treatment of) all the other miasms apart from sycosis. Just as *Thuja* is an energy of separation and split, it is an energy that stands between the miasms and can act as a conduit, so to speak, from one to another. It is not unusual to see on a prescription sheet that *Thuja* was given between doses, say, of *Medorrhinum* and *Syphilinum* or *Syphilinum* and *Psorinum* – even if the timescale shows some months in between. *Thuja* is often a natural stepping stone for those who are using their treatment for medical archaeology; to delve down into the system to mitigate the effects of negative hereditary influences. This should not surprise us when we consider that the miasms are influences that can disrupt us from our sense of purpose just as easily as they can seem to enhance it.

Here is something quite different.

A young man was referred by a music therapist. The therapist felt that there was a hidden or undeveloped cause for his pupil's inability to produce the top range of his voice. When he tried to sing forte in his higher register, his voice cracked and wobbled. This rather anxious eighteen-year-old, Peter, found it very difficult to articulate what he wanted to say. He apologised for not being clear but said that he was nervous. He had great difficulty, it transpired, in facing up to making decisions, to dealing with people he did not know very well, to coping with exams or tests. This was partly why he had gone to singing lessons and music therapy; he felt they would encourage him to be more confident. He was doing theatre studies and drama and it was hard for him to stay calm when he went on stage. And yet it was what he really wanted to do.

Peter was pin neat; dressed casually but immaculately; there was not a hair out of place. He spoke in short words and short sentences and answered questions with an unqualified "*Yes*" or "*No*" where he could. He did not, he said, have many friends; he spent a lot of time in his room listening to music or watching videos. He liked to practise his guitar and he composed songs which he was too diffident to let anyone else listen to. There was very little else that he seemed willing or able to discuss and it seemed precious little on which to base a prescription.

In order to make differentiations between remedies that might have been chosen to 'open' the case, he was quizzed about the usual things such as diet, digestion, sleep patterns. What emerged was a picture of *Lycopodium*, a remedy that not only covers lack of self-confidence and a sense of anticipatory anxiety when faced with an ordeal (such as he might experience when appearing on stage) but also a tendency to flatulence and bloating (especially after eating) and flagging energy in the late afternoon – all of which Peter suffered though he would not have bothered to complain of these things unless asked. He was given *Lycopodium* 100 and it did next to nothing. He thought he was getting a cold once or twice – he had been advised that he might as a result of the remedy – but nothing had come of it. He did feel that his singing lessons were getting better but he spoke as if this were wishful thinking.

However, he began to open up a little more about his emotions. He had experienced a difficulty that he felt he should talk about but he did not know to whom. He tentatively described what had happened and how it had affected him. He had met a girl who was older than him and had become friendly with her. She was, he said, very quiet and not like the other girls at the college who put him off with their loud clothes and raucous laughter. One day she had taken him back to her flat and she had made a pass at him. They ended up having sex and this event had made him feel uncomfortable. It had been physically painful for him and he had felt thoroughly inadequate. He made no criticism of the girl at all; he said that she had been very gentle and kind about his awkwardness.

"*Nevertheless, the whole episode has made me realise that I need to look at the fact that I may be gay.*" He went on to say that he had been befriended by a couple of men in their thirties who had invited him to go to Portugal with them. He had hesitated. He guessed that they were gay though they did not live together. "*They hunt as a pair,*" was his comment.

He had eventually decided to go with them at the last moment but felt unsure of his ground, not knowing what was expected of him. He had, only a couple of days before, got back home from the trip. "*I don't know what I expected. It was just a holiday. We drove around looking at places. We swam and walked. There was nothing else to it. I'm really glad I went...but it has left me no better off about knowing me. I'm really confused. I don't want to try and work anything out with the girl I told you about...though she is keen. I just want this whole sex thing to go away. It keeps coming up in my mind. I can't get on with the course. My mum...I don't know if she worries about me...if she's guessed. It's all such a muddle. I don't know if she'd mind. I keep on thinking she'll be hurt. One minute I think, 'So what if she or anyone knows!' and then I see myself as this person going off and being something different. I'm scared...no, not scared, shut off, maybe...I don't know.*"

He went off with *Thuja* 1M. He never came back for his next appointment. Some time later he was seen in animated conversation with another young man in a van in sluggish traffic. This cameo reminded the homoeopath of their last meeting and he wondered what had been the result of the last prescription so it was fortuitous that just a couple of days later Peter's music therapist should have called about another matter.

"Peter? Yes, he's doing very well. His singing is really improving though I don't think he could ever make a career of it. He's much better since he moved out of his home; he shares a flat with some other young man and the independence has done him the world of good. He's so much more relaxed now."

The exchange of energies

The following case raises a rather more controversial premise that might be called the 'exchange of energies'; the way in which energy generated by one person can affect or, indeed, *infect* another. Not only can this occur on the emotional level but also on the physical level as well. The sycotic miasm is peculiarly susceptible to this, being yin orientated and the subject easily 'invaded' by outside influences.

Perry, a young man of seventeen, came with a problem he found acutely embarrassing. He was very familiar with homoeopathy, having been brought for treatment for at least the previous seven years by his mother. It was only this familiarity that helped him to explain the extent of his condition. He had genital warts. On examination these were raised, red warts on the underside of the foreskin. They tended to itch but only very mildly. He said they did not cause him any physical distress but they worried him because he feared that he had developed some incurable condition that would compromise his chances of having children or of being able to form relationships.

"I haven't been with anyone since they first came up," he exclaimed as if *answering a policeman. "This won't get back to anyone, will it? I mean it's all confidential, isn't it?"* It transpired that he had had sex with a girlfriend for the first time some three to four weeks before. They had made love on two or three occasions in the following week but, when he discovered the appearance of the warts, he had been too scared to continue. He had not had any other physical relationships before and he was certain that the girlfriend had not either – *"actually she's not quite sixteen"*. He had used a

sheath each time; he was adamant that there had been no direct genital skin contact and the condoms had been intact afterwards.

"*It's enough to put you off for life! I don't understand. I thought that you had to go with someone who already had something before you could get anything like this.*" Perry was close to tears and he was clearly scared, mortified and despondent. He was desperate for help though he did his best to maintain as much composure as he could. This was his first visit to the clinic on his own. He was built to become quite a big man but on this occasion he seemed more like a crushed schoolboy.

He had always done well on *Pulsatilla* in the past and, with some other general symptoms that were present, it was clear that he needed it again now – though not just for those physical representatives of sycosis, the warts; more for the acute psychological state. The warts required a different remedy and one that would complement the *Pulsatilla*. He was given *Thuja* LM1, the liquid form, and he was asked to take a single drop each day. He was also asked to report back within a week to ten days if there was no improvement. Perry phoned back in two weeks to say that he was "*much better thank you*" and should he finish the drops? As there were no symptoms at all, he was asked to leave the *Thuja* and to keep in touch if there were any further trouble. Which there was.

Some eight months later Perry came again to the clinic and with the same problem. This time the warts were different in that they were only two in number and were a little larger and had far more body to them. They were still beneath the foreskin but they were on the glans itself this time. In addition, he felt that he smelled bad; he was aware of a sickly, rank smell to the sweat he was exuding in the groin area. Another difference was that he had had sex with a different girl, one that he felt more strongly attached to. He was not as frightened this time but he was very concerned that it should have happened again.

"*I really don't understand. I thought condoms were supposed to be a protection! But that would mean that Holly had something but I'm sure she doesn't. I didn't ask before we did it but I did afterwards and she was very hurt to think that I could ask her such a thing – or so she said.*"

"*Do you doubt it?*"

"*No! Well, I don't know. I did wonder. She says that I've become all suspicious and introverted since this blew up.*"

It was certainly true that Perry no longer needed any *Pulsatilla*. He was confused and filled with self-disgust; he was angry and, far from being a crushed schoolboy, was rather belligerent. In the last eight months he had definitely grown up a lot. Now he was given *Thuja* LMII, the next level of potency, and *Medorrhinum* 200, to be taken once each week. He was advised that the warts that he now had would take a little longer to go. It was then that he mentioned that he also had them around his anus. This did not warrant a change in prescription. He was also asked to consider that infectivity was not necessarily to do with direct contact or contagion; that it was quite possible that something in his own energy make-up had matched the energy make-up of the two girlfriends with whom he had had sex and that, somehow, their sexual contact had sparked off the manifestation in him of the sycotic miasm (the hereditary disposition to produce such warts). He went off with a somewhat quizzical expression on his face, as much as to say, "*Well, I'll believe you but many wouldn't.*"

Perry did not contact the clinic again until his regular appointment came up which was some three months after the latest prescription. He strode into the consultation with a beaming face and a broad grin. He had grown and had filled out across the shoulders. He looked and sounded very confident. A man was talking, no longer a boy.

"*Those warts were amazing! They did some weird things. They itched like fury to start with – as soon as I took the first one of those weekly remedies. In fact, every time I took one the itching got worse but each time it was progressively easier. That awful smell went quite quickly. The warts themselves turned a funny colour, a sort of greyish, reddish…a bit like the colour of a rasher of bacon that's gone off. They grew a bit more and became quite stalky…and then they just shrivelled up! It was fascinating.*" He paused and then sat forward on his seat, "*Now, is it going to happen again?*"

He was well in every other way, he thought. He appeared happy and lively. He had a sense of direction. He was still with the same girlfriend and they had, he confessed sheepishly, resumed their physical relationship. "*I just couldn't resist, I'm afraid. It doesn't seem to have caused us any more trouble…at least, not so far.*"

He did have dry skin; was hot in bed – and hot most of the time; he appeared to be a little disorganised and unkempt; he also spent some of the consultation time talking of all his future plans that did seem rather high-flown. He was given *Sulphur* 1M and it is possible to say that Perry has gone from strength to strength since.

This case is positive for more than its happy, not 'ending' perhaps – continuation would be better. It is important because it illustrates how a miasmatic disease energy that is dormant can be brought to life in a physical form through sexual contact – *even when flesh does not meet flesh* – but that this revivifying process can, if treated correctly, be of inestimable benefit. Consider what would have happened to Perry if he had chosen to go a different route. He would have had the warts cauterised or lasered off. They were *of his body*; he had generated them. Cauterisation would have suppressed their energy instead of allowing them to complete the process of coming out of the system and withering. The suppressed energy would then have to start again in the same place or, worse, in another and probably deeper place. His system, in its effort to rid itself of as much of the sycotic miasm as it could at one go, had found its true form of expression. Many a patient who has had genital warts radically removed has to return to hospital to see the rheumatologist, the gynaecologist or the oncologist. Suppressed warts do not always manifest again in their original guise but return in a different form – polyps in the bowel, cystic tumours in the ovaries, rheumatism, cardiovascular trouble and the like.)

Leaving aside moral considerations, it is important to see that even casual sexual relations often occur for a *greater* purpose than simply gratification. Though compulsive masturbation and gratuitous sex are frequently like a drain overflow to the sump of sycosis, any physical relationship that has any deeper meaning also holds greater potential than just physical sensation. People are qualitatively changed by sexual contact. This is not simply an emotional issue; on this level, people are aware of any such changes. It also occurs on the physical, mental and spiritual levels as well. To exchange energy at the level of the pelvis is of greater consequence to the whole body than it might appear. This is why promiscuity or prostitution are so negatively charged. If personal energy is exchanged with each sexual encounter, enough to alter qualitatively the partners' lives, then frequent switches of partner can turn life into a bazaar of mixed and potentially clashing energies. Frequent partner changes leave no time to assimilate the energy exchanges of previous relationships. Many people become tremendously confused about their emotions if they have had a series of such encounters even if it takes years for them to be aware of it. In Perry's case, he grew into manhood through his experience and subsequent treatment. The trouble and, sometimes, the tragedy is for those who do not take one of the alternative routes to recovery.

This is not a lecture in morality; though it could be used as ammunition by those who have a moral axe to grind. The premise of 'energy exchange' through sexual contact is more a tenet of alternative medical philosophy; what is more, it is a tenet of homoeopathic medical philosophy; no other system of medicine witnesses the miasms in the same light of hereditary influence that *needs expiation through hereditary evolutionary development*.

The gene pool is not only a blueprint for the individual; it is also a deck of cards that needs to be played out in sequence so that whatever was dealt can, if the correct attention is paid, lead to a healthier constitution. If much of this type of work is addressed in childhood and adolescence then that person will pass on to his or her children all those evolved strengths. It is almost universal that for young people who come for treatment through their childhood and their teens (and especially if they come during the time of their earliest pubescent relationships) *Thuja* will feature strongly on the list of prescriptions. *Thuja* is one of the most commonly required remedies for starting the process of getting back in touch with the clean slate of one's original energy – even when the basis for that is absent from the physical and emotional bodies and locked up in the gene pool.

To help you understand these points it is now the moment to reveal that Perry's parents were sycotic by nature. Both his mother and father had received treatment over the years and they had displayed physical symptoms that were absolutely typical of sycosis. Though neither had had gonorrhoea, both had been children of the 1960s, 'flower power' and dope-smoking hippies. They had become successful business people with gradually evolving ideas – largely materialistic – about the way they wanted their lives to run; they had even decided to send Perry and his sister to private school, the very thing, they later recalled, that they had always sworn they would never do because their parents had done it to them. The mother had early symptoms of the menopause due to fibroids; she had swollen finger joints and stiffness in the sacrum; she was very catarrhal. All this is known to be sycotic and was helped, over the years, by sycotic remedies such as *Sepia*, *Thuja*, *Lachesis* and *Medorrhinum*. Perry's father was prone to sycotic asthma and he had occasional bouts of gout. His face was punctuated by lumpy moles. He had needed and progressed well on *Natrum Sulphuricum*, *Thuja* and

Medorrhinum as well as *Sulphur*. He had recalled, at one point in his treatment, that his hands had been covered in warts when he was a boy.

Perry's medical problem could easily be dismissed as an example of any young man 'sowing his oats' – and being left with the bill. It is not so simple. He had grown physically and emotionally in stature as he went through the treatment. He also emerged from the whole episode with a much greater sense of direction and purpose – the spiritual aspect. He was able to cut the apron strings which had become constricting and even threatening to his self-worth – he had previously been slightly intimidated by his mother's powerful drive. The *Pulsatilla* boy shed his childhood straitjacket. The catalyst had been the two sexual encounters which triggered his system to produce the warts of two different types on two separate occasions. One of the greatest benefits is that Perry, having been given the energy to throw out the warts, will not pass down to his children so strong a genetic imprint of sycosis.

When syphilism uses sycosis for its own ends

The final case to illustrate sycosis continues the theme of energy exchange and introduces another piece of the same jigsaw. This case is about the interchange of sycosis and syphilism and the agencies each one uses for its own ends. It is important here to remember that when sycosis and syphilism are mentioned in this context, it is not the actual acute diseases that are referred to but the state of 'miasmatic mind and body'; the hereditarily influenced being. So, 'agencies' are those means by which miasmatically affected people manifest the condition that both affects them and which needs healing. In the chapter on syphilis, alcohol and heroin were referred to in this light; money as well. In sycosis it is (among other things) *Cannabis indica* that insidiously works on the human condition to enhance the sycotic state. The desire for uninhibited fun is only natural but when the release is artificially engendered then the body is put into disharmony.

This is a case of a young woman who worked in a bank. She had a responsible position and gave the impression that she knew her professional worth. She was neat and well groomed. She had very long blond hair which was dark at the roots; she was dressed in Prussian blue but only because that was the uniform; she had absurdly long fingernails that were painted shell pink; she had an almost imperceptible lisp. Her name was Cathy. She gave her name, address and phone number in precise, short phrases, sitting slightly forward with her knees together and her clasped hands resting on them. She appeared eager and determined yet tense. Her wide-eyed gaze was curiously false and a little unnerving, as if she were struggling to maintain eye contact at all costs. When she was asked in what way she could be helped, this odd ambience she had created changed. Everything seemed to lose its focus.

"*Well, I don't know if homoeopathy can help at all. I feel rather odd being here really. I have a number of problems but they all seem trivial when I mention them. A friend recommended that I should come so here I am.*" She made a number of false starts such as this, avoiding the original question. Each time she started to develop her theme she became more vague. Her gaze could not hold its intensity for long and would wander off to the pot plants or the mantelpiece or the cushions. Finally she said that she had eczema in the groin. This was mentioned without the faintest hint of embarrassment so it was not modesty that had delayed things. This condition, she said, was around more or less all the time but in varying degrees of intensity. Some times she was hardly aware of it; at others it would drive her "*bananas*".

When she had exhausted the symptom picture of the eczema, she again found it difficult to focus on what she had to say next. It seemed as if everything she wanted to say about herself needed to be guided into place. Her professional air had completely slipped; instead there was a confused and inarticulate girl. She was not lost for words exactly; she was lost for meaning or sense. She began sentences and they petered out. She started to say something about one subject and then moved into another subject area without a break so that it was difficult to follow the train of thought. After an hour, the timespan of the first consultation, some fabric had to be woven with all the threads that she had spun out. This was her story.

She was living in a certain amount of fear. She was in trouble with a company of moneylenders who had threatened to call the police as they had received a cheque from her which had bounced and was, they claimed, forged. She said that it only looked suspicious because the account was in her maiden name and, while she was married, she had been called Anita; so the suspicion rested on the fact that she continued to use her erstwhile name and a style of writing that had changed over time.

"*He hasn't got a leg to stand on,*" she said in a rare flash of clarity, "*I think he's just using that as an excuse to put the squeeze on.*" She had found herself in this situation because of her ex-boyfriend. He was an American, ten years older than herself, who made frequent trips to the UK she knew not for what purpose other than "*business*". She was obviously in awe of this character and confessed that he had been able to twist her will to suit his needs. She had originally borrowed money in order to "*pay off a friend of his in London*". She said that she had suspicions at the time that she would never see the money again and that she would be left to pay it all back.

"*It was stupid of me but it didn't seem to matter at the time. It was only afterwards that I realised that he was into pushing. Smack was his thing,*" and she wandered off onto another tack. She spoke of the American a little more. She described him as being charismatic, attractive and exciting. He was, she said, always on the move. He spoke Italian like a native and had seemed completely at home when he took her on a trip to the north of Italy some two years before. He would ring up at all times of the day or night from wherever he happened to be and leave messages on her answering machine about when or where to meet him. She found him to be mysterious and "*a bit spooky*"; it was only later that she found out that he was dangerous too.

"*When he had money, things were fine but when he ran short, he became frightening. At first he would just bawl his head off at me. Then he began hitting me. Afterwards he would make a big show of apologising but he really knew where to hit so that it would hurt. My friends all said that I was mad but I was the one he always came back to. It was, if I'm honest, probably the sex that kept us together. I never knew anyone like him.*"

It emerged that he had been arrested at some point and this had shaken her into realising that she had to make a break. She changed her name (it seemed for the second time) and moved out of her parents' home, where she had been staying since her divorce, and into a flat on the other side of London. Now she was afraid that he would find her; one of her friends had seen him around. "*The only stable thing in my life is my job.*"

Because of her inability to stay focused on what she was saying, to establish any continuity in flow of thought, she was asked, just before the end of the interview, if she had ever taken any recreational drugs. "*Oh, yes. I must have done the lot at some time or another. I've had speed, acid and then there's Ecstasy. I've had crack but that's not my scene at all. I wouldn't touch heroin. Amphetamines I've had but they're not all they're cracked up to be. Pot, of course. Why? Does that make a difference? I've stopped all of them now except the odd Ecstasy at a party and the odd bit of grass from time to time."*

It was explained that recreational drugs tend to antidote homoeopathic remedies; that the effects of the drugs change the energy generated by the nervous system so that self-healing is compromised. It was added that she might find that treatment would be less effective because of the history of having had so much; that it was necessary to try and 'clean up' her system before remedies for physical ailments would do their work. She promised to stop taking the drugs and only to take the remedies. She knew, really, that they were *"no good for me"*. *"I'll go down to the Indian and get a vindaloo instead,"* she said with a smile, clearly not meaning to be funny.

She was given *Nux Vomica* 30, one twice each day for five days to be followed by *Thuja* 1M, one to be taken each week for four weeks. She was asked to return in six weeks. *Nux Vomica* is well known for its ability to encourage the body to rid itself of toxicity from drugs – not just medical ones but also recreational drugs. It helps to clarify the mind as well as the body. It is a remedy with an affinity for the liver, which stores so much toxic waste, and for the nervous system, which acts so readily on the influence of a toxic liver. She was warned that the eczema might flare and that she might experience some distressing mind symptoms. So *Nux Vomica's* job was one of *drainage* rather than making any long-term constitutional changes. Strictly speaking it was not 'homoeopathic' to Cathy, the person; it was, rather, more homoeopathic to her state of toxicity. (Such toxicity is, in itself, not part of the essential disease product of the whole person; it is incidental and superimposed.)

Thuja is also a remedy that treats people with symptoms arising from having been on drugs too long. The split between reality and unreality that drugs create is often exactly suited to the energy of this tree. Often, the drug-induced effects of unreality are not cleared away with the initial drainage remedy. The energy of the drugs remains even if the chemicals and their effects on the physical body are drained away. *Thuja* can treat both the energy results of drugs on the psyche (the split) as well as the underlying state that fostered the need to explore this (which can be anything from *"This is fun, let's have some more!"* to *"Life is so shitty it doesn't matter anyway"*). No-one should forget that the use of recreational drugs not only *creates* a symptom state but *is* a symptom state in its own right.

This is not a moral view but a medical one; Man's *survival* is not improved, let alone dependent on hallucinogens.

When Cathy returned she claimed that she felt much better. Her eczema had flared up; she had been violently sick; her hair was falling out; she was developing acne all over her chin and along the jaw line; she could no longer rely on her bowels being regular and her motions tended to be loose. "*Apart from that I'm fine! My head is just so much clearer. I can think straight. I'd got to the state where I didn't know that I wasn't thinking clearly.*"

She then recounted how the American had found her address. When she had returned home from work a couple of weeks before, she had found her neighbour's front window smashed in the flat below. Wrapping an obscene message round a brick, he had hurled it into the wrong room. Cathy did not appear to be particularly frightened, just upset that the neighbour had had such a shock. She had handled the police well but still was frightened of Marc; she never knew what he might do.

"*He can always find me. God, it's so hard. There's such a pull but I absolutely know he's just no good. I have had a few weeds actually. Just to steady my nerves. I drove and drove one day and found myself in Cliftonville. I sat on a hill near there and just relaxed. It was as good as a holiday. It did me the world of good. That was the first time I'd had any since I saw you. Then I did have an Ecstasy one night at a party. I know what you said,*" she held up her hands to ward off any words of criticism, "*but I have been very careful and that was my one lapse. Do you think it's done much harm? I feel the remedies are still working. I really am ever so much happier.*" Cathy appeared to be bubbly. Her words had been punctuated by chuckles and giggles.

The next prescription carried no words of warning or advice. She was already excited that homoeopathy could effect changes such as she had experienced; she wanted to find out more of what it could do. There was a naivety and a sense of intrigue that would not let her stop exploring this new form of sensation and self-discovery. She was using homoeopathy as she might have used cannabis. This is not uncommon for drug users who come to alternative therapies. She was given more *Nux Vomica* 30 to be alternated with *Cannabis Indica* 30, one at night and one in the morning. She was then given a single dose of *Ayahuasca* 1M, to be taken ten days after starting the drug clearing. *Ayahuasca* is a curious and relatively recent addition to the homoeopath's medicine chest. It is as described made from a liana from the jungles of South America; it is a hallucinogenic drug in its raw state but as a homoeopathic medicine it is making a name for itself as a major remedy for those who have difficulty

integrating mind and body (especially after pleasure drugs) where there is
an underlying thread of anxiety from strong emotional attachments. (This
symptom state brings *Ayahuasca* into the list of sycotic remedies but it is
distinguished from *Thuja* by some of its other attributes. Incidentally, it is
a major remedy for the eradication of warts.)

   "*I haven't touched any tablets, I haven't had a weed, I've not even had a
cigarette,*" she declared on her return, "*I chucked in my job. I'm unemployed
and I'm living on my savings. My complexion is bloody awful but the eczema is
completely gone and my hair has stopped falling out. I thought I'd feel elated
when I left work – I realised that all I was, was good at it; I didn't really like it.
It wasn't creative. I feel a bit deflated even though I know I've done the right
thing. It's a bit scary really, seeing things in the cold light of day. I don't know
what I'm going to do. One thing I do know I'm going to do is to go to the States. I
have an auntie who lives there on the east coast. She doesn't have any kids of
her own though she's got a stepson who's nearly her age. I know she's quite
lonely and it would be a chance to explore and perhaps get some work.*" And
that is what she did.

Cathy illustrates the sycotic who is *used* by a syphilitic for their own ends.
The man is not always the syphilitic partner though he was in this case. She
found him irresistibly attractive and allowed herself to be thoroughly
abused by him. Drug use helped to cloud her judgement and prevented her
from seeing a way out and forward. He dealt in cocaine and heroin which
are syphilitic drugs; she used cannabis which is sycotic and Ecstasy which
can be either in its effects. It is not uncommon for sycotically orientated
people to be subjected to and influenced by the manipulation and abuse of
syphilitics. They often respond by subsuming their personalities to the
aggressive partner whose hold over them is often one of fear, sexual attrac-
tion and confusion. Hard drugs, like syphilism itself, are destructive, cruel
and expensive; soft drugs, like sycosis, are easily available, socially acceptable (on some levels) and promote a party atmosphere. What they have in
common is a loss of identity.

Sycosis and the loss of identity

It is this loss of identity that is the territory of both *Thuja* and sycosis; so like
a black hole, that the patient in a *Thuja* state often needs the assistance of

related and complementary sycotic remedies to ease the person into the condition of 'whole-bodiedness'. This 'deep' does not necessarily occur only as the result of taking recreational drugs; hallucinogens are only one agency of engendering it. All that is needed, sometimes, is a powerful personality holding sway over a weaker one. Alma Mahler, whose extraordinary life might have been the invention of an expressionistic novelist and one of the most sycotically gifted women in the first half of the twentieth century, became more famous for her adulterous love affairs than for her talents. Had she had *Thuja* and *Medorrhinum* it is unlikely that her husband, the neurotic, tubercular/syphilitic composer Gustav Mahler, would have been able to prevent her from writing her own music or from leaving him much sooner.

Thuja is a clarifier of the mind and, as it sets about its work, it integrates the mind that has become splintered, confused or disorientated; the mind where the creative force has become diverted from its purpose. This state is peculiarly sycotic and, because of the vulnerability that goes with it, the sycotic falls prey to the influence of those who, single-mindedly in pursuit of their own distorted ends, need to witness their power and perpetuate the destructiveness of the driving force of syphilism. For those with a shaky perception of their identity, syphilism is potentially a creeping evil. This is truly bleak but bleakly true.

Look at Cathy who found it so difficult to grasp that cannabis and Ecstasy prevented her from seeing through her boyfriend clearly. Think of Joan who married an alcoholic jazz musician whom she thought she could reform; she spent almost ten years threatening to leave him after she realised that she could not change his nature and, in the process, she became addicted to red wine, drinking up to two and a half bottles each day which, in turn, brought on high blood pressure and lung trouble. Witness Marion who, married to a hypochondriacal religious bigot, spent years supporting his every whim and carrying out his every order – such as sitting in absolute silence through a meal while the children read aloud in turn from the Bible and then being permitted to speak only of spiritual matters for twenty minutes afterwards – only to find that it was she who became mortally ill rather than her grim spouse.

Making the most of sycosis and syphilism

Ultimately, *Thuja* and *Medorrhinum*, standing as they do for sycosis, are about returning the mind and emotions to a state of integrity with the body; about returning from a mental state of unreality to one of truth; about restoring the sense of purpose through creativity that has been lost or buried by outside circumstances and influences. Just as gonorrhoea is the galloping proliferation of a dual bacteria that has been planted within the generative organs (the site of physical creativity), so sycosis is a similar process of energy working on the system of the *whole* body through heredity. There are many more remedies than *Thuja* that treat sycosis and they all share something of the attributes mentioned. Not everyone who needs their sycosis treated will need *Thuja* (though most of them do sooner or later); some will even need those remedies described under syphilis: *Mercurius* and *Nitric Acid* – both of which are capable of producing sycotic pus and catarrh or anxiety about being removed from reality – though this will occur in those sycotics who are close to tipping into the syphilitic state. *Ayahuasca* and *Cannabis* have already been mentioned but there are also others such as *Calcium Carbonate*, *Iodum*, *Kali Sulphuricum* (potassium sulphate), *Lachesis* (the snake venom), *Lycopodium*, *Pulsatilla*, *Sepia* (squid ink), *Silica*, *Staphysagria* (delphinium) and *Sulphur*.

It may seem confusing, at first, that *Calcium*, *Lycopodium*, *Sulphur* and the like should be useful in sycosis as well as in syphilism and psora but some of these remedies have universal use; they are multifaceted and capable of great plasticity – just as the human system is. (What assists us in recognising when they are indicated is understanding how, though their core symptoms remain unaffected, each of these great remedies is expressed differently within each of the miasmatic states – something that is gained only through experience as the *Materia Medicas* make no such differentiation clearly.)

These energies are available to us to restore the system by matching the energies of those influences that have diverted the proper course of creative purpose in each individual. It matters not that the perverting energy is a drug like cannabis or a manipulative relationship, a grief, a threat to livelihood or a dubious semi-religious conversion; there is a remedy or, more likely, a clutch of related remedies that will trigger the self-healing power to nurse back to health and order all that has been distorted. This is always dependent on how badly damaged the system is; patients often go so far down the road of sickness that their physical bodies are racked by disease and too changed to be restored to a condition that might allow us to use the word 'cure'. The same is true of psychotically damaged people who have spent long years on mind-changing drugs that are prescribed to effect nothing short of a lobotomy.

Nonetheless, whatever the condition under consideration, the pursuit of *'quality of life' through continued personal evolution* is always the best possible reason for the patient to seize the initiative and claw back self-motivation and self-determination. What can make this so difficult in sycosis is the yielding, confused, addictive nature. When a homoeopath treats a sycotic with an addiction, be it to junk food, cannabis or to a relationship, the practitioner is obliged to work against and alongside the power of the 'agent', in itself abstract or inanimate but, when taken up by the patient, a living force to be reckoned with. The patient, in other words, brings the controlling 'agent' to life so that it takes over part or most of the psyche of its willing host.

We are a long way now from the scabies mite: man's awareness of his 'nakedness', his separation from the security of his accepted place in nature, of his perception of self-motivated determination. His curiously ambivalent relationship with God or a higher spiritual force, is far behind us when we consider the sexually driven inheritance of syphilism and sycosis. If psora forces us to question our very foundations then syphilism and sycosis oblige us to struggle with the seven deadly sins, all of which are generated from our baser and more materialistic motives. If we can turn our syphilitic or sycotic illnesses to our advantage by viewing them as signed pathways to return to the more straightforward – but just as difficult – road of psora then we are using sickness for a positive purpose.

This is much easier said than done. If man were only subject to these three miasms then he would be a simpler creature. However, the deeper into his nature he digs, the more complex he becomes. With psora we witness what happens with a creature that lives out its life on the surface of man's body even if the effects drive deep into his psyche. In syphilis and gonorrhoea we see what happens when man plays host to apparently simpler bacteria *deposited* on or within the body, at first near the surface but then further into the system. Now we come to a curious anomaly. We arrive at the description of a disease and its miasm that is, like the others to which it is related, a constant struggle to maintain balance but which is neither as hopeless nor terrible as its reputation leads us to believe. It is as if nature herself, finding syphilis and gonorrhoea to be the unremitting scourges that they are, has invented a way of highlighting the best and the worst of both so that man could, by treading a straight and narrow path, survive – and survive splendidly.

What we are about to look at is a miasm and its disease that have paradoxically benefited mankind through their enormous influence on human expression through culture and art. Though in its acute form it has been just as much an instrument of death over the millennia as its two relations, syphilis and gonorrhoea – probably more so – it is nevertheless a condition that can lead us back to psora, in its simplest and healthiest manifestation – of holding a position of trust in the natural order of things.

CHAPTER 23

TUBERCULOSIS

A preliminary comparison of tuberculism with the other miasms

So far, in this survey of the miasms, we have seen how humanity is:

a) primarily psoric – the tendency to a basic state of anxiety and inadequacy – susceptible to general disease conditions in which the body slows down, dries out and cracks up;

b) secondarily syphilitic – the tendency to violent and/or self-destructive patterns of thought and behaviour – susceptible to general disease conditions in which the body is open to tissue, blood and nerve damage and destruction, characterised by insidious, creeping and ultimately malignant development with terminal consequences;

c) thirdly sycotic – the tendency to addictive, overindulgent excesses of mind, emotions and body – susceptible to general disease conditions of inflammation, overgrowth and morbid manufacture of mucus and pus.

We have seen how each miasm is, before anything else, a state of being which gives rise only *eventually* to any physical manifestation. Each state resides initially in the psyche and only gradually develops through stresses, strains and suppressions of life, to the emotions (where psycho-somatic symptoms appear) and then finally to the physical body (where physiological symptoms appear). The eventual physical pathology mirrors, mimics or becomes a metaphor for the disturbance to the other two bodies.

Each of the inherent miasmatic states has an associated disease – scabies, syphilis and gonorrhoea. The agents of these diseases – the scabies mite, the spirochete and the diplococcus – might be seen as parasitic; simple life forms that exist *before* entering the body, finding a new congenial habitat. It is a fact of homoeopathic philosophy that none of these diseases would be possible *without the prior states of being* to cause susceptibility to the physical disease, parasitic though the disease agents might *appear*. To this canon we need to add TB.

Viewed as a miasm, TB at first has no difficulty in fitting neatly into the scheme of things. It follows the criterion of being a very characteristic general susceptibility to a wide range of disease conditions as the result of a tendency to particular patterns of thought and behaviour. It is also an acute disease that is the physical *end* product of that particular state of being. As a frank, miasmatic influence it is instantly recognisable to the trained eye. As with psora, syphilism and sycosis, the tubercular miasm (tuberculism) may be evident in behaviour patterns of the individual who, nevertheless, is unaware of its presence (in the form of physical symptoms) or its influence (in emotional ones) and, therefore, unaware of the need for treatment.

In its *physical* manifestation it is apparently the result of the depredations of an invading bacteria though the bug would be innocuous without the receptive state of the psyche. It will become clear that TB may be suffered in the acute, physical manifestation while the patient and the physician remain unaware of the presence of the bacillus that is specifically associated with it. When the acute disease, in its obvious form, is left untreated it can be quicker in its devastation of the physical body than any of the other miasmatic diseases. Yet TB differs from the other miasms in at least two ways and they are essential to a more complete understanding, not only of the miasms but also of the way homoeopathy views health in general.

Firstly, as a *miasm*, tuberculism is very much an offspring of psora – and therefore a close relation of syphilism and sycosis. As we shall see, the characteristics of tuberculism are already evident in both its 'siblings' and, continuing the analogy, any tubercular type of illness will often display partiality for one or the other. Patients exhibiting tubercular conditions tend to veer towards either the excesses of sycosis or the destructiveness of syphilism. Nevertheless, tuberculism has its very own unmistakable personality. In being directly related to syphilism and sycosis, it is automatically part of the great psoric picture as well.

Secondly, the acute disease TB is not a contagion, like scabies; not an invasive infection of aggressive spirochetes, at first *deposited on* the body, nor bacteria *deposited within*. It is apparently an infection by specialised bacteria within the lungs or, through its transference via the blood or lymph, to any other part of the body. No physical contact is necessary for someone to develop the acute disease. The progression from mite to spirochete to diplococcus to single bacterium shows that as the structural simplification of the disease 'agent' continues, so does the 'internalisation' of disease.

> Scabies – lives on the skin and is 'animal' by nature;
> Syphilis – sophisticated, mobile bacteria that it is, starts on the skin and burrows its way in;
> Gonorrhoea - the double bacterium, starts its life inside on a mucous membrane (i.e. an inside surface), simply lives by multiplication and, when the body is left to its own devices, has its gross pathological productivity thrown out of one or other orifice through the system's habit of excreting what is alien to it;
> TB – a single bacterium, has its inception within the closed and vital organs of the body or in the skeletal structure. For the first time, we come across an acute disease in which the physical symptoms appear immediately and apparently without preliminaries, in the soft tissue, the blood, the lymph or the bones of the body.

There is a third difference between TB and the other miasmatic acute diseases but it has nothing to do with the course they run. In the first three conditions we have no intellectual or rational difficulty in laying the blame for our suffering on the 'agent' of the disease – which is a paradox when we consider that they are only ever the *result* of direct human contact. Even if we subscribe to the homoeopathic idea that infection will not occur unless there is a predisposition, it is still easier for our *rational* minds to invest the invading bug with powers of parasitic malevolence that it does not actually possess – we can blame something other than ourselves. Scabies, syphilis and gonorrhoea are almost lumped into our collective unconscious along with rats and death-watch beetle; things which are considered not much more than social nuisances that nevertheless can be seriously disruptive and should be eliminated. Humanity has never made the same mistake with TB. (In the sixteenth century when the initial epidemic was at its raging height, syphilis was accorded rather more respect. Antibiotics have changed our perception of it with disastrous consequences.)

The 'White Plague' has never been relegated to the level of opportunistic vermin. It has always touched our deepest fears. Possessed of a rational mind, man has always most feared what his ingenuity has been unable to combat. Even now that we have antibiotics to kill off the bacteria, we still hold TB in terrified awe. With scabies, one can continue, for the most part, to function in spite of the irritation. With syphilis, unless the susceptibility prove fatal, the original lesion and its acute results do not stop the patient from functioning more or less as usual. It is only later, in its third stage, that insanity can set in or tissue damage might create a cripple. With gonorrhoea, the results of infection are often seen as purely local, intermittently affecting glands and the urinary tract so that symptoms do not (immediately) interrupt the patient's career – though subsequent crippling rheumatism and some forms of cancer are typical late results of suppressed gonorrhoea.

Acute TB is not so easily dismissed; it affects the whole being permanently through debilitation, tissue destruction, emotional trauma and psychic imbalance and it can do this before the physical symptoms are obvious. With syphilis and gonorrhoea there is the almost mitigating fact that their 'agents' are only able to create the havoc they are deemed to create because of depravity. TB is not the consequence of any venal activity and it seems to strike indiscriminately: rich and poor, old and young.

Some vital statistics

TB is the most widespread disease in the world. Some eight million cases are diagnosed each year. Some three million TB patients die each year. One third of the world's population is infected. One person is infected every second that passes. In spite of optimistic views held in the middle of the twentieth century about the satisfactory decline of TB since the advent of antibiotics and sulphur drugs, the race is definitely on to discover why it has never been remotely threatened with eradication. Science is desperate to know why it returned with a vengeance in the First World and in new treatment-resistant forms and then, later, in association with other diseases such as AIDS, and why it is in no way in sight of the illusory winning post – and all this despite the widespread BCG vaccination programme.

Playing the statistics game is scary. It is just one of the reasons why we have to be able to put TB into a compartment in our collective mind in which we can find comfort in knowing that the experts, since the coming of age of microbiology, have always found ways of keeping up with the pace of disease evolution. We *know* that medicine only came out of the Dark Ages in the eighteenth and nineteenth centuries with the discoveries made with stethoscope and microscope. We can cope with the thought that our Victorian and Edwardian forebears suffered terribly from the ravages of TB because they were the last generations to be without the miraculous treatments available since the 1930s and 40s. Having some inkling of the varied resources at scientists' disposal we mostly leave the experts to wonder why TB should be back and in such virulent forms. At heart we know that, armed with the 'germ theory', scientists will find a way. For TB seems to be all about a germ - the *Mycobacterium tuberculosis*. Would that it were so simple.

The orthodox view of TB

The official life history of the TB bacteria starts with a cough or a sneeze; a spray of sputum and saliva is released into the atmosphere and the unfortunate passer-by breathes in the germ and 'catches' the infection which is borne off, via the trachea, into the lungs. The primary infection causes the local lymph nodes to be enlarged. There may be an accompanying fever, even a night sweat so that the whole episode appears to be a feverish cold. Though it does not tie up with the death rate quoted above, it is considered that at least 95 per cent of people recover from this without further acute symptoms though subsequent X-rays would reveal 'shadowing' on the lungs and the Mantoux or Heaf test (the five-pinprick test on the arm) would show 'positive'. The unfortunate remaining five per cent might go on to bronchiectasis (basically, holes in the lung tissue in which purulent mucus collects), tuberculous bronchopneumonia or TB of any part of the body.

The 95 per cent (if you buy into the statistics game) who recover from the primary infection have their immune systems to thank. The enlarged lymph nodes were activated to produce white blood cells to deal with the 'invading' bacteria. The shadow on the X-ray is the evidence of the struggle; the site shows where the multiplying bacteria caused some local tissue damage before they were killed off. This does not seem much of a medical disaster so far. Unfortunately, TB has a habit of lying dormant.

Further attacks of the infection can arise; they can be increasingly frequent, virulent and debilitating. Between acute crises there are common infections of colds, 'flu, bronchitis and pneumonia. The patient is almost never free of illness, a state that virtually promotes the growth of the mycobacterium. The bacilli may never have been eradicated by leucocytes during the primary infection but just held in check; the original mass of proliferating bacilli would have been surrounded by white blood cells which would have formed an imprisoning 'cheesy' (caseous) mass – known as a tubercle. When a patient's immune guard becomes lowered and weakened, the trapped bacilli stage a 'break out' and continue multiplying in other pockets of the lungs (or any surrounding tissue).

With the acute onset comes the typical symptom picture of TB: initially there may not be much more than a hard dry cough with the taste of blood or bright red blood that would appear on the handkerchief; then follow bouts of racking cough which bring up purulent, bloody sputum, night sweats (cold or hot), fever and delirium with tiredness and weight loss. (The old name of consumption came from the wasting away aspect.) There can also be joint pains, swollen lymph glands and the pallor so beloved of the heroines of Victorian novels. (This pallor can cause the patient to appear to have translucent skin or even to be a sickly shade of green. This was known as chlorosis – a condition that is still common enough today but which is often put down to junk-food consumption and consequent poor nutrition.)

The result after many acute episodes is the destruction of the breathing apparatus and an utterly depleted immune system. (If the tubercles form elsewhere in the body the function of the affected organ is compromised to the detriment of the whole constitution or, if they form in bone, the result is deformity.) The whole process may last for months or years depending on the strength of constitution of the patient and their willingness to participate in their own healing – not always a foregone conclusion. In 'old cases' – those who have had TB and recovered – damaged tissue becomes fibrous and old areas of caseation become hardened into 'stones' through calcification. These can remain *in situ* without causing further symptoms.

This view of TB leaves us in a state of fear, not just about the disease, but that we might not have adequate protection. As a result, we trust in the immunisation programme, the pasteurisation of milk (because bovine TB was at one time very common in Europe and, if reports are to be believed, is making a determined comeback in Britain), antibiotics and the principle of sterilisation generally. Though we subject our bodies to the injection of tuberculous material into the bloodstream, drink chemically adulterated milk, take antibiotics at the slightest sign of a chest infection and clean everything with antibacterial cleaners, TB has not gone away. For our tidy minds it is inconvenient that it is *not* only immigrants and those who live in squalor who contract TB even though such a comparatively large proportion of such people do. It is inconvenient that it is not only the thin and peaky who develop the symptoms; it used to be thought that those with scrawny necks and scarecrow frames were the only ones to be susceptible. In truth, it was the disease that caused them to become this way.

Rationally speaking, it is inconvenient that some sufferers contract the disease in isolation from others similarly infected, while there are those who have spent their lives caring for tuberculous people without showing the slightest sign of infection. These ideas raise questions that have never been satisfactorily answered for a very good reason – the germ theory, first expounded in 1546 by an Italian poet and physician and made popular by nineteenth-century scientists, gives us such a clear and rational explanation of how we come to suffer acute disease that we imagine we need look no further. The bug and the disease are so obviously associated that we do not have to question whether there is any deeper causative factor. The theory simply confirms that we live in a hostile environment. We know that already without being told; our psoric ancestors have handed down that piece of information very convincingly. The questions remain though. Is the germ theory enough to explain how ill we can become with bacterial (and viral) diseases?

The germ theory and microbiology

The germ theory states that we are all indiscriminately susceptible to invading bacteria (and viruses) that are airborne and simply waiting to be picked up; this has turned us all into complacent hypochondriacs. 'Knowing' that we have to keep our hands washed and spray the houses we live in with germ-killing cleaning fluids in order to escape infection, we can do and think as we are taught and become doctor-dependent – because if a germ slips under the door we can always consult the people who know how to kill germs once they are inside our bodies. The theory is true for the common cold as much as for TB, they are just at opposite ends of the same pole.

By appealing to our rational mind, the development of microbiology and the germ theory has inevitably altered our general perception of disease and how to treat it. It is now 'shoot to kill'. If there is a bug on the slide and the means of eradicating it has been developed, then bumping off its brethren in the body would seem the obvious way to deal with the problem, swiftly and terminally. Gonorrhoea and syphilis come into this category. So does pneumonia. Certainly this has been the preferred method of treating TB since the advent of antibiotics.

There are other ramifications though. By being able to identify particular bugs, the emphasis on observation of the *whole patient* is at once removed from the general symptom assessment to the pathologist's laboratory report – even though it is the presenting *general* symptoms that may have caused the physician to send the samples for analysis in the first place. Nineteenth- and twentieth-century advances in technology have enabled pathologists and chemists to determine what procedures to follow in the treatment of threatening diseases. Years ago, doctors lost their diagnostic supremacy to those who went in search of the microscopic causes of patients' suffering. Paradoxically this began to happen just at the time that homoeopathy was beginning to be taken more seriously and some of its philosophical tenets were becoming accepted. The doctrine of similars, though scorned by many, began to be officially taught in some of the leading European medical schools of the period (the middle years of the 1800s) and the idea that the patient was the source of his own healing was given more than a passing nod by influential writers of the time.

Nevertheless, the discovery of the miniature world of microbes forestalled any widescale acceptance of a theory and practice of medicine that took so long and so much experience to master as homoeopathy. Nothing less than mastery of this malignant world of bacteria has been the goal ever since.

For diseases like TB, syphilis and gonorrhoea, conventional practice has now been somewhat reduced to 'medicine by numbers', almost entirely due to the revelations of the microscope and the proliferation of killer drugs. But this brief description cannot, and very clearly should not, be dismissive of microbiology. In the absence of any other general alternative approach, it has contributed invaluably for legions of suffering individuals and has led to their *immediate relief* from appalling conditions through drug intervention. This was made possible because the *perceived* causative factors – be they tubercular bacilli, treponema, streptococci, staphylococci, pneumococci or any one of a host of others – have been identified. 'Immediate relief' is italicised here because it should be clearly understood that no 'cure' takes place through the identification and execution of the disease agent – only the cessation of obvious acute symptoms. 'Perceived' is italicised because the causation, as will be shown, is actually within the patient. The patient's underlying, constitutional susceptibility to the disease remains – though its future form may be changed into something else. TB is nothing if not protean in its ability to assume an infinite variety of aliases.

Up until the development of chemotherapy from the discoveries of nineteenth-century microbiology, acute and recurrent diseases were quite often unwittingly left to the immune system of the patient's body to cure. Not that the average doctor realised that this was happening. The physician between the sixteenth and eighteenth centuries, having been largely taught to base his practice on logic (rationalism) rather than the accumulated wisdom of experience plus a determination to observe patients objectively and subjectively (so called empiricism), may have advocated any number of different activities to limit the suffering of the sick: cold baths, hot compresses, herbal infusions, leeches, bleeding, the curette, diets, a trip to Bath or Tunbridge Wells – yet healing (particularly in the towns) quite frequently took place by default. The patient got better by himself, relieved of his symptoms, the treatment and the physician's fee. Without the benefit of knowing whether they were dealing with causative agents or the pathological results of 'humors', dangerous 'miasmas' and vaporous lurgies that blew in from swampy marshlands or just plain hysterics, physicians were encouraged to speculate as to what they were dealing with.

In the early years of the nineteenth century, the stethoscope and the increasingly sophisticated microscope between them did for medicine what Darwin did for the Church. Increasingly refined medical instruments and technology meant that no scientist could ignore the hard evidence of the world of microbiology. Man's spiritual and emotional bodies need not be consulted or observed further for evidence of causative factors of ill health![1] No-one in the orthodox field, with one vital, small-voiced exception, asked the question: *"Could the bacteria be the* result *of the disease rather than the cause?"*

So, morality and medicine were finally divorced almost as soon as Pasteur (1822-1896), science's most successful spin doctor, and Robert Koch (1843-1910), inventor of the first and, it turned out, deadliest TB vaccine, erupted onto the scientific stage.

TB and the germ theory: the questions that won't go away

TB is described as being spread by droplet infection, the introduction of the *Mycobacterium tuberculosis* into the system via the mouth or nose after an infected person has coughed or sneezed. However generally true this may be – and it is undoubtedly a means of infection – it simply remains inadequate to understand the nature or natural history of the disease or man's susceptibility to it. Too many questions are left begging. For example, why should a person (unvaccinated) living amongst and nursing TB patients for a considerable time not contract the disease while another, living in isolation and far away from obvious infection, does so and dies?[2] Why should one person develop TB in the lung and another in the kidney? How is it that one member of a family might succumb to TB and not the siblings living in the closest proximity? (Although heredity does play a vital part in the story of TB; witness the unfortunate Brontë family.) Why should some who suffer bronchopneumonia, whooping cough or diphtheria go on to produce TB so readily while others do not?

We need to go deeper in order to cope with the idea that TB *already exists* in some form or other *within* the system, within the *whole*. It is not enough to say that TB is in the air. It is not sufficient to study the *effects* of a disease on the human body to understand more than how to *alter* those effects. It is never sufficient to remove physical symptoms in order to say that the disease is cured. TB is a disease that exemplifies many diseases that are initiated within the body (rather than from an obvious outside parasite), therefore it becomes imperative that the very process of *susceptibility* be understood comprehensively. The germ theory has completely obscured our vision of susceptibility. In the case of TB, scientists either frankly admit that they do not know why some people are affected and others are not or they ignore the facts and blithely say that everyone is potentially susceptible.

We know why we accept the concept of invasive germs – it is easier to understand rationally that something out there is looking for a victim. What we do not generally appreciate is what led up to its adoption and what else happened (in the middle years of the nineteenth century) that might colour our view of the way in which germs behave.

Pasteur and his colleagues

Louis Pasteur is credited with the first modern exposition of the germ theory – *Germ Theory and its application to Medicine and Surgery* (1878). This treatise was actually addressing anthrax, a disease problem that he determined to tackle after a colleague had isolated and cultured the bacillus. He gained enormous prestige (and great wealth) from the development of a vaccine that he tested on sheep.[3]

He is known to have carried out experiments that proved bacteria were airborne and that they proliferated when introduced into a congenial environment. He is also credited with the discovery that certain disease germs can live and multiply *anaerobically*, that is without air; further, in his study of the fermentation of wines, each brew of bacteria had its own specific enzyme. This led him to expand the ideas of prophylactic treatment of specific diseases with specific curative agents – such as the anthrax vaccine or cholera vaccine. Through his work on wines he was led to recommend the heating of wines and milk in order to kill off bacteria; this led directly to the reduction of TB cases resulting from the drinking of untreated cow's milk.

He is hailed as the discoverer of the principle of inoculation; that a *weakened* form of a bacteria can be introduced into the body so that when a more virulent one should attack the system, it will be recognised and dealt with by dint of the artificially 'acquired immunity'. We have come to think of him as a benefactor to humanity. The German, Robert Koch also achieved fame when he isolated the TB bacteria; he called it tuberculin and he proceeded, tentatively, to recommend that it could be used, under certain conditions and circumstances, in the treatment of tuberculosis. (This precipitate move was quite out of character. Koch was a thoroughly diligent and conscientious scientist who designed exhaustive protocols for laboratory experiments which are the models of present-day procedures.) The idea of using the weakened bacillus in a sterile medium was basically similar to the homoeopathic view that *like treats like*; the gaping difference was that Koch did not prepare the material into a homoeopathic medicine first nor 'attenuate' the bacteria sufficiently before prescribing it. (Pasteur at least perfected the 'attenuation' or dilution of his anthrax and rabies vaccines even though he dispensed material, albeit weakened, doses.)[4] Koch had to disappear to Egypt for a while, when the devastating results of his 'cure' came to light; there were many hundreds of deaths. He retired with a tarnished reputation still trying to establish the efficacy of tuberculin.

Paul Ehrlich (1854–1915) has his place in the story of the germ theory because he established the use of aniline dyes to stain tissue samples which show up changes in the presence of bacteria. He succeeded in staining the TB bacillus in 1882, the same year that Koch cultivated the bacteria in his laboratory. His firmly held belief was that medicinal drugs, like the aniline dyes, create a chemical bond with their target organs through direct contact thus enabling the drug to kill off local infection.

Then, in the early 1900s, two Frenchmen, Albert Calmette and Camille Guérin, discovered that by the multiple 'subculturing' of a culture of highly virulent bacilli in a medium of glycerin, potato and bile, they could weaken the strength of any bacilli and render it safe enough to inject into an animal without causing any appreciable symptoms. At the same time, the animal's immune system was stimulated into producing antibodies that would kill off anything that looked like the TB bacillus. It took many years for their vaccine to be taken up by the medical profession. (This was, not least, due to the suspicion in which vaccines were held after the debacle arising from Koch's precipitate experiments.)

Calmette and Guérin gave their name to the anti-TB vaccine that is known throughout the world as the BCG. It has been a routine inoculation given to the vast majority of children born in the second half of the twentieth century and seems set to continue into the twenty-first. It is either given at around the age of twelve or thirteen or, wherever there is a hereditary or immediate environmental threat, to infants of only weeks or even days old.

So why is TB still with us? Even if immunisation were partially successful, why does TB still behave in the way it always did by coming in a wave pattern of epidemics yet still picking off individuals from all walks of life at any time? Does TB work to another germ principle that differentiates it from other diseases? Why is it that so many patients who suffer the full-blown disease in middle years have a history of childhood or teenage pneumonia or bronchopneumonia, severe whooping cough or frequent bouts of throat infections and tonsillitis? What is it that has made them so prone to this type of disease and when did the TB bacillus dig in? Was it there all the time? Could it have evolved *in situ*, from those pneumococci or streptococci that multiplied during the early acute episodes of pneumonia or tonsillitis? And if mutation is a possibility, what could cause one bacteria to evolve into another in the way that we know viruses can? And a question more immediately contemporaneous: why is AIDS so closely identified with TB?

In spite of the evidence of the microscope, the essentially parasitical view of bacteria is inadequate to explain epidemic disease; it is based on *assumption* – that the introduction into the body of a bacterium sets up the characteristic symptoms of a disease specific to that vector – because no-one has ever 'freeze-framed' that instant when infection is conceived naturally within the body. Studying bacteria in a Petri dish is not the same as studying the diseases associated with them in the bodies of patients. The bug on the dish is divorced from the 'whole body' context and not necessarily subject to the same influences. It is easy to see how the myth that bacteria are the *origin* of acute diseases, rather than their *product*, has been perpetuated when they are studied in isolation; this notwithstanding the disease experimentation on animals that has marked research since World War II. Animals in captivity and far from their natural habitat, however closely related genetically they may be to ourselves, are not suitable subjects to make judgements on about the way disease works, not least because such animals are in a false environment and do not have the same emotional history or miasmatic history that we do.

Pasteur exposed?

An interesting book was published in 1923 called *Béchamp or Pasteur?* The main thrust of the book is devoted to the detailed accounts of the experiments carried out by the former. These experiments, carried out with the utmost rigour and meticulously documented, had a profound bearing on the future of medical science. Yet it is clear, from all the documentary evidence that the author was able to secure, that these experiments and their results were misrepresented to a public desperate for hope about the frontiers of medicine. The diligent and painstaking scientist who did these ground-breaking experiments was Antoine Béchamp.

The author, Ethel Douglas Hume, had been inspired to write by a Dr Leverson. He had been enthused by the writings of Béchamp and met him just before the latter had died. Leverson had been convinced that a monumental miscarriage of scientific justice had occurred. Miss Hume began her work during the First World War once she had found Béchamp's writings in the British Museum and spoken with his remaining family and old colleagues. What she discovered and wrote has never been taken up by the scientific establishment. Her book did not sell very widely and ran out of print shortly after the publication of the fourth edition in 1947.

Pasteur was a chemist and not a doctor at all. He only had, it would appear, the most rudimentary knowledge of anatomy and physiology. His knowledge of pathology was restricted to epidemic diseases, such as anthrax and rabies with which his name became associated through his work on vaccines. What is more it appears that he was a plagiarist; he drew on the painstaking work of Béchamp for his own claims. If that were not enough, it seems that his plagiarism was inaccurate, that he only partially understood what he was plundering and that, as a result, posterity has been left with a legacy of scientific half-truths. Posterity has never seriously questioned his word even though there were contemporaries within his profession who did at the time and most vociferously – only to be bulldozed by his hectoring manner.

So entrenched is our thinking about pathology and the germ theory that Pasteur continues to enjoy his honourable place posthumously. To shake the rationalist equation of [malevolent bug + opportunity = acute disease] approximates to a heresy. Yet herein lies a deeply disturbing anomaly. The original work that Pasteur seems to have plundered continues to languish uninvestigated even though it contains so much that truly contributes to a thorough understanding of bacterial diseases such as TB.

Miss Hume sifted through many reports on meetings of the French Academy of Science and found that Béchamp had reported all his major experiments well in advance of any of Pasteur's and that, in comparing the parallel experiments of the two men, not only did Pasteur's efforts fall far short of the technical excellence and exhaustive thoroughness of Béchamp's but his conclusions were substantially different and seemed to be based on assumptions.

Béchamp

Antoine Béchamp (1816-1908), the doctor of science, and of medicine and professor of chemistry was engaged for a number of years (in the 1840s, 50s and 60s) on certain experiments that seemed to inspire Pasteur and were shadowed by him. The nature of these experiments is central to understanding the role of bacteria in disease and in seeing the flaws inherent in our concept of the germ theory.

It all began with 'fermentation' which was, for so long, seen by the majority of medical scientists as the origin of disease. Fermentation is the characteristic compositional changes wrought on organic substances through the introduction of a fermenting agent (such as yeast). The resulting changes can be qualified by terms such as *acetous* (souring by conversion into vinegar), *lactic* (the souring, through decomposition, of milk) and *putrefactive* (rotting).

Between 1854 and 1857 Béchamp conducted his 'beacon experiment'. He dissolved pure cane sugar in water in a covered jar that also contained air. Alongside this he had other bottles that contained the cane sugar dissolved in water with different chemicals such as sulphates of zinc and mercury. The bottle with air but no added chemicals was the one that showed fermentation in the form of moulds. To explain the presence of moulds, Béchamp set up more flasks full of cane sugar dissolved in distilled water; some had no air whatever while others had creosote added. In the flasks with no air, there were no changes at all. In the two bottles into which air had been allowed, there was abundant change. In the bottles in which changes had begun and to which creosote had been added, there were further changes but a slower growth rate.

While Béchamp experimented with cane sugar and distilled water, proving conclusively that fermentation was due to airborne moulds and yeast that came in contact only with the medium which was exposed to air, Pasteur experimented with sugar *already* in a solution of yeast which guaranteed fermentation whether the medium were in contact with air or not. While Béchamp drew the proper conclusion that fermentation occurred only when the medium was 'sparked off' by airborne particles, Pasteur claimed that *his* medium sprang into life spontaneously. The former had proved the significance of *aerobic* micro-organisms while the latter subsequently found it convenient to forget his own first experiments, publicly claim Béchamp's results as his own and conclude vociferously that airborne organisms were indeed part of the process of fermentation.[5] (If the experiments had been left there then we should never need to doubt that all disease bacteria behave like those mould spores, carried in the air we breathe and causing us the diseases associated with each type.)

Béchamp's efforts may have proved that albumenoids (chemical compounds that form the bulk of tissues of plants and animals) would develop and grow in sugared water that had been in contact with air but they also showed that, once the process of fermentation had begun, the *continued* fermentation was self-generated by the mould through absorption, assimilation and excretion. The generation of a life form initiated a life cycle. Béchamp was throwing a spotlight on the whole process of digestion and the action of enzymes.

Béchamp repeated his original experiment with the cane sugar dissolved in water; this time he added common calcium carbonate (chalk) – which he took from a block of ancient limestone, some eleven million years old. In the earlier tests, the water that had contained potassium carbonate had shown that fermentation had not been allowed to take place. With the calcium carbonate, which had been introduced to the medium without air (and therefore *without the possibility of airborne bacteria*), there was abundant fermentation. Béchamp had discovered that fermentation was *not solely* dependent on air or airborne bacteria. (When, in a further experiment, he heated the calcium to over 300 degrees, it lost its power to initiate fermentation.)

Then Béchamp examined the chalk under the microscope and discovered that it contained what he termed 'little bodies' that he eventually called *microzymas* [6] – the word being based on the Greek for fermentation. He further found that microzymas were absent from the heated chalk and the potassium carbonate. What was more, these tiny organisms were capable of movement – a fact that showed, incidentally, that they were possessed of (electrodynamic) energy. The significance of his experiment was that it demonstrated that it was *not the invading, airborne bacteria or spores that determined what form the fermentation would take but the microzymas*. Rather more controversially, Béchamp went on to speculate that the chalk microzymas carried a 'memory', that they bore the life potential of the fossilised creatures that had gone to form the compact mass of chalk from which he had scratched the mineral material. (This was a suggestion that the chalk microzymas would, in a congenial habitat, set about reacting to their environment in the way they had when they were first part of a living organism.)

Béchamp and his collaborator, Professor A. Estor, found that all organic matter, whether healthy or diseased, is invested with microzymas which they considered to be 'molecular granulations'. They found that they were 'indestructible' – except at high temperatures; that they were what remained after all the *living* matter of a substance had decomposed. Wherever they were, they were associated with bacteria. Through exhaustive experimentation they came to the conclusion that microzymas were cell *builders* and that *bacteria were evolved growth from microzymal activity in a congenial environment.* Béchamp and Estor believed that all living organisms included congregations of these minuscule particles which were vital to the comp- osition, growth and repair of cells. Bacteria only occurred when decomposition took place as part of the natural process of recycling. They went on to prove and claim that airborne 'germs' were simply microzymas or bacteria that had been freed of their original living habitat after compositional breakdown. Bacteria, in other words, are not basic, single-celled structures that *initiate* life processes themselves – as is so widely believed today – but they are a development from the characteristic catalytic activity of microzymas in a congenial habitat; they are the *result* of the initiation of life processes begun by microzymas. The physics of the microzymas makes possible the chemistry of bacteria. Here is the very beginning of the science of cytology: the study of cells and their formation.[7]

In an experiment that took them over seven years to conduct, Béchamp and Estor used the decomposed body and parts of a kitten that had been steeped in carbolic acid to rid them of all extraneous bacteria and placed in airtight containers with carbonate of lime. The matter decomposed to the point that all the original cellular life was expunged while leaving a teeming abundance of microzymas as well as some bacteria. Because of the extreme measures taken to remove bacteria at the very beginning of the experiment, it was shown that the bacteria present at the conclusion were the result of microzymal activity.

It would appear that microzymas are little short of *'energy seeds'* and that essentially Béchamp – without the aid of an electron microscope – was tentatively beginning to unravel the mysteries of not only cytology but also the atomic energy of cells. Once supported by a congenial environment, the energy seeds would show their potential as purposeful initiators of an evolutionary process. An analogous example of this would be how a particular plant, many times greater than its original fertilised seed, achieves its mass by interacting with heat, water and nutrients from the soil.

The nature of his experiment with the kitten carcass led Béchamp to conclude that microzymas were capable of dormancy. He had left untouched the glass jar of lime and its body for six years. When he opened the flask, discovered the mass of microzymas and then subjected them to a further fermentation test, he found that they performed in exactly the same way that they had in his first experiments. Thus Béchamp was able to explain how it is that animal and vegetable bacteria are capable of lying dormant for indefinite periods within the soil and remain so until activated by environmental changes. The interaction of microzymas with animal and vegetable matter creates bacteria that hasten the process of breakdown. When that breakdown is complete and there is no further 'food' for the bacteria to live and work on then they, in their turn, return to their basic microzymal form; inert until reactivated by a new life 'initiator'. This point is of particular significance when looking into the life history and heredity of patients with TB.

Béchamp also went in search of microzymas in the different organs of the body. He found that each organ – liver, kidney, pancreas and so on – had microzymas that were differentiated. In other words, the cell builders of each organ were programmed to create cells for specific functions in specific parts of the body. Today, 'microsomes' are vital to the acceptance of transplanted organs; there are companies that trade in the sale of specific microsomes so that they can be introduced into the tissues of transplanted organs to promote the ready growth of correctly differentiated cells.

> 'Matter, whether albuminoid or other, never spontaneously becomes a zymase (i.e. that which would create a chemical change) or acquires the properties of zymases; wherever these appear some organised (living) thing will be found.'[8]

This is very close indeed to Hahnemann's Vital Force; the chemistry of matter is nothing without the physics of a living, dynamic entity. He also wrote,

> 'The microzymas can only be distinguished by their function which may vary even for the same gland and for the same tissue, with the age of the animal.'[9]

Here he is pointing out that microzymas are 'programmed' and that the programming is even influenced by the passing of time; perhaps, even, that the history of the life force that dictates the essential purpose of the microzymas is experientially held by these tiny energy seeds. (This is as if microzymas were to the Vital Force what DNA is to the physical body.) Béchamp and Estor found that human blood contained microzymas and that they differed from one subject to another. Not surprising, then, that he found microzymas in vaccine material and syphilitic pus as well. The implications of this are enormous when considering inheritable states of sickness.

Pasteur, meanwhile, contented himself with the discovery of pathogenic bacteria and their isolation and artificial generation in the laboratory. By stopping short of Béchamp's full experiments he never noticed that microzymas had a vital role in the *formation* of the bacteria that were causing so much stir. Inevitably, without this link, he drew the wrong conclusion that bacteria were *responsible* for our sicknesses rather than being the product of them. Neither he not his rival, Robert Koch, would have realised that microzymas informed with the susceptibility to a disease such as TB, *would predispose a system which was carrying them to encourage the spontaneous manifestation of bacteria associated with the specific disease.*

As a doctor, Béchamp had unique opportunities to confirm his observations in the local hospital. A patient, who had incurred a severe accident and whose forearm was already becoming gangrenous, provided Béchamp with the amputated limb. The surface skin had turned black and the patient had reported complete insensibility below the exposed bone of the elbow (decided symptoms of gangrene), before losing his arm. However, on examination under the microscope, Béchamp found no gangrene bacteria. There were only signs that the microzymas were beginning to institute changes. On observing this, Professor Estor declared,

'Bacteria cannot be the cause of gangrene; they are the effects of it.'[10]

This is to stand the germ theory on its head. Béchamp and Estor were not denying germs existed; they were saying that germs, in the host, came *after* and not before infection. Nothing that Béchamp and Estor discovered denied that bacteria, in coming after infection, were capable of initiating fresh infection; bacteria resulting from a disease reaction in a patient is redolent of the electrodynamic energy of that sick person. Airborne droplets containing bacteria are quite capable of spreading and perpetuating an epidemic. Yet, each fresh infection in any individual is the individual's response to the dynamic energy of the ingested bacteria and if there is *no susceptibility* to reacting to those bacteria then *no disease will result.*

Pasteur, having eventually been convinced that chemical changes in the body were not spontaneous, nevertheless clung to the belief that the body was a chemical factory that was subject to constant bombardment by bacteria from the environment. The germ theory, which was given such a tremendous boost by Robert Koch when he isolated the TB bacillus and later cholera, has the merit of being simple and immediately comprehensible – on the level of 'If you walk into a river infested with crocodiles, you won't come out in one piece.' We all keep our distance when someone starts sneezing not thinking that we might be miles away in the barren wastes of the Sahara, far from all civilisation, and still 'catch' a cold – which, if neglected while in a poor state of health, might develop into pneumonia.

Béchamp shows us that bacteria will form in the body *only* if there is microzymal activity to promote them. For this to happen negatively the microzymas must be programmed via heredity to produce a personal illness type. Someone with a tubercular family history will thus be inclined to produce bronchitis or pneumonia or fevers with aching joints and night sweats. Someone with a sycotic ancestry would be more likely to produce inflammations, pus and other gross discharges. Those with a syphilitic taint would produce conditions that led to bleeding, emaciation and tissue destruction. (Thus, pus-inducing staphylococcus is an essentially sycotic bug; the flea-borne bubonic plague bacterium is decidedly syphilitic.) It is here that we find the origins of like cures like; producing a set of symptoms that mimics a hereditary disease state has to be the only way for the microzymas to be reprogrammed.

If microzymas are *'energy seeds'*, invested with electrodynamic energy, then they must be influenced by the physical, emotional and spiritual condition of the living patient; *if that influence is negative then disease bacteria can result.* If the internal conditions are not right for negatively charged microzymal activity then no infection can occur – however virulent the epidemic raging on all sides. Therefore, several things are explained:

i)   how a patient's environment, mood or circumstances can be determining factors in susceptibility; this is 'the stress factor' in disease and it can work in both chronic and acute states;

ii) how two patients with the same identifiable condition can have their own variations on the general symptom picture and thus require different remedies or even different types of treatment;

iii) why allopathic drugs are incapable of curing anything by their chemical activity as they are unable to eradicate the negative charge of the building block of the disease state, the microzyma. They are only capable of stopping the *effects* of the microzymal activity: the symptoms. (It must be recognised that drugs can and often do alleviate symptoms while the patient sets about changing the negative state for himself.)

We create our own germs.

A word of experience

Florence Nightingale was certainly not one to be complacent about the origins of disease in her field hospital. Seventeen years before Pasteur claimed an idea that had been extant for over three hundred years, she said:

'Diseases are not individuals arranged in classes, like cats or dogs, but conditions growing out of one another. Is it not living in a continual mistake to look upon diseases as we do now, as separate entities which must exist like cats and dogs instead of looking upon them as conditions, like a dirty or a clean condition and just as much under our control; or rather, as the reactions of kindly nature, against the conditions in which we have placed ourselves?

'I was brought up by scientific men and ignorant women distinctly to believe that smallpox was a thing of which there was once a first specimen in the world which went on propagating itself in a perpetual chain of descent, just as there was a first dog – or pair of dogs – and that smallpox would not begin itself, any more than a new dog would, without there having been a parent dog.

'Since then, I have seen with my own eyes and smelled with my own nose smallpox growing up in first specimens either in closed rooms or in overcrowded wards where it could not by any possibility have been 'caught' but must have begun. Nay more, I have seen diseases begin, grow up and pass into one another. I have seen, for instance, with a little overcrowding, continued fever grow up; and with a little more, typhoid fever; and, with a little more, typhus and all in the same ward or hut. For diseases, as all experience shows, are adjectives not noun substantives.'

She further added:

'The specific disease doctrine is the grand refuge of weak, uncultured, unstable minds such as now rule the medical profession. There are no specific diseases; there are only specific conditions.'[11]

Part of our animalistic condition is to inherit the characteristics of forebears, including their susceptibility to disease generation – but, as we have seen with gonorrhoea and syphilis, though the characteristics are consistent, the *form* of the disease is not a constant. As we shall see with TB, it has a multiplicity of forms both as disease and as influence while remaining constant in its characteristics. And such characteristics are only possible *because of their human context.*[12]

Béchamp, without the benefit of Crick and Watson's work on DNA, postulated after much experimentation, that microzymas carried a hereditary link from one generation to another and in so doing they carried the information for disease susceptibility from one generation to another.

There is much more to the story of Béchamp and Pasteur; all of it along the same distressing lines. The history of these two has had the net result that contemporary medical thinking is based on half-right truths. One half of the truth is that, yes, there are germs associated with specific conditions and they are more often than not present in acute disease; one sneezing, coughing individual can set off infection in another; germs can be airborne, waterborne or lie dormant in the soil or elsewhere. But to know this is not enough. Bacteria are the result of whole-body changes in reaction to environment, emotion or trauma (as Florence Nightingale so graphically observed at first hand) and these *can and do* happen irrespective of others having become infected beforehand. It is the susceptible individual's reaction to the *energy* of a sick patient producing bacteria that is important – the bacteria themselves are not a vital ingredient; people can become acutely (and chronically) sick by being in a sick place or a sick mood or amongst sick people. It is Béchamp who shows us on the microcosmic level that 'fermentation' principles exist not simply for digestion (positive, beneficial enzyme activity) but also for disease, with bacteria being a *by-product* of the body's reactions. Microzymas, when negatively charged due to adverse circumstances and hereditary influences, transform themselves into disease inducers. This is due to an unsuspected purpose of the body – to recreate conditions that will goad the body into cleansing itself; purging itself of the disease influence. Add to this the idea of hereditary disease patterns and we come up with the outrageous idea that the body is capable of reproducing even fatal diseases such as TB in order to set about dealing with the past influence in a present acute form. The ultimate purpose of this is far from outrageous – the survival of the cleansed gene pool.

The gene pool can only be cleansed of hereditary taints of diseases like TB, gonorrhoea and syphilis if the body is allowed to reproduce a symptom picture that represents the particular disease – like cures like, again! – and then receives *curative* rather than suppressive treatment. Cure then comes about through retraining the body's innate skills at self-healing, that which it had lost by neglect, wrong treatment or suppression. To avoid the appalling risk of producing TB, many of us produce other, perhaps less dangerous conditions that look similar enough so that the body can recognise what to do if and when the energy of TB is about.

Just as we hatch chickenpox to relieve ourselves of psora and psora/syphilis or psora/sycosis and we produce measles to retrain the body to recognise and eliminate the depredations of syphilism and mumps to lift the burden of sycosis, so we produce other conditions to deal with the inherited taints of TB.

Whooping cough and diphtheria

These two diseases are essentially tubercular by nature; diphtheria also has syphilitic overtones and whooping cough can lean that way when it is extremely severe. It was common enough, before the advent of antibiotics, for patients with either of these two diseases to go on to develop TB – just as it was so after pneumonia. Whooping cough is usually considered to be one of the childhood diseases while diphtheria, rare these days, is not.

What makes whooping cough – or pertussis, as it sometimes called – a tubercular condition? The symptom picture has parallels with TB; it begins with a few cold symptoms – runny nose and sneezing – and a mild fever; this is followed by a cough that becomes increasingly severe and every paroxysm is followed by a 'whoop' as the patient struggles to recover breath. In addition there are often other characteristics: cyanosis – blue lips from lack of oxygen – and nosebleeds; bloodshot eyes and headaches; retching with the effort of coughing and vomiting which brings up, on occasion, quantities of mucus that have been swallowed. The situation can last for anything from two to twelve weeks. Occasionally, blood vessels can burst in the brain. With coughing and mucus production lasting this length of time it is not unusual for the patient to suffer damage to the lung tissues – bronchiectasis. This is serious as the tissue does not repair and holes are left in the lungs for mucus and pus to collect in; the patient is therefore in constant threat of renewed infection from pneumonia and bronchitis. If these do arise they are often accompanied by high fever and night sweats.

All this is very similar to acute TB. Not only does pertussis precede TB in some very sick individuals and look like some of the milder characteristics of TB but, in homoeopathy, it is treated with medicines that have a reputation for treating patients suffering from acute or chronic TB. It is very common to find that a patient who has been suffering from whooping cough or a pertussis-like cough, requires *Tuberculinum* (the homoeopathic nosode) before their constitution becomes thoroughly well again.

What about diphtheria? This is a very serious acute bacterial disease that can also precede TB. Its characteristic picture is of initial headache, sore throat and fever. The glands of the throat swell, sometimes dramatically. There is difficulty breathing as the throat closes up. This causes dysphagia (difficult swallowing) and reflex gagging and vomiting. The mucous membranes of the pharynx and throat become covered by a thick, grey, gelatinous membrane which further restricts breathing and drinking. The mucosa of the sinuses often manufacture quantities of thick, foul mucus as well. The colour of the throat can vary from white through grey and red to purple. Associated toxins can cause subsequent heart pathology.

Here the parallels with TB may not be so obvious. The swollen glands, the acute fever and the excessive mucus production are the chief ones. There can also be a croup-like cough, vomiting of swallowed catarrh and a change to a feeble pulse rate. Night sweats often persist. In very severe cases, there can be bleeding from the membranes of the throat which also occurs in TB. (These cases are often dealt with by snake venom remedies such as *Lachesis* or *Crotalus Horridus*, from the rattlesnake. The bite of these snakes causes tissue destruction and coagulation of blood in the arteries of the throat and head.) Convalescence is long and there can be complications; the whole constitution can be weakened so that septicaemia can set in along with conditions of the circulatory system and the nervous system.

There are plenty of cases of severe sore throat that are characterised by swollen lymph glands of the neck, swollen tonsils that threaten to close up the throat altogether, thick, foul mucus that is difficult to cough up or out, and feverishness. While the patients initially respond to indicated homoeopathic remedies, the symptoms only resolve completely when the patient is given a dose of the nosode, *Diphtherinum*, made from the infected mucus of a diphtheritic throat. (This is surely another indication that vaccinations do nothing more than mask the presence of the diseases that they are meant to eradicate.) The kind of case where this prescribing is not only expedient but necessary occurs in patients who have very tubercular histories and who only stop reproducing the diphtheritic sore throats after being given *Tuberculinum* and, in some extreme cases, *Syphilinum*. (The use of *Diphtherinum* to clear the symptoms of quinsy does suggest that diphtheria could be regarded, like malaria and cholera, as a minor miasm.)

This excursion into the descriptions of whooping cough and diphtheria is intended to draw attention again to the idea that Béchamp might have been keen to prove: that such acute conditions can imitate a greater and more threatening disease in order to prepare the body to deal with its own heredity. It also tentatively supports Béchamp's conclusions about the activities of the body's microzymas: that it is microzymal activity in a severely depleted constitution that engenders the production of bacteria such as the TB bacillus. Microzymas, perhaps, could also be the initiators of the steps taken by one bacterium in its metamorphosis into another.

Uncomfortable questions

Surely, such a serious and life-threatening disease as TB cannot be allowed to express itself in a patient without drug intervention? Isn't the first priority to eradicate the bacterial infection? Shouldn't patients be isolated in case others are infected? Wouldn't the ideal be to eradicate TB worldwide? To think like this is to think like Pasteur and other chemists; those who only look at the supposed activity of the bacilli. These are questions that are rational but only in so far as only *some* of the facts are known and accepted on which to make any judgements. Each question needs a qualified answer; each implicitly carries a hidden burden of meaning.

To start with, every culture in the world has had to find methods of dealing with the disease; the resulting treatments are not all the same and none of them should be ignored because they do not involve the use of bacteria-killing drugs. Next, eradicating bacterial infections is not always a priority when the bacteria are dormant; acute infection must be prioritised but so often in TB the acute episodes are simply phases of a deeply chronic state – begun long before any evidence of tuberculous bacteria were present. Isolation is often what a tubercular patient seeks anyway though in a rather different sense than the question implies; isolation in a sanatorium will only reduce the likelihood of infection in others *immediately in danger of their own susceptibility* – a condition that does not go away just because there are no coughing TB sufferers in the vicinity.

The last question has its origins in wishful-thinking humanitarianism. It is inconceivable that the efforts made by science in the last century could lead to the eradication of TB. The disease is part of our *nature* and, unpalatable though it might be, it has contributed a dual legacy, both negative and positive, through every successive generation. It is important to realise that in focusing so much on the *acute* disease we are in danger of losing sight of the *whole* picture of the tuberculism. There is a vast canvas to explore and we need to call on some key witnesses to show us the way.

Keats

John Keats' mother died from consumption when he was fourteen. He had devotedly nursed her to her death. His brother, Tom, died at nineteen of the same condition when Keats was just twenty-one. Keats himself was only twenty-five when TB killed him in 1821. Tom, the gentle brother, had faded away in spite of the love and devotion of his family. It took John only five years to write himself into history with the most extraordinarily passionate poetry before pain, coughing and emaciation relieved him of his life too. They were intense years crammed with fervour, frustration, ardour, confusion, bitterness, imagination, jealousy, vitriol and love. He was inflamed by life and he burnt himself out.

The first physical signs were evident from his tendency to catch chills. Then in early 1820, after a period of apparent good health and creative spirits, he became chilled to the bone after travelling on top of a coach without a coat on. He rapidly developed a high fever with delirium. On coughing he brought up blood which, with the knowledge he had gained as a medical student, he knew to be the arterial blood of a consumptive. The surgeon who was called then bled him, after which he was starved on a vegetable diet and forbidden to exert himself by reading or writing poetry – all of which was likely to hasten the speed of decline. For some months he languished in various lodgings, writing despairing, bitter letters to the love of his life, Fanny Brawne. Despite his engagement to her, Keats made it hurtfully plain that he had equivocal feelings about the state of marriage. The more the disease gripped him, the more he made himself out to be the bleak outsider looking in at the cheerful merrymakers round the hearth. Yet he would also be full of remorse and grief that he could write to her in such terms.

He tried to stave off the inevitable by travelling in search of a better climate than the cold, damp winter of Britain. He went, in the company of his great friend, the artist Joseph Severn, to Italy. He eventually came to a halt in Rome. After months of spewing blood from his lungs and with a sense that he had no more strength left, he wrote: 'I have an habitual feeling of my real life having past and that I am leading a posthumous existence.'

Joseph Severn, always in attendance, watched his patient go through high fever, delirium, teeth-chattering rigors and debilitating sweats while intermittently vomiting cupfuls of blood. One of the great Romantic poets died a shrivelled wraith in the fraternal arms of his faithful friend. When they opened up his chest to see the extent of the disease, they could not understand how anyone could have lasted so long with so little lung tissue left. Joseph Severn, in spite of being in the poet's potentially lethal company for so long, never contracted TB. He died 61 years later and was buried beside his friend.

D. H. Lawrence

Lawrence took quite a bit longer to die. Born in 1885, two weeks later he developed bronchitis and was not expected to live long, being a child with a weak and fragile constitution. Throughout his childhood he suffered repeated colds and hacking coughs. He twice developed pneumonia and the year after the second bout he spat up blood for the first (recorded) time. By 1916 he was 'so far gone with consumption' that he was exempted from military service. Like Keats and many others, he went in search of a more suitable climate for his lungs and travelled restlessly, trying out Europe, Ceylon, Mexico and America. To worsen to his appalling health, he contracted malaria while in Asia and had recurrent bouts of it in Mexico (for which he was given quantities of quinine), as well as typhoid fever that crippled his gut. He also suffered but amazingly survived the 1919 'Spanish' flu epidemic that killed more people than the war.

As if this were not enough, he was at one stage persuaded to inhale radioactive spring water and on another prescribed a cocktail of phosphorus and arsenic which left him feeling poisoned and thoroughly worsened. Having initially refused to admit any belief in the fatal diagnosis and having avoided for years the exile in a sanatorium suggested by several of the umpteen doctors who examined him, Lawrence finally came to a grinding halt in France where he traipsed between lodgings and a sanatorium. In the final act of his life he weighed not much more than six stone; he had hallucinations and a sense of detachment from his physical body – at one point mentioning that he could see himself 'over there, on the table'. He spent long hours of the night, restless, awake, shivering and sweating by turns.

Intriguingly, one of the last doctors to examine him, later to be an eminent specialist in chest diseases, pointed out that, while Lawrence had probably suffered from TB for ten to fifteen years and there was extensive scarring in the lungs, there was only one small cavity – a surprising fact for someone so far gone with a disease that creates holes in the lungs by destroying tissue. The doctor went on to say that it was Lawrence's general condition that was so poor. 'His resistance to the disease must have been remarkable to have enabled him to survive so long while doing all the wrong things...'

Strict rest was ordered though the physician knew that it was probably in vain to tell such a man to behave like a convalescent. Lawrence died at forty-four after months of miserable suffering and having shown an extraordinary degree of quiet stoicism for a man known for his diabolical rages.

Lawrence had met his wife, Frieda, when he was twenty-six. In spite of their violent rows and intermittent separations (when Frieda was unfaithful), they had remained inseparable. Frieda was a strong, vital woman who had given up her children to be with Lawrence. For eighteen years she lived at close quarters to and shared a passionate if somewhat curious and turbulent relationship with this tuberculous man. She survived him by 26 years, dying on her seventy-seventh birthday as the result of a stroke. She smoked like a chimney and had lungs like bellows.

What Keats and Lawrence can tell us

There are almost as many differences between these two great men as there are similarities. Keats came from a family riddled with TB. The hereditary element is direct – even though Fanny, his sister, and brother George never contracted the disease. Lawrence came from a mining town that would have been rife with TB but, while his father was a miner of robust constitution, David Herbert never went down the pit where conditions were known to be conducive. Lawrence's mother was slight and sensitive but she was known more for her vigour and determination. (She died hideously of stomach cancer – the causes of which might be found in Lawrence's partly autobiographical *Sons and Lovers*.)

As a child Keats was reputed to be short of stature but tough; he liked fighting games and seems to have had a reputation for athleticism. He had none of Lawrence's feeble constitution; he did not succumb to frequent bouts of coughs or feverish colds until later, in his teens. What he did have, though, was a furious temper which erupted suddenly and frequently ended in tears. His moods swung between extremes bewilderingly fast. Lawrence, on the other hand, remained as delicate as Keats was initially robust. He found physical fights intolerable and he could not stand arguments as harsh words seemed to be almost physically painful.

Keats' TB had come on after a severe, feverish chill – whether the disease was already there but dormant can only be surmised from the emotional background to its development; Lawrence's TB had apparently developed from a bout of pneumonia. The speed of Keats' decline was far more rapid than Lawrence's. Both men suffered deprivation, poor housing and indifferent treatment – though Keats had to suffer appallingly from being bled while Lawrence refused to accept specific treatment for quite some time. While Keats' lungs deteriorated so quickly, it was Lawrence's insistence on living intensely and in a significantly unhealthy manner that ultimately caused his constitution to succumb to the TB. (Though some of the appalling treatment that he did accept would have contributed to his demise.) Keats' lungs were completely destroyed by the activity of the bacteria while Lawrence's lungs only had one small cavity and some extensive scarring. Lawrence complained that it was his bronchus (the main airway into the lungs) that was the seat of his condition. At their deaths, Lawrence died comparatively patiently while Keats fretted that his friend and the doctor would not help him to take his own life by supplying laudanum.

So much for the differences; it is in the similarities that we find the essence of tuberculism. Both men were of the utmost sensitivity; they felt emotions to an excruciating pitch and they were left exhausted, weak and vulnerable by the turmoil. Both were prey to anger which could erupt with lightning speed and was expressed in any form from impatient irritability to towering rage. These furious feelings were vented on those dearest to them and on those who impinged negatively on their lives – publishers, politicians, even friends. Both suffered the direst pangs of jealousy, characterised by irrational imaginings of faithlessness – though Frieda Lawrence did give her husband just cause. Both could be charming, delightful and witty and had the keenest perception about others. Yet, while they could empathise to an extraordinary degree, they could be unremittingly intolerant and capable of downright cruelty. Both men demanded absolute devotion and loyalty from their loved ones even to the point of self-sacrifice as both had an ideal of what a love relationship should be – all or nothing. Both formed friendships that endured even the harshest criticism that seemed to be based – at least from the friends' point of view – on the flagrantly vital quality of life of which these poets were possessed. They were both incandescent life forces that proved irresistible to those attracted and intrigued by their passion.

Both Lawrence and Keats suffered a common symptom: *restlessness*. Neither could find comfort or satisfaction in any one place; they had to keep moving. It was not just the need to find a suitable climate that made them shiftless; it was the disease that engendered an inner sense of dissatisfaction. Lawrence frequently arrived at a place which he felt would be ideal for both domesticity and his muse but the feeling did not last long. As a result of failure to find what they were ever in search of, they were both prone to fits of deepest melancholia. Their letters are full of despair, grief, bitterness, remorse, guilt and hopelessness. Idealism was common to both men. Lawrence, particularly, drove himself and others to distraction with his schemes for a Utopian communal life based on friendship and simplistic communism. They pursued their image of perfection indefatigably and the stores of passion they invested in it contributed to their deaths. So much powerful and intense emotion is unsustainable for any length of time. It becomes pathological.

We can see that even before there was any outright evidence of TB, both men displayed characteristics of the disease. The typical mood swings, emotional outbursts and exhaustion were all there early on. Both felt intensely about relationships but were involved in those that proved unsatisfactory, partly or mostly due to an ambivalence in their natures. Both felt intensely the sense of restriction at being tied down by any institution – such as marriage – even though both so wanted to enjoy a sense of 'belonging'; both felt that they were 'outsiders'.

Then there was the fevered imagination; both had intuitive insight which at times exaggerated and illuminated their irrepressible powers of invention. This tapped into their already combustible temperament with the result that they were weakened physically enough to be susceptible to producing infections. Both knew the symptom of short but intense physical exertion causing a disproportionate loss of energy. These are all well recognised symptoms of the disease. At the same time as the onset of physical acute symptoms, the sensitivity to climatic conditions began – though Lawrence had felt these all his life. In spite of the discredit that clean, crisp mountain air [13] has fallen into as a prescribed treatment for TB, both men did suffer from lowland climates of cold, damp weather or oppressive, hot humidity. Both complained that they felt such weather conditions had a deleterious effect on their health.

Robert Louis Stevenson

It is interesting to compare R. L. Stevenson with Keats and Lawrence. He too was born a sickly child. He developed frequent colds and had the same hacking and racking coughs that Lawrence had. He had a vivid imagination that, at times, disturbed him and left him wondering whether his inner visions were part of a dreadful childhood – though they were not. He had a bout of diphtheria which left him further weakened and later, while living in America in penury and poor health, he had pleurisy. Illness for him was marked by cold sweats, prostrating cough, bouts of total exhaustion, loss of voice and fever. He knew he had consumption. Yet, before he left the USA to travel restlessly round the South Sea Islands, a sputum sample taken by a doctor whom he consulted showed a negative reaction; no bacteria were found. (This is reminiscent of Béchamp's case of gangrene where no bacteria were found.) The same thing happened to Lawrence while he was a teacher in Croydon and in danger of losing his job because of the suspicious symptoms that looked so much like TB.

Stevenson's mind seethed as tumultuously as Lawrence's and Keats'; not only did his imagination boil over with fantastic stories but his intellect was deeply involved with religion and philosophy. He had powerful moral principles and, like the two other poets, he had a burning sense of righteousness and a loathing of injustice. Idealism was common to them all and is almost a given state of mind amongst all tubercular people and those touched by inherited tuberculism.

Comparing acute TB with the miasm

The comparison of the acute disease with the chronic inherited miasm is just as instructive here as it was with syphilis, gonorrhoea and scabies. TB has a signature and it is readily witnessed. Before there is evidence of bacterial invasion, there are mental and emotional changes that take place. They are often concomitant with the frequent susceptibility to colds, 'flu, bronchitis, pneumonia, pleurisy and or tonsillitis. Mood swings, irritability, irrational bouts of anger followed by abject remorse; sensitivity to all external stimuli and to atmospheres, daydreaming and flights of imagination are all part of the picture. Sleep is often punctuated by horrific nightmares which can seem frighteningly real and continue into waking. As with Lawrence, who only developed his persistent rage with puberty, children can be so sickly that they do not show the mental and emotional activity so soon but remain quiet, cautious and studious as a method of self-preservation. This often leads them into conflict with other children who see them as reserved and haughty or as a butt for their jokes; they are frequently treated as victims. No wonder that many of them become 'outsiders'.

There is also a heightened degree of angst over relationships. This can appear in small children, no less than in adults. Children can be possessive about their mothers and deliberately antagonistic towards their fathers; they can be piteously insecure about both parents which can lead them, in their manipulative moments, to play one off against the other. In their intense state of lack of confidence due to the swings in temperament the goal is to survive the emotional storms. Tantrums erupt from frustration at not being able to perfect what they are doing. (In a TB tantrum there is almost always a trigger to be found; this is not necessarily so in a sycotic one.) In very delicate children, harshness of any description can be physically painful and these people might, if their underlying state is more passive than active, turn into family peacemakers, to the detriment of their own creative spark.

In adults, relationships are idealised. The character of love becomes one of yearning and pining; love becomes a focus for emotional pain. Puberty is often early and complicates an already difficult emotional life. Passions run high and often in the wrong direction. It is common for tubercular people to become involved in full and physical relationships before resolving those with their parents. Consequently many of them feel pulled in different directions or still eaten up with hate and guilt while experimenting with adolescent love. Inevitably this can lead to confusion: about self-confidence; about expectations; about sexuality.

Children cannot stay still; they cannot concentrate; they constantly fidget or interrupt. Adults pace about; they fidget with pens or rings; they cannot concentrate on learning anything for extended periods; they find it difficult to settle. Restlessness affects the future: careers are marred by many and varied false starts; sudden ambitions prove to be unsatisfactory; nothing comes up to expectations, least of all the other people with whom there is continued contact. There is a wanderlust that becomes imperative to answer, especially when everything else becomes heavy going.

If the patient is exceptionally gifted then the scenario can be slightly different. There is extraordinary concentration on developing the gift. The tubercular person excludes all extraneous superfluities and devotes every ounce of energy to the task of learning their craft in order to become the mature and fully fledged artist as soon as possible. (There is as much ruthlessness about this as the screaming toddler demanding absolute attention for all the waking hours of the day.) Such people usually command a marked respect from the rest of us by dint of their rare degree of self-assurance and self-determination – which is often only as deep as their chosen discipline. What else there is of themselves is a shambles in constant need of propping up by more practical people.

Their sensitivity leads them to a natural understanding of other people's difficulties and suffering. There is an overflowing empathy which causes them to feel emotionally involved and can lead to entanglements in the lives of others that they eventually might come to regret. The person who will watch, enthralled, a tear-jerker film is just as likely to listen to the sob story of a neighbour or the heart-rending news item of refugee children from some war-torn country, with tears running down their face. Overemotional reactions are more common than not; while they can lead to generous feelings of joy for others' happiness they can also be expensive by depleting stamina when the emotions are spent on other people's traumatic lives.

Tubercular people have great difficulty in preventing themselves from becoming sucked into emotional whirlpools.

There is a downside to this. Our willingness to be drawn into the emotional maelstrom of other people can lead us to wish to go beyond contributing positively and charitably and to start to interfere with their lives. By seeing ourselves as better off than those who are suffering we assume a protective role. Our feelings get the better of our common sense and the tubercular missionary zeal tempts us to tell and show others how things ought to be. The result is often disastrous, domestically, culturally and politically.

The effects of tubercular susceptibility

The chest is the most common focus for ailments. The child catches cold as soon as the weather changes; as soon as the east wind blows; as soon as his hair is cut and washed; as soon as he goes back to school. Along with chest trouble or throat problems there is the high fever which can burn all night and, if it breaks, there is sweating and delirium with the vision of monsters or soldiers or black dogs. When a cold starts, there is bronchial congestion, rattling, bubbly breathing with infected mucus, yellow, green or khaki. It runs from the nose, it blocks up the sinuses and the Eustachian tubes and it runs down the back of the throat causing eventual vomiting – a decisive moment that can sometimes resolve the acute symptoms by expelling everything at once. This is often followed by a persistent cough – dry, tickly and spasmodic or rough, hacking and paroxysmal. These days, if the cough continues, it is called asthma even though it isn't. It is a tubercular type of bronchospasm. Or, if there is a 'whoop' to it, it is probably an undiagnosed case of whooping cough, virus or no virus; vaccine or no vaccine. What is often missed is that these acute episodes can be preceded by a storm of temperament. They are equally often followed by weakness, poor appetite and lack of willpower. The period of convalescence can be a lot longer than one would expect. The parent might even be suspicious that the child is malingering.

Weak-chested individuals often do not have much flesh on the ribcage but this is by no means the only sign of the tubercular state. What is of far more significance is if the chest is sunken; fat or thin, tubercular patients may well have a tendency to concave ribs with an inverted sternum. This goes with a pallor which can cause the skin to appear that translucent, somewhat greenish colour, especially when ill. Hair is fine and often lank. Nails break easily. There is a tendency to fungal infections such as athlete's foot. Posture is round-shouldered and slack and they are inclined to lean, droop over furniture and slouch at meals. This description might make it seem that all tubercular individuals are rickety, weak and feeble. However, even strong, fit people may show the tendency by not growing as broad shouldered as their hips would lead one to expect. The result is a less robust upper half with a strong and muscular lower half. The tendency is always there to any or all of these details in someone who is susceptible to producing TB – even if it were to take years for the acute disease to manifest. This description is, with infinite variations, one that fits a vast proportion of children, young adults and artists throughout the western world.

Almost all children go through a tubercular phase; a time when their tuberculism is to the fore. They have these acute episodes of fevers and infections and we think little more of them than that. The vast majority of cases are treated by paracetamol or antibiotics or by letting nature take its course. It becomes worrying only when they persist. It is the not knowing why there should be susceptibility to these frequent acute illnesses that is difficult to cope with. There is no orthodox label or clinical diagnosis for susceptibility. The labels start being applied only when suppression of the frequent acutes causes the patient to produce a chronic condition such as so-called asthma, allergic rhinitis or otitis media; frequent childhood fevers, recurrent nosebleeds or tonsillitis.

Actually we do have a diagnosis for this susceptibility – it is the TB miasm and it has come up to be treated. There is a purpose in it happening during childhood: so that the patient will arrive at sexual maturity equipped to pass on genes *less tainted* by the inherited miasm. Now think of how many must be missing the opportunity to treat this naturally.

So what if children do go through this tubercular phase without holistic treatment? They usually grow out of it and all the sore throats and chest infections do not reappear – despite the fact that most of them have been suppressed by antibiotics. Yes, children very often do appear to grow out of the frequent acute episodes and grow up into puberty without suffering fevers and colds. Then they grow up into restless, rebellious teenagers who want to kick against their parents' upbringing or leave home at fifteen or drop out of their examinations. They have terrible acne and rotten digestions. Girls have trouble with their periods and boys lose their focus. The childhood years of preparing the immune system by having acute illnesses that enhance disease resistance are over. The body is doing other and more hormonally orientated things after puberty sets in. So, instead of being able to produce physical symptoms to express tuberculism, the whole body expresses this state through the psyche and produces complex patterns of emotional imbalance. Those acute flare-ups do return; they begin to be a nuisance at just that time when the person has settled into a life routine in the thirties or forties. By this time that person has had children and the tainted genes have been passed on yet again.

The only difference between a toddler with an angelic face and a filthy temper and someone like D. H. Lawrence is that the former is unlikely to go on to produce full-blown TB while they live in congenial surroundings, are given loving care, nutritious food and creative prospects. Change those positive conditions to negative ones and some form of tubercular pathology will inevitably follow. It is a salutary fact that in the practices of busy homoeopaths a very large majority of child patients require *Tuberculinum* as part of their treatment before they achieve really good health.

A closer look at the TB signature

One of the chief characteristics of TB is the restlessness; the need to break away from routine, from restriction. It is not hard to find a parallel in the acute disease. The bacteria that develop and multiply once they have found a convenient spot are tackled by the immune system which sends white blood cells to surround the foreign bodies until they are thoroughly encased. In those whose immune system is compromised, there develops a stalemate; the bacteria are not killed off and excreted, they are held in perpetual check. That is until some new event lowers the body's resources and resistance to the point where the bacteria can muscle their way out and start to spread all over again. The caseation breaks apart, releasing bacteria that are associated with purulent material and damage the surrounding tissue. This process accounts for the fact that many TB patients have periods of remission which are then followed by renewed and worse bouts of disease. It is this process of imprisonment and breakout that is reflected by the tubercular psyche.

The fine balance between holding the bacteria in check and the breakdown of resistance is also reflected in the miasm. The mood swings are characteristic. Many people – and especially children – are frequently described as being like an angel and a devil or like Jekyll and Hyde; it is no accident of nature that it was Stevenson who wrote this tale. Cherubic children who have 'the terrible twos', sudden outbursts of furious temper, are displaying this tubercular lack of balance. The distance travelled at lightning speed between sweetness and rage is pathological.

The bacteria, once they have broken out of the cheesy mass formed around them, set about destroying their environment. It is not a deliberate act; bacteria do not have an intelligence with which to cause the damage. Similarly, once seized with fury, a tubercular patient will become destructive, not as a syphilitic would with deliberate and calculated purpose to wound or to destroy, but to relieve their pent-up emotions, blindly and indiscriminately. They will throw things and smash them; they will kick or lash out; they will slam doors, stamp feet and run away. They will not notice danger; small children in a temper might run away from the restraining parent straight into the road or into unknown territory and get lost.

By the same token, the powerlessness of the patient's immune system to stop the bacteria from breaking out is reflected by the feelings of powerlessness in relationships that are restricting. Lawrence spent his whole adult life combating this. His frightful rages with Frieda were about his inability to be her stronger half. Their conflict turned to threatening behaviour and physical violence – he would strike her; she would retaliate. Such episodes would always end in the same way: he would be thoroughly weakened and become pathetically dependent.

None of these characteristics depends on the presence of the bacteria though. One does not have to be suffering TB acutely to experience these emotions to some degree, either in oneself – for we are almost all affected at one point or other – or in others of our acquaintance. It is only necessary to be aware that the tubercular miasm is uppermost and in need of attention. Knowing how to read the signs means that the miasm can be balanced before it becomes out of hand and turns to physical expression.

TB and higher matters

What of the spirit? Where do idealism and romanticism come from? These two great matters of the heart and of the spirit are of the very core of the TB miasm. In the miasms discussed so far we see the following spiritual traits and how to use them to a positive end:

Psora
– there is the unworthiness to be fit for God's purpose; the positive way forward is to learn our limitations and to operate within their confines, exploring every potential of which we are possessed.

Syphilism
– there is the sense that there is no God to be worthy for;
– it is the acceptance of the ultimate benevolence of the universe and that there is a place for each and every one of us in it without the need to seek control for our own security or the domination of others.

Sycosis
– there is a confusion of identity and a sense of something missing, of something other-worldly and mysterious that draws us off into a cloud of separation from our grounded, purposeful selves.
– the life lesson is in seeking the integration of body, mind and soul.

In TB there is something quite different yet it is something of a mixture of the others. In tuberculism, where we are at any moment soon begins to feel insufficient and unsatisfactory; it is as if we must move on to find a more exciting or productive place. We are driven to explore our environment (mental and emotional as well as geographical) to its limits and beyond in a search for the ideal place to settle, but each place proves as inadequate as the last. What is missing is contentment. Whatever faith in whatever god we might hold dear is not enough for us to be content with our lot. We become spiritual and emotional nomads. The problem is not the external environment but our internal one. Yet we are always loath to find fault with ourselves so we blame the external. (This is a mistake that we do not make in psora.)

Tubercular subjects, being of a highly imaginative nature, often visualise their dream place before they reach it. This has two disadvantages: what they find can rarely match their expectations and they become waylaid by surface glamour and only look into things skin-deep before dissatisfaction creeps back in. So, in their pursuit of the ideal they fall short of it, often because of a lack of psoric thoroughness in doing the groundwork. For tubercular people are also sensationalists who are seized by the thrill of pursuit: of excitement, of pleasure, of novelty, of the eccentric. The act of discovery becomes an end in itself; there is always the need to know more.

Romance is one of the most attractive aspects of tuberculism but it is often accompanied by an urgent need for sensuality which can draw people towards the excesses of sycosis and the destructiveness of syphilism. Not for the tubercular is courtly love; they might pay lip service to it but such tedious formality is basically psoric and quite beyond the impatience and questing ardour of a tubercular person. The TB miasm is the story of the struggle and interplay between high ideals and adrenaline-driven desire. It is the story about romantic love that stops at the bedroom door but would continue in the divorce court. It is the history of our creative imaginations, shot through with a curious mix of spiritual and libidinous fantasy, running riot, plotting our own gratification and glory but falling short of what we need in order to achieve it all. Fulfilment is always just out of reach.

In tuberculism, lust becomes the double agent of love. Not surprising then that early promiscuity is a symptom of its miasm. The desire to experience everything leads to sexual experimentation. Even with primarily lustful relationships there is a longing search to find the ideal mate that is thwarted by the ever-present sense of dissatisfaction. The one-night stand is not exclusively a tubercular trait but, when it is part of an unacknowledged quest, it most certainly is. Our contemporary habit of eschewing marriage in favour of unfettered partnerships is distinctly tubercular as the back door is always on the latch if not open for escape. The *reality* of the Lawrencian ideal of a combined mystical and sexual union is quite beyond the scope of any tubercular person as their unbalanced temperament creates too much stress within any relationship – but they are driven to try for it; a 'tuberculean' effort. It is, however, not so very far from the hedonistic revelry of bacchanalian sycosis; sex for sex's sake as a means of lifting oneself out of the drudgery of everyday life. It is a bit further off from the cynical, chilling and calculated sexual exploitation that is one of syphilism's characteristics though a disappointed tubercular person can easily slip down this route. It is a long way from the straightforward, practical, down-to-earth, procreative union of friends that is the healthy aspect of psora.

Many tubercular people mistake their idealism for spirituality. Despite the positive characteristic generosity of spirit and of personal sacrifice that is peculiarly tubercular, there is a tendency to proselytise and cajole others, often with emphatic intensity, into joining them in thinking, feeling and acting in their way. This is the essence of Cervantes' Don Quijote de la Mancha, one of the greatest tubercular characters of fiction. The escapades of the eccentric knight with his fantasies of love and honour, bound up with an impossible ideal image of the perfect woman, encapsulate the once brilliant but now fading vitality of all that is essentially tubercular.

This is also the trail of missionary zeal and it commonly ignores and is generally impatient with what has existed satisfactorily up to the moment of contact with those it seeks to influence. It is redolent, too, of the art world since revolution erupted at the end of the eighteenth century when the Classical and the Baroque gave way to the Romantic. This is the world of Byron, Shelley, Chopin and George Sand: the restless, transient world of sweeping passions and endless travelling from Italian villa to mountain shack and back. It also informs the character that medical research has assumed since Pasteur and his contemporaries began exploring the world of microbes. Tubercular people can have an extraordinary spiritual arrogance and conviction that their path is the right one and this miasmatic tendency has led many otherwise (psorically) painstaking scientists to believe that their profession can improve on nature.

Yet it is not always so. Others have faced the temptations that could just as well have led to disaster though they have had the strength of purpose (or lack of stamina) not to be sucked into the dark pit of no return. Jane Austen's world may be mistaken for the genteel pastoral idyll suggested by her happy endings but there is no doubt about the strength of passion that rocks the lives of her characters. In *Pride and Prejudice* Elizabeth's father, Mr Bennet, did not feel impelled to drown his sorrows in drink or take a lover or to contrive a fatal accident to be rid of his exasperatingly silly wife. His good humour and self-effacement are very psoric traits. The eponymous Emma's naive ebullience and snobbery is tempered by an ability to accept her errors of judgement once she sees them. Not for Mr and Mrs Knightly are the tempests of tubercular or sycotic passions.

But all we have said so far, about the miasmatic influence of TB, is a generalisation. Not all miasmatically tubercular people (and that is, sooner or later, most of us) are so easily categorised. There are inevitably subtle differences from one individual to another. The scale can range from the weak and dependant 'victim' to the dramatically powerful personality of a 'leader' or 'aggressor'.

The end of the tubercular road

'Burn out' is a particularly tubercular problem. Those redolent of the miasm are especially susceptible to stress. The extreme sensitivity, the restless anxiety to achieve and the sense of dissatisfaction with everything all contribute to the easy sapping of vital energy. This means that those who do not know how to temper their creativity with discretion, with balance, with harmony and with compromise break down physically, emotionally and, eventually, spiritually. Just as it is perfectly possible to survive the ravages of acute TB so it is possible to survive the torrential outbursts of creative inspiration characteristic of the miasm that might otherwise lead to susceptibility to the disease itself. Lawrence never compromised and his pathetic, etiolated body paid the price. The rest of us have time to learn from our disabilities and shortcomings. TB and its miasm are all to do with striking exactly the right balance while sustaining creativity. The same is true of psora but the purpose behind this miasm is to become deserving of a place in the family, in society, in nature; a proof of adequacy. Psora is content, at a profoundly healthy level, to 'be'.

621

With tuberculism, the sustained creativity is the end in itself; 'doing' equates with 'being' and 'being' ceases when there is no more energy to 'do'. Nobody really of the tubercular miasm is ever truly content simply to 'be' – unless they have learnt its lessons. One such was Igor Stravinsky, iconoclast of twentieth-century music, who suffered TB as a young man but by dint of a routine of hard work and the sustained rigour of self-discipline survived well into his eighties. Like all great artists he set himself to reinvent his creativity constantly; his musical journey nevertheless bore the unmistakable stamp of the tubercular in its extraordinary, almost bewildering diversity of style. By balancing his tubercular nature with the psoric resources of one willing to keep his nose to the grindstone, he lived long and productively.

Tuberculinum, the nosode, and other tubercular medicines

At this point it is worth turning to another form of 'evidence' in the search for understanding of TB and its soil in the psyche – the medicines made from tuberculous material.

There are several nosodes of TB. This is confusing for homoeopaths who sometimes have difficulty in selecting which one to prescribe when the remedy is indicated.[14] That which is called *Tuberculinum* bears the name of Robert Koch who had first isolated the *Mycobacterium tuberculosis* in the laboratory. What he had done was to raid the Hahnemannian philosophy books – as did several of his contemporary colleagues – and create an 'isopathic' medicine.[15] What he failed to do was to understand the principle of potentisation through succussion; patients were therefore treated with *live* material of TB. In fairness it should be mentioned that Koch's discovery was eventually used to help some patients who suffered from TB of the skin (lupus) and it was also put to use later on by those who realised that it could be used to diagnose cases *prior* to any development of symptoms.

Homoeopaths have been very grateful to Koch ever since. Tuberculin was potentised and proved, mainly on tuberculous patients; so the homoeopathic clinical evidence is based on cases treated and cured by this remedy in its homoeopathic preparation. Dr Clarke's dictionary has been a primary source for the information since it was published a century ago.

Before looking at this extraordinary medicine in depth it is worth mentioning the other TB nosodes.

i) *Bacillinum* is made from the infected sputum of a tuberculous patient. It is very similar to Koch's preparation but it was not 'prepared' in any way before it was potentised, there being no glycerine content or suspension.

ii) *Tuberculinum Bovinum* is made from the tuberculous tissue of cattle. This is commonly used by homoeopaths today, not least as the connection between bovine and human TB was (and in the third world still is) very strong.

iii) *Bacillinum Testium* is prepared from the tuberculous tissue of a testicle. As with *Bacillinum* we have Compton-Burnett to thank for this remedy as he was the first to describe its value in the clinic.

iv) *Tuberculinum Aviare*, as its name implies, was prepared from the diseased tissue of a chicken. It is not a particularly well-used remedy which is a pity as, amongst other things, it has a remarkable effect on post-influenza patients who do not get better quickly.[16] (They tend to suffer poor appetite and a persistent cough.)

TB in the mind

Dr Clarke tells us only the basic details about *Tuberculinum*'s mental symptoms. Patients were *anxious, gloomy* and in a *melancholy humour*. There was a disposition to *whine and complain*. There was dejection and *nervous irritation* with an aversion to any form of work, *especially mental work*. There was *sensitivity to music*. Also noted was a dislike of being *disturbed by people*. With a century's experience of using the remedy we can expand on what he tells us.

Tubercular children are unmistakable: they are often bright as a button and quick-witted. The parents will describe them as Jekyll and Hyde, one moment they are happy and extrovert and the next they are brittle, irritable, negative and introverted with a tendency to throw tantrums. Little things can trigger off this change: being asked to complete a chore or to finish dressing; being given the wrong pencil or too much mashed potato.

In a tantrum, they are furious and unreasonable. They will stamp their feet, slam doors, drum their heels on the floor, bang their heads on the wall and throw things about. They might lash out with a swift kick – usually at someone whom they know would not strike back, such as a younger sibling. They might escape to another part of the house or the garden or out of the supermarket. They are oblivious to anything except the moment and there is usually a degree of bloody-mindedness about getting their own way. Such a storm of emotion will leave them weeping and probably exhausted. They very often cannot explain why they went into the tantrum; they have forgotten what it was all about or they dissemble and pretend not to remember because they do not want to have their emotions discussed.

Such tempers can be displayed by anyone of any age though older people are usually more subtle in their behaviour patterns. The aim is the same – a discharge of emotional tension brought on by hypersensitivity and/or frustration. It is there from the 'terrible twos' to second childhood. Mothers complain of their infants who seem to be not just crying for attention but really angry with it. Teenagers become restless, anxious and irritable and their school work suffers. They slack off and flounce or slouch about; they seem far less energetic and are preoccupied. Parents wonder if it's boyfriend or girlfriend trouble; which it may be. They become morose and monosyllabic. They are at their most cheerful when they are with their friends, going to parties or out on trips. Anything that hems them in feels like a restriction. This is typical teenage behaviour but if there is a pathological loss of energy, motivation and *joie de vivre* then it is distinctly tubercular. People in their twenties or thirties who do not settle down to a career but need constant change are beginning to dip into the TB miasm. They will travel nomadically from country to country. They will try doing something here and another thing somewhere else but nothing holds them for long. To be tied down would make them fret and chafe; they would become uncomfortable to live with; those who try to settle feel that they cannot understand what makes them tick. If a tubercular person felt that the ties were becoming too tight then they would 'do a bunk' – escape is easy; they do not hang around to give explanations.

The miasm might well surface in early middle life. Here it would be the cause of sudden decisions to break out of a mould. Snap decisions about career or relationship changes might not actually be so snap; they are often preceded by depression, anxiety, irritability and intolerance. In a household where everything might have been running smoothly, tempers begin to flare; words of explanation are not spoken but kept back; atmospheres develop which are pregnant with suspicion, worry and hopelessness. Resolution often comes in the form of sudden changes that seem to satisfy the ego – but usually it is only temporary.

The miasm can arise with and complicate the menopause – for both women and men. With all the necessary hormone changes it is more physiologically obvious in women but men will display the typical patterns behaviourally, even if it is in the mildest and most subtle forms – such as sudden anxiety about their health accompanied by an urgent desire to take up some activity that would help keep them fit; golf is a favourite. Rather more disturbing is the demand by menopausal women for HRT which, apart from the dubious medical reason of preventing osteoporosis, is essentially an internal cosmetic to put off ageing naturally.

Cantankerous, eccentric old people with short tempers are often tubercular; this is especially true if they are restless, anxious and given to wandering off in their minds. They become petulant and hate being fussed but they are very demanding of company which tends to tire them out more quickly than they care to admit. Like their grandchildren, they are often prey to quick mood changes that they find difficult to disguise. The restriction of infirmities is what frustrates them most just as with the younger generations it is the restriction of parental control or the school system – or even just nappies and bedclothes. They tend to become saddened by all the things that they imagine they could have achieved. They may be given to fantasising about what might have been. Reminiscing does not belong to any particular miasm but when it is tinged with regret, sadness and anxiousness then it can be typical of the tubercular state.[17]

Apart from the temper there are other aspects of the psyche that are very characteristic. Fear is very prevalent, especially during childhood. There are fears of anything that might restrict them or impede motion. Some children can be fearful of closed places (claustrophobia) and almost all tubercular children prefer to be out of doors. (There are exceptions and they are likely to be those who have some traumatic reason for preferring to be in enclosed spaces – such as a difficult birth and a consequent separation from the mother for a period afterwards.) There is a fear of animals in spite of an urgent wish to be with them. The most commonly cited example of animal fear is of those that are black. This is a very real problem for some children and it has a connection with dreams; tubercular children who have either nightmares or high fevers with delirium might 'see' black dogs approaching them aggressively – though they are quite as likely these days to refer to monsters or to dinosaurs. Also associated with this are irrational, sudden fearful dislikes which take the parents by surprise; they are unaware that the child has developed an instant negative reaction to something witnessed in a dream – express trains, soldiers, woodland, the milkman.

A seemingly insurmountable fear is that of the night. All those children who need night lights, well into their primary-school years and even beyond, are simply expressing something of the miasm – though sycosis can have this trait strongly too. This should not surprise anyone as tubercular patients will imagine anything out of the weird shapes that can come at them out of their mind's eye in the dark. Furthermore, this is the miasm of 'the bright lights'; that need for company, light and the business of living things. There is the fear of being alone which contrasts so curiously with that need to escape.

There is a fear of poor health – hypochondriasis. In children there is a fear of any little hurt; a thoughtful explanation will usually temporarily dispel the anxiety. They only want to know what they cannot explain for themselves. In the teens there is a fear of the physical body not appearing or performing at its peak. There is a great preoccupation with the cosmetic; acne becomes intolerable; eczema also. Such problems can cast them into despair out of proportion to the condition – and explanations will not do. Later on there is a fear of infection; anxious parents, particularly of tubercular children, become obsessed about the threat of quite simple conditions such as colds, tonsillitis and minor chest complaints. There is the fear of ageing and of heart disease. Both these have to do with the increasing inability to move. There is frequently despair at the imprisonment of old age.

The Jekyll and Hyde pattern is not restricted to infancy. Later on it comes out in mood swings and contradictory behavioural patterns. A timid child can throw a monumental tantrum and be completely obdurate about getting his own way. A tearful, clingy child might suddenly become aloof, cold and sarcastic. An independent, self-confident lad might become nervous and dependent and lose all his self-esteem. Quite usual stresses might provoke these switches of mood and behaviour. The underlying common factor, however, will always be that some form of restriction is being imposed. This might be parental control, school rules, unremitting bad weather, suppressed instincts, workload or some form of stifled self-expression. While daily routine is what most supports a psoric person, is manipulated to best advantage by a syphilitic, ignored as far as possible by a sycotic, it will seriously upset a tubercular one. The constant desire for change has to be met. One of the ways this is expressed healthily is for the person to set himself goals and challenges. Each achievement is a spur to create more. This can get out of hand as can any other facet of the miasm. Recklessness is a major mental indicator of *Tuberculinum*. (They often have a history of accidents and broken bones from the sports they love playing; they tend to be spendthrifts as well.)

The need to broaden horizons can be academic and intellectual, emotional or geographical. Part of the challenge of life lies in experiencing the sensation of changes as well as the change of sensations. The desire for travel burns in the physically adventurous; the wish to explore the mind can glow in someone who is physically timid and who would not dream of travelling further than the next bus stop. Both might be expressing the restless spirit of tuberculism; both feeling the joys of discovery. It is when there are impediments to discovery and change or when weakness catches up with the person so that they are unable to carry through their plans, that ill temper or sickness erupts. Little ailments become the cause of anxiety; there is fear of something impending; there is the loss of concentration. Soon the irritability explodes into abusive language, vicious thoughts, sudden impulsive reactions; cruelty is not far from the surface – this is the adult's version of the child's tantrum.

It was noted by Clarke and Compton-Burnett that TB and its effects were strongly related to insanity. As Clarke notes insane patients who suffer acute infections characterised by high fevers often experience an improvement in their mental condition. High fevers (such as might be dealt with by *Belladonna* or *Stramonium* – both tubercular remedies and both useful in treating some forms of insanity) are often if not always tubercular in nature. This fact suggested that the use of *Tuberculinum* in cases of insanity would be beneficial. The results reported by Clarke showed that '...though the decidedly favourable [i.e. curative] symptoms soon disappeared after the fever subsided, still there was a steady clearing of the confused sensorium'. Compton-Burnett recorded a case of insanity entirely cured after he had been led to administer *Bacillinum* to the patient by dint of his suffering ringworm – which is a tubercular, fungal, skin eruption.

Insane patients do not, as a rule, consult homoeopaths. Long before the idea of seeking alternative help for psychical conditions arises, such patients are sectioned and prescribed drugs. In the present medical climate there is simply no idea that homoeopathy might be of service. Yet it is not so very far-fetched to think that someone in need of *Tuberculinum* (or remedies that are closely related) might be bordering on the insane. It is not normal for the mind to be so easily tipped one way or the other by slight causes. To watch a five-year-old in a tantrum in which he is banging his head against the floor or the wall in a manner that would obviously be painful and distressing is a temporary insanity. For an outgoing, optimistic self-confident teenager to become withdrawn, morose, belligerent and prey to suspicions and frightful anxiety is a temporary insanity. For a pretty girl with no material worries and bright scholastic prospects there may be no obvious reason to become anorexic; this is a peculiar form of insanity that is not always simply hormonal and not always just a temporary episode.

Insanity is a form of expression even if it is taking abnormality beyond the socially acceptable and it is also a form of release – from the appalling difficulties of fitting into normality when 'normality' to the patient is severely warped from either experience or heredity.[18] A person who might, conversationally, be described as 'mad as a hatter' – a mildly insane person and not one who requires restraining – and comes (or is brought) for treatment, may do reasonably well on their prescriptions. Yet, overall there is the sense that the mental world they live in is more comfortable than the real one; there is so often the sense of escape into unreality. As with so many deeply held conditions, there is an unwillingness to face healing changes.

Tubercular in mind and body

The mind symptoms of the *Tuberculinum* remedies (for they all share most of the symptoms mentioned above in some degree) are not too often witnessed in isolation, without physical manifestations. It is not unusual for the physical symptoms to be the deciding factor behind a prescription. It can be difficult to decide, based on the mental symptoms alone, whether the patient needs *Tuberculinum* or *Medorrhinum* or *Syphilinum*; the three medicines apparently share so many aspects of behaviour. (We shall see why this is when we come to make a more detailed comparison.)

One of the most common instances of the use of *Tuberculinum* is in cases of children who have recurrent high fevers. These fevers often respond well to *Belladonna* but there are cases where, in spite of all the indications: red face, cold extremities, throbbing arteries, glazed eyes, hot head, *Belladonna* does nothing at all. Or there are cases where *Belladonna* does work but the fever returns with above average frequency. Often the child has the typical mind picture (alternating mild and furious moods, alternating truculent and silly behaviour, a tendency in the fever itself to become delirious) to go with the intermittent fevers. *Tuberculinum* deals with both the fevers and the difficult behaviour. It is common for the parents to report that the child has a sudden burst of growth and learning after the remedy.

> A girl of five was reported to be having nightmares. She would wake up screaming and terrified. She would be inconsolable but, the parents explained, she would appear not to be awake; she failed to recognise that her mother was there, consoling her. She would sit up in bed and twist her fingers; she would weep and point out things in different parts of the bedroom. Eventually she would become exhausted and fall asleep again but only if the light was left on. The nightmares would happen two or three times a week but the girl was unable to say what she saw in her dreams; it was as if the memory of them was blocked. She was only aware

of the fear. In the daytime she was well but she had taken to being extremely unkind to her younger brother; she would pinch him and bite him and then run off, leaving him to cry. This situation had begun after she had had a high fever some four weeks before. The mother had given *Belladonna* with no effect. After 48 hours the temperature had come down with cool sponging and Calpol. Since then, apart from the nightmares, she had very flushed cheeks. She had also been rather clumsy which the parents had particularly noted as she was normally a very well-coordinated child. One other thing – the girl had developed a very peculiar high-pitched, rather manic laugh that the mother felt was *"false"*.

The child was given *Stramonium*[19], a remedy made from a highly hallucinogenic plant, *Datura* or the thorn apple which covers just this curious mental condition; one that is surprisingly common. The nightmares stopped altogether; the behaviour returned to normal and she became her usual well-coordinated self. There was no return of the fever even though that had been predicted. Some ten days later the mother reported that her daughter was again showing signs of the vicious temper towards her baby brother. She was also very restless and, in spite of the cool weather, wanted to take most of her clothes off. At this point she was given *Tuberculinum* with the almost immediate effect of a raging fever. The temperature peaked at 104°F but by the following morning had completely disappeared. No further symptoms were reported. The terrifying dreams and the distinctly insane behaviour pattern may have been typical of *Stramonium* but this remedy had not dealt with the underlying miasm exemplified in the beginning by the original *Belladonna*-type fever. (It is not uncommon for TB patients to have wild delirium in their feverish episodes which might well respond to *Stramonium*.)

Tuberculinum is sometimes called for to deal with acute fevers. For example:

A mother phoned to say that her son (aged nine) had a very high fever and it was climbing. It had started in the afternoon (it was now 9 p.m.) and she was worried about going through the night without any advice. The picture that emerged was of *Belladonna*. The mother had given *Belladonna* 30 several times but it had done nothing. She was directed to give the same remedy in the 1M potency and report back within an hour. There was still no change after the higher dose and by now the child was showing *"worrying signs of delirium"*. At this point she was asked to give the boy a dose of *Tuberculinum* 200. In the morning there was a message on the clinic answering machine to say that the boy had gone to sleep within a few seconds of the *Tuberculinum* and, though he had had no appetite for several days, had woken wanting breakfast.

In both these cases the underlying tubercular miasm was responsible for holding the patient back from complete cure. Neither patient was particularly threatened constitutionally by their illness. There are more chronic conditions in which the nosode is vital.

A boy of twelve was brought for treatment. He had suffered from bouts of tonsillitis for a long time. His tonsils were so enormous that they appeared to close up his throat, only leaving the narrowest of apertures for air – and when he was examined he was not in an acute episode. The left tonsil was worse than the right and was of a dark red hue. The other was paler but looked pitted, rather like the surface of a golf ball. The lad was tall and thin, pale and peaky but he had a very cheerful expression and appeared to be completely unworried about his problem. He said that he was used to having sore throats; he developed them every six to eight weeks. There was a long history of taking antibiotics.

In taking the case of such a patient it is always advisable to find out not only the general constitutional picture but also the common symptoms of the acute flare-ups of the throat infections. Constitutionally, he appeared to need *Silica* a common childhood remedy for those who are thin, pale, chilly and prone to glandular problems. This was confirmed in his case by the tendency to suppurative processes (his tonsils produced quantities of pus) and profuse foul sweating of the feet (he did not need to remove his shoes for this to be evident). For the acute throats he needed one or other of the mercury remedies; it often depends on which side of the throat is affected as to which one is prescribed. He was sent off with a supply of three different mercury medicines, each one labelled with indications and instructions. He was also given *Tuberculinum* 200 to hold in case of need. This was one of those cases where physical reactions were almost a foregone conclusion – and he was warned to expect 'aggravations'. *Silica* is a remedy well known for its ability to galvanise the body into its centrifugal habit of expelling from within all that needs to come out. And come out it did.

Within 48 hours of the *Silica* the throat became extremely sore and the tonsils inflamed. There was a filthy, metallic taste in his mouth, the glands on the right side of his neck were swollen and like a string of beads. His tongue was a repulsive shade of yellow and thickly coated. He was very light-headed and he felt excessively bloated and full of wind. He was given protoiodide of *Mercury* 200 (*Merc-Iod-Flav.*, for short, which covers this apparently disparate collection of symptoms) which made him feel less dizzy and easier in himself, caused the digestive symptoms to ease off and brought down the glands in the neck. Then the left tonsil flared up; his neck became stiff and he was unable to turn his head; he became inordinately thirsty, the glands below his chin swelled and he produced foul mucus from the back of his nose. For this he was given a different mercury, the red iodide (*Merc-Iod-Rub*, for short). This remedy also did its work. The grossly swollen, dark red tonsil on the left went down, he could move his head and speak more distinctly. Again he felt better in himself. He reported that he had sweated profusely all over on both the nights after the remedies. Though he did not get much sleep he said that he felt as if the perspiration had been to the good. Throughout this episode his temperature remained slightly below normal. After the second lot of *Mercury* he found that his left tonsil had exuded white pus which came away when he hawked and spat. Because he said that he felt so well he was not given any further remedies for the time being.

Within the next three months this type of acute flare-up happened three more times; each one slightly different in that the order of the acute remedies was not the same. In addition to the mercury remedies, he also needed *Hepar Sulphuricum* at one point. After the third episode there was less pus from the tonsils and the pain in the throat and neck glands was much less severe than before. It was evident that each successive bout had been less of a problem. Nevertheless, he was left with permanently swollen tonsils and sublingual glands and he felt as if he had a permanent cold, one that was just lurking below the surface and wanting to 'come out'. He kept sneezing and had a persistent post-nasal drip. His mother also reported that he had become very easily bored, was far less able to concentrate, was disinclined to do his homework and was getting poor reports from the school. She felt that he was becoming a 'typical teenager', rebellious and independent, full of "*backchat*". This was a propitious moment to prescribe *Tuberculinum*. The result was that the cold came out without the usual tonsillitis. He poured mucus from his nose for three days after which it gradually dried up. He felt well with it. Within two weeks he reported that the glands were far less swollen though his tonsils remained enlarged. (They went down somewhat over the following two years.) The following year, at the same time, he developed another sore throat. He was given the appropriate *Mercury* and was asked to take a dose of *Tuberculinum* 10M when the acute problem had resolved. He has remained well ever since; he is no longer thin, peaky and pallid.

In this case the affinity for glandular trouble is illustrated. It is extremely common for one of the tubercular nosodes to be given for illness involving tonsils, cervical glands (back of the neck), submaxillary glands (under the chin), glands of the external throat, axillae (armpits), the breasts, the abdomen and the groin. Children who complain of tummy ache when they have a fever are often feeling pain in the mesenteric glands of the abdominal wall. Women with painfully swollen breast glands before their periods are quite often in need of *Tuberculinum* even if they do not otherwise feel physically unwell. (Though they may well complain of premenstrual tension with some or many of the typical behavioural symptoms of the remedy.)

Hypersensitivity and allergies

One of the most common conditions of hypersensitivity and allergy is hay fever. It is becoming a nuisance of epidemic proportions even if it is not regarded as a particularly serious problem. Two myths need to be dispelled about it. The first is that it is only a seasonal problem. It might appear to be so in some but it can be a perennial condition in many others. The second myth is that allergens, be they grass seed, pollen or any of the host of others, are the cause of hay fever. They are not the cause; they are the triggers for the symptoms. The underlying cause is the hereditary mixed miasmatic influence of psora and tuberculism. Look into the family history of any hay fever case and there will be links in the past generations that show TB to have been there before – and psora is always lurking.

Hay fever is commonly linked to eczema and asthma. It is usual to find either or both these problems in the relatives of a patient who comes for treatment complaining of watery, itchy eyes, copious sneezing, running and itchy nose and dry skin on the face. Eczema and asthma are linked and both are profoundly tubercular diseases. Hay fever makes up the trio in that eczema of childhood often diminishes or even disappears – one is said to 'grow out of it' – only to be succeeded by hay fever which in its turn can be succeeded by asthma (though for those with a stronger inheritance of TB the hay fever step is frequently missed out). This progression is all too commonly the result of allopathic suppression.

Sometimes hay fever comes out of the blue. It can come in a wide variety of symptom combinations. Some have no trouble with their eyes whatsoever but suffer terrible irritation in their throats instead. Others have only chest and nose symptoms. Yet others are to be seen rubbing their faces with the exasperating itchiness of the facial skin. What is more, the same allergen can illicit different symptom pictures in two different people. So dog's hair can bring on tickling in the throat and wheezing in one but streaming eyes and profusely running nose in another. The allergen is simply an agent of irritation that sets up the individual's unique response and it has no determining factor that dictates what that response will be.

The range of symptom combinations is relatively limited and it is not too difficult to select the remedy that is most likely to ease the symptoms. Patients produce hay fever pictures that conform to the energy pictures of a well-known group of remedies. It is easy to spot a *Euphrasia* (eyebright) patient or an *Allium Cepa* (common red onion), a *Natrum Muriaticum* (rock salt) or a *Nux Vomica*. In fact, patients who might be sceptical of the efficacy of homoeopathy can be won over by the apparent success of taking the appropriate remedy for their intractable condition for which they are so used to having to resort to antihistamines and decongestants.

Yet it can take up to three or four years for someone to be relieved of their hay fever entirely. The reason for this is that the indicated remedies for the hay fever symptoms are never likely to be anything more than that; they are not 'whole body' remedies, homoeopathic to the patient. They are palliative remedies for an irritating condition. To eradicate the tendency to hay fever it is necessary to treat people constitutionally and on a deep level.

A woman of thirty-five complained of a congested head, a feeling of something lodged deep within her nasal passages, itchy ears and a sore mouth. Worse than these was the feeling that her throat was swollen, that the pharynx was dry and prickly and that the roof of her mouth had an itch which she simply could not reach. She had had recurrent bouts every year for the last five years, ever since the birth of her last child. (Hormonal changes can be a factor in setting off hay fever.)

She was given *Wyethia*, a remedy made from an American plant that produces just this symptom picture. It worked well and she was much relieved that she could take a pill every time the symptoms began to get the better of her temper. She did not come back for any constitutional treatment in spite of being advised to do so.

The problem was that in the following year, the symptoms were different and the *Wyethia* no longer did anything for her. The case was taken again and a new picture emerged. Now the focus was on the eyes and the nose. There was burning and rawness in both with much foul, yellow mucus. Her symptoms needed *Kali Iodatum* (potassium iodide), a vicious chemical in its raw state. This remedy did a lot to relieve her again but this time she agreed to return after the hay fever season was over for some constitutional treatment so that the following year would affect her less.

During the following months she came twice and was given remedies that covered her general state. She had *Nux Vomica* – she was an ambitious businesswoman with a keen sense of purpose and a very intolerant attitude to inefficiency which she had no compunction in demonstrating. She was also, a little later on, given *Thuja* as she became concerned about her ability to function due to feeling detached and rather separated from what she felt was her normal reality. When the hay fever season came round again she began to have allergic reactions but they were somewhat milder than the previous years. For this new attack she needed *Arsenicum Iodatum*. Her eyes were watery and sore, her nose produced quantities of yellow, burning mucus and her throat was dry. Though the new remedy worked well she reluctantly agreed to continue to come for the out of season treatment. She was given *Tuberculinum* 1M. She had no further attacks of hay fever at all.

Not all patients are so responsive to treatment. The more chronic and the more perennial the problem is, the longer it will take to deal with. Some hay fever sufferers need 'strategic' doses of all the nosodes before the problem will resolve. Allergy trouble can be evident in any of them. Irritation and restlessness will mark out tubercular allergies; profuse, foul catarrh, compromised breathing and violent histamine reactions will characterise sycotic allergies; raw, sore, excoriating mucous membranes that produce thin, burning and sometimes foul-smelling mucus are typical of the syphilitic allergies. Anyone might and most do produce a combination of these. The original soil in which all this occurs is psoric. This scheme of things also holds true for eczema.

Eczema

Eczema is a profoundly uncompromising expression of heredity. It is thought of as a skin disorder but if we limit it like this then we gravely underestimate it. Eczema can express our deepest nature. It can also – and usually does – assume responsibility for some of our inexpressible emotions. Skin diseases are so often an overspill from our unspoken minds and hearts. Tuberculism is probably the most common reason for a case of eczema not to clear up. This is not surprising given the extraordinary degree of sensitivity and emotional seesaw to which all tubercular patients are subject.

A small boy with weeping, bleeding eczema of the backs of his knees, his ankles and his wrists was brought for treatment. He was a chubby child with ample folds of skin and it was in the folds that the problem was at its worst. Every morning he would have scratched his limbs till they were raw, sore and bleeding. Sometimes the result became infected and he would be given antibiotics. He was a hot child and always threw the covers off his bed at night; sometimes his mother would find him on the floor sound asleep – she had learnt to leave him there.

The symptom picture of this child's condition added up to a prescription of *Sulphur*. He was given *Sulphur* 6 to be taken on a daily basis. He responded well initially and the parents were pleased to see a more marked improvement than they had done when they applied topical steroid creams. The improvement came and went, came and went. When he had bad skin, they reported, his temperament improved dramatically; when his skin was calm and healing over, his mood became intolerable. They noticed this development over an eight-week period. When this symptom swing was added to another feature of this boy's case – his tendency to throw high fevers quite frequently with a subsequent outpouring of copious catarrh – it was clear he needed *Tuberculinum*.

This he was given with the result that his skin flared dramatically for 48 hours (though he remained happy). This was followed by a gradual improvement of the eczema areas as well as the general quality of the skin which had been rather coarse, especially on the cheeks and the upper arms – common places for tubercular roughness. His fevers grew less dramatic and further apart and without any flood of mucus. His temperament evened out until tantrums, headbanging, biting and truculence were a thing of the past. His skin has always been inclined to show how he feels 'in himself'. Now that he is older and able to speak for himself he says that, whenever he is anxious or lacking in confidence about anything, his wrists begin to redden and feel sore and the sides of his fingers begin to itch. He feels that it is a signal for him to 'take things easier'.

From these cases (which are far from isolated) it is clear that *Tuberculinum* has the ability to clear miasmatic blocks in the same way that *Syphilinum*, *Medorrhinum* and *Psorinum* do. It is used as a remedy of resolution when the indicated remedies do not complete the action of cure.

Tuberculinum as a constitutional remedy

It is so common to find hay fever, asthma and eczema within the family history of patients who require *Tuberculinum*. Emotional turmoil amongst such families is also to be expected; there is always a deep seam of untapped angst that has never been resolved. It is often the case that patients presenting for treatment of physical pathology that is tubercular in nature will reach a stage of using the consultation more like a counselling session. As they talk about themselves, in terms of their physical symptoms, they begin to stray into explaining how they *feel* within themselves. They often apologise for going off the point but this is because it is not obvious to them that they have begun to express their familial emotional processes. Though their history of emotional turmoil and grief is their own, they are as much a genetic product of their parents and other forebears *in their emotions* as they are in facial features – though remaining unique individuals. It is usual for someone of one generation to reflect in their history something very similar in emotional effects of a person from a previous generation *where the forebear found it impossible to resolve the painful issues*.

If a mother carries the burden of guilt that she ran away from home to marry an 'unsuitable' man or that she had an abortion after an affair, it is common enough that her daughter will mirror this in some way when she reaches a similar age. The act may not be precisely the same but there will be an echo in the emotional effect. The later event can even spark off in the parent a healing reaction as she relives her own grief through her offspring's trauma. In cases of unresolved emotional trauma, *Tuberculinum* is a very important remedial agent. It will not expunge history but it will help the patient to discover within whatever healing resources there might be; to accept the past and encourage understanding and self-forgiveness. Though we have few details of the mother's emotional history before her daughter was born, the following story can serve to illustrate the point.

A young woman came for treatment. She was seventeen years old and only came because her anxious boyfriend persuaded her. She appeared nervous but she only needed a few minutes to settle into the unaccustomed surroundings in order to find her voice. *"I have eating problems. I can't eat. I don't have any appetite and when I try to get anything down I just feel sick. Sometimes I do vomit."*

She had had this problem for several months, ever since her mother had taken a new boyfriend to live in the house. *"He's OK really, not my type but he doesn't bother me. It's my Mum. She makes me so angry. We're always rowing and she wants me out of the house. I spend most of the time at my boyfriend's house; his Mum's nice. She just leaves me alone. She's always let Mark and his brother come and go as they please; she calls them latchkey boys. My Mum always has to know where I am and what I'm doing. It wouldn't be so bad if she really wanted to know because she was anxious or something – but she's not. She's been like that since Dad went. He left about eight years ago; he found out that Mum was having a relationship with someone else. He just upped and offed; later we found out that he'd been having an affair with one of the dinner ladies at the school. She was nice, I always liked her. I'm not surprised that he liked her. They're still together; married. I don't see him that much."*

After a diversion in which she spoke of her school days and of how she was now on the point of leaving school to find a job, she went back to the subject of her home life. *"I don't remember much before I was five or so. My older brother was always off with Dad – he sees him much more than I do, and Mum was always in the kitchen or doing the books – she did all the money side of things – or making curtains or covers; that's what she does. Things were different after Dad left though. It was weird, somehow. It wasn't a good time. Mum was always busy; she was afraid of something, I think."*

She had begun to fidget. Her talking seemed to become elliptical; she was not hesitant at all but it was as if she were speaking around something rather than stating what was on her mind. Quite suddenly, after making some unremarkable comments about her brother and mother, she said, (referring to one of her mother's lovers) *"It wasn't nice when Charlie was there; my Mum was afraid. I hated him; he had such a mean look. He thrashed her when she found out. I didn't tell anyone; she guessed. He made me swear not to tell anyone; every time he made me swear. I don't know how many times; I lost count. It stopped after Mum found out but it had gone on for months, years it felt like. I used to hear him say that he'd be happy to babysit. It was about the only time he could have been happy to do anything. The rest of the time he'd be swearing and hollering all the time. I don't think my Mum ever forgave me. We never talked about it and then Charlie was gone. Funny, I used to have trouble eating then, too. Mum used to try and force me to eat everything on the plate but I wouldn't even when she threatened me with the doctor. If I'm at home now, I have to get my own meals. She said she gave up trying."*

The girl gave a sense of isolation and distance; the feeling of an 'outsider'. Though her emotional history indicated *Tuberculinum* – and sexual abuse is a distressingly usual historical reason for this remedy to be needed – there were other symptoms that confirmed it. She did have a craving for crisps and ice cream. These were the two foods she could guarantee to keep down. *Tuberculinum* covers the craving for salty foods as well as ice-cold things. She was able to drink quantities of milk; another tubercular craving. She was intolerant of being indoors too long; there were times when she had to get out of the house – wherever she was – and walk, whatever the weather. She was prone to fits of anger which she took out on her boyfriend; she would want to hit him and had done so on occasion. She was desperate to leave school; she wanted to travel.

She was given *Tuberculinum* 1M. When she returned in ten weeks she was quite different. She had lost that 'outsider' look and sense. She was open and frank and looked extremely well. She was back to a normal eating pattern and was actually enjoying cooking. She had moved back into her mother's house more permanently and had decided to do another year at school. She still wanted to travel – *"more than ever"* – but she realised that she needed qualifications, if not to go abroad then to come back to when she wanted a more settled job. She was also getting on better with her mother and she had decided to see more of her father. She also stopped seeing her boyfriend, at first gradually and then altogether. When asked what she felt the treatment had done for her she replied, *"Apart from a stinking cold, I'm not sure but I suddenly somehow knew that it was no good being angry all the time; it was so exhausting. I knew other people weren't going to change just because I wanted them to."*[20]

Typecasting tuberculism

It is possible to pick out from a crowd those who would *seem* to be the most likely people to be susceptible to tuberculism. Like Lawrence and Franz Kafka, who died of TB of the throat, they would be thin, wiry, etiolated and drawn. (Think of Modigliani's paintings of women.) The quality of the skin would be poor; it would be thin and sensitive. The hair would be lank. They would tend to sweat and feel damp from it. They would have a tendency to take cold easily. The eyes, when well, would be brighter than most people's but, when ill, they would be dull, sunken and lifeless. Generally, they would give the impression of being tense and restless; they might fidget with their hands. If nervous and timid, the restlessness would be in the eyes alone; watching, observant, looking as if searching for a suitable escape route. (A tubercular person's visual and aural acuity can be phenomenal.) When they become animated there would be a flush to the face; or the ears might be suffused with blood. But this is not the only kind of person who develops signs and symptoms of the inheritance of TB.

The typical tubercular child might have many or all of the above features but, if so, they would be likely to be rather more ill than otherwise. There are children who are relatively well and yet, like the case of the *Belladonna*-fever child, need the miasm treated. Thin, fair and precocious would describe many of them. Frequently such children grow fast and have sturdy legs but thin, weak musculature of the chest. They might even be pigeon-chested. If they grow into their teens like this they can appear to be pear-shaped. There is often a fine blond down on the back from the top of the spine to the mid-back. In babies and very young children the whites of the eyes are more of a translucent bluish colour; like porcelain. (This is not to be confused with the normal blue colour of the eyes of newborn babies.) Such children are often easily startled and can have reactions bordering on the hysterical to anything unexpected. Every change of weather can bring on a cold or a chest problem. They might have a permanent runny nose. They can be prone to frequent nosebleeds. Wounds take a long time to heal.

Precocity is often academic or physical or both. Yet there is often a downside to this. Though it might be a source of pride to a parent that their child is exceptionally talented, it would behove them to consider that the child might be susceptible to tuberculism. Many bright children advance rapidly in one area but lag behind in others; the achievements mask the lack of progress in less obvious aspects. The boy who is gifted at maths might not be going through the normal steps of childhood. He might demonstrate this by lapsing into silly behaviour – thumb sucking and tantrums – at twelve or thirteen. The girl who is prodigiously gifted at playing the flute might dissolve into floods of tears when there is too much pressure and then not be able to face going to school – all of which might lead to frequent bouts of, say, tonsillitis. (Or, as in one case, severe tenosynovitis; an inflammatory condition of the tendons of her wrists and elbows that prevented her from continuing to play her instrument.)

Such children often benefit from their remedies in a peculiar way. The reactions to the medicines, which almost always include *Tuberculinum*, are a cessation of the physical symptoms and a regression of behaviour patterns. The parents complain that their son or daughter had not done this or that for years; there might have been tantrums or bed-wetting, thumb sucking or clumsiness. By leaving such deep-acting remedy reactions alone and asking the patient and the parents to wait until they have finished, it is as if the remedies cause the child's system to go back in time and complete a stage of development that was never experienced at the appropriate time or not fully resolved. The energy that had been invested in the development of the major talent tended to divert the whole system away from an even development through the normal stages of childhood. Remedies allow the bit that had lagged behind to catch up.

Increasingly it is becoming obvious that many children with learning difficulties have strongly miasmatic tendencies.[21] 'Learning difficulties' simply means what it says; it has little to do with intelligence except in specific cases. Many children who have the utmost difficulty in reading or writing, concentrating or computing are attempting to use brains compromised by awkward wiring. Such 'faults' do not constitute illness even though parents are often heard to say "*I don't know what's wrong with him!*" – before they realise the nature of the problem. Yet what they are complaining of is the nature of the child's behaviour. This can include any or most of the typical behaviour pattern of the tubercular state. Few children, brought for homoeopathic treatment, who are labelled hyperactive, ADD (attention deficit disorder) or ADHD (attention deficit hyperactivity disorder) are not in need of *Tuberculinum* sooner rather than later (though, as has been seen, they often need other nosodes as well). The remedy will often cause the child to regress to a time when the imbalance between the emotional, mental and physical bodies first began to manifest. This occurs too early in the patient's record for even most parents to be aware that such a thing might be happening. There are definite signs that can be looked for: early talking but late walking; bottom shuffling; slowness to be involved in group activity – instead there is a tendency to hang back and observe; difficulty in holding small, light objects; refusal to read despite obvious intelligence etc. Such signs suggest that the origin of the learning difficulties began not just in the toddler or infant years but in the womb.

It should not be supposed from this that *Tuberculinum* is ever prescribed in order to put right such learning difficulties – dyslexia and dyscalculia (difficulty computing numbers) being the best known. It is prescribed because the general symptom picture of the patient calls for it. The learning difficulties are not the *cause* of the need for *Tuberculinum*; they are incidental to it. Nevertheless, as part of the 'picture' of *Tuberculinum* there are symptoms that include the apparent making of 'errors'; mistakes in calculation, in connecting words, in spelling, in the ability to concentrate and so on. Other remedies also cover such 'mistakes'; *Lycopodium* and *Thuja* are just two of them but they are very commonly prescribed before (and after) indicated doses of *Tuberculinum* which supports their action.

A boy of six was brought by his mother because he was having difficulties at school with his work and his social relationships. He was also very small in stature for his age. The mother was worried because she felt that he was a bright boy who was being held back by his problems. He was always exhausted by the time the school day had finished at 3.30. He would come home extremely irritable and hungry; he would be insolent to his mother and vindictive to his younger brother; he would go straight to the television and remain glued to it, seemingly oblivious of anything going on around him. Supper would improve his mood, almost instantly. (The mother had, at one stage, resorted to giving him a chocolate bar as soon as he came out of school so that he would not display such filthy temper. This had not worked as he became hyper on the chocolate.)

He had become truculent towards the teacher of whom he had been very fond. He often refused to involve himself in work tasks she set and he would never commit his work to paper, preferring to answer questions aloud. He frequently flew into a rage; he might become furious with another child or he would demonstrate his frustrations by ripping up all the work that he had done. This included many of his drawings, which particularly distressed his mother as this was an area of his work for which he was always praised and which he enjoyed.

"He's always been such a self-confident little chap. He never had any problems when he was in the pre-prep. He had lots of friends and he was always popular but now he's being isolated. I'm not surprised because he's frankly so beastly to the others. One or two of the other mothers have said to me that they have been a bit worried because he's been bullying their children. Nothing dreadful but it's not right. I have tried to talk to him but it honestly hasn't made any difference. To start with he's mortified and he says he's so sorry and it will never happen again. Within a few days he's back to being just the same. It's been like this since he started doing full-time proper school work."

When the mother was asked what seemed the most troubling aspect of her son's situation she replied that it was his behaviour.

"He's so rude and beastly. He hates everything and he must be in such a torment to have such a 'down' on everything and to wear such a dark expression on his face all the time. He swears like a trooper. He knows all the four-letter words! Frankly, I'm exhausted."

The picture of the child's behaviour was that of the remedy *Anacardium*, a nut from South-East Asia that has a heart-shaped kernel that is black; neatly appropriate in a homoeopathic sense. He was given three doses of the 1M potency. Within days his behaviour was quite different and he was back to what his mother felt was normal. However, he developed a severe cold and cough which his mother felt was threateningly like a chest infection. During the course of it he threw a high fever for which he was given *Belladonna* 200. He recovered and returned to school before the week was out.

His teacher reported that the boy was back to his usual cheerful, friendly self but that he was now given to bursting into tears when he could not complete work within the time allowed. He still had moments of frustration during which he would destroy his work. He could still be very loud and vociferous even though the other children were now not avoiding him. There were times, still, when he would become quiet and withdrawn. He would look pale and have dark rings under the eyes. The *Anacardium* had worked well but only on the top layer.

643

The boy did not shake off a cough that had lingered from the cold. He had a runny nose and found it difficult or impossible to blow it. He developed tummy aches which came on after lunch, as he was getting tired. He would go home complaining of them. They would be gone by the late evening by which time he had had some food and managed to evacuate his bowels. "*I have to say that the bathroom is very smelly after he's been in there. He does seem to have got an awful lot of wind.*" As an afterthought his mother added that he had had a growth spurt which she felt had contributed to the tiredness and being easily run down.

For this general state he was given *Lycopodium* [22] as it covers this ragbag of symptoms: sensitive, tearful but at times loud and brash; snuffly nosed and windy with a bad time in the mid to late afternoon. It is also a tubercular remedy as it has a strong affinity for the lungs and larynx and the production of quantities of mucus. The boy was given *Lycopodium* 1M with the result that the cough, the windiness, the snuffles and the afternoon tiredness all vanished. So did a lot of loudness. The teacher reported that he was producing more work than ever and that his spelling had improved.

So far so good except that he was unable to maintain the improvement he had achieved on these two remedies. Odd symptoms resurfaced from time to time. Along with this came a gradual wearing-down process that seemed to undermine his general health. Within six months of the *Lycopodium* the mother brought him back and reported that her son had a tendency to excessive bouts of tiredness, a constantly runny nose and flips of mood. In addition he had experienced several nosebleeds. It was the moment to introduce *Tuberculinum*. The lack of resolution, the switching of moods, the changeability of symptoms from one site to another all indicated it, as did the spontaneous nosebleeds. He was given a dose of *Tuberculinum Bovinum* 200. Not only did his physical symptoms resolve but also his school work improved considerably. He no longer avoided doing written work though his efforts were not as neat as they might have been. His reading and writing skills rose to a level commensurate with his age. Furthermore, he had a growth spurt again.

In statistical terms, such a case in isolation has no significance. It does suggest, however, the potential of homoeopathically treating children with learning difficulties.[23] Experience shows that one cannot succeed in such cases by taking the symptoms of the specific difficulties and prescribing on them. As always, it is the whole picture of the individual at any given time that needs to be considered.[24]

If we left the descriptions of 'types' at this point we would be doing an injustice to the tubercular miasm. One should not be left with the impression that the miasm only surfaces in those who might appear in a Lawrencian novel or a Kafka story; nor that it only influences bright, precocious children who could well be geniuses with attitude; nor those neglected children, misunderstood and misdiagnosed who struggle against the flood tide of the curriculum – one of the most severe stress factors ever imposed on young minds that do not conform to the academic norm. The fact is that any and all of us are likely at some point in our lives to manifest tubercular problems. We may have missed it in our infancy, our teens and even in middle age but it will come up at some point even if it is only evident in arthritis of the extremities in our dotage. Heavily fleshed people can be just as prone to chest infections that bring on TB-type symptoms as anyone else. Those of less than average intellectual grasp who might be slow of pace can also produce the typical picture. It is not necessary to display the whole gallery of symptomatology to deduce that tubercular remedies are needed.

The main tubercular remedies

What one is looking for is *similarity* and it is never really hard to find. This is borne out by the number and nature of the remedies that have a reputation for treating not just the miasm but the actual disease itself. Some of these we have met before: *Calcium Carbonate*, *Arsenicum Album*, *Lycopodium* and *Sulphur* among them. Throughout the literature on the subject it is common to read that none of them completes a cure of acute TB on their own; there are stages through which the disease develops, each one needing remedies to hasten and lessen the process. Two remedies that are tubercular as well as profoundly constitutional (in the same sense as are *Calcium* and *Sulphur*) are *Phosphorus* and *Silica*. Both of them are easily recognisable when they manifest in a symptom picture. It is a cliché that homoeopaths speak of a *Phosphorus* type or a *Silica* type; they are simply acknowledging that someone appears to be tubercular in one or other of two ways. (It would be a profound mistake to think that either *Phosphorus* or *Silica* is only tubercular;

they are great influences on all the miasms.) To draw these portraits will help to see how both the disease and the miasm have become so completely absorbed into our everyday lives; in the case of *Phosphorus*, one of the reasons for finding all things tubercular culturally acceptable and even attractive.

Phosphorus

Phosphorus, the element, is strange. Trapped in a space without oxygen it remains dull and apparently lifeless. Exposed to oxygen it ignites into activity with a bright and hungry flare. Its intense energy is soon over; burnt out. This description encapsulates the 'signature' of *Phosphorus*, the remedy. A '*Phosphorus* person' is one who illuminates whatever they are doing or whomever they are with. They are bright and sparky, effervescent and essentially good-humoured. They bubble with brilliance, both in activity and ideas. They are often remarkably attractive physically – or good at making the impression of being so. They love being with people because what they enjoy most is stimulating company. Stimulation is a key word for this remedy type for it is needed on every level, physical, emotional and spiritual. They are the 'touchy-feely' people who crave being stroked and massaged. They become enthralled by drama and enter into the spirit of any theatrical event. They love talking about themselves but not exclusively because what really grabs them is to feel included. They may want to be the centre of attention (when well) but they would want that more if they felt it was benefiting everyone else too. They can be generous to a fault.

This is too good to be true. The downside is that phosphoric people become exhausted very quickly. Like champagne they can be bubbly after the cork is out but it all goes flat quite quickly. Phosphoric people tend to burn themselves out because they do not know how to pace themselves. The pretty, pink and white, dairymaid complexion goes pale and wan; the crisply wavy hair goes lank and greasy; the sparkling eyes look as if a light has been put out; they become limp. Their mood changes to one of irritability, of nervousness, of changeability. They can be snappy and not want to have anyone near them. They become tense and easily startled. The slightest exertion causes them to relapse. They suffer from headaches, nausea, digestive upsets, chest complaints and skin irritations. If they are careful and know when to stop they might find that short but frequent rests will restore their flagging energy. (Just to contradict this, if a healthy phosphoric is truly involved in a creative enterprise they can pursue it for as long a time as any other would. However, it is likely that they would need a considerable recovery period afterwards or else they would come down with some physical condition as a means of expression of exhaustion.)

Many things can cause a phosphoric to collapse into the remedy's particular pathology: anger, fearfulness, grief, anxiety, excessive mental stimulation or keeping up long hours of study, strong musical experiences or psychic experiences that cause a degree of shock. They can also be highly sexed individuals and excessive sexual activity can seriously weaken their systems. Though they react to having all the five senses stimulated, they suffer from hypersensitivity to the point that if they are exposed to noxious things such as gas, strong odours (like drains or flowers) or, specifically, general anaesthetics they suffer egregiously. They can also be susceptible to conditions arising from being 'allergic' – on a cellular level – to a sexual partner; erosion of the cervix or irritation of the glans penis can arise from relations with those who are physiologically incompatible.

They can be swept away by their enthusiasms. They can be so stimulated by something that they indulge in it to excess. This includes careers, hobbies and love affairs. So dedicated to experiencing sensation are they that they can lose all inhibitions. This makes *Phosphorus* a remedy often needed by actors. Their force of personality should never be underestimated in spite of their tendency to weakness. They can hold their audience in thrall or in stitches; being innate performers they respond to their audience in turn and can sustain their performance for a long period. The film industry would be a poorer place without their make-believe, their beauty, their sheer bravura or their infectious sense of fun. Think only of Errol Flynn, Rosalind Russell, Fred Astaire, Maureen O'Hara and Judy Garland – all of whom have aspects in common with *Phosphorus*.

It is not too hard to see how the phosphoric temperament fits in with a susceptibility to TB. Their physical welfare can as well.

Dr Clarke lists for us the body types who are likely to need *Phosphorus*:

i)   Tall, slender persons, of sanguine temperament, fair skin, blonde or red hair, quick, lively perceptions and sensitive nature.

ii) Young people who grow too rapidly and are inclined to stoop; chlorotic [of greenish tinge]; anaemic.

iii) Persons of waxy, translucent skin, half-anaemic, half-jaundiced. (Such persons might well be rather overweight and not fit in so well with the usual image of the slender and spare-fleshed individual suggested by i) and ii).)

iv) Tall, slender, narrow-chested, phthisical [tubercular] patients; delicate eyelashes, soft hair.

v)   Tall, slim, dark-haired persons, especially women, disposed to stoop.

vi) Nervous, weak persons who like to be magnetised [stroked or caressed].

vii) Haemorrhagic patients; slight wounds bleed profusely.

He might have added: those who relish salt, salty foods and smoked meats; who enjoy ice cream especially when unwell (it is sometimes the only thing the patient will eat); who are excessively thirsty for cold water (which, when unwell, they might vomit once it has warmed in the stomach); those who feel every atmospheric change. These are generalisations. What of particulars?

Phosphorus has an affinity for the left side. Chest infections tend to cause symptoms in the left lung, especially the lower lobe. Thick, yellow or green mucus can be formed and be difficult to cough up. The cough is hard, hacking and painful. The larynx and throat is dry, sore, rough and tight. The whole chest can feel tight and constricted. The cough is often brought on by a tickling sensation in the chest, behind the sternum. It can cause nausea and vomiting and, if mucus is brought up then it can be a rusty colour or blood streaked. A change of room temperature, talking, laughing or taking a breath to speak can all be causes of a paroxysm of coughing – which will leave the patient weak and breathless. With the coughing there can be a pallor that changes rapidly to a flushed face or, more typically, to reddened, circumscribed patches on the cheeks such as a puppet might have. If the chest infection is serious enough to be called bronchitis, pleurisy (or even pneumonia) the *Phosphorus* patient will have sharp, stitching or burning pains in the chest; feelings as if the very tissues of the lungs are tearing.

There will a strong thirst for cold water – the patient might even, like *Mercurius*, want ice in the drink. This would be quaffed down but it might make them feel nauseated. They will have a fever that comes and goes and that will be marked by shivering and shuddering because, despite the raised temperature they are chilly and cannot get warm. Any heat comes in waves and flushes and is only transient. Diarrhoea can be a concomitant symptom of chest trouble. The pulse of a *Phosphorus*, either well or ill, can be very rapid and sometimes feeble. They can be covered in a clammy sweat.

This picture would be familiar to anyone who had nursed TB patients. *Phosphorus* has a reputation for being used to beneficial effect in the acute disease in the mucosal and haemorrhagic stage, that is before the tubercles become consolidated or calcified. *Phosphorus* is one of the great 'bleeders'. It has a wonderful track record for staunching the flow of blood in more or less any circumstance (when the other indications are there) including TB.

Being a remedy of extraordinary sensitivity it is found of enormous value in treating conditions of the spinal column and the central nervous system. Numbness, tingling, twitching, neuralgia, poor control of motor coordination, sciatica and paralysis all come under its influence. Dr Clarke has also recorded that it has healed people who suffer from brain conditions. It covers vertigo, headaches and, rather more serious, petit mal and epilepsy – all when the rest of the symptom picture corresponds to the general state of *Phosphorus*.

In a generally healthy constitution, *Phosphorus* will heal on its own account a vast and multifarious collection of symptoms whenever its core symptom picture is there. In those phosphoric people who do not have basic good health, it is more or less inevitable that *Tuberculinum* will be needed to promote or complete a 'cure'. This is not to say that *Phosphorus* is never needed in cases that call for *Syphilinum*, *Medorrhinum* or *Psorinum*. It is a multi-miasmatic remedy and is in everyday use. It is, though, most often associated, in chronic cases, with tuberculism because of the *likeness* it bears to the state of incipient and primary TB, in all its aspects – or rather, the other way about because *Phosphorus* was *of* the Earth long before man or his domesticated animals produced the TB bacillus.

Silica

One fine spring day, when many in the street were already in their shirtsleeves, a patient came for treatment. He was tall, gaunt and stooping. He was untidy with tousled hair and peg teeth. He was in his fifties but his age was indeterminable from his appearance. He wore a woolly hat and a scarf which he had wound twice around his throat. When he sat down, his trousers rode up his leg a little and it was evident that he was wearing long johns. He was worried that he was continually getting so many colds. He had one at least every two months but his nose never really stopped dripping and there was always catarrh in his throat.

His story was not a particularly unusual one. He worked in the council offices as a clerk. He had gone into the job after his national service and there he had stayed. He did not terribly care for the post but it paid the bills and gave him time to indulge his hobby. He was a philatelist; he had an extraordinary passion for stamps and had a vast collection. He said that it gave him enormous satisfaction to arrange the stamps into categories of country of origin, value, date and so on. *"It saves an awful lot of money on travelling; I do all my travelling with the stamps."*

He had once been married and had a son who now lived in Scotland with his own family. His wife had left him but they had remained on affable terms until she had died of cancer some years before. The patient had a history of severe childhood illnesses. He had had whooping cough badly enough to be taken into hospital and pneumonia twice. Then, at twenty-four, he had developed TB of the left lung. He had been sent to a TB hospital where he had made a 'full recovery'. *"Since then I've more or less been OK except that I've had all these colds and sore throats. I have tried homoeopathy before and with some success but I think I need some professional help now."*

Everything about this man shouted *Silica* as the remedy that would do the most good. He was pale, thin, debilitated and undernourished. His hair was lank; he was a chilly mortal who had to protect his head and neck from cold draughts or winds – he even said that he wore his woolly hat in bed. (This is a gift of a symptom as *Silica* is the only remedy listed that will do this.) Yet *Silica* was not given.

The textbooks state that one should not administer *Silica* to old cases of TB in case the remedy reactivates it. *Silica* has a reputation for causing tissues to allow foreign objects to pass through them on their way to the surface to be expelled. *Silica* is the primary remedy for the expulsion of splinters, fish bones, shrapnel, bullets and whatever else might have become lodged within. TB tubercles are packages of bacteria that amount to foreign objects. *Silica* has the reputation of activating the body's response to them which means that *Silica* might encourage the body to set up an attempt to rid itself of the bacteria; this would have to be diagnosed as active TB as the result would be the expulsion of tuberculous material.

This patient was given several remedies (including *Tuberculinum*) over a number of years. He suffered far fewer colds as a result and when he did have one it lasted only two days and left no residual problems. He also found that his stamina improved. He became more outgoing and optimistic. He went up to Scotland to see his son regularly. He found a 'female companion' with whom he enjoyed evenings of doing complicated jigsaws or going to the cinema. However, he still had an underlying sense of "*not feeling 100 per cent well.*" His digestion left something to be desired; he still got out of breath if he exerted himself too much; his sleep was often disturbed; he was still a very chilly person who wore his woolly hat in bed.

Eventually it was obvious there was no other remedy that was remotely indicated for his general state than *Silica*. He was given *Silica* 30c to be taken three times per week for four weeks. When he returned in just over two months he seemed no different at all. Nothing seemed to have changed in any outward appearance. He said that he was well and that he had had no colds at all. He felt that he was sleeping a little better but that his digestion was not really very satisfactory as he could only pass a motion every third day. After thinking, he corrected himself by saying that every third day was better as he had only "*been going once a week*" before.

Almost at the end of the consultation he suddenly remembered there was something else. He had had a spot on his chest which had got bigger and bigger. It had come up between the lowest ribs on his left side and eventually become the size of a small walnut. He thought it was a boil so he had simply covered it with a plaster and left it alone. After some days he had a further look at it and saw that the head of the abscess had split open and was revealing a pale lump of what he took to be pus until he touched it and found that it was hard. Not wishing to interfere with it he had left it for a few more days. By this time the lump was very visible and he encouraged it to come away. "*It was hard as stone. It wasn't smooth but a bit knobbly. It looked like a round chip of concrete more than anything else.*"

(Silica is, after all, sand.) Shortly after this the eruption had healed over and there was not even a scar.

Silica had caused this man's healing mechanism to eliminate the old calcified TB tubercle in the most expedient manner possible – by thrusting it to the surface directly above the point at which the TB had created its acute manifestation some 30 years before.

It is not surprising that, if *Silica* has the ability to inspire a body to do this, it should be regarded as one of the great remedies in healing abscesses, whitlows and carbuncles. It is a remedy for cleansing of the blood as it will encourage debris to gather in the form of pus at one site so that it can be ejected. As TB involves the collection of pus in pockets in the lungs or other organs and tissue, *Silica* therefore has its place in the canon of remedies that are used for its treatment. Similarly, *Silica* will get the body to shift thick and yellow mucus from sinuses, airways and orifices. It will, when indicated, obviate the necessity for antibiotics in cases of tooth abscesses. Deeper into the system, it will encourage the clearance of the lymph system. *Silica* is one of the greatest remedies for the healing of swollen and painful glands – in any part of the body. It even has its use in such dire pathologies as lymphatic cancers where it will afford the body the chance to release blockages in hard and swollen lymph nodes – other indications being present.

However, as the last patient's story suggests, there is far more to *Silica*. There is also the constitutional picture which the patient exemplified so well. It is a major remedy for the treatment of children who are puny and malnourished; who are timid and bashful and who cling to their mothers' skirts and hide their faces; who are prone to snivelling colds and earaches and who do not grow well. Silica children are pale and have dark rings under their eyes. They are not always dark-haired as the books would have us believe but can be of any colouring. They do not eat well but have very small, picky appetites. Though they are always chilly they prefer cold foods (like sandwiches or salads) and only drink cold drinks – an example of a strange, rare and peculiar symptom. They also defy their mothers' understanding by being able to go out in the winter's cold in just their tee shirts in spite of their general low body temperature. They may be meek and shy on one hand but they can be unbelievably stubborn on the other.

If they get a bee in their bonnet about something – say, that they take a dislike to a particular vegetable on their plate that they may have eaten many times before – there is absolutely no moving them. They become silent and truculent, dark-browed and intractable. When something goes wrong, the *Silica* child will be pathetic and tearful, clingy and whiny. (This picture looks very like *Pulsatilla*; *Silica* and *Pulsatilla* are very close remedies and often follow each other. *Silica* is found in the stems of plants to provide strength and uprightness; the *Pulsatilla* plant, however, is a flower that tends to bend to every wind that blows – and survives thereby.)

Children with such constitutions are not uncommon even in our nutrition-conscious age. (It is quite usual to find that babies who are born prematurely or who were born by Caesarean section require *Silica* sooner rather than later. It is as if the experience is enough to foster the '*Silica*' energy.) As they are so susceptible to coughs and colds, ear infections and chest infections,[25] it is not difficult to see how epidemics of TB have carried off so many throughout history. Though *Silica* may not, any more than *Phosphorus*, be exclusively a tubercular remedy, it is a most important medicine that is of great use among patients who are manifesting the tubercular miasm.

The stamp collector had been born a *Silica* person. His tubercular nature had kept him working at the same sort of pathologies for his adult life. He never lost the habit of wearing long johns or a woolly hat in spite of being given *Silica*. Nevertheless, he no longer suffered the same degree or frequency of troubles. *Silica* never activated a moribund TB – indeed, it helped him rid his body of the calcified deposits of it – but it did rejuvenate him.

When is tuberculism not tuberculism?

Let's look at asthma for a moment. It is an interesting condition because it is so misrepresented and so badly misinterpreted. Part of the reason for this is that so little attention is paid to its origins and its variety. It is a tubercular condition because it manifests in forms that can so easily resemble the state of acute TB. It is a lung condition in which there is usually profuse production of mucus, considerable coughing, difficult respiration, night sweats,

653

potential fevers and debility. In severe cases there can be considerable damage to the lungs that resembles TB. Asthma is a disease with an emotional origin; all tubercular patients, as we have seen, are emotionally highly charged and most susceptible to mood swings that 'rock the boat'.

If this were all then asthma might be relatively straightforward to treat. To begin with there are more ways than one for the condition to start. Though the favourite is deeply suppressed anger sometimes from very early childhood or even from the womb, it can also be brought on by grief, anxiety or even euphoria. Beyond these there are other triggers such as a difficult birth, vaccinations and suppression of acute or chronic diseases such as chest infections or eczema. Whatever pushes the button for its manifestation, there will always be an element of the tubercular in the case because this will be the underlying and fundamental miasmatic root.

Yet we are not much nearer to healing asthma by knowing this. It is necessary to acknowledge the subtlety of the individual's body in producing its own particular signature in this disease. One asthmatic will have 'dry' asthma; another will have 'wet'. One will have difficulty breathing at night; another in the day. One will produce quantities of green mucus from the left lung; another will be affected only in the right. One will be seasonally affected; another will suffer all year round. One will cough between 2 a.m. and 5 a.m.; another will only cough in the evenings. In spite of the enormous diversity, the tubercular traits remain constant. But is the miasm constant?

Not really. We can take a brief look at two contrasted cases to illustrate the necessity of relating miasms to pathology.

In the first case there is the thin, debilitated man who suffers terrible asthma at night. He looks gaunt, dark complexioned, almost grey with it, and thoroughly depressed. He has 'dry' asthma in that his lungs produce only small quantities of mucus that he finds so hard to remove. He coughs like someone out of a Tolstoy novel and sweats profusely till the bed is soaked. He is anxious, restless and a bully. His wife ministers to his every need but the disease makes him unkind and possessive. He takes *Arsenicum Album* for his condition and knows that it gives him considerable relief even though the damage done to his lungs is irreparable in the long term; he has coughed for 40 years. *Tuberculinum* only gave him short-term benefit, respite from the last infection that he struggled to throw off. His lymph glands reduced in size for a little while until the next cold came on. Then he was given *Syphilinum*. This made the most significant difference to his well-being that he had yet experienced; this was after some two and a half years of treatment. He felt as if his whole being *"had been given a huge lift"*; it was *"as if a weight had been removed from not just my chest but all over me"*. While he would never really be well in the accepted sense, he felt so energised by this remedy that he experienced *"the worthwhile-ness of living again"*.

The second case is very different. This is a woman whose attacks come and go. She has aggravations at the time of her period so that there is a hormonal element to complicate matters. She is hot, overweight and sluggish. Apart from her cycle, the weather also triggers her asthma. When the weather is damp and humid or damp and cold then she will start to wheeze. She produces quantities of green mucus from her lower lungs, especially the left and she finds it impossible to exert herself. She becomes completely enervated. Her remedy is *Natrum Sulphuricum* (sodium sulphate) and it does relieve her symptoms considerably. They return, though, with unfailing regularity. That is until she was given *Medorrhinum*. Since this 'intercurrent' remedy, which she has every so often, her asthma attacks are much reduced in severity and frequency. Having had asthma for more than 30 years she is aware that it is unlikely that the chronic pattern will be eradicated. She is content with the relief the remedies give. It was with the *Medorrhinum* that she achieved this philosophical approach; she is immensely grateful that she feels more at peace with herself. She now feels that stress, which also played so big a part in the attacks, is less of a factor in her condition.

Both patients had generally tubercular symptom pictures. Both *Arsenicum* and *Natrum Sulphuricum* might be called for in treating cases of acute TB. Yet the principle disturbing and underlying factors were the buried influences of even deeper-held miasms. Syphilism can look so much like 'dry' TB. Sycosis always underlies a 'wet' asthma. In the first case we have a depressed man whose nights are miserable with destructive coughing and sweats. In the second we have the stress- and hormone- affected woman whose days are intolerable when the weather changes for the worse and who finds night-time worries only marginally preferable to coughing up foul catarrh all day. These two cases graphically illustrate the close relations between the three miasms. We have used asthma as an example but this is certainly not the only state that demonstrates the relationship. The parallels are evident in pathologies as diverse as chronic sore throats, diverticulosis, cancer or AIDS. They are there not just in the physical symptom pictures but also in the mental, emotional and spiritual ones. Tuberculism, syphilism and sycosis are woven into an intricate tapestry with psora as the canvas.

A curious union

The tubercular miasm is a strange amalgam of influences. It seems to have many similarities of expression with the other miasms described. In its negative aspect tuberculism can mirror sycosis in its mucus and pus formation; its inflammatory states of flesh and joints; its explosive, filthy temperament; its vagaries of mood and the gullibility. It can mirror syphilism in its tissue destruction and physical breakdown; its despair and tendency to hopelessness. The difference between the two influences goes some way to explain the marked differences between D.H. Lawrence and Keats in their TB and deaths. (Keats was far more syphilitic than Lawrence. The destructiveness of the disease on his tissues was far greater, much more associated with blood loss, more rapid and devastating.)

The similarities between the miasms are the cause of much deliberation for the homoeopath who has to differentiate between them all in order to prescribe. The difference between a *Medorrhinum* and a *Tuberculinum* tantrum is sometimes hard to spot. A tubercular rage always has a reason underlying it, generally frustration; a sycotic fury is usually unreasoning and unreasonable leaving observers to wonder 'what was that all about?' (A syphilitic tantrum is obvious by its coldness and the calculated malignancy of the person's intentions.) The difference between a tubercular/*Calc. Carb.* eczema and a psoric/*Calc. Carb.* eczema [26] might be slight in physical appearance (though the former would be quicker and more inclined to become infected) but is obvious in its effects on the patient's psyche: both would be itchy, flaky, red and inflamed but the tubercular patient would be restless, anxious, irritable and quick to flare while the psoric one would be quietly anxious, dulled and relatively slow in reaction.

To know whether to give a dose of *Syphilinum* or *Tuberculinum* is sometimes a dilemma that only the result of the prescription will confirm or
refute – the only reason for giving one above the other being, perhaps,
apparently the slightest of symptoms: the patient is always much worse at
night or he can only find relief during clear, frosty weather. Quite often a
dose of *Psorinum* seems to do more for the patient after a string of remedies
such as *Phosphorus*, *Tuberculinum*, *Pulsatilla*, *Medorrhinum* and *Calc. Carb.*,
say, than all the rest put together! Actually, this is common and simply
reflects the fact that the patient required all the remedies, probably in this
sequence and it was the *Psorinum* that completed the cycle and therefore
seemed to deserve the most credit. A body on the path to positive change
tends to follow its own logic; it is only by observing cycles of remedy 'events'
that we can see how a patient weaves in and out of remedies that nevertheless have relationships with each other and that reflect, in their sequences,
the body's strategies for dealing with its history.

The truth is that the TB miasm is not simply related to the others but is a
state that holds characteristic elements of all of them while being its own
unique self. If psora is the root of all miasmatic activity and syphilism and
sycosis are the yang and yin that grow out of it, then tuberculism is their
further development. As we all have all the miasms deeply ingrained in our
make-up, to a greater or lesser degree, sooner or later we are going to manifest them. It is unusual for those with pathology not to need treatment for all
the miasms at one time or another through the process of healing. (After all,
the purpose of treatment is not to heal the pathology but to heal the
person.) What mitigates this process of cyclical miasmatic manifestation is
that it is extremely rare for more than one miasm to arise for treatment at the
same moment. For them to arise one after another over a single course of
treatment that might cover anything between some months to several years
is more common than not.

As the asthma patients demonstrate, in tubercular cases of any description there will always be an underlying current of one, two or all three
miasms even if they do not necessarily become obvious by virtue of frank
symptoms. If a tubercular patient manages to tread a narrow, steady path on
which he may encounter trials and tribulations but is able to maintain

equilibrium and purpose then there is little reason for sycosis or, worse, syphilism to rear their heads. It is as if tuberculism, having sycosis and syphilism already inherent, is yet close enough to psora for us to return to our solid basic foundations of the psoric root. The positive side of our tubercular nature has enough for us to remain purposeful, creative and happy in a way that is extremely difficult to maintain in either sycosis or syphilism – by dint of their very one-sided natures. If once we slip or tip the balance and fall from the positive tubercular state (or from the psoric, for that matter) into syphilism or sycosis then we will express those parts of our nature that being in the tubercular (or psoric) state was not enough to resist.

Miasms as strata

It is only by viewing things as an archaeologist would view his 'dig' that we become aware, over time, of the strata of health history – present, past and ancestral – and we see just how far and deeply the human body is prepared to go in its quest for positive change towards optimum health. The tubercular miasm, no less than the others, is imbued with emotional, mental and spiritual aspects as well as the physical ones that become manifest as metaphors for disturbance at the level of the psyche. Therefore it is even more apparent that the nosodes – medicines carrying the essence, so to speak, of the miasmatic tendencies – should be part and parcel of everyday practice and seen as tools in the medical archaeologist's bag. This is also to say that the miasms are not to be thought of in the same negative way that we think of the acute diseases that give them their names.

This is a very contentious way of viewing the human condition. It suggests that no philosophy (medical or metaphysical) could ever be complete without compartmentalising our nature and labelling the various bits with the miasms. This would only be true for the homoeopathic philosophy of *healing* and its exponents. In the healing philosophies of the East where *disease* terms for the underlying ills of mankind are not considered, people are very adequately described in their negative health states by means of the expression and interplay of the eminently neutral elements: earth, water, fire, air and ether. (To which wood and metal should be added in some cultures.) The advantage of this is that no reference is made to diseases that have become 'taboo' or that carry negative connotations. Ayurveda and the variations of oriental medical philosophy elegantly express our ills without reference to specific diseases – which reflects the refined cultures they come from.

Yet, because of the nature of homoeopathic medicines and their relationship to the disease nosodes, we are obliged to use the specific labels of the relevant, chronic and inheritable diseases as terms of reference. They are the motorways on the route map for the journey back to health. Yet it is the use of the particular labels that make this area of homoeopathic philosophy so uncompromising, controversial and conversationally intimidating.

So, at the risk of repetition, any arbitrary categorisation such as we are engaged in here should be limited to a study such as this for the purposes of explanation. It would always otherwise be a severely limiting exercise. Whilst constantly bearing in mind the fact that the miasms can be defined by 'portraits' of states of being, the origins of which predate any subsequent specific disease that has grown out of them, they show us the *patterns of influence* on the growth and development of both the collective and the individual human psyche. They do not describe the inevitability of diseases – only the form of their likely outcome when disease eventually becomes manifest after spiritual, mental, emotional or physical suppression.

It is worth underlining this whole aspect of the study of the miasms in relation to TB because it is certainly true that the tubercular state can be one of exciting creativity and productivity and not necessarily through the extraordinary fire that burns so fiercely in those who are suffering from TB itself. That fire can readily ignite in anyone sufficiently gifted with creativity and purpose without any health problems becoming evident – at least, not until they overstep that invisible line that is the threshold of their limitations. In other words, we should not object to being categorised as being in one or other miasm for the purposes of healing – to visit any one of them is providing us with the opportunity of developing on every level of our being.

In examining the two major miasms we have left, it can be hard to hold onto this point of view. One is so elusive and poorly represented even in homoeopathy, the other so complex to the point of utter confusion that at times it seems we are reduced to dealing with sweeping generalisations. Still, bear in mind that the nosodes of both are made from the disease material taken from human bodies and as such are representative of the sick energy that we all might be capable of producing should we be both functionally disturbed enough to fall ill *and* influenced by one or other particular miasm.

CHAPTER 24

LEPROSY

It is something of a surprise, perhaps, to find a chapter on leprosy. It is a condition that very few of us in the First World have much cause to think about as it has not been newsworthy in Europe for several generations. We are very unlikely to know any physician who has had anything to do with it, let alone any patient. Most people are unaware that it is a disease that once created as much fear for our island population as TB or syphilis or, indeed, as AIDS today. We consider leprosy to be a disease of the tropics or the desert, of poverty and squalor.

Leprosy is still a severe and expensive problem that causes great concern in Africa, the Americas, South-East Asia, the eastern Mediterranean, the western Pacific, Arabia and even small pockets of Europe. There is still a lot of research being done on the disease and treatments are comparatively frequently revised and updated in an ever more sophisticated effort to eradicate it. The WHO is actively involved with funding, research and information dissemination. There are many charitable foundations dedicated to the welfare of patients – even in Britain where there is no evidence of the disease whatever. At least, not at the moment.

So, what does leprosy have to do with a western European population or with a patient or a student of homoeopathy? The answer is that leprosy must be counted as one of the miasms. While it is *apparently* nowhere near as prevalent as those we have described already, it is undoubtedly a condition that fulfils the criteria of all miasms. It is a chronic disease that has profound implications on heredity and that has grown out of a state of being that primarily exists within the psyche of humanity but which has its physical manifestation in a condition of a destructive nature.

The biology of leprosy

What would greet the eye at the end of the microscope is a rod-shaped mycobacterium that looked extremely similar to the TB bacterium – to which it is related. *Mycobacterium leprae* is pervasive by nature and behaves much as a fungus might, insidious and uncompromising in action – a bit like dry rot. No-one has convincingly established just how it is transmitted though it is generally regarded as an infectious disease; the most accepted idea is that it is transmitted via particles of dust. It is not, apparently, as easy to contract leprosy as one might cholera or typhoid; it is statistically more likely that one would succumb to TB than to its crippling cousin.

The incubation period for leprosy is a matter of conjecture too as it might take as much as 40 years for the symptoms to manifest or as little as a few months. Such time spans make it impossible to be certain of the moment of initial infection but they confirm that the progress of the disease is governed not by the bug but by the patient's constitution and circumstances. An enormous majority of leprosy patients today come from societies that subsist at levels below the poverty line. It is commonest amongst young people between the ages of ten and twenty and it affects males more than females. It is estimated that more than half a million new cases are diagnosed each year. There are different and conflicting statistics of the number of patients in the world: the figure is likely to be somewhere between one and two million. The mathematics of these odd statistics means that Third World medicine is constantly struggling to keep its nose above the flood water.

There are two main kinds of leprosy – lepromatous and tubercular. (The first is sometimes referred to as multibacillary and the latter as paucibacillary. The former is characterised by an invasion of huge numbers of bacilli; the latter by comparatively few.) There is also a less easily defined version that is dimorphous and combines characteristics of the other two.

Lepromatous leprosy

In this form there initially appear skin lesions called macules. These are raised, reddish patches that can have a shiny appearance. They are most common on the ear lobes and the facial skin though they can be freely disseminated over the body. The affected areas of skin have sensory loss. The onset is very gradual. There are episodes of acute fever. Pain occurs in the peripheral nerves though there is little evidence of neurological damage in the early stage. The affected skin becomes coarsened and corrugated with a tendency to be oedematous. The outer half of the eyebrows and facial hair fall out and nodular tumours appear on the skin surface where the bacilli collect and multiply in the lymph nodes. Internally, there is a general break-down of the mucous membranes with consequent ulceration. This is particularly marked in the mucosa of the eyes and the nasal cavities. There is heavy production of mucus from the related sinuses. Iritis and blindness can result. For those who remain untreated, deformity of the nasopharyn-geal mucosa creates the characteristically hideous appearance sometimes referred to as 'leonine'. Loss of sensation leads to injuries to limbs that even-tually become necrotic; the body is gradually 'eaten away'.

Tubercular leprosy

The tubercular form is only a little less alarming. There are similar macules which are well defined but less widely distributed. The lesions have raised edges that lend the skin a pebbled appearance. The skin generally becomes dry, hairless, scaly and depigmented. Lesions appear on the legs, particu-larly on the shins; they are erythematous in character – reddened from local congestion of the capillaries. The peripheral nerves are affected and become thickened and palpable – almost as if ganglia were being formed. Neuritis at the extremities develops and any sensory or motor changes are the result of the destruction of nerve fibres. The surface of the skin loses sensation and it becomes generally inelastic, shiny and incapable of releasing sweat. Muscles become fibrotic and contracted; the face is palsied. The nasal sinuses become chronically active, creating a lot of mucus, and perforating ulcers appear at pressure points. Tubercular tumours occur along the nerve lines. These become caseated and cold abscesses are formed – indolent collections of pustular matter that do not erupt with heat.

This description serves to show how closely related the tubercular and leprotic *mycobacteria* are. It also shows how close the lepromatous form is in its effects on the human constitution to those of syphilis: the formation of bacteria-filled tumours and nodules is similar to the syphilitic gummae; the destruction of mucous surfaces and the tendency to ulceration; the gradual deformity of the body; the susceptibility to opportunistic infections. Where leprosy differs is that it is not the ultimate cause of death; that is an infection such as pneumonia or TB. (There is now talk of AIDS being a fatal potential complication.) Leprosy kills by proxy.

It is interesting to note that anyone with TB is likely to be immune to leprosy. The reverse is sadly not true; there is a tendency among lepers to develop TB. An extra twist to this is that research has shown that the BCG inoculation has an influence on the promotion of immunity to leprosy in some geographical areas. The determining factor seems to be in the variations among local environmental bacteria; some act in harmony with the BCG and some antagonistically. What this implies is that bacteria mutate and evolve to suit their local environment just as all other forms of life do. What, perhaps, now needs to be examined is the way that bacteria energy can transmute within the environment of the body itself. It has been suggested that the TB bacillus itself has some specific role to play in the occurrence of leprosy. (This is not very far from the premise that a bacterium energy such as diphtheria can transmute itself into a TB bacillus. It certainly echoes Florence Nightingale's words – see p. 600.)

A historical look at leprosy

Leprosy is a very ancient disease with its origins lost in prehistory. Sanskrit authors who practised Ayurvedic medicine described the disease and discussed its earliest treatment. It was to them *Kushtha*; a word derived from *Kushnathi* which means 'eaten away'. From some time before 600 BC hydnocarpus oil (from the crushed seeds of a gum tree) was the favoured treatment and it continued to be so until 1941 when it was superseded by a newly discovered group of drugs called sulphones.

From the earliest times it was considered to be a hereditary disease. This was, perhaps, due to its habit of affecting families isolated from areas where infectious diseases might have been expected in epidemics due to denser population. Later, when organised religion began to spread across the globe, leprosy was held as a sign of God's displeasure; meted out as divine retribution to sinners. Sufferers became ostracised and outcast. They were forced to live the humiliating life of scavengers. By the early Middle Ages this picture had been expanded (chiefly by Rome) and lepers were imputed with being degenerates, followers of Satan, prostitutes, homosexuals and heretics. This was supported by the misapprehension that the Bible seemed to point the finger at the disease. It was believed that leprosy was described in the Book of Leviticus where instructions for dealing with contamination and rituals for purification are given. It is unlikely that leprosy was what the authors referred to at all. When the Alexandrine scholars translated the Old Testament into Greek, the original Hebrew word *Tzaraat* was given as *lepra* which means 'scaly'. (*Tzaraat* actually referred to ritual ablutions and purification of skin diseases in general.) Then, once the Greek word *elephas*, which the Alexandrines coined for a particular form of the disease, became associated with leprosy, the divorce from the original Hebrew meaning was complete. The disease gradually became invested with connotations of evil. Leprosy took on the stigma that, as we shall see, might more appropriately be reserved for syphilis.

Descriptions and paintings tended to lump disfiguring skin diseases together. Medieval depictions show 'lepers' with what was more like story-book measles – blots of rosy red rash scattered across the body. Before the enlightening advent of the microscope, God or the gods were convenient excuses for any destructive disease force; it was more digestible for an ignorant, fearful and easily persuaded populace to associate a virulent rash with the stigma of heavenly wrath. But the wrath was not just from above. Kings were known to have condoned or even ordered the execution of lepers by sending them to the stake or having them buried alive, though royal touch was at one time considered curative. Priests drove lepers from their parishes and denied them any contact with anyone but their spouses. Forbidden to touch others or their belongings, lepers were forced to point to any food they might want so that it could be thrown to them; they were made to carry bells or clappers so that they could be avoided.

It was not entirely a black picture. Leprosaria were set up across Europe. These were hospices for lepers run by religious organisations on a charitable basis. They became self-sufficient as a direct result of their inmates being denied interaction with·the world outside. As these establishments knew no class barriers a particular culture grew up within the colonies based on a need for mutual support in a situation that took for granted an inevitable fate.

The first evidence of leprosy in Britain seems to come from about 600 AD in literary sources. The disease advanced steadily through the next 800 years and on its way claimed some memorable victims. Henry II's daughter-in-law, Constance of Brittany, and his cousin Baldwin IV (the so-called Leper King of Jerusalem) both succumbed. Another famous victim may or may not have been Robert the Bruce of Scotland. He too was thought to have suffered terribly from the disfiguring effects of leprosy but, as it only took two years for the disease to dispatch him, it has been suggested that he contracted syphilis though it might be difficult to square this idea with the generally accepted history of the 'great pox'. Robert having died in 1329, it would be another 165 years before the first great epidemic of syphilis swept across Europe. (Syphilis and AIDS share an intriguing mystery – did they both have a presence long before their official debut dates? It seems to be increasingly likely.)

It is generally considered that leprosy in Europe began to decline by the end of the Middle Ages. From the Renaissance onwards the threat of leprosy was overtaken by the concern over syphilis and TB. It is debatable whether what might be termed European syphilis (the acute disease) is an offspring of the leprotic miasm and yaws, imported by Spanish explorers. (Yaws is surprisingly similar to leprosy in its effects on the body.)

Father Damian and the Hawaiian leper colony

Joseph de Vuester was born in 1840 in Belgium. He is better known to us as Father Damian. He was a Roman Catholic priest who found himself on a mission to the Hawaiian islands. Father Damian fulfilled his role as a missionary for some nine years until, in 1873, an ecclesiastical conference on missionary work was convened. One of the points of discussion was what could be achieved for the local leper colony. Father Damian volunteered to join the colony on the island of Molokai. He discovered the appalling plight of the inhabitants. They lived and died in squalor; there was no sanitation, no shelter, little food and certainly no medical care. Father Damian became doctor, counsellor, builder, plumber, carpenter, undertaker and friend to these benighted people. Their initial hostility towards anyone from the outside world turned to undying gratitude for his extraordinary selflessness. The rest of the world remained ignorant of what was happening on this tiny piece of scorched earth in the middle of the Pacific – despite the good father's repeated pleas for help.

Then, in 1885, washing his feet in hot water he noticed that the skin of his feet was blistered and that he was unable to sense the temperature of the water. At some point in the previous twelve years he had contracted leprosy. He had four more years of work before he died in 1889. He was buried under a tree on Molokai. Though it took his untimely death to create any effect, it was as a result of his life that the first charitable society dedicated to the victims of leprosy was formed. It set about educating the world to a greater understanding of the disease and the conditions of its sufferers.

The search for treatment

Ironically, it was in the same year as the conference that became the turning point of Father Damian's career that the 'cause' of leprosy was discovered. It was G. A. Hansen who identified the *Mycobacterium leprae* in 1873. It was not to be until the late 1940s that the antibiotic dapsone was discovered as an alternative to hydnocarpus oil – but only against the tubercular or paucibacillary form. This new drug was used for some years until it became ineffective against the bacteria. Since then the WHO has advocated a multidrug approach. This means that a cocktail of drugs is administered until the bacteria are no longer in evidence. This has proved very effective in controlling the disease and, though deformities cannot be reversed, patients can be restored to health if treatment is begun soon enough.

It is intriguing that leprosy should have disappeared from northern Europe without vaccines or satisfactory drug therapy. It might support the idea that, with the advent of yaws from the Spanish dominions, leprosy became subsumed by the far more virulent and lethal variant of the tropical disease we now call syphilis. It is also fascinating that it took so few years for dapsone to become redundant. In the relatively short time it was in use it would have been unlikely for the bacteria in all parts of the affected world to become so accustomed to this that it was able to render it useless.

The World Health Organisation's avowed intention of eradicating leprosy by the year 2000 was always doomed to failure. With leprosy and TB so rife in the poorest countries of the world and not in competition with each other but apparently in cahoots, there is little prospect of humanity ever being rid of such ancient diseases in one form or another. Orthodox science may well find a way of killing off the bacteria but they will never be able to prevent the basic susceptibility through the use of drugs.

Leprosy dies hard

The last vestiges of leprosy in Britain were to be found in the Shetland Isles in the eighteenth century,[1] while on the European continent Norway was its final bastion with the last hospital for lepers being closed only in the 1950s. The last 500 years may have seen the demise of this frightful disease in Europe (though there are cases reported in Portugal and around the Mediterranean) but it is not difficult to find echoes throughout language and literature of the stigma attached to leprosy. The very word 'leper' is pejorative and always means 'outcast'. Other words that are associated are 'untouchable', 'unclean' and 'beggar'. Images include groups of poor, slow moving, white-robed, homeless people resigned to wandering aimlessly and without hope. It is worth holding these ideas in the mind when we come to look at the miasm that is the legacy of this extraordinary disease. Its physical manifestation may not trouble us directly now but its influence on the psyche is not far beneath the surface of each of us. And whatever is in the psyche that can become a negative energy will sooner or later manifest in a physical pathology.

The leprotic psyche

We have seen how psora, syphilism, sycosis and tuberculism can all be identified in terms of psychology – even though to separate them out is no more than an arbitrary exercise.

> – Psora encapsulates the essence of inadequacy with its consequent sense of anxiety;

– Syphilis holds the essence of self-destructive behaviour that can be characterised by manipulativeness, deviousness, passive aggression – any of which can even extend to downright evil;
– Sycosis has to do with dissociation of body, heart and mind;
– Tuberculism is all about breaking away from boundaries due to an uncontrollable sense of dissatisfaction and restlessness.

Leprosy defines quite a different psyche though – as you would be able to predict by now – it is imbued with aspects of the others.

It was said about psora that man felt unworthy of God's divine protection. It was man's self-awareness that led him to feel spiritually out of favour with whatever was his idea of the Almighty. Leprosy has a more rational and retrograde variation on this theme – there is a sense of being outcast by society. The way to survive this ostracism is to turn to God (in one guise or another) or some other form of institutionalised social group for succour.

Many people have a strong sense of rejection which they cannot blame on any particular person or institution. It is an innate feeling that they do not belong to the family or to the community or to the culture into which they were born. They are 'outsiders'. This should not be confused with the tubercular outsider – they are people of a profoundly restless *artistic* temperament who are loners. They are hypersensitive to external impressions, to criticism, to their environment. The leprotic outsider is rather different; such people seek others of their own kind for support rather than isolation in which to ponder their muse. There is deep sympathy within the leprotic psyche for others in the same condition while the tubercular psyche is far more selfish.

Leprotic people go in search of company that is congenial but as the general world threatens rejection they look for comfort amongst other outsiders who are in need of company. Tubercular people who come together spark off each other; they make fire. The leprotic temperament would feel scorched by such combustion. Leprotics need a plateau of peace and harmony where little ruffles the surface. The artistic energy of the tubercular is too rarefied and extravagant for them; what they want is what matches their own quiet, characteristically meek temperament. The leprotic nature does not seek to change the world; it does not want to make waves. Rather there is the need to lead a quiet and orderly existence; one that allows them to pass by unnoticed. What this community life feeds on is a fervour for the guiding force of the social group.

Inevitably certain religious communities come to mind: Amish, Pentecostal, Seventh Day Adventist among others. These are all apparently gentle groups of people who seek to lead a life that is determinedly not like the majority. The culture of these communities is one of mutual support, restraint and self-sufficiency. Most of their numbers are content to lead uneventful lives in which ambition is fulfilled through service to others within their socio-religious group. This does not prevent members (more tubercular than leprotic – for no group is ever exclusively of one miasmatic persuasion) of some groups from going out into the world and seeking to persuade others to join them. There can be a powerful (tubercular) missionary zeal[2] within some organisations to draw others into the community to add to the fervour from which they gather strength. They face rebuff from the rude majority that views them with anything from amusement and arrogance to disdain, suspicion and intolerance.

What often happens though, is that recruits are found among those who have recently faced emotional trauma, privation and poverty or some spiritual crisis. Such people, finding that they are no longer able to face the world on equal terms, are in a state that is characterised by the 'leprotic outsider' mentality; stress has ripened the leprotic influence. They need a place of safety and communion. They need a simplified, communal and homespun spiritual connection.

Nonconformist religions are not the only ones coloured by the leprotic psyche. Most religions have adherents who wish to follow the code and principles of their faith in a quiet and unspectacular manner. When they are in difficulties they turn to their maker and their immediate community for support and comfort, feeling that they cannot find the resources to override their troubles from within themselves. A syphilitic might appear to do this too but there would always be a degree of exculpation and manipulation for a selfish gain or a need to draw others down into their own despair. A sycotic might do the same but the approach would give them away: there would be a display of pitiful self-indulgence that could not be missed.

A tubercular person would be too narcissistic to enter into the spirit of the community wholeheartedly and would accept some assistance but remain on the fringes in case they were drawn into something from which there would be difficulty escaping. As always with the tubercular state, there is another side; the person, temporarily too weak to stand alone, might enter into the spirit of the community and gradually rise to the 'top of the heap', enjoy the brilliance of the limelight for a while and then leave.

The most politically powerful denominations in the world have also got aspects that might appeal to the leprotic psyche. What would obscure this from view is the clout wielded by the leaders of these religions. Few within the Vatican would qualify for the leprotic label; there is too much worldliness to the business of running Roman Catholicism for that. Neither could the hierarchy of the Church of England produce many who might be seen as leprotic because there is too little unity among those with heated passion within the General Synod. Billy Graham, the charismatic proselytiser of the 1950s and 60s, was no leprotic. His ego was not sufficiently humble for that. A true leprotic nature does not seek the limelight nor favour hierarchy. Surely it is no accident that the selfless Mother Theresa should have spent her life, most of it in obscurity, working in a country that supports the largest population of leprosy patients?

And what of fundamentalism? There may be many with the essential leprotic characteristics within religions that have a face of cruelty and violence but the aggressive arm of such a body would be syphilitic and tubercular, without doubt. Those leprotic souls behind such a front would have no communication and little contact with the driving force of manipulation and destruction. The leprotic nature asks to be guided by a sense of community and directed spirituality but the essentially closed society it engenders seldom knows or notices (or wants to) that *secular* and, often, political power is actually in control.

Particularly in the West, where organised religion has caused widespread apathy and disappointment and is on the retreat, there are those who find no succour within a church. They might instead turn to an alternative culture or even to spiritualism. The leprotic is a sucker for the sycotic medium who produces messages from dead relatives. Where the tubercular mind would want to know what it felt like to be 'on the other side', even to experience being there, and would savour any message for its novelty, the leprotic mind would be content with the simple fact of communication.

The 'victim' state

The leprotic state is potentially so liable to rejection that it is also liable to feel victimised. The 'victim' state is above all leprotic wherever the mild individual feels the need of sympathy and empathy from a larger group of similarly minded people. This exposes them to being taken over by syphilitic types with axes to grind. (Not all 'victim' types are leprotic; some 'victims' are manipulative and destructive – another aspect of syphilism – some are hostage to their desires which is sycotic.) Leprosy is about 'small' people who are easily shamed or otherwise emotionally maimed. It is about meek outsiders bonding to survive and even prosper, and syphilitics are masters at marshalling those who fear standing alone.

It is not too far-fetched to apply these aspects of leprosy to political and social groups. The essentially nonconformist inspired renewal of socialism that took root in Europe after World War II and blossomed after the Cold War, appeals to all those who want to see social, political and cultural levelling. The extraordinary thing is that so few see that the combined power-brokering syphilitic/sycotic psyche lies behind the mask of spin doctoring. Herein lies another aspect of the leprotic psyche: *numbing of the awareness of self*. Even in psora, so humble a state, there is still an acute awareness of self – only it is so often negative hence the feelings of inadequacy. In leprosy the self is abdicated eventually to the dictates of fate or the common cause of the community. Their sense of choice and self-determination is weak or absent. The name might change so that one reads God, Allah, Buddha or even education for fate but the effect is the same. There is the sense of being singled out and isolated away from the mainstream of human activity.

Such a 'them and us' mentality appears in the other miasms too though with subtle differences. The victim/syphilitic feels 'the whole world is against me' and the aggressor/syphilitic senses the advantage of 'it's me against everyone else'. The former manipulates from the vantage of passive aggression; the latter aggressively sets out to destroy others' potential, to eradicate competition for their own material gain.

The tubercular variation is one of arrogance; they create their own distance through feeling that everyone else is not as refined, perceptive, sensitive or creative. They can be egotistical to the 'nth' degree. This can be apparent in the most subtle and disarming ways – many do-gooders are thoroughly tubercular and convinced that their charity is essential even when the long-term consequences are unfortunate.

Psorics have as strong a sense of community as leprotic subjects but they feel less ostracised from *other* people than separated from the kind of person they expect themselves to be or to become.

Sycotic subjects, who can be as victimised by syphilitics as any, are often unaware of the 'them and us' syndrome; they suffer so profound a separation between body, emotions and soul that they have little concept of order in groups or society except in a purely intellectual way. (The typical image of the hippie characterised by freedom from convention, freedom to wander and freedom to experience drug-induced 'other states' is tubercular/sycotic.

Essentially, the leprotic psyche is mild in nature. Little is expected from the rest of humanity (though much from the chosen saviour – wherever there is a tradition to adhere to). The leprotic has a sense that no-one should suffer the isolation and rejection he feels while at the same time holding destiny (his own idea of it) responsible. This is not surprising as destiny is a nebulous affair and easily blamed by those without power.

In sickness too, the patient has a sense that the illness (and there are many leprotic disease states) was somehow inevitable. He feels that he could not have avoided the problem and resigns himself to the course of the disease. There can be a remarkable patience that is not present in any of the other miasms. (Psorics can display patience but not in disease; they are too anxious when ill to be 'laid back'. Syphilitics can appear patient but are almost always using their condition, even when comparatively well, subtly to undermine others. Tubercular patients are impatient and inclined to sabotage their healing process by dashing off and doing something else before treatment is complete.) For the leprotic, with the patience comes a curious hopefulness of recovery, even in very serious conditions.

He does need sympathy and empathy – though he will not show it – but he does not need pity. Being pitied by well-wishers is anathema. It causes him to retreat and become uncommunicative. (Leprotics cannot abide handouts; they are thoroughly averse to the concept of begging – a paradox, given the history of the disease.) The patient needs to be led with attentive advice; common sense encourages him as he feels it is close to the truth. Living with a sense of the inevitable means he is receptive to the harshest truth; there is 'acceptance'. Perversely, having heard the truth, he may well go into a passive denial of the seriousness of the condition. Nevertheless, even the grimmest of prognoses will not destroy the deep sense of self-sufficiency held by the individual and fostered by the supporting group.

Shame runs deep in leprosy. This can be crippling. The patient will hide and prevent anyone knowing his situation or his illness to avoid both pity and rejection. Despite the mildness of his nature, the leprotic can be angered. Apart from charity, the other thing that will rile the patient into irritability is questions intended to find out the underlying causes of the condition. To dig too deep might uncover reasons for rejection; better to leave things be so that anything that might be seen to deserve rejection cannot become the cause of isolation. This is especially true in those who find that their illness draws them back into the fold of humanity. Raynaud's syndrome, a relatively common example, is a chronic but comparatively uncomplicated problem that is nevertheless often intractable and resistant to orthodox treatment. Many can empathise with the patient as the syndrome can cause distressing symptoms that do not elicit repugnance in the way that, say, psoriasis can. Both conditions can have strongly leprotic energy but Raynaud's is more successful psychologically as it fosters empathy.

An interesting aspect of the psyche that is related to the paradoxical hopefulness of recovery and the conviction of the influence of destiny is that suicide is not an option. There is a strong moral code borne out of the sense of community and strong religiousness that prohibits thoughts of taking fate into their own hands. Psorics might commit suicide from utter hope-lessness; they are most likely to swallow pills. Syphilitics, amongst whom the suicide rate is by far the highest, would throw themselves from a height, shoot themselves, slit their wrists, jump in front of a train or hang them-selves. The result is often messy and designed to leave deep reverberations in all those connected with the deceased. Sycotics would be more inclined to kill themselves slowly by indulging in all their harmful habits such as eating, drinking, smoking, drugging and debauchery – though they might choose a quicker way by taking a leaf out of the syphilitics' book – a mixture of alcohol and barbiturates. (Unsuccessful suicide attempts are usually sycotic; more of a *cri de coeur*.)

This is a long way from the leprotic psyche. Despite the slowly and insidiously destructive side of this miasm, it does possess a strong work ethic and a sense of purpose. It might be thought of as the obverse of the tubercular coin. The life force in both can be positively charged for creative ends though in the leprotic the group dynamic subsumes the individual while the vital tubercular subject is always ego orientated. Talking to a leprotic one can get the sense that he or she puts the family or the community first. They seem unaware that there are choices that can be made without reference to anyone or anything else. The only time a tubercular person would come across like this is if he or she were in a relationship that fulfilled all the romantic criteria so essential to the adventurous and idealistic nature that is redolent of the disease state.

The miasm starts early

Those who feel isolated and marginalised by society or by an institution are legion. Yet even while such people are together they can feel cut off, not only from their peers but also from those who could help. A good example of this is the dyslexic child. Though the problems of developmental learning difficulties are far better recognised than they were, the afflicted child can still feel mentally and emotionally crippled. He or she can spend so much energy on hiding what are felt to be inadequacies (and even more in inventing methods of compensating for them) that it seriously lowers their physical energy and compromises their immune system. Many children with learning difficulties are subject to health problems that seem simple childhood conditions: eczema, asthma, tonsillitis, growing pains, sinus congestion, intermittent mild fevers, allergies and headaches. Each condition might well respond, as it arises, to the chosen form of treatment. Yet, while the child is in school, struggling to make sense of the situation, unable to perform as well as the peer group yet bright and often more articulate, the underlying cause remains untouched. It is a situation that can waken the leprotic miasm in some children. It is often characterised by reluctance to admit that there is a problem. The child compensates by not having much to do with his own age group but plays with younger children or remains amongst adults, holding conversations on topics normally thought to be beyond his years. This is unsatisfactory as there is a profound sense of not fitting into either group comfortably.

While it has already been suggested that learning difficulties can be strongly related to the sycotic and tubercular miasms, this does not preclude the involvement of other miasmatic states. While such remedies as *Thuja* and *Medorrhinum* are invaluable in treating the 'off the planet' state, the anxieties and the obsessiveness so often inherent in learning impediments, leprotic remedies also have a role in relieving the effects on the psyche of those who, through being long misunderstood or misdiagnosed, suffer isolation and marginalisation in the classroom or even the school in general.

Leprosinum, the nosode made from leprotic material, can be useful as a remedy to support the constitution of a dyslexic who suffers frequent acute bouts of ear, nose and throat illnesses, frequent colds, headaches and allergies (especially aggravated by the sun), mild gum disease, chest infections with copious amounts of catarrh, growing pains, knee conditions and tendonitis. It is the underlying psychical state that causes the remedy to be indicated. Such illnesses are quite as likely to be found within the orbit of *Tuberculinum* or other tubercular remedies. But those remedies will only deal with the conditions if the tubercular psyche is uppermost – hence the vital importance to be able to make the subtle distinctions between the miasms. This is particularly true when treating those with learning difficulties as their psychological state can swing so dramatically from one miasm to another.

The physical appearance of the miasm

Another area of study can help to distinguish between the leprotic and the other miasms. The physical appearance can be quite telling.

i) The face can be waxy looking; the skin can have an oily texture even though little sweat is evident; it can also be coarse and thickened.

ii) The nose can be broader and slightly flattened at the tip in those who harbour the miasm strongly.

iii) The ears can appear to be 'rat bitten'; they are either misshapen or nodular.

In extreme examples the facial features might appear to be almost ape-like with heavy jowls and broad forehead. Ugliness to the point of deformity can be characteristic of the miasm – though this is far less in evidence in the West as the more dominant tubercular miasm ensures that the fine featured, more delicate bone structure of tuberculism predominates.

iv) The eyes might appear heavy, baggy and with a tendency to look swollen; the lids sometimes do not close fully; it is not uncommon for there to be a squint.

v) The skin generally wrinkles easily and looks prematurely aged.

vi) The outer third of the eyebrows, in older patients, tends to fall out and the hair greys too early.

vii) A common characteristic is lumps and nodules (indolent and benign tumours) that appear on the skin, especially on the face and hands; ganglia appear close to tendons (particularly around the wrists and knuckles) where there is little flesh.

viii) Lips may be swollen or misshapen or tend to cracking and peeling.

ix) Facial palsy or anaesthesia occurs.

x) Alopecia, sometimes an intractable problem that defies swift resolution, is another tendency and can affect not just the head but also the beard or body hair.

xi) Congenital deformities, especially with the foreshortening of limbs or missing digits, might also sometimes be attributable to the leprotic strain.

Such a list of signs, either physical or psychical, is not exhaustive but it gives a fair idea of the potential range of the miasm. As with the other miasms, it should not be supposed that a patient would need to display a majority of such an unfortunate picture before needing it to be taken into account at some point during long-term treatment, through the use of leprotic remedies.

An example of the leprotic energy could well be James Merrick, the famous Elephant Man. His deformities were truly hideous and their cause is not fully recognised though there have been suggestions as to the name of the condition from which he suffered. Elephantiasis, a condition of swellings and obstruction of the lymphatic system has been dismissed. Nearer the mark is neurofibromatosis which is a congenital condition in which the growth of nerve cells is altered. The result is the development of tumours that distort tissue, muscle, bone and skin and that are associated with changes in pigmentation – any of which could indicate the miasm. However, this disease is not necessarily confined to the head and one arm as was the case with Merrick. More interesting a suggestion is that Merrick suffered from the rare disease, Proteus syndrome, which is characterised by overgrowth of bone, cartilage and other tissue. Whatever the label of the disease, he might have been considered to be affected by the leprotic miasm.

Remedies that look like leprosy

We have given examples of common remedies used to treat the acute diseases of the other miasms. With leprosy the situation is rather different – in northern Europe at least because there is no acute form of the disease left to treat. As affluence spread and professional people gave more credence to physicians than the clergy, so leprosy was kept within limits that eventually led to its isolation – whether or not leprosy contributed to the rise of syphilis and thereby its own retreat into hereditary obscurity. It means that no physicians in general practice in Britain have any experience in treating the disease. Nor do homoeopaths unless they have served some of their apprenticeship in a country where it is endemic. Even those who have travelled extensively in India, where homoeopathy is used in treating leprosy and related diseases, would not necessarily have had any first-hand experience. It is thanks to the work of Dr Prakash Vakil, a professor at the Government Homoeopathic Hospital in Bombay, that we have so much information about the miasm and the nosode.[3] Nevertheless, in accordance with all the basic principles of homoeopathy and with the knowledge that remedies are used in treatment in India, we can select remedies that would undoubtedly have curative effects on the disease.

We only have to study the *Materia Medica* of certain remedies to see that they have a 'likeness' to the symptom picture of leprosy. Certain textbooks written by Indian practitioners, who do have the necessary experience, give us a substantial number of remedies recognised as curative. *Calcium Carbonate* and *Sulphur* come high on the list. This is not surprising given that both remedies have a reputation for treating fungal conditions generally as well as those in which the skin erupts and peels; in which mucous membranes become chronically active, energy becomes depleted with a consequent lowering of the immune system and both the nervous system and the lymphatics are compromised. Both also have a mental attitude that is common to many of the remedies listed in the leprosy rubric: either mental lassitude and a disinclination for work or the opposite: a strong, 'nose to the grindstone' work ethic. (Other symptoms, specifically characteristic of one or other remedy, would determine which would be the curative remedy.)

Bearing in mind that in these days with such a deeply chronic disease there is no single remedy likely to heal the body entirely, it is instructive to look back at some of the medicines that have a proven track record in the treatment of leprosy. Dr Clarke's dictionary presents material from many sources including practitioners who wrote of their experiences. He mentions *Hoang-Nan*, from the bark of tropical bindweed that contains strychnine, and had a reputation amongst natives for the cure of leprosy, hydrophobia, snakebite and skin diseases. Apparently they used to roll pills out of the reddish powder mixed with a little vinegar and the resulting medicine would cause a reaction that brought about a cessation of those symptoms commonly felt by the local population. The symptoms included malaise, lassitude, malnutrition, malignant ulceration and tingling of the extremities.

Hura brasiliensis, a member of the *Euphorbia* genus with its virulent, milky sap that so affects the skin on contact, was subjected to a proving. 'Two of his provers had been affected with leprosy but under homoeopathic treatment they seemed to have got well.' Better known and still widely used is Indian pennywort, *Hydrocotyle asiatica*. Though it also covers symptoms that seemingly have little to do with leprosy, it does have many of the hallmarks of the disease in its effects on the body. It has the raised, scaly spots; intermittent feverishness with malaise; wandering pains in all the muscles; weariness and heaviness of the limbs; contractions of the tendons; the weakened, croaky voice; oppressed breathing in the lungs that have difficulty in expectorating mucus; nasal congestion and the sense of constriction in the back of the skull. It has the mental attitude too – misanthropy and need for solitude. What might mark it out in a case of leprosy is if, in addition, there were constriction and irritation at the neck of the bladder – a very characteristic symptom of this remedy. Interestingly, *Hydrocotyle* is another remedy with a reputation for not only curing leprosy but also syphilis; remedial agents thus draw us to the similarities between the two diseases.[4] *Calotropis gigantea*, a tree we met before in discussing old-fashioned cures for syphilis, is a remedy for tubercular leprosy but also has use in the treatment of the related lupus vulgaris.

Such remedies are not often called for in present-day prescribing in Britain (though *Hydrocotyle* should be part of every homoeopath's tool kit). There are others, though, with a reputation for healing aspects of the actual disease that are enormously important to everyday homoeopathic practice in any part of the world. Amongst others we have the ubiquitous *Arsenicum Album*, most of the carbon-related remedies, *Graphites* (pencil lead!), *Secale* (a deadly black fungus that grows on ears of rye), *Sepia* (squid ink), some of the salt-related remedies and *Silica*.

There is another, from the plant kingdom, which is worth describing in a little detail as it is used to heal psychological states that are very similar indeed to the predisposing *mental* condition of leprosy. Even if we do not see this particular physical disease any more, we do see physical pathology that can derive from the leprotic state of mind and that also mimics the original blight – though in the case of this remedy it is more common for us to be asked to help the patient in need of it before the pathology works its way towards any physical manifestation. It is called *Anacardium*.

Anacardium

This is a remedy that is most frequently thought of in treating people who have psychological difficulties in fitting in with society – particularly young people; remember how leprosy most frequently affects youth . (Yet it is almost never considered in relation to the leprotic miasm when prescribed in the northern hemisphere.) This remedy comes from a part of the world where leprosy is rife – the East Indies. It is made from the layer of skin between the shell and the kernel of a particular nut which is heart- shaped and black. The indigenous people use it to mark their laundry.

Anacardium has a 'personality' that is unique. If you were to ask a homoeopath, you might be told that it is a great remedy for exam nerves or that it is useful for digestive troubles or that it is a 'head case' remedy; even that it was the remedy that many of the Nazis needed. If you find it hard to credit that *Calcium* or *Silica* or *Phosphorus* could hold the energy most similar to the personalities described in the *Materia Medica* then you may find it impossible to believe that a nut in the shape of a black heart could hold the same energy as someone who suffers waves of mind-blanking anxiety before a test; or as another who would have little compunction in carrying out the murderous orders of a psychopathic political regime. Yet *Anacardium* has a vast range that can cover psoric, syphilitic and leprotic areas. 'Exam funk' can be seen as psoric; vicious hatred with murderous intent is undoubtedly syphilitic. So what is leprotic about this nut?

In Indian textbooks it is recommended as indicated where the guiding symptoms are: 'numbness, feeling of pins and needles in the parts which are cold (with) patches of raised, hardened skin'. This is expanded to include the affected skin 'on the face and arms; perfect anaesthesia of affected parts; weakness and prostration'. These are the signs of tuberculous leprosy. Add to these the possible psychological picture that accompanies anyone needing *Anacardium* – a sense of being less able than others; of being unable to establish a place in the pecking order; of being the object of others' pity; of being without personal courage enough to take matters into one's own hands – then the remedy will contribute to cure on every level.

There are other physical symptoms that might appear in both the disease and in the remedy: loss of the senses of touch and smell; tingling or fleeting pains in the limbs; trembling and sensations of pressure on different parts. Although it is, classically, the *psychological* picture which is the main determining factor in the choice of remedies, sometimes, in prescribing for a profoundly chronic disease state like leprosy or TB, the *physical* symptom picture is so obviously indicative of a remedy that it is possible from that alone to predict what sort of emotional and spiritual picture might emerge from detailed questioning around the psyche.

In the case of *Anacardium*, no-one is ever in need of this remedy alone. Being a plant remedy it is never going to be as constitutionally profound as a mineral such as *Sulphur*, *Calcium Carbonate* or *Silica* – remedies that can establish permanently a degree of constitutional *physical* health that surpasses even the most extraordinary powers of remedies from among the plant and animal kingdoms. It is a remedy that constitutes only one aspect of a person's general make-up though it might be so exaggerated that it takes over the whole. It is always a state that has developed out of a deeper level; a *Calcium Carbonate* constitution might produce the picture of *Anacardium* when in particular distress. Nevertheless, when *Anacardium* is called for by a leprotically compromised body then nothing else will do.

Take the example of the sixth-former about to take her A-level exams. She became irritable with the family who sought to help with revision; she complained of losing her memory; she worried about her health; she was filled with dread at the prospect of the exams. She wept and shut herself in her room; she avoided going out with her friends. Then she would become quiet and resigned and say that she knew she was going to do badly. *"What can I do about it?"* was the attitude. She had swollen neck glands though there was no other evidence of ill health apart from a constantly mucus-filled nose. She was given *Anacardium* 200. She took her exams feeling far less troubled and without complaining of poor memory.

She passed with flying colours. Just as importantly, she came back into the family fold and began meeting her friends again. The burden of the examinations had caused her psyche to produce a state somewhat akin to the mental and emotional aspects of the leprotic miasm. *Anacardium* lifted this. It was no more than just a thin 'layer' brought about by a temporary situation and might well have been no long-term trouble anyway. Many feel as this girl did and still succeed well. After the trauma of the examinations is over the 'layer' lifts and they are back to normal. (The advantage of having the treatment is that the situation is less likely to happen again or, if it does, then it is less severe.)

However, the layer can be a deeper seam in the personality's bedrock. The psychological state can be so ingrained that longer-term treatment is required to relieve the system of a chronically 'adopted' bad habit. The layer can have several strands that are inextricably entwined. Imagine the man who has spent his life doing the same mundane job year in, year out. He is of average or above average intelligence and was known to have potential (though he is unlikely to put this to you). It seems as if he has either deliberately restricted his vision or that life has conspired against his seizing every opportunity. (He would probably suggest that the latter were true.) He is filled with apprehension. This is most obvious when he is expected to do anything out of the ordinary and in front of others. His reluctance to put himself forward and 'perform' is what has delayed any promotion. He is also unsure of himself socially. He is tongue-tied and easily embarrassed. He might not admit it but he is ashamed of his inability to speak his mind – or he used to be for now it has become a habit. He is better in his own company even to the point of spending ages in the bathroom. (He might well have difficulties in passing motions and sit reading the newspaper while straining sporadically. He might soak for hours in a hot bath.)

On his own he can fantasise about his life. In his imagination he becomes far more heroic, more powerful, more expansive. There is no hint of slavery to any institution or to family. He becomes a free spirit with extraordinary visions. That is unless he has been so cowed by circumstances that the imagination has atrophied. In company he contributes encouraging phrases so that others will do the talking. He is afraid of initiating any conversational gambit as he might be asked to expatiate on ideas that he could not develop aloud without becoming confused. He prefers to cultivate a sense of vagueness as he doesn't trust his memory – especially for the names of things. He is fearful of making mistakes as he is afraid most of all of the disparaging opinion of others. Though he hides it as well as he can, he believes that everyone else looks down on him and sees him as not worth their while. He can feel this so acutely that he takes carelessly spoken words amiss and feels slighted where no rebuff was intended.

He would so like to be able to take a more dynamic role amongst people; he so wants to be well thought of yet it is completely out of his reach. He is too passive to feel more than resentment and bitterness. If he starts to express active dislike or even hatred then he becomes agitated and confused and then he goes into retreat. Where he can score, though, is if he is responsible for anyone else in either the family or the office; then he might impose his own form of subtle, even passive revenge to the point of making life difficult for those under his influence.

Such a man spends much or all of his life doing the bidding of others who seem to him to make use of him but who make him feel that he is of little consequence. He is powerless to control his own destiny and feels trapped in the sidelines where he passes his days unnoticed. The original cause of this is buried in the past. Many factors may have played a part: an unfeeling father who brutally told him too often how inadequate he was; a failure to achieve academically because of undiagnosed learning difficulties; being born into a large family of bright and extrovert children where the competition was too great. The heart blackens slowly but the die is cast early. This is fertile soil for the beneficial effects of *Anacardium*.

Forms of chronic pathology of the leprotic miasm
This is not an uncommon condition. It is a *passive* state and it is *depressed*. It is one that in strong but leprotic constitutions tends not to cause illness too early and too severely; anyone else would have produced, before too long, physical pathology as a practical means of expressing their problems. Eventually physical pathology does occur but it takes a considerable length of time to manifest – just as leprosy can. When it does it can take the form of neurological symptoms or trouble with the liver, gut, mucous membranes or musculoskeletal system or skin.

Peripheral neuropathy is a chronic, general condition of the central nervous system that mimics the anaesthesia of lepromatous leprosy. The nerves of the extremities become numbed so that picking up objects becomes difficult and the gait changes till they walk with a curious 'slap'; with no feeling in the toes or sole, the foot is put down without any flexion.

Another condition is scleroderma, an autoimmune condition in which skin becomes hardened and swollen. Sometimes the lungs, oesophagus, heart muscle and kidneys are also involved. Where the skin is thickened it becomes characteristically waxy in appearance. Where the skin is affected around the joints they become stiff and the muscles are painful.

Lupus is increasingly common and has similarities to both the tubercular and the lepromatous forms of leprosy. It is a systemic skin disease that takes one of many forms but it is basically a condition where the skin has lesions with a characteristically eroded surface. It is frequently to be found across the bridge of the nose, spreading across the cheeks in a butterfly shape. The skin can be flaky and reddened. In some forms, this is the extent of the problem but in others the symptoms can be worse. There may be deep ulceration of the reddened macules (lupus exulcerans); the surface skin might produce nodules all over the eyelids, the nose and the lips (lupus miliaris disseminatus faciei); bone cysts may be associated with soft, raised lesions on the surface (lupus pernio) which affect not only the face but also the hands. It is associated with sarcoidosis which is a tubercular and precancerous condition of the inner surfaces of the internal organs. Lupus vulgaris is regarded as TB of the skin.

Psoriasis around the face, head or ears can be particularly distressing, leaving high-tide marks of dead flakes of skin on the collar and threatening infection and unpleasant, dry-caked discharges from the ears. Another example, less severe, would be chronic sinus trouble with inflamed and even ulcerated mucous membranes of the nasal passages. The tubes feel plugged up. The symptoms can cause headaches, eyestrain and frequent bouts of laryngitis. There is a tendency to develop frequent colds or bouts of 'flu either of which would involve the mucous membranes of the lungs.

These different guises of what is essentially similar to symptoms of leprosy may develop as the result of being in an *Anacardium* state for a considerable length of time. What will help the practitioner decide that *Anacardium* is needed are the symptoms that are peculiar to it: a sensation in any affected part or organ of pressure as of a plug fixed into a bunghole; a sensation of a band or a hoop around a part. If these are accompanied by nervous dread of failure in any enterprise and a feeling that the memory might let one down *Anacardium* will act curatively.

Other major remedies have their own slant on the leprotic state. *Graphites* has a picture of abject dejection borne out of a chronically timid disposition. The patient can feel as separated from society as *Anacardium* but expresses it differently – with much grieving, complaining and lamenting with fearfulness about the future and life in general. She (it is more frequently useful in women) becomes confused and indecisive and cannot judge what she should best be doing for her welfare. She is anxious to be amongst her family, to feel part of a whole; in a place in which she can feel supported and anonymous in her distress. Physiologically, the hardened, flaking skin lesions with cracking and tendency to suppuration of honey-coloured exudate that are characteristic of *Graphites* are all typical of the miasm as are the remedy's shortening of tendons, arthritic nodosities and emaciation of limbs.

Making a miasmatic connection
Before we leave *Anacardium* it is worth mentioning that it has a darker, more malevolent aspect that is relevant to the leprotic miasm. The intellectually capable but emotionally crippled subject – the square peg in the round hole; the one who feels constantly at war with himself – might turn to hatred in his inability to find his place in the pecking order. He might be filled with intolerance, invective and rage which bursts out from time to time. He becomes a petty tyrant with a foul mouth and vicious habit of meting out physical abuse especially to those close to him who are defenceless. The cause of this can be just the same as that which produced the milder portrait of misery – physical or emotional abuse in one form or another. There is many a gang member who needs *Anacardium*. There is much of the destructive syphilitic miasm here, though; the syphilitic engrafted onto the leprotic. This is the type that seeks out victims and treats them abusively; they vent their aggression on others as a reflection of their own deficiencies – just as the Nazis did to the Jews; all that is needed is the suppressed creative individual who feels ungovernable feelings of rage and somewhere to invest the responsibility outside the self.

Himmler was an extreme example: organiser of the concentration camps; author of the drive to prove the historical truth of the Aryan purity of German blood (a particularly syphilitic activity!); a man obsessed by the deluded notion that he was the reincarnation of a medieval Teutonic king; yet, he was Hitler's lackey. Just as syphilis can reflect the worst and most destructive elements of leprosy (in the destruction of flesh and the nervous system), the frighteningly black and hideous side of *Anacardium* can terrorise the other, apparently meek refugee from an alien society. In other words, there is a relation between syphilism and leprosy that can be reflected in the nuclear energy of a small nut from South-East Asia that has been invested by nature with opposite but complementary aspects.

This is less absurd than it seems. Whatever negative force comes out of nature has a balancing positive force. What might seem strange, is that the positive force should be invested in a nut. And yet, after years of studying the *Materia Medica* one becomes used to reading of the bizarre and twisted personalities of metals, plants, trees and animal poisons that have not one face or two but sometimes a whole range of complicated, interrelating expressions – just as the human psyche has – which reflect the different miasmatic layers that we all have. The psyche in its departure from the norm is what principally guides us to the source of the appropriate natural healer. The fact that we do not at present produce leprosy as one of our common pathologies does not mean that the disease and its miasm are finished. It means that we have to use skill and intuition in observing the typical patterns of the condition in order to identify it now that it has 'gone to earth'. In the West, leprosy is hidden by dint of its being buried deep in genetic memory and obscured by the richer, more obvious TB and syphilis miasms.

Practitioners miss the leprotic miasm to the detriment of patients' health; it can be so hard to spot because information on it and the nosode have only recently been given. We may have remedies that can draw a leprotic patient back into a normal relationship with the world, society and the family but often we base the prescriptions of these remedies only on the *presenting* psychological state without considering the depth of and connection with *the miasmatic roots of the condition of the psyche*. It is not always enough to identify a disease state by the name and prescription of the indicated remedy.

What makes things more difficult is that all of the polychrest remedies are 'multi-miasmatic'. It is comparatively easy to see the syphilitic, sycotic, psoric or tubercular aspects of most remedies. The physical manifestations of these miasms are still with us so we should expect to be able to see the roots from which grow the mutant branches of chronic disease. Yet it is hard to see the differences between a weakened tubercular patient and a leprotic. Then we have the character of the miasm's psyche which is shy, retiring, in retreat and reluctant to be identified. It is a measure of this that there are no famous characters as examples of this miasm.[5] Leprosy does not produce egos; *it humbles or destroys them*. Herein lies a keynote of the miasmatic tendency that can be used in the clinic as a practical guide for the homoeopath: where a patient's ego is threatened with suppression or extinction through a weakened ego meeting overwhelming circumstantial odds then the underlying leprotic state should be suspected of being active.

But homoeopathic practitioners have a distinct problem in the case of treatment versus the leprosy miasm. Practitioners who know the background and use it to inform their healing approach are working, for the most part, on assumptions. They are in the same position as Hahnemann when he began his experiments. He based his work on observed provings and an intuition of remarkable acuity. Homoeopaths now have the work of practitioners 'in the field' such as Dr Prakash Vakil to add vital clues to buried troubles. In western society leprosy is well and truly interred; the contention, though, is not that it is not dead but that it is dormant. Interestingly, a characteristic of fungal life forms is that they can remain in a state of limbo for any length of time, waiting for their opportunity to waken into a slow and gradual but ineluctable crescendo of activity.

Leprosinum – the nosode

This brings us to the nosode of the remedy made from lepromatous material. Two different types of the remedy – known variously as *Leprominium* or *Leprosinum* – were developed in India. One was made from the leprous nodule of a patient's ear. The other was made from the bacilli cultured on the foot of an armadillo. (Armadillos are the only other animal to suffer leprosy; a fact that has given rise to speculation that humans 'caught' it from them in the way AIDS was supposed to have been 'caught' from green monkeys.) It was the latter remedy that was used by Dr Prakash Vakil in his proving.

Leprosinum is not like the other nosodes. It is not that it was made in any manner different from the normal procedure, the curiosity lies in the fact that its effects on patients in the West seem to be frustratingly nebulous. With *Psorinum*, *Syphilinum*, *Medorrhinum* and *Tuberculinum* we have nosodes that are vitally effective and necessary on a daily basis; they are familiar remedies to every homoeopathic prescriber in Britain. We could not practice effective homoeopathy without them. In India (and probably any other area where leprosy is endemic) *Leprosinum* seems to be potentially just as useful. Dr Vakil quotes cases where it is used with startling efficacy.[6] In a case of gout he based his prescription of *Leprosinum* 1M on just a few symptoms: increased irritability, greater religious devotion, early ejaculation, resistant but sensitive skin, a history of TB in the family and an aversion to wearing black clothing. In addition the man had oily skin and premature ageing.

He cites three other cases where *Leprosinum* was instrumental in creating health in patients suffering from a range of diverse conditions: anxiety neurosis complicated by a peptic ulcer, a recurrent, chronic sore throat and lupus vulgaris. Through his experience with using the nosode Dr Vakil speculates that *Leprosinum* would be of use in many other conditions that have symptomatology in common with leprosy: from acne vulgaris to AIDS.

This experience is from a country where leprosy is rife. In Europe, we only have the buried miasm and our judgements on that are essentially speculative, though based on the empirical knowledge of how miasmatic energy works in the other chronic hereditary diseases. We are left with our subjective observations of how patients who suffer under the 'victim' state characterised by leprosy, tend to metamorphose into more self-determined, proactive people who have a better and more balanced sense of ego after remedies such as *Calcium*, *Graphites*, *Anacardium*, *Sulphur* and *Causticum*. We can observe in these remedies the similarity between them and the leprotic state of mind (and body). We can observe the *effects* in people as 'like' cancels out 'like', revealing a more balanced constitution.

Because these remedies are associated in their other aspects with the other miasms, we do not at once associate the curative metamorphosis with the fact that the patient may have shed (or partially shed) the leprotic miasmatic chrysalis. This is a pity because there are occasions when the indicated remedy fails to fulfil expectations and it becomes necessary to prescribe the nosode as an intercurrent 'bulldozer' to remove the genetic influence of the deeply entrenched miasm or to underpin the good work of the chosen indicated remedy. As we have seen, this is necessary when the genetically-banked miasm is more powerful than the disease condition.

Unfortunately, as leprosy has been so long absent in any physical mani-festation from our northern shores and has been superseded by such a malignant agency as syphilis, not to mention the ever-present tubercular miasm and the ever increasing cancer miasm, we often fail to recognise the need to give *Leprosinum* or even to know that it is an available option. But then if *Leprosinum* is used, frustratingly it so frequently appears not to spark off either the expected response in the patient or any reaction at all.

Comparatively speaking, *Leprosinum* has not been available for anything like the time that the other nosodes have. We are in need of a great deal more time for clinical experience. Nevertheless, we should not be discour-aged from using the nosode; it is our lack of experience in *observing* the effects of the remedy and not the *absence* of effects that makes this medicine difficult to use. A homoeopath treating a patient on a long-term basis tends to lurch from one appointment to another in search of the curative effects of the last remedy given, often forgetting to take a longer-term view of the mi-asmatic path the patient is taking. Yet when *Leprosinum* is indicated (usually as an intercurrent remedy) and then given, though the immediate effects may not be as spectacular as those of *Syphilinum* or *Tuberculinum*, *Medorrhinum* or *Psorinum*, it nevertheless creates within the patient's system a climate ready for a subtle and profound change. This change is most easily observable in attitude, body language, choice of words, facial expression and choice of activity. The shifts are slow to occur and happen very often without the patient's awareness. As the metamorphosis takes place over a long period it is all too easy to dismiss the nosode as having been ineffective and conclude that it was the other remedies with a greater track record of success that produced the curative, positive, creative changes. The energy of *Leprosinum* is only betraying the essential nature of the disease from which it is derived.

The prescription and the timing of this remedy therefore depend largely on the intuition of the practitioner – much more so than would be the case with *Syphilinum* or the others. This can be an insuperable stumbling block to those ruled by a strictly rational mind. Issuing a patient with a remedy based on the idea that they may be suffering from the hereditary miasmatic effects of a disease that began to die out at the beginning of the Renaissance is decidedly unscientific. Nevertheless, a practitioner who senses that the leprotic state is an underlying influence would be perfectly justified in prescribing *Leprosinum* particularly where indicated remedies fail. After all, if Hahnemann had not experimented according to the dictates of his intuition and imagination we should not have *Psorinum*, *Medorrhinum* or *Syphilinum* nor, indeed, homoeopathy as it is today.

An artist came for treatment; a sculptor who worked with wood and occasionally stone. He suffered from allergies that plagued his sinuses and throat (he believed that this was caused by the materials he used) and other allergies that affected his gut. He was pitifully thin and had a stooping posture. He was fifty-eight but looked more like seventy. His arms, that one might have expected to be muscular, were scrawny and covered in liver spots and the veins on the back of his hands stood out proud and purple. He complained that he could never put on any weight and that he had been losing pounds at an alarming rate since the latest bout of diarrhoea had begun a week before. He explained that if the gut was playing him up then his sinuses were better and vice versa.

His story was complicated further by a history of medical examinations that had led to mistaken diagnoses and wrong treatment. He had taken every conceivable antibiotic for sinus and chest infections and he had taken steroids, anti-inflammatories and painkillers. He had been through an exploratory colonoscopy, a barium meal, sinus 'washes' and an exclusion diet. He had also consulted practitioners who had put him on nutritional supplements, liver 'detox' diets and a regime of five litres of water each day. The man was heartily sick of talking about his symptoms and with experts telling him what was wrong with him. His greatest trust was in his osteopath who had treated him with cranio-sacral therapy and had now recommended homoeopathy.

Apart from the physical condition it proved useful to hear of his history. He had been born before the war. He was six in 1940 when his parents sent him to relatives in Scotland. His younger brother and sister remained with their mother and his father went to fight. While he was an evacuee he persistently had tonsillitis and sinus infections. His tonsils were eventually removed (he could vividly recall the chloroform) and he was operated on six times to clear the mucous membranes of his maxillary sinuses. He was not at all happy with his distant relatives who appeared austere and forbidding; they were cold and loveless and had no children. They were in their fifties and the man was an embittered invalid. In the two and a half years that he stayed with them he never saw his mother and he only had half a dozen letters each year from her.

The man came over several years for treatment. Remedies were used to treat the acute episodes of diarrhoea and sinusitis, to detoxify the lymphatic system and the liver of the history of drugs and to support his constitution that had been so depleted. There were many emotional issues to address and not only to do with his dismal childhood. He was married to a woman who took no interest in his sculpting. She led a separate existence involved with the Women's Institute and certain charitable organisations; she was a local JP and had more than a passing interest in local politics. In the last twenty years she had only been to one of his exhibitions *"and that was because one of the guests at the opening was the minister of transport"*. He loved her dearly and was very proud of her as he was of their three children who were now grown up with their own families. Nevertheless, he admitted to feeling abandoned by her. *"She seems to have no further use for me; she hasn't had since the children went off to university, really. I am de trop. She tells me I have my bits of wood to keep me happy and that she couldn't compete with them."*

Treatment was frustrating but because progress was marked by small successes with remedies that hastened any acute problems to a speedier resolution than he had hitherto experienced, he was happy to continue. (The osteopathic treatment also continued to his benefit.) He was a willing self-prescriber: he quickly learnt that certain remedies slowed down diarrhoea and others followed that would clear it up; he found that there were remedies that loosened thick, offensive- smelling catarrh and that there were some that would stop a potential sore throat dead in its tracks. He had a first-aid kit of some fifteen to twenty remedies which he could employ for himself. When he came for his appointments he would bring his exercise book of notes and recount, blow by blow, what had gone on in between. This meant that remedies for his general constitution could be given fairly regularly. Bearing in mind that emotions affect the whole constitution, many of the main remedies were prescribed based on what he had to say about his feelings. He would gradually lose interest in what he had written, lose his place in his notebook and start to talk of his doings. This inevitably led to his exploration of feelings that always had a bearing on both his past history and on the treatment. He would often say, in an embarrassed and apologetic way, that he should not be using the session for psychotherapy. *"It's so unfair to expect you to listen to all this."*

Over the years he went through phases of needing remedies to address the tubercular history in the family – his allergies were typical of this miasm – as well as syphilitic and sycotic aspects. There were emotional issues about his mother and about his father that he expressed at different times. Most especially when his mother died he needed remedies to assist him to deal with feelings of guilt and grief and what he described as *"an unexpected anger"*. He also had an episode when he had a series of acute sore throats and earaches which reminded him of his childhood traumas with specialists and surgeons; he responded well to both acute remedies and those for going through deep fear – fear and shock that he had held in his system for so many years.

There came a point when he began to express his sense of isolation not only from his wife but also from his family (who were scattered over the British Isles) and from society in general. He felt that his physical condition prevented him from enjoying company – he was always afraid his gut would start rumbling and that he might be obliged to dash to the lavatory which he would fill with putrescent smells. He became melancholy about his work which he felt was stale and lacking in inspiration. He wanted to go into retreat. He was not in the least self-pitying; on the contrary, he spoke in a matter-of-fact voice. He felt no-one was to blame but that this was how things were to be. *"I really don't have any cards to play this hand but I'm sure that it will all be the same in a hundred years."*

Added to the mental state were physical symptoms; he had developed a ganglion on one wrist and he had athlete's foot, a fungal condition. At this point he was given *Leprosinum* 200. The results were not immediately apparent. Over the next few months he needed other remedies for a cold and a sore throat, an episode of difficulty in swallowing and a stye. His gut had been quiet for some time. Gradually it was clear that he was becoming more decisive, less tolerant of impositions, increasingly irritated by his wife's lack of respect. He spoke with a more determined and less drifting tone of voice. He no longer worried about his work; he just got on with it when his stamina would allow. He coped with his weakness – now less of a problem than it had been – by working on pieces that were of a more manageable size. At the same time his wife suddenly began to take more notice of him. She was still not interested in his work but she did want to know where he went if he left the house and she did ask him if he wanted to accompany her to various functions. Rather more alarmingly, his doctor became interested in him after meeting him in the street. He called him in for tests and referred him to specialists. He was given appointments with experts that reminded him of all that he had been through in Scotland in his childhood – all without his having lifted a finger let alone the telephone to arrange anything. He felt confused but abused and this time he did not *"feel particularly inclined to stand any nonsense"*.

"They can do all the wretched tests but I shall decide what sort of treatment I'm getting whether they like it or not!" It appeared that *Leprosinum* contributed to a transformation from someone who let things happen to him to someone who was prepared to take the initiative. This is one of the most self-empowering events that can happen. Nor was it lost on him that history repeated itself, reproducing the situation in which he had to confront his old dragons: hospital, the ignominy of medical tests, white coats, the smell of chemicals, waiting rooms and lofty doctors talking across him to his wife just as they had done years ago to his guardian relative. He spoke of these things with wry humour as if the dragons were now toothless and breathless.

This man would never be able to restore his former vitality; he knew that his constitutional health had been severely compromised by so many years of mismanagement. He remains frustrated by his tendency to gut problems though his sinuses are very much better. He seldom develops a sore throat or earache. He has a cold no more than twice a year and it never causes his chest any bother. He knows how to use his remedies before anything like that can happen. His digestion lets him down if he overexerts himself or eats anything related to wheat or dairy foods and he still finds it difficult to maintain a weight suitable for his frame. Nevertheless, he works and knows that his work is good and that it is sought after.

Another twist to add to the confusion

This case demonstrates the use of *Leprosinum* as an intercurrent remedy. It was based on the fact that other remedies, given for their similarity to physical, mental and/or emotional symptom pictures, were not 'holding'; they would effect a response but not make much difference before the body succumbed to another bout of illness. *Leprosinum* was selected because of the deep isolation of the patient and his virtually mute acceptance of his situation – a status that was seen as the cause of a medical stalemate.

To confuse matters – or perhaps to confirm what we already know – many patients who appear either to be in the leprotic state of mind or have phases of displaying leprotic characteristics, produce physical conditions that require *tubercular* remedies. We know the connection between TB and leprosy: the similarity of the bacilli; the susceptibility of the leprous to TB and the immunity of the tubercular to leprosy. It is intriguing that intercurrent doses of *Bacillinum*, one of the TB nosodes, should be so useful in skin diseases that have common symptoms with leprosy – ringworm and athlete's foot, for example. *Bacillinum* seems far more useful in treating them than *Leprosinum* which appears to be largely ineffectual in these conditions – though its effects may contribute to these conditions not reappearing.

The interest here is not so much in *which* remedy is potentially curative as *why* it should be so. Intercurrent doses of nosodes are prescribed because of the similarity of the patient's *underlying general* condition that has been preventing the body's satisfactory response to otherwise well-indicated remedies. Even in those cases where the mental and emotional characteristics – always given precedence when deciding on any *general* condition, underlying or not – are typically leprotic and the tubercular aspects are entirely absent, *Bacillinum* will often appear to work better than *Leprosinum*. It seems that the likeness of the physical symptoms produced by *Bacillinum* and leprotic remedies is enough for *Bacillinum* to be curative.[7] But this doesn't explain why *Leprosinum* should be less effective especially when the proving of the remedy showed such a rich variety of physical symptoms (thereby suggesting that it would have great curative potential). In particularly intractable cases it is not unknown to prescribe *Bacillinum* and *Leprosinum* in alternation on a weekly basis for a short period.

One reason might be that the tubercular miasm is generally far more prevalent in our western society than the long-buried leprotic miasm. Comparing the mental and emotional sides of the two, shows us that tuberculism is very much more in evidence in Europe. It is always easier to select examples of it from any casebook. Of all the miasms, tuberculism proclaims itself more readily than any of the others by dint of the nature of those under its influence. They are more vital, interesting, exciting, fickle, irritating, attractive, humorous, mischievous and superficially talented than all the other miasms and, often, rather more obviously ill. Leprosy is the most shy, retiring, humble, uncomplaining, easily victimised and forgotten and, often, quite the least interesting type of patient. If the patient belongs to a religious group that objects to any form of therapy that might be construed as having anything to do with spirituality then he or she would be highly unlikely to come for treatment in the first place.

Leprosy indubitably exists in our history and it seems to have created within the collective psyche of our ancient forebears a terrible fear and loathing. So, too, did bubonic plague, cholera and typhoid but these are diseases that have relatively short-lived albeit fearsome historical episodes. Though we fear such epidemic diseases they have been unable to take root in our genes to anything like the same degree as psora, syphilism, sycosis, tuberculism and cancer. The plague, cholera and typhoid are not diseases that affect the psyche so vividly as the acute conditions that give us the names of the major miasms so it is not surprising that they do not impinge so readily on our heredity. We may not see the leprosy miasm so easily or anywhere near so often but that is to do with its nature and its being subsumed by the prevalence of the others. It does not mean that it is not there.

What can be done with what we know about leprosy

It is up to the future generations of homoeopaths to discover the full potential of *Leprosinum*. To do that it is necessary to understand the psyche of the leprotic state as well as knowing the *Materia Medica* of the remedy and that of others with similarities to it. If we limit such research to a hunt in the filing cabinet for all those patients who never got better on well-tried remedies, to see if any of them could fit the leprosy bill, then much will be lost. Leprosy has been a universal problem in its time and is still endemic in many parts – areas, too, from whence many immigrant populations come. So the relevance of our efforts may not simply be historical.

If we spread the net a bit wider it will not take much to see the leprotic miasm's relevance to at least two major diseases. One is seen as the end of the road and the other is one of the most publicised ever known – cancer and AIDS. Both have things in common with the leprotic psyche:

i)   there is the possibility that the patient feels a 'victim' or an outsider;

ii)   there can be the sense of being marginalised and ostracised;

iii)   patients can feel as if they have been destined to suffer in this way;

iv)   patients can become melancholy at the hopelessness of their state and feel resigned to their fate;

v)   patients can feel that they are beyond the reach of orthodox channels of help;

vi)   there can be resentment at the intrusion of official expert advice and treatment.

Both diseases ask that their sufferers go through many stages and each of them will be characteristic of one or other of the miasms. This is because both AIDS and cancer are multi-miasmatic conditions. Both diseases have many variations on their central themes but there is no doubt (among homoeopaths, at least) that they are conditions that ask patients to face all the miasmatic, spiritual, emotional and physical problems that they have never been able to resolve before. It would not be surprising to find that any cancer or AIDS patient would go through a time in their disease process when the leprotic state would arise and thus the need for *Leprosinum*.

CHAPTER 25

CANCER

D on't let the word above put you off. It may be redolent of fear: of disease, of pain, of loss of dignity, of hospitals, of loss of control and of death. These are acute responses to a state of being that exists long before any physical manifestation. They are fears fuelled by television programmes and medical journalism which attempt to chronicle the constant war being waged against the disease with only the least notion of what really lies beneath. This chapter is about recognising that the seeds of the disease lie within both the psyche and heredity no less than in the other miasms. It is about understanding that this miasm is a 'journey'; one in which we have the opportunity to unravel the tangle of suppression, trauma and 'wrong path' decisions of the past. The miasm is about absolving the past through returning to the beginning; the disease is the imperative call to set one's own record straight; to set one's house in order. Before going any further, let's start this survey with just the word, 'cancer'.

It comes from the Latin for 'crab'; hence also the name of the zodiac sign.[1] The crab's characteristic sideways movement and its distinctive red flushed streaks along the limbs gave the Romans the idea for calling ulcers and malignant growths that spread and creep through tissue 'cancer'. After the Normans colonised Britain in the eleventh century we acquired a similar word with which the Latin became confused – *cancre*. Later (in seventeenth-century France) this became *chancre*, a word still in use though mostly as a medical term. The word 'canker', of which Shakespeare made much descriptive use, derived from the Norman spelling. It did not mean 'cancer' as we recognise it today. A 'canker' in Middle and late Middle English (1150–1450) signified an eating, spreading sore or ulcer; a gangrene. A 'canker' today usually refers to mouth ulcers or herpetic eruptions in and around the mouth. (In America a 'canker-sore' means an eruption of herpes simplex.) A 'chancre' specifically means a venereal ulcer and is associated with syphilis. Whatever the etymological niceties, these various words bear the burden of meaning associated with spreading growth that corrupts normal flesh, destroys tissue and leads to a morbid condition of the whole body.

It is no accident that syphilis has been mentioned within the first paragraphs of this chapter. The aspects of cancer most loaded with fear belong to what we shall refer to as syphilitic cancers: insidious, fast-growing malignancy that uncompromisingly leads to chemo- and radiotherapy, radical operations and ultimately to the painful (or medicated) death that everyone had been fighting to avoid. But this is a very limited view and gives us no panoramic perspective of a disease state that can appear quite different. Strange as it may seem, even here in something so many inappropriately perceive to be terminal, there is a positive note to be struck. Before there can be cancer, the disease, there must be cancer, the miasm – a state of mind and body and spirit that, if given the right stimuli and circumstances, can lead us back into well-being through a journey of self-discovery.

Cancer and the other miasms

– Psora is about the susceptibility to playing host to either parasites or notions that cause an unbalancing degree of anxiety and feelings of inadequacy.
– Syphilism is about being susceptible to the depredations of either an aggressive and invasive bacterium or destructive emotional and spiritual negativity.
– Sycosis is about the effusive proliferation of either congestive mucus and pus or the disturbance of mind caused by separation from reality that creates the confusion of duality.
– Tuberculism is about the need to express life in as brilliant a way as possible under increasingly physically, emotionally and spiritually challenging circumstances. At the same time it is about the need to find equilibrium in a body which is either ravaged by a

malignant bacterium or charged by a dissatisfaction with the past
and present and illuminated by a false dawn of idealised hope.
– Leprosy is about either the creeping and destructive activity of a
fungal bacterium or the abdication of individuality altogether.
– Cancer can be about any or all these things because each of the
other miasms has its own route into the cancer miasm and will
pervade, inform and colour the physical pathology that may result.

But this is not all for this great miasm has more to say about the human condition than simply being an extension of the others might suggest.

Cancer is not only about the multiplication of cells that have lost their
genetic integrity. Let's imagine that we are like those diagrams in geography
textbooks of cutaway mountains showing all the different strata of rock and
soil. By the time a patient's whole body has reached the state of cancer, the
complexity of historical symptomatology is extraordinary – some of it even
belonging to family history. The interweaving of different causes and triggers, all held in place by the stasis of having no resolution for pain, trauma
and sickness, is as potentially dangerous a state as it would be to have a
home on shifting tectonic plates. Like many who live in the shadow of a
volcano, we can fall into a condition of complacency, unaware that the underlying negative energy of all that we have allowed to be buried is
disturbing our well-being. The efforts we make to avoid the pain of expressing grief – sometimes by indulging in fruitless and enervating hatred or
refusing to acknowledge the source of pain - lead us away from our life purpose; away from our creative spirit. Cancer is thus also about the *breakdown*
of all the efforts we make to sustain our whole bodies in denial by superficial
and artificial means that we employ in our determination *not* to seek resolution for suppressed spirit, emotions or physical symptoms. It can so easily
be the result of shoring up our lives with possessions, position and the pursuit of unreal goals. It is about maintaining the status quo for fear of having
to face painful change. It is about the *loss of purpose* of the whole where 'purpose' is intended to mean the creative, forward-moving spirit of life. The
cancer miasm is about facing and dealing with the collective damage to
one's gifts from *negative experience* that we have failed to resolve. This is true
even of young people who, one would have thought, might not have lived
long enough to look into such a dark well.

In terms of the diseases that are related to the different miasms it is immediately evident that the scabies mite, a parasite, is at the very opposite end of the pole from the undifferentiated, rogue cell that sets about reproducing itself against the collective programme within the the body. The inward process of self-destructive disease has reached its apogee with cancer having advanced by means of an inverse sophistication: animal mite (psora) to self-propelled bacterium (syphilism) to an indolent diplococcus (sycosis) to an *in situ* replicating mycobacterium (tuberculism) to perversion and malignant multiplication of the cell structure.

On the microcosmic level it is the evolutionary journey from parasite to the chaos of undifferentiated cell proliferation. What started with the innate sense of inadequacy on a spiritual and mental level has reached the point of actual inadequacy of the body; its inability to prevent it turning against itself. Rather than seeing this as the end of the road we need to recognise we have come full circle. Cancer may be a potentially terminal disease involving the basic cellular structure but the state from which it develops is about recognising that we can go back to the beginning. We can heal ourselves by stripping away all that is not essential to life and yet still have purpose despite our deepest feelings of inadequacy.

Just as tuberculism is a variation on the themes of syphilism and sycosis (and therefore of their parent, psora), so the cancer miasm is a set of variations and fugue on them all. Just as tuberculism is a unique state with its own characteristics, so too is the cancer miasm. The miasmatic state of cancer is not the same thing as the disease itself. It is the 'soil' from which the disease can eventually emerge. The soil can be of different qualities according to the individual's predisposing miasmatic history; the carcinogenic soil can be predominantly syphilitic, sycotic, tubercular or psoric. If the disease were to become manifest then its form would be shaped by the predominant miasmatic quality of the soil. However, the disease is only one aspect of the miasm and not necessarily the first to be considered in treatment. It is very common for people to be in a carcinogenic frame of mind, emotions or spirit without manifesting anything of the physical disease at all – which, as we have seen, is true of all the other miasms.

The predisposing frame of mind

The triggers for waking the cancer *miasm* are legion but the underlying predisposition is relatively simple and singular. If we accept that each of us has a unique purpose in being incarnated and that one's life can be a never-ending exploration of opportunities and experience then the predisposition to this miasm is the limitation and suppression of that purpose. It is not natural or healthy for our emotions or spirituality to stand still. All life, in whatever form, must keep moving. The moment it stops its restless forward drive there is stagnation and decomposition.

> – In psora movement is maintained by constantly exploring one's potential through harnessing experience to routine.
> – In syphilism stagnation can be held back by the person's ability to manipulate other people and circumstances to their own ends.
> – In sycosis it is achieved, albeit temporarily, by escaping into unreality, often a place rich in fantasy and humour.
> – In tuberculism the individual is driven to eventual exhaustion by the need to move for its own sake.
> – In leprosy, the miasm, the individual is governed by the urge to create movement through finding support from social massing.
> – In the state of cancer there is no self-motivation that results in creative movement. *The focus of self-determination is absent.*

At one time or another most of us experience being balked in our objectives. We learn ways of overcoming frustrations and may think nothing more of those events. "It'll be all the same in a hundred years." We might be able to cope with far more serious issues such as redundancy, the breakdown of relationships or the death of a relative. We 'learn to live with it'. All would be well if we were able to express ourselves appropriately through communicating and sharing with like-minded others. Unfortunately, the more 'civilised' we are the less we do this satisfactorily and with honesty. Our efforts at expression are often woefully inadequate or nonexistent – or they are blocked by those we would communicate with if they have a hidden agenda and a stronger negative purpose in doing so.

Eventually the *physical body* has to express what the heart and mind no longer have the capacity to hold without externalising. Even this would not necessarily be enough to wake the cancer miasm. We would more likely produce minor pathology first: *frequent colds due to a lowered immune system* (psoric/tubercular); *cold sores* (sycotic/syphilitic); *bladder infections* (sycotic); *haemorrhoids* (psoric/sycotic/tubercular); *migraines* (psoric/tubercular); *gallstones* (psoric/sycotic/tubercular); *diverticulitis* (sycotic/tubercular); the list is endless. The more insistent the pathology, the stronger our need to suppress the discomfort. The worse the symptoms, the more powerful the agent of suppression. The more fearful we are of the *apparent* breakdown of the body, the more we hand control to experts who claim greater knowledge of our bodies. The greater the suppression, the nearer we get to the cancer miasm.

There are some people who do not operate on this level. Instead of physically manifesting symptoms of hurt and anger they learn to shut down on painful emotions so effectively that no-one could guess that anything might be amiss. They appear healthy and energetic even though this is a façade. They may feel fatigued at times or they may become less tolerant of heat or cold (though heat is commoner) or alcohol or other factors. Those who know them really well might see them as emotionally distant. Such a state of emotional suppression is acquired conditioning, usually from parental influence. It is a virtue, in the British at least, not to display emotions. Yet the cost is great for those schooled in the nursery to control their natural feelings. Little signs betray the way things can go – perhaps, to start with, nothing more significant than early evidence of ageing. There might be greying of the hair; wrinkling of the skin on the neck; failing eyesight; more frequent need to visit the dentist; trembling of the hands; a weaker bladder; an imperceptible increase in the lack of confidence; a rise in blood pressure. More trivial instances tend to cause greater anxiety. The ability to cope becomes more of a struggle. (Some people make a name for themselves as great 'copers'; not a good sign.)

There is another path that seems to come from the opposite direction but still leads to the same narrow corridor. There are those who are perpetually angry. They are driven by aggression. They are often workaholics. They tend to put pressure on others. They live in a state of constant combustion which they might fuel with rich food and drink. They do not notice that anger, wine and deadlines all stoke the liver to dangerous levels. We might think that we are dealing with someone who speaks his own mind and who 'lets it all hang out'. The risk for such people is to feel the softer, gentler emotions. The suppression is of warmth and cherishing. They have lost the ability to nourish the spirit with loving kindness.

There are those who are trapped in a world of deadened emotions, like the princess in the story whose tears were jewels and who was beaten so often that she could cry no more. Such people appear calm and demure or cold and uncaring. Their reserve hides little for they have been rendered speechless to express the void in their hearts. Look into their eyes and you will see an empty well. People in this state become 'doormats' for others.

The contrast to this is the bright, bubbly character with the almost hysterical laugh that they would like to control but which bursts out of them. They cover their timidity with an avalanche of gabble; they find amusement in a shopping list. They become exhausting company even if they are attractive to start with. For them, life might have begun in a genuine state of delight but, for whatever reason, the suppression of some part of their life force has meant the assumption of a desperate mask of false jollity.

After years of suppression comes the fear. There is fear of inadequacy that undermines their ability to cope (psora). There is the fear that everything is futile (syphilism). There is the fear they may be losing control and becoming confused to the point of mental imbalance (sycosis). There is the fear that something is missing, that unless that vital thing is found fulfilment will be swamped by guilt and despair (tuberculism). There is the fear of having to stand up and be counted, of taking responsibility for oneself, of discovering the essential loneliness of being a sick human (leprosy).

Most of us at one time or another have felt we could answer to more than one of these states at the same moment. Most of us, much of the time, have the resources with which to lift ourselves out of them. We change our patterns of energy. We might go shopping; go away for the weekend; swap the furniture around (a favourite device of children); change jobs; tell someone what we really think of them. Or we might become ill with an acute condition. A bout of 'flu will change your energy and will do you good if you allow it to work its way through your system without suppression. Strange as it may seem, people often have accidents when they are in this mixed miasmatic state. The accidents, though calamitous at the time, invariably work out to have curious advantages. (Frequently patients will report that they had a life change after a serious accident and though they suffered – sometimes horribly – they realise that the forced change was positive.)

There are times when people find it virtually impossible to overcome their feelings of inadequacy, despair, confusion and lack of grounding. It can happen just as much in acute situations as in chronic ones.

A woman came without an appointment. She was ashen coloured with fright. She could think of nothing else but that she was due to see the dentist that morning. She was paralytically afraid of the drill and the hypodermic and she was about to have a filling replaced in a molar. She was breathless and hot; her hairline was damp with sweat. Her speech was made up of half-sentences and questions that began with "*What?*" and "*How?*" almost whispered in a breathy voice. She was ready to be told what to do. She knew that she should be in control and she felt that her condition was "*so silly*". But it was not silly. It was torment. It was suppressing her whole being.

Acute states of being out of control can be settled acutely. Chronic ones need more time and effort.

Josie, a woman of forty-two, came with a list of complaints that could not be written on one page. She was in a state of complete exhaustion and depletion. She had difficulty breathing, difficulty in digesting her food, in staying awake, in consecutive thought. She was a strange colour. What little hair she had left was dyed blond but her face was the colour of *café au lait*. She had acne and was vastly overweight. She had water retention and constipation. (She needed to pass water every half an hour or so but could not pass any motions at all without suppositories. On one occasion she had not passed anything for three weeks – an assertion that would be greeted by most doctors with disbelief.) In spite of this appalling condition her main complaint was that her breasts were excruciatingly painful. They were engorged, hard, lumpy and agony; she was forced to cradle them to avoid the pain that came with every step.

Josie had been born prematurely to a single mother. She was put up for adoption immediately and had no contact with her natural mother. She remained in hospital in an incubator until any threat of infection had passed. (Her breathing had been compromised from a great deal of mucus in her lungs.) Eventually a foster home had been found. This cannot have been satisfactory as over the following ten years she experienced eight different foster homes. When she was not with foster-parents she was in an orphanage. At twelve she went to yet another set of foster-parents. They were older than she had been used to but she was glad to get out of the stifling and competitive world of the orphanage. Within a few weeks she discovered that the orphanage was perhaps a better situation. The man locked her in the cellar without food or water for twelve hours. This was punishment for something she had no recollection of doing. The same thing happened again though this time he shut her in the dark without sustenance or bedding for several days. At the earliest possible moment she fled back to the orphanage and refused ever again to be fostered.

At sixteen she left the home and soon became pregnant. She was advised to have an abortion which she agreed to. She attempted suicide shortly after. She took a bottle of wine and lots of pills down to a beach. Ramblers spotted her and called an ambulance. At twenty she married a man who turned out to be alcoholic and a wife beater. She had two children by him.

At twenty-three she had a car accident and lost her spleen which had been ruptured in the collision. She was told that she would have to take antibiotics for the rest of her life as anyone without their spleen had lost an important part of their immune system. She left her husband and took her children with her; they never saw him again. She *travelled around a bit*” until physical symptoms began to worry her and threaten her ability to care for her children; she had attempted suicide again but this was thwarted by her son who discovered her. She was taken into hospital where tests revealed that she had an underactive thyroid. The thyroid was removed and she was put on 200 mg of thyroxin permanently.

Shortly after this she met her present husband who *“swept me up and whisked me off from all that – he’s my angel.”* Her troubles had not finished though as she developed uterine fibroids which caused heavy blood loss and her two teenage children began to express their own troubles. The daughter began mutilating herself with pieces of broken mirror and the son began playing truant from school and shoplifting. Josie underwent a total hysterectomy that brought on an early menopause. She was put on HRT which violently disagreed with her. Since taking the drug she had suffered monthly from the breast pain, water retention and inability to control her temperature; she was either very hot but unable to sweat or freezing cold and clammy. Though she had taken herself off the HRT she had been too afraid to drop the antibiotics or the thyroxin.

This is a story of suppression on every level. There was acute and chronic suffering. The patient had no energy to be sad or angry. Her story was related in flat, emotionless tones of tedium. The only spark of life was when her husband was mentioned.

Both these cases, though completely different in character, are examples of the way that some people depart from normal equilibrium and head into the cancer miasm; that state where there is stagnation of self-determined movement. It is the *whole* system that is so profoundly disturbed that it can be hard or apparently impossible for the patient to re-establish the balance. The balance must be restored in the physical body. The organs must work in harmony so that the liver maintains control of distributing nutrients to the cells; so that it can work to discard toxicity; so that it can store and release carbohydrates, fats, some of the essential vitamins and iron; so that it can create urea and maintain its communication with the kidneys. The kidneys, in turn, need to maintain the fluid balances in the body without which nerve function, digestive functions and circulation are all affected. The endocrine system, of which the liver is just one part, has to be in concert so that each of the different hormones is secreted into the body at the right time. The central nervous system has to be balanced in order to manage the sympathetic and parasympathetic nerve responses.

The emotional body has to be balanced. The emotions are only attuned when heart and mind feel as one while the whole feels grounded and in control through a sense of self-confidence and well-being. Anyone who finds that they are *giving* all the time and not *receiving* or vice versa (rather more difficult to judge subjectively) is not emotionally balanced. Anyone discontented with their career or their relationships but who does nothing to change anything is not emotionally balanced. Living in doubt or fear for any length of time will create the same stagnation of purpose.

With the emotional and physical bodies in such a state, the spiritual side of things is not going to be in any sweeter harmony either – if by the 'spiritual side of things' is meant that inner resource which assuages all negative thoughts and feelings from a point of acceptance, understanding and loving. To reach that point requires a journey; a journey that usually begins with physical pathology and emotional pain.

The longer we remain without any internal solution to such mixed levels of disharmony, the more likely it is we raise the cancer miasm. Of all our besetting sins it is the inability to 'let things go' that harms us most. Few of us have the requisite sense of composure. That extraordinary storyteller, Laurens van der Post, related the tale of the young monk who, falsely accused of a petty but antisocial crime, was obliged to leave his village. Years later, when he returns as an older man and is greeted with embarrassment and shame by those who have since discovered the real culprit, he is able to say truthfully that he has no bitterness. He was able to accept even as a young man that it was his destiny that such an apparently terrible thing should happen to force him to go away and create a successful life elsewhere. Would that we could all be as well composed as this.

The predisposition to raising the cancer miasm includes not just fear and suppression of the physical, emotional and spiritual bodies but also lack of harmony between the parts of the three bodies. The three bodies become fragmented. This can be in danger of happening whenever we are strongly influenced by any of the individual miasms but the body's survival mechanisms maintain sufficient integrity for most of the time to enable us to cope with the negative aspects of the imbalance. We have safety valves. They always take the form of discharge, either emotional or physical. Suppression of discharges stops up the safety valves. Grief, fear, anger, guilt, hate, humiliation and many other disrupting emotions can affect the physical body so profoundly that important organs no longer function satisfactorily. It is accepted that the immune system is compromised by negative emotions. Add this to the poor performance of vital organs and allow the situation to go on for long enough and the result is that the whole is negatively affected right down to the basic cellular activity of the body. This is the state that is ripe for the development of abnormalities of cell structure. How long it takes to reach this point is dependent on the inherent quality of the constitution. It is imperative that whatever strength we begin our lives with should be preserved and encouraged by every means.

A summary of the carcinogenic predisposition

The body that is turning toward the carcinogenic state is one that is physically suppressed. It probably has been for years. To be too long on antibiotics (and some people are asked to remain on them for years) or steroids (and some are on them for life) can eventually break down the constitution dangerously. To have repeated minor surgery for benign conditions such as cysts and fibromas is going in the same direction. To have polyps and warts and any other excrescence systematically and repeatedly removed does the same. Such intervention is tantamount to telling the body that it is getting its sums wrong. It may take many years for any sinister changes to come about but this is more a reflection on nature's consummate skill than on our *rational* understanding of how to treat ourselves.

The emotions that turn towards the carcinogenic state are those which are allowed either no expression, too prolonged a period of inappropriate expression (such as impotent rage) or that are absent through total denial. In providing us with awareness, feelings and interpretative intuition, nature gave us a double-edged sword. It can cause self-inflicted wounds if we forget that there are positive as well as negative aspects to being selfish. So many of us take too long to discover that the true healing of emotions is part of spiritual growth and therefore part of our life's purpose.

The spiritual body that is turning toward the carcinogenic state is one that has lost its aspiration to fulfil its purpose or that was denied this from the very beginning through the undue influence of parents, family or society – or, dare one say, as a result of a long line of ancestors refusing to face cumulative results of an original 'wrong path'. (Young children who develop cancer are often expressing ancestral miasmatic disease that has a profound positive emotional and spiritual effect on their families.)

If we can frame the essence of the cancer miasm in a few words it would be 'suppression, fear and the loss of purpose'. The long-term results of this state do not necessarily lead directly to the development of cancer, the disease – it can equally readily lead to serious heart conditions. What it almost always leads to is a moment in one's life where one has to stop, take stock, and make a choice about the 'now'. The choice often boils down to whether one puts oneself first or not. All too often the decision is put off. What engineers this moment of decision, if we pay no heed to the whole body's call for nurturing, is usually an illness (acute or chronic), an accident or a trauma.

The case of the woman on her way to the dentist and the case of the woman who had spent so long in foster homes are examples. Both people needed to alter their circumstances so that they were in control of their lives. In the first case, the extreme nature of the disturbing fear and in the second the extreme emotional and physical suppression illustrated the *miasmatic energy* that was evident and in urgent need of addressing. The confirmation of this was that both patients were given the same treatment. Both received *Carcinosin*, the nosode of cancer made from cancerous tissue. However appalling this might seem it is an invaluable medicine and one that is very frequently used.

Treating the cancer miasm

The woman on her way to the dentist went for her appointment. She experienced no fear, having sat for half an hour in the clinic after taking the remedy and before setting off. She reported feeling comfortable in the dentist's chair and remembering that she had wondered why she had been in such a panic. Josie, needed far more than simply one dose of one remedy. However, the initial dose of *Carcinosin* made her feel "*so much more together*", comfortable in herself and comparatively more energetic that she felt inspired to pursue the homoeopathic route. This would not be enough in itself to claim that the remedy had achieved anything as she might have felt relieved after simply relating her story. (Though she had recounted her biography to others before without any similar relief.) What was more convincing was that she also felt free of pain in the breasts for the first time in years. (She was even able to sleep without the support of a bra.) If such results were isolated then there would be no merit in relating these cases but they are not.

A boy of five was brought for treatment for his asthmatic breathing, profuse catarrh and tendency to throw high fevers. He had been in this state for most of his life; his symptoms had first become manifest when he was eleven months old. Since then he had been on steroids, Ventolin syrup and frequent courses of antibiotics. He seemed to have a permanent cold and his problems were evident from the loud, wheezy breathing. He was given treatment over several months designed to limit the need for antibiotics, clear his chest of phlegm, relieve his liver of overdoses of chemical agents and to improve his immune system. The mother reported that he was less susceptible to coughing spasms, to infected mucus (it had always been green before but was now yellow or clear) to night-time asthma attacks or to high fevers. He went through a period of profuse, yellow discharge from the eyes and he had two 'ear infections' – which were, in fact, acutely swollen eardrums that burst and released a lot of pus from the Eustachian tubes. However, the boy was still not growing; he was considerably undersized for his age. He was not progressing in his learning development particularly well. Furthermore, he consistently had an above normal temperature; his mother had noticed that he was hot all the time and his temperature was hovering around the 99°F mark.[2]

At this point the boy was given *Carcinosin*. The change was radical. He threw a very high fever within hours of taking the remedy – not such an uncommon reaction to this medicine amongst children. It lasted only two hours and needed no treatment other than a cool sponge. From this point on the boy began to grow, his vocabulary increased dramatically, his usual state of raised temperature left him and he began to feel the cold for the first time. His bowel motions became regular and normal (having been bordering on diarrhoea) and his colouring became clear and pink instead of pale and wan with bright red ears. His breathing gradually improved and he was able, over the next few months, to dispense with all allopathic drugs. Why had there been this need for *Carcinosin*?

The answer lay in the degree of suppression to which this child had been subjected, albeit for the best possible reasons. However, the suppression had not simply been due to the drugs. The child's first symptoms had manifested themselves shortly after being given the DPT injection. The mother had initially put it off as she had felt unsure of whether to have it done but had been persuaded by her family. Within a few hours of the inoculation the boy had thrown a high fever, become delirious and had breathing difficulties. His mother had sponged him down, given Calpol (just as she had been advised to do by the doctor administering the jab) and waited. Within a week or two the boy was having breathing difficulties for which he was given antibiotics – and so the cycle began: high fevers, repeated chest infections, severe coughing, a permanent round of cold symptoms and earaches.

The inoculation for DPT is one of the most common culprits for this situation – see p. 302. Homoeopaths are not only familiar with this kind of result of the vaccination but have been treating the conditions set up by it ever since the problem first arose. While *Thuja* is regarded as the most commonly needed remedy, it is seldom the only one. *Thuja* was one of the remedies the boy had already taken; it had improved his health generally and somewhat reduced the asthmatic condition but he still needed the *Carcinosin* to complete the healing process.

As more generations are given the DPT vaccine, it goes deeper into the genetic make-up and requires deeper and lengthier periods of treatment. Remedies such as *Thuja* and *Silica* [3] were once enough to do this job on their own. Now *Carcinosin* has become very well known and invaluable as a remedy to heal an immune system compromised by inoculation. This, incidentally, does not only apply to the DPT injection. *Carcinosin* is sometimes called for in treating people who have been inoculated frequently for going abroad or who have been given multiple jabs for being in the armed services or for frequent hepatitis B inoculations given to hospital staff.

Allergies

Another condition that is deeply associated with the cancer miasm is that of multiple allergies. We saw how the other miasms – and particularly tuberculism – play a significant role in the problem of allergies and how the character of the manifesting symptom picture illustrated whether the patients were producing tubercular, sycotic, psoric or syphilitic signs. However, there are increasing numbers of people who are intolerant of not just one or two allergens but a whole range. Included in this are wheat, gluten, yeast, dairy products and sugar.

The onslaught of symptoms that are caused by these substances is bewildering. Though the allergens primarily affect the gut, they are capable of compromising every department in the body. They affect the body chemistry and in the process cause thrush, bloating, abdominal discomfort, constipation or diarrhoea (or both), mucus discharge and haemorrhage from the bowel, vaginal discharge, urethral and anal itching, menstrual disorders, liver malfunction, stomach pain, profuse mucus secretion which can lead to asthma, muscle weakness, sinusitis, headaches, nervous disorders, depression and obsessive-compulsive behavioural disorders. Any of these conditions can be misdiagnosed and the wrong treatment given for them.

It is, paradoxically, very easy to miss multiple allergy syndrome. Not uncommonly it is accompanied by hay fever which is more to do with being ultrasensitive to all sorts of other airborne allergens. The patient is not only subject to eating and digestive troubles but also to chronic sinusitis and oedematous membranes of eyes, nose and throat. The profuse production of phlegm in the head leads to an impaired capacity to think or to remember much. The normal general functioning of the body is suppressed.

If the system is so sensitive to these irritants that it produces profoundly disturbing or even incapacitating symptomatology then there is clearly something fundamentally wrong with the defence system. The body should be capable of dealing with these outsiders without producing any noticeable symptoms. Just as a healthy person is usually capable of dealing with a 'flu virus or a stomach bug without showing any sign of chronic illness, so each us of should be – and still most of us are – able to despatch dust mites that get up our noses or tree pollen that gets into the lungs. These ubiquitous bugbears do not miraculously miss out well people. They are simply swiftly and silently dealt with. Those who have a broken-down defence system show symptoms of the body's stress at being obliged to harbour irritants. They might produce copious quantities of mucus in an attempt to flush them out but there is no ability to set up a permanent body-watch to recognise the invaders and repel them automatically without alerting the rest of the system. Such a situation with the body's chemistry so out of sync is, by its very nature, of the cancer miasm.

There are many remedies employed in the treatment of multiple allergies. All the nosodes are often used at strategic intervals over the long time it takes to treat the condition. (It is a peculiar and frustrating state to treat in that its focus of debilitating symptoms frequently switches sites – going from gut to skin to lungs and back.)

The deeper and more intractable the problem, the more likely *Carcinosin* will be called for. It is one of the most common remedies in the treatment of patients with myalgic encephalomyelitis,[4] ME, which can be associated with allergies and a history of glandular fever. It is also one of the noted remedies for helping children who suffer from compulsive behavioural disorders that can sometimes accompany the allergies. (The behaviour patterns can be present without any sign that the child is allergic to anything very much.) These children frequently have that hallmark symptom of a permanently slightly raised temperature that indicates the need for *Carcinosin*. (It is a sign that the liver is distressed and cannot cope and that the spleen is weak and cannot replenish the supply of fresh blood cells to the body or support the immune system as it should.)

Nervous disorders

The cancer miasm is riddled with nervous conditions. This is not surprising when we consider fear and suppressed emotions are at the root of it. Here is a typical example with which many homoeopaths would be familiar:

> A woman in her fifties complained of ME. She had suffered weakness in all her limbs – particularly her legs – for some five years. She explained that she was of a nervous disposition and frequently felt as though life was too stressful. Her diction was precise, hurried and clipped as if she needed to be absolutely clear but in the shortest possible time. She seemed flustered beneath a hasty but ordered exterior. She sat forward on the edge of her seat and kept brushing strands of hair away from her eyes even when they were not there. Between taking breaths and delivering words she would smile in a toothy grimace that had little humour. She needed no prompting to describe how the problems had begun.
>
> She had received a phone call from her father six months after her beloved mother had died. He declared he was going to come and live with his daughter and that she should get the spare room ready. He would move in one month. She was left speechless and furious. She disliked her father intensely and blamed him for her mother's death, feeling that he had bullied and harried her to her grave. *"He bullied us all. He has always been impossible. He treated my mother like a slave; I can't think how or why she put up with it. We three girls left home early just to get away. He was always angry. We were so afraid of him. Our mother was our ally really."*
>
> The father had come and for a while was ensconced in the spare room. He had not changed since his wife's death. He merely transferred his attitudes onto his daughter and her husband, a mild-mannered man who kept his own counsel. This situation lasted a few months until her father decided that his room was cold and damp. He bought a house further down the road. He moved into two rooms and left the rest empty. From then on he made his daughter's life a misery by phoning her, up to

six times a day, with lists of demands and to recount to his catalogue of complaints, both bodily and social. It was now at the stage where she began to shake whenever the phone rang. She had to spend long periods of the day resting. She could no longer do gardening or go shopping because any effort would cause her to feel faint, breathless and weak. If she fell over she would not be able to raise herself. She had developed nervous tics at the corner of both eyes and the fleshy space between thumb and forefinger. She had episodes of internal trembling and others of pins and needles. She could never count on a good night's sleep because she would jerk awake with a violent start or lie restless unable to control the twitching in her legs.

"I was never able to say anything to him. It seems so awful to say to one's father that he's not welcome but that's how I feel. How do you explain to your own flesh and blood that they are slowly draining you of everything? It makes one feel so guilty even to think it but one has questioned whether one loves them. You see, I'm not sure he knows quite how frightful he is. He's never been anything else really so he's not going to change now, is he?"

This woman's otherwise very happy existence – with a much loved husband and two children – had been brought to an abrupt halt and suppressed. Her guilt and fear about her father consumed her every waking moment. She had no respite and no assistance beyond the devotion of her husband. (He was by no means a feeble person; he had been unable to prevent his father-in-law from buying a house so close or to convince his wife that she should not answer the telephone. She was too afraid of the consequences of not responding.) One of her sisters lived in America and the other was an invalid so she could receive no help from them. With what she felt was great courage, she eventually told her father that she would only be able to see him once a week as his attitude and presence made her feel so agitated and unwell. He responded by telling her that she was totally unreasonable and suggesting to mutual friends that his daughter was possibly getting early signs of Alzheimer's.

The woman began to make a slow recovery. She was fully aware that although her symptoms were physical in sensation and reality, she would only get better as she was able to come to terms with her father and rebuild her own life without his interference. It was possible to measure her growing physical strength by the increase in her self-confidence and her self-assertive attitude to her father. She felt guilty but elated when she changed the phone number and went ex-directory. She allowed herself a small smile of triumph when she booked a brief holiday in Scotland with her husband and laid no plans for anyone to check up on her parent. She was now confident that he would be all right left for five days to fend for himself. After over a year of treatment she was able to do about twenty minutes of gardening in a day and to have a couple of friends round to tea. The remedy that initiated these tiny improvements was *Carcinosin*.

"*Since that first remedy I noticed that I no longer have those feelings as if I'm coming down with 'flu. I don't get those fearful bone aches and shivery feelings.*" This was significant as influenza with bone aches, swollen glands and shivers is to the cancer miasm what whooping cough is to TB; what mumps is to gonorrhoea; measles is to syphilis; and scabies is to psora. It is an acute condition that is there to teach the body how to cope with more chronic disease. She was, before treatment began, never quite free of the underlying symptom picture of 'flu as her system had never discovered how to cope with the periodic glandular swellings, the pains in her back and long bones and the general feeling of malaise.

The *Carcinosin* also greatly improved her other nervous disorders. The tics left her and only returned when she had pangs of guilt which did come back but less frequently. The pins and needles stopped, the internal trembling lessened and only bothered her when the telephone rang. (She had to school herself to remember that only her husband and children knew the new number.) Her sleep was far more restful and the 'restless leg syndrome' bothered her not at all. What persisted were the symptoms of weakness, breathlessness and the faintness whenever she felt overheated or agitated. The return of her pleasure in her family and all their activities was what she most treasured. Though she needed some eight years of treatment to arrive at this point there was now no going back to the abject misery that she suffered before.

Carcinosin, the remedy

Carcinosin was first given wide coverage in homoeopathic circles by a Dr Foubister and his colleague, Dr Lees Templeton, both of the London Homoeopathic Hospital. Their extensive knowledge came from clinical assessments at the hospital in the 1940s and 50s. They compiled details which covered mental, emotional and physical symptomatology that come under the positive influence of this bizarre remedy. The origin of the preparation they used is not exactly known, only that it came from the USA and was more than likely from a sample of epithelioma of the breast.

Just as *Tuberculinum* is representative of tuberculism and the other nosodes are of their respective miasms, so *Carcinosin* is of the general state that leads to the cancerous diathesis or state of being about to produce cancer. The remedy is a polychrest in its own right; it has its own peculiar 'picture' as the cases and examples mentioned above suggest.

i)   It is one of chronic and deep suppression, fear, guilt and an inability to express oneself fully, appropriately or at all.

ii) It is one of nervousness or anger or both. (Patients in need of its healing power may therefore be shut down and inexpressive or volatile and voluble.)

iii) It is one of curious and uncontrollable nervous signals given off by a nervous system under the severest strain.

iv) It has the third dimensional aspect, as well, of a chequered family history; anyone with any or some of the following list amongst their forebears might be likely to need help with this miasm: cancer, TB, syphilis, gonorrhoea, depression, alcoholism, insanity, suicide, violence and abuse.

This is not to mention a patient's personal history that might reveal bad reactions to vaccines, severe whooping cough with lung complications, a long series of childhood fevers that had no particular explanation, a history of accidents with broken bones and the allergic conditions referred to earlier.

In addition to the 'history' there are also physical characteristics:

i)   the appearance of or change in character of moles;

ii) the appearance of naevi (red birthmarks);

iii) the development of curious symptoms such as a craving first for salted foods and then sickly sweet foods;

iv) a seemingly chaotic array of symptoms that keep switching emphasis from one part to another.[5]

The 'picture' of *Carcinosin* is invaluable as a guide to whether a patient is heading towards that time when his or her body might begin to lose its integrity on a cellular level. *Carcinosin* can be and is often used as an intercurrent remedy to support a system that is heading for this sort of breakdown. Even someone suffering from haemorrhoids who does well on *Sulphur* might need *Carcinosin* to complete the healing process if the piles are the product of perpetual suppression of anger, fear and the self. *Sulphur* on its own might not be able to lift the patient out of a learned habit of keeping violent emotions locked in. Though piles are a long way from cancer itself, it can be the thin end of a wedge that leads in that direction. Suppressed piles can lead to hiatus hernia. Drugs for hiatus hernia can lead to digestive disorders and liver function suppression. This can lead to ulceration of the stomach or duodenum – because the body has to find another site to express itself. Drugs for internal ulcers can further affect the liver and bring on high blood pressure and other changes to the digestive tract. This is a threshold that once stepped on carries great risk of cellular changes.

So the judicious use of *Carcinosin* (where it is indicated by a patient's symptom pictures or any lack of response to well-indicated remedies or when the family or personal history suggest it), can redirect a patient away from the risk of stagnating; of remaining too long trapped in a suppressed condition. It can be seen as a prophylactic in treating a patient who would otherwise head towards developing cancer, the disease. Because the picture of this remedy is at first sight both confused and confusing with its appearance of being a cocktail of the other nosodes, it took the profession some time to follow Dr Foubister and prescribe the remedy on its indications with confidence. It has now taken its rightful place in the canon of remedies.

The lessons of history

It is worth witnessing what occurred to one or two historical figures whose lives and deaths can illustrate the progressive process for us.

Catherine of Aragon, wife of Henry VIII, was just fifty when she died. She had been born in 1485 to Ferdinand of Aragon, a loving but inflexible father and spouse, and Isabella of Castile. Five of Catherine's siblings died very early – probably as a result of inadequate hygiene and nursing during years of military campaigning. Of the others, none but the lunatic Juana had satisfactory marriages from the point of view of carrying on the family line; their offspring were stillborn or died as a result of unidentified childhood illnesses. Juana managed to produce an heir to the throne while Catherine, out of her six pregnancies, was only able to produce one healthy baby girl though even she, Mary Tudor, became chronically sick.

Catherine was despatched to England at the tender age of sixteen. She was first married to Arthur, Henry VII's eldest son, who died of a lurgy at sixteen leaving a wife who spent the rest of her life denying that she and her young husband had ever consummated their marriage. This hotly contested matter was without doubt one of the stresses that contributed to Catherine's health problems because the validity of her subsequent marriage to her husband's brother, Henry, hung on just this point.

Catherine, older than Henry but sweet natured and pretty, had genuinely won the young Henry's affections and she was never to lose the genuine love she bore him. She was faithful to him to the end of her life. She offended him by not producing a son and heir, so after 24 years of marriage she was dismissed as a wife, demoted as a queen and humiliated as a woman.

Catherine was prone to stress-induced illnesses. She would frequently go down with fevers and stomach complaints. It was put down to the inclement English weather but this did not explain how quickly she managed to recover when something occurred to lift her spirits. The fevers and other symptoms were genuinely physical. Once she was banished from court, Catherine devoted her life to prayer and seclusion. She suppressed her naturally sunny and open disposition and became serious and unsmiling. She aged quickly as she pined to see her daughter and felt all the frustrations of being cut off from the man she regarded as her lord and husband. She remained stoic, though, even in the face of the obvious attempts to find any excuse to have her executed.

She died still trusting that her monstrous husband would be forgiven. The postmortem revealed that despite her physical agonies her vital organs were sound with the exception of her heart. On the wall of her heart there was a black growth and the inner walls of the organ were black as well. She died of cancer of the heart. It had taken some 34 years to progress from a succession of viral maladies to terminal disease. Only her unusual disease betrayed her inner expression of anguish and how appropriately her body tells the story! All the ingredients were present: an enfeebled family tree decorated with madness, stillbirth and disease (quite likely syphilis); separation and abandonment[6]; humiliation and injustice; repeated fevers and viral infections; repeated pregnancies with stillbirths; suppression of natural expression with oppression of the spirit.

Catherine's daughter Mary did a great deal worse. Mary was brought up in an atmosphere of suspicion, distrust and downright threat to her life. She was forcibly separated from her mother whose maltreatment she was well aware of. She was kept away from her father whom she was desperate to love. She was married to her cousin, Felipe II of Spain, who all but abandoned her after a short interval of what to Mary was conjugal bliss. She suffered torments of religious fervour. She endured the agony of false pregnancies only to realise that she would never produce the heir to her Roman Catholic throne which would keep Spain and England united. In addition to her mother's unfortunate genes she also inherited her father's rather more dubious ones – it is possible that Henry had already contracted syphilis before his daughter was conceived. She undoubtedly carried the tubercular miasm in her blood as her grandfather, Henry VII, died of the disease as did her half-brother, Edward VI. Mary often suffered colicky pains. She probably had difficult menstruation. She definitely developed ascites or dropsy which is swelling of the abdomen from excessive water retention. Her symptoms demanded that her doctors bleed her and give her quantities of 'physic' which may not have suppressed anything but certainly could have made her more ill. As she was also given to coughing up 'black bile' it is possible that she had some ulceration of the stomach. Her illness and death were not inconsistent with someone suffering from terminal cancer of the digestive tract. With the tremendous bloating of her abdomen this would have described her mental and emotional state well for her abiding obsession in life beyond her faith was that she should become pregnant and be delivered of a healthy child.

Another woman of royal blood whose story illustrates this miasm well is Victoria, daughter of Queen Victoria and Prince Albert, wife of Kaiser Friedrich III of Prussia and mother of Kaiser Wilhelm II. She was born in 1840 to doting parents. She was married at seventeen and it was very much a love match. Her marriage, though, meant political exile in Prussia.

'Vicky', as she was known to her family, found herself isolated in an inhospitable palace, reviled by much of Germany who responded to gossip put about Bismarck. She watched with impotent rage her husband's political influence being slowly emasculated. She suffered the ignominy of being constrained by the strictest protocol in respect of her communications with and visits to her family in England. She buried two of her eight children; she lost one to meningitis and the other, when he was eleven, to diphtheria. She watched and nursed her husband through the illness that eventually killed him – cancer of the throat; the condition that also deprived her of her brother, Alfred, when she herself was mortally ill and their mother was dying. In addition to her other tragedies, Vicky endured the repellent behaviour of her eldest son. Once he became emperor he even denied his mother anything other than the briefest contact with her grandchildren and she remained *persona non grata* in his household.

Vicky's disposition was such that, though she might write self-indulgently to her mother or sisters about her feelings and symptoms, she remained a stoic to the rest of the world.[7] She received the confirming diagnosis from her mother's own physician that she had breast cancer. She told no-one but her mother and her faithful Lord Chamberlain whom she forbade to repeat the news.

In fact, Vicky lasted for a little over two years from the date of the diagnosis. There was metastasis to the spine which caused her 'lumbago' and 'neuralgia'. As her health declined her emperor son ignored her and refused to believe that she was as ill as reports made out.[8]

The hallmarks were there from the beginning. Vicky came from a royal line riddled with inherited disease. The most exotic was porphyria, most famously displayed by the scion of another house, George III who suffered bouts of apparent insanity as a symptom of what is essentially a liver disease. TB, cancer and haemophilia were also threads that ran through the various family lines that led to Queen Victoria and this is not to mention the tendency to disease resulting from overburdened livers and libidinous living.

Vicky's ideal marriage was damaged irreparably by social and political circumstances so that, despite being a highly intelligent woman she was unable to find an emotional and spiritual resolution to her experience of trauma. As a child who left her mother before she was ready and as a mother who lost her husband and two of her children to illness and her eldest son to a form of madness, Vicky's own disease state need not surprise us. It is in no way uncommon for women whose sense of nurture and nurturing is suppressed or hurt, to produce carcinoma of the breast – and particularly the left breast, on what is regarded as the yin side of the body. The breast may be composed of glands and fatty tissue but it nevertheless represents the physical form of nurturing energy.

Symptoms as symbols of a different malady
These three cases of royal women might seem not to apply to the rest of us. Yet we all have traumas and tragedies to cope with that might be just as desperate as anything these people had to face. Their upbringing would have focused their lives towards playing their particular roles and this would have restricted their spirits' expectations of life. So that they would have been less able to contemplate making changes in their lives that would have been necessary to transmute their grief away from the physical body and into acceptance, understanding, forgiveness and equanimity of mind and emotions.[9]

But the roles they played are only one aspect; these women were human beings with as vulnerable emotions as the rest of us. Brought up in a culture in which Church and State had ensured the profound separation of spirit and emotion from the body physical, nothing could have taught any of these queens how to process their grief, anger, fear, shame and defeat in any other way *but* through the physical body. They were denied any other expression. But notice the word 'expression'. The body expresses in physical symptoms just how it feels. Catherine's blackened heart, Mary's tumulus of a belly and Vicky's hardened breast graphically describe their mortally stricken emotional and spiritual bodies. While it is contentious and not always possible to draw any generalisations from this, many patients suffering from one or other of the many forms of cancer *do* illustrate their states of mind and spirit in what might be termed a 'symbolic symptomatology'. Percy Grainger, composer, pianist and arranger of English folk music, provides us with one further if rather bizarre example.

Grainger was born in Australia in 1882 to parents who proved to be incompatible. His father, an alcoholic, contracted syphilis shortly after his son was born, during a period of intense debauchery. His mother, after contracting the disease from his father, was so appalled and disgusted that she shut out her husband and never physically touched her son again. Instead, possessed of the firm conviction that her son was more than merely gifted, she devoted her days to promoting his career. Though she never touched her son through tenderness it is reported that she did so as a means of correction and put to use a horsewhip when she considered Percy might be slipping into his father's ways or he seemed to skimp his piano practice. It is probably to do with her methods of inculcation that he became a sadomasochist. Grainger left a letter saying that if either he or his wife were found dead as a result of the violence they inflicted on one another, it should be accepted that this activity was to him the highest expression of love. Furthermore, he left a clutch of photographic and written material which, ten years after his death, was to be given to the museum that he had founded in Melbourne.

Grainger's mother developed neurosyphilis, a condition that affects the spine and causes pains, paralysis and dementia. These symptoms along with the creeping rumour that mother and son had an incestuous relationship, were enough to cause her to throw herself off an eight-storey building. This left Grainger with a guilt complex that he never assuaged. Instead he married Ella in Hollywood in front of 20,000 people and devolved onto her not only his sexual cravings but also his other emotional needs.

Grainger, composer of 'In an English Country Garden', was a keep-fit fanatic. People would see in him the picture of health; with boundless energy and bursting with enthusiasm. All of which was true but it was only one layer of a very complicated man. He was also narcissistic and self-absorbed as his warped diaries and photographs suggest. His preoccupation with deviant sex he allowed to spill over into material that he wanted the public to witness. This is also a deviation from mental health. When he was seventy his physical health began to show the strain by producing an appropriate form of cancer. Prostate cancer is relatively common. It is a condition that can be very slow to develop with few initial signs other than restricted flow of urine. It is also a disease of an organ that is intimately related to the sexual organs. Grainger had prostate cancer for quite a long period. It was diagnosed eight years before his death when it was found to have metastasised to the rest of the pelvic cavity – which means that it might have been brewing for ten or more years. He had an operation to remove the prostate gland followed by radiotherapy which gave him considerable relief at first. However, he began to have painful retention of urine which required catheterisation and the metastasis to the bony tissue caused pain into the testicles. When the chemotherapy no longer afforded pain relief, he was castrated. Grainger had his testicles preserved in formalin and packed off to the museum.

In spite of expert medical attention – his surgeon became a great friend and champion – Grainger could not hold back the tide of the cancer which proceeded to his spine and then his brain causing him symptoms that his mother would have recognised in herself – similar pains and mild dementia. With metastasis to bone and the cerebral haemorrhage that killed him, Grainger ultimately expressed the essentially syphilitic nature of his disease, his sexuality and his family history. That his prostate should have been the initial site of disease is not surprising given that the focal point of the expression of his emotional energy was in his pelvic organs. That the disease then moved to his spinal column and brain further demonstrates its *likeness* to the syphilis that slew his parents.[10]

The esoteric nature of symptoms

The symbolism of site and symptom in cancers is not rare for those who 'look laterally' at patients. If one confines one's study to the textbook and lab reports such ideas are fanciful at best and misleading at worst.

Thyroid cancer

> the patient is in a chronic state of feeling 'When is it going to be *my* turn? When do *I* get a chance in life?' (The thyroid is the glandular organ esoterically most associated with vocalised self-expression.)

Kidney cancer

> almost always there is an issue with 'family', the origins of which might be buried in the past. (The kidneys are associated in other medical cultures with 'ancestral energy'; the quality and character of emotional and spiritual energy inherent in the forebears.)

Pancreatic cancer

> the patient is bound to be terminally suffering from 'lack of joy'. (Other cultures view the pancreas as the physical site of joy since it

is the organ that allows us to process sugars and is therefore associated with 'sweetness.')

Lung cancer

so often patients are expressing their fear of releasing their true but thoroughly suppressed emotions. Their fear is warranted very often because the rage and anguish would be truly frightful to witness. (The lungs are traditionally viewed as the organs of stored emotions and emotional experience and are closely allied to the heart in this respect.)

Ovarian or uterine cancer

there is likely to be an unresolved background issue to do with children, childbirth or their essential femininity.

Liver cancer

suggests that rage remains unresolved or that the patient's will has been thwarted too deeply. (The liver is, esoterically speaking, the physical aspect of the will.)

Bone cancer

so often a secondary stage, it almost always turns out to be representative of the loss of fundamental structure and security in the life of the patient, and not simply because he or she is so very ill.

Cancer of the blood

suggests the souring of the life force and lack of happiness through grief.

Cancer of the lymphatic system

is associated with the inability to clear old hurts or the inability to give expression to fears about one's sources of love. It often occurs in those who are addicted to destructive relationships.

Causes or triggers?

Most people think that the *causes* of cancer, the disease, are not in the body at all. There is little perception that the body's parts – and by extension, the cells that make up the parts – may resonate with the energy of abstract emotions. This is in spite of age-old associations such as heart and grief, gall and bitterness, spleen and anger, stomach and fear. It is less problematical to associate the onset of cancer with external stimuli. So, what about smoking? What about pollution? Isn't there a case to be made against the Pill or HRT – can't they cause certain types of the disease? What about dietary and nutritional factors? Isn't it true that a lack of fibre can contribute significantly to bowel cancer? Then there is the sun – isn't it the cause of so much skin cancer? There are power stations and other sources of radiation, lead, nitrates, asbestos and industrial waste products; the list is interminable.

Our willingness to participate in 'Hunt the Cause' is because we can, by doing so, avoid the main issue - that *we inherit and create our own internal environment for disease*, whatever its manifestation. By believing that smoking *causes* lung cancer we do not have to look at the emotional and miasmatic predisposition that precedes the desire to take up smoking and prevents smokers from seeing the reality of the dangers. The same is true of mobile phones and brain tumours or leukaemia and living next to a nuclear power station. The true cause of cancer is really no different than any other chronic and potentially terminal disease – it is the 'soil' that we prepare for it to develop in by not being able to process *experience* into a positive light. And this includes the inherited 'experience' of the miasms and negatively charged family energy. Anything else must be seen as a trigger that *contributes* to the negative development of the disease. Yes, the Pill and HRT can indeed be implicated in the development of breast cancer and probably testicular, ovarian and uterine cancers as well. Yes, exposure to radiation can initiate tumour growth and probably blood cancers – why else would doctors remove themselves from the room when X-raying their patients! Yes, the surgical removal of warts and polyps can trip start malignancy. Yes, the continued suppression of deep visceral ulceration with steroids and antibiotics can lead to ulcerative cancers in vital organs. Yes, poor nutrition with excesses of certain types of food can lead to cancer of the digestive tract. But we are talking about trigger factors here and *not causes*.

We can and ought to do as much as possible to eliminate these triggers. But to stop smoking or taking the Pill will do nothing for the constitution's *predisposition* that is rooted in heredity and personal emotional and spiritual experience. What the opportunity of life offers us is the chance to find

methods of resolution for all that ails us within any or all of the three bodies
that make up our whole.

> Physically we have *acute diseases* that encourage our systems to discharge
> – and influenza is the one most concerned with the cancer miasm.
> Emotionally we have verbal and gestural display mechanisms – one of
> which is the unique ability to ask questions[11]…and to answer unspoken
> ones from the heart. (Both of which we fail so miserably to do when they
> are most warranted by highly charged situations.) Spiritually we have a
> refined sense of connection to God and/or to the Earth which allows us
> the capacity to feel compassion, forgiveness and loving kindness that can
> transmute all that is potentially negative. At least, this is the ideal. If
> only…

Not all of us are given the capacity to find such finer feelings in sufficient
abundance that we can alter to the good our miasmatic inheritance. It is a
lifelong struggle for most of us to keep our emotional heads above water, let
alone our spiritual ones. So we become susceptible to the miasmatic
tendencies that are in our make-up; which, as we have seen, can be influenced by emotions and spirit just as much as by the physical direction of
disease.

Differentiating cancer according to the miasms

The cancer miasm is peculiar in its habit to appear in the guise of one of the
other miasms when it reaches its *physical* manifestation. This is why
homoeopaths talk of sycotic, tubercular, syphilitic or psoric cancers. It is
possible to differentiate between the forms of the disease in terms of the
miasmatic characteristics that describe each of the chronic inherited disease
patterns. Unfortunately, when cancer progresses towards its terminal stages
the body tends to show increasingly how syphilitic it can be.

Percy Grainger's illness was probably sycotic initially and only in its
later stages – possibly after the radical surgery – turned to a more sinister
and syphilitic malignancy. This only mirrors the man; a person of extreme
excesses with parents who suffered syphilis. Sycosis tends to encourage
tumour growth that is (initially, at least) somewhat indolent and spreading
with altered organ function or, where there are adjacent mucous

membranes, concomitant symptoms of foul but bland discharges. It is implicated in disease of the pelvic organs and the breasts, mucous membrane surfaces and lung tissue. Sycosis is also often the underlying factor in the formation of cysts and fibrous tumours; benign forms of tumour that can be a physical symptom that connects the patient's sycosis with the cancer miasm. These can remain indolent for years or come and go seemingly at random or they can just disappear. They usually cause no serious trouble unless they are interfered with. If other excrescences are removed often enough then the body will produce increasingly syphilitic and malignant versions. One of the reasons that the practice of 'zapping' such growths with laser treatment or surgery is still favoured is that few have noticed that the patient who had their genital warts removed by the gynaecologist's laser now has to see the oncologist about potentially malignant polyps in the bowel – necessitating a visit to a different department in the hospital.

George Gershwin died young of a malignant brain tumour that went undiagnosed for many months because its presenting symptoms were of a purely psychological nature. He suffered malaise and loss of concentration as well as lack of energy and depression. By the time he started to produce physical evidence of his condition – blackouts, headaches and weight loss – it was too late. This gives us a good example of a syphilitic cancer. Syphilitic cancers manifest themselves in insidious, creeping and rapidly destructive disease, just as one might expect from what we know of the miasmatic state of being. Any discharges are likely to be foul and destructive enough to cause local ulceration. Tumours are always invasive and quickly shut off vital blood supply or close down vital functions; they can also compromise the nervous system by affecting important nerves in the spine or cripple the skeletal structure by affecting bone tissue.

Gershwin's contemporary, the composer Bela Bartok, was another musician who died of a syphilitic cancer – chronic leukaemia. He suffered from a severe reaction to the smallpox vaccination as a child. He also seems to have had TB at some time as he had a shadow on his lung. He was prone to melancholy especially after the invasion of Europe by the Nazis whom he abhorred and from whom he escaped by exiling himself to the United States; for him a country full of noise and confusion and far from his beloved Hungarian countryside. He was profoundly discontented in America where he was disagreeably affected by the medical attention he received – multiple blood transfusions. Nevertheless, he managed to rise above his predicament and produced the ravishing music of his last years.

The form of leukaemia he suffered from is a disorder of the blood-forming organs in which the red blood cells are replaced by vast numbers of white blood cells that pour out of the bone marrow. It creates a situation of very low resistance to infection, a tendency to fevers and enormous fatigue. The patient wastes away and usually dies from an acute condition such as pneumonia – which demonstrates leukaemia's affinity with the tubercular miasm as well.

Psoric tumours tend to be very slow growing indeed. Often these are the cancers that are never diagnosed until a postmortem reveals that the patient who may have died from something like a heart attack, had also several well-defined, neatly contained tumours that simply did not impinge on any body functions. When psoric tumours are diagnosed and removed surgically the prognosis usually remains good. Calcified masses are usually psoric or psoric/tubercular in nature.

Tubercular malignancy combines the characteristics of the syphilitic and sycotic varieties. We should note how closely TB, the disease, resembles the cancerous state with the formation of tubercles (tumours) which the body attempts to isolate but, when resistance is lowered, break open and release bacteria to form new tubercles (metastasis). The tubercles can damage local blood vessels and mucous membranes (haemorrhage and ulceration) and cause the body to attempt to eliminate the problem (mucus and pus production). Tubercular remedies are frequently needed by patients who produce cancers. One of the origins of the cancer miasm can be found in the inheritance of neglected or suppressed TB.

Leprosy should not be forgotten in this context. Even without the clinical evidence, what we know about the miasm should be enough to suggest that quite a few cancer patients might fall into this miasmatic category. At the very least, skin cancers and cancers of the eyes, lips, mouth and throat could be, in part, leprotic in nature. So too might cancers where painlessness is a feature and those that involve nerve tissue that induces numbness and paralysis. As leprosy can so affect the glandular system, lymphatic tissue cancers might also be coloured by this miasm.

But cancer, the disease, in whatever form it takes, is ultimately multi-miasmatic. It is not uncommon that a patient will 'brew' cancer for a long time before being physically troubled by symptoms that require treatment. Once there is an obvious physical manifestation the disease progresses more rapidly and will show signs of changes in character: discharges might change colour; pains might shift location or switch in character; anxieties become depression. The variations in the character of its presentation often reflect a particular miasmatic pattern. The more proliferative and exuberant the form, the more it is sycotic. The more sinister, destructive and inescapable it seems, the more it shows the mark of syphilism. The more it goes into remission, slows down, hardens off into calcification, the more typically psoric it is.

Or one could see it another way. The more restless, dissatisfied and self-critical one is, the more likely the cancer will manifest in a tubercular fashion. The more self-deluded and separated from one's reality one is, the more likely that the symptoms will be tumescent or proliferative – sycosis. The more self-destructive, emotionally eaten-away and negatively motivated one is, the more the disease will become insidious and terminal – syphilis. The closer one gets to dealing with basic solutions to life that involve facing all the deepest held anxieties, the more likely it is that symptoms will slow down, ease away and leave only a memory of the spiritual and emotional journey that one has made – psora.

Self-awareness

The cancer miasm is a territory we find ourselves in when we need to explore our whole being; to explore our present selves in the light of our pasts and the reality of our potential for the future. It is a terrain in which each of us is asked to become more self-aware. If we fail to do this then we have the negative potential to produce a form of the disease that most represents our whole body, mind and spirit. We find ourselves in this predicament when our forward driving motivation is outweighed by fear and loss of purpose. Many people see chronic disease as a life test that one has to come to terms with on a personal level. The so-called incurable chronic diseases are those in which there is no escape from a situation; for which there is no internal solution. While MS, motor neurone disease, and advanced heart disease, for example, are all as threatening as cancer, it is the latter that holds the public imagination in the most abject fear – with reason.

Cancer is beyond all others a *learning* disease. It demands that the person go back to the very beginning to re-examine everything – in the general and the particular. This is often very threatening – and no other disease state seems to have this attribute so strongly. We not only have to question hard-won values but relationships past and present, career and upbringing. It can mean visiting old wounds, sometimes from the deepest past. Sometimes it means letting go of feeling responsible for a dysfunctional relative or family; by letting go of the guilt one hands back to those who have unwittingly 'dumped' their own 'stuff' on the most willing 'host'.

Jean, sixty-seven, came for treatment. She had been a practitioner of Chinese medicine and acupuncture for years. Despite being familiar with alternative therapy in general she had come to a block in her own treatment. Homoeopathy was the one thing she had not tried before. Her complaint was tennis elbow and she had always been able to resolve any symptoms with acupuncture and reflexology in the past. However, when the case was taken it was apparent that she had a chequered health history involving severe menstrual symptoms and hysterectomy, suspected TB and hepatitis. She complained of pains in her right elbow and foot but was otherwise *"very well"*. Yet she was nervous as she spoke. Her 'body language' was defensive and her speech was breathy, hasty and full of false starts as she looked for adequate words.

To cut her long story short, tennis elbow was not really her problem. She had been married to an alcoholic wife beater from whom she had escaped, taking her two very young children with her. She had lived for some years in terror as he had sworn vengeance. She fled from Scotland, changed her name, went out to work and put the children through grammar school. In leaving her native Scotland she not only abandoned her marital home but she also incurred the wrath of her father who said that he never wanted to have anything to do with her again. (He had been more concerned about the family prestige than his daughter's welfare.) However, none of this emotional biography came from her mouth. Her story was related by her son when he came for his own visits.

She did well on homoeopathic remedies and she maintained regular appointments. In a dozen appointments she felt that she cleared a chronic lung condition (which she neglected to mention on her first visit), several minor ailments and in between was able to deal effectively with 'flu and a poisoned toe.

One day Jean phoned to say she was going back to Scotland and asked if it would be possible to continue consultations by phone. Within three months of settling into her new home – not far from where she had grown up – she rang to say that her new doctor had diagnosed a suspicious lump in her breast. He was concerned and was sending her to the specialist. A biopsy followed and malignancy was confirmed though the carcinoma was well differentiated[12] and described as Stage 1. She asked for support with remedies as she went through the process of a lumpectomy. This was duly given; *Arnica* being one of the most important as it helps patients recover from the trauma of the general anaesthetic and, in mammary surgery, to the soft tissue of the breast.

Jean felt that she "*sailed through the whole thing*". What is more she found that being back on her own stamping ground she was "*more earthed*" and felt much more comfortable about her relationship with her two children who had been to visit her several times. She was feeling less guilty about what she had put them through as children and was able to come to terms with her son's homosexuality, something she had never mentioned before but that she now admitted had caused her untold grief.

In the operation the surgeon had removed all the lymph glands from her armpit "*as a precaution*". The result was that her left arm tended to swell significantly as the drainage system had been affected. Remedies, she found, helped to reduce the swelling and prevent any infection and pain. She refused to have radiotherapy or chemotherapy from the start which the oncologist did not contest as the general prognosis was good.

Ten months later, in spite of an excellent diet, plenty of rest and exercise, lots of meditation and yoga and several life changes that had made her feel "*on top of the world*", Jean suddenly developed cancer of the pancreas. She was told that the original cancer had metastasised which would have been prevented by radiotherapy. When she told them that she "*did not believe a word of it*", they did admit that they could not understand why things had taken such a turn for the worse.

Jean's condition worsened but her spirits did not. She allowed them to do "*countless tests*" but refused to take any medication other than painkillers. She also found that certain remedies relieved the symptoms considerably – *Arsenicum Album* being the main one[13] but so did the remedy made from *Emerald*. She adopted a very philosophical and calm attitude that her family found inspiring. However, as she became more seriously ill she began to be querulous and tetchy. Her son phoned one day to say that the painkillers were not helping and though morphine kept her drowsy it did nothing for her stomach pains. She also had mouth ulcers that were very painful and prevented her from speaking.

Jean was given *Nitric Acid* 30. According to her son, within an hour of taking this his mother began talking of her brother whom she had not seen or been in contact with for over 30 years. She explained that he had taken her father's side when she left her husband. He had tried to make contact some 20 years ago but she never responded; she felt too bitter and resentful, especially as they had been so close as they had grown up. He had not tried again to get in touch but Jean had always known that he still lived in the locality. She asked to see him and he came. Jean's son gave a simple description of the reunion saying that few words were spoken, quiet tears were shed and they held hands. Jean died peacefully in comfort and without any pain the following morning. One of the last things that she had said was that she was so grateful for the opportunity to set her mind at rest about her brother. It had lifted the years of unspoken anger, bitterness and regret. Jean's son said that he too had found the whole time uplifting and healing; he felt that he at last understood his mother in a way that he had never been able to before. Such a passing has an ineffable healing quality for all who witness it.[14]

Where does treatment begin – with the cancer or the patient?

This case illustrates many things, not least that homoeopathy and allopathy are not necessarily incompatible even in such serious pathology and that a patient can still maintain their independent choice about their treatment. The case also shows that cancer is not simply about the malignant changes in the cells of the body. It is about far wider issues that are not always apparent from interviewing the patients, certainly on the level of any clinical investigation but even in the broader context of interviews in which patients have space to express themselves emotionally. Jean so effectively shut away her feelings about her brother and father that her body produced a situation that demanded that she release them. (Such a theory might be anathema to some but those who have witnessed patients struggling with and then releasing such 'emotional pathology' – whatever the physiological outcome – would have no doubt of its validity.)

No-one should claim to treat cancer for there is no cure from outside the body; nor will there ever be. Drugs never cured cancer or any other pathology; nor will they ever. Surgery and radiotherapy never cured cancer or any other pathology; nor could they ever. Drugs, surgery and radiotherapy are three different methods of stemming the tide. This can go one of two ways. The invasive approach can accelerate the disease process and exaggerate the malignancy, or the manifesting symptoms can be expunged, *giving the patient time* to set in train those changes necessary to effect their own healing. The intervention by conventional means can create a delay in the advance of symptoms so that a temporary respite is afforded. This pause (which can last for weeks, months or even years) is sometimes all that is needed for the patient to make adjustments in his or her life; the precious time to come to inner understanding. But the *healing* belongs to the patient.

Prognosis for cancer patients in conventional medicine is limited to a prior knowledge of statistics – only these keep changing and are, anyway, subject to different interpretations from one hospital to another, from one oncologist to another. The degree of invasiveness and aggression with which the cancer is treated depends on which category, described by the statistics, the patient falls into and on the personal view of the consultant.

The treatment of patients with cancer from the orthodox point of view – which amounts to the relief of symptoms – should never be condemned for falling short of cure but the view that it is contributing to the *cure* of cancer should be taken with some circumspection. When it is used with respect it can make all the difference. Tumours that threaten the function of vital organs do need to be removed. The problem is that doctors, having such powerful resources at their disposal, so often overplay their hand. In treating the cancer, the wholeness of the patient is forgotten. A doctor prescribing cytotoxic drugs is thinking primarily of killing off rogue cells and has forgotten (or is obliged to ignore) that there is nothing that the drugs can do about the *original cause* of the disease [15] – if it was ever recognised.

Patients who go through orthodox treatment and survive are justifiably grateful to the extraordinary skills of their consultants. Nevertheless, those who continue to flourish know that it is their own efforts that prevented any return of the disease – only they themselves can deal with the cause.

This might sound like cavilling but it is simply putting cancer into a more truthful perspective. So many who go through the agonising anxiety of discovering malignancy place excessive faith in orthodox medicine. It is nothing short of abdicating responsibility for their condition. Those who meet their practitioners on equal terms, who ask advice as someone determined to make informed choices and who find the inspiration to institute creative changes in their lives have, by far, the greatest chance of quality of life for the rest of their days, however long that may be.

A quarter of a century before the last millennium doctors declared war on cancer. They determined that cures would be found that would put paid to the disease that causes more fear than any other. This was a naïve hope that will always be doomed to failure – because they are either looking in the wrong place or at too small a part of what is a vast canvas. A measure of the desperation felt by scientists is that they have turned to genetic research in the hope of finding solutions that drugs, surgery and radiotherapy have failed to supply. What they fail to see is that the spirit, the mind and the emotions are beyond the scope of genetic engineering. The life force is not housed within the double helix. To attempt to cure anyone through gene therapy (in whatever form it might eventually take) is similar to attempting to treat a failing business by tinkering with its computer system. What is always needed is to look at its personnel.

Though the hereditary link has long been acknowledged, it is only one (albeit vital) aspect of cancer – indeed, of any chronic disease. Science is on the trail of kinks in the gene pool that represent all sorts of pathologies. No doubt there will be a huge assortment of incidental discoveries that will be of enormous benefit to humanity. However, attempting to hunt down rogue genes, developing associated 'cytotherapy' or vaccines and pumping them into people as prophylaxis takes absolutely no account of the fact that in all chronic disease there is a psychosomatic element that requires expression.

In cancer, probably more than in any other, this element is stronger than anything else – and much further from being expressed because of the years (or even generations) of emotional suppression. Someone who might have the kink in his gene pool that indicates susceptibility to bowel cancer might well, once the technology is available, choose to have a vaccine to eliminate the risk. Yet what would his body do to express any emotional symptoms that he could not then express appropriately? If the bowel were denied the ability to produce symptoms his body would have to put them elsewhere – and the symptoms would not appear in any place less serious than the bowel; suppression will always push disease inwards.

The same is true for women who have already been found to hold the gene recognised as 'causing' breast cancer. The grotesque solution of radical double mastectomy is tragically valueless. If the patient were to go into a state in which she produced cancer, her body would find an alternative site to express its disease. The truth is that the gene path is no less of a cul-de-sac than other disease-orientated therapeutic approaches. Scientists involved in genetic research are still not looking at the whole person. The empiricism[16] of the alternative approach demands that practitioners look into all three bodies to find whatever it is the patient needs in order to create their own healing that will inevitably lead to life changes that are creative and developmental.

The use of homoeopathy in the treatment of people with symptoms of cancer
Dr James Compton-Burnett published a brave little volume in 1893 entitled *Curability of Tumours by Medicines*. This great homoeopath was anxious and took pains to explain that tumours could be removed from and by the body by means of homoeopathically prepared remedies. (This would seem to imply that he took a therapeutic approach and prescribed only on the diseased part – which is in contrast to the philosophy expounded above. As we shall see, this would be a simplistic and erroneous interpretation of Burnett's methods.)

In his book he acknowledges that he was not only at odds with the leading allopaths of his generation but also with most of the homoeopaths as well. He accuses the latter of being too quick to consign patients with cancer to their local surgeons; they were in error, he felt, in always believing that the pathology had gone too far beyond the reaches of their help. Burnett proceeds to support his contention by quoting cases from his own files. His style is almost cursory as he strips the cases to the essential details. It is clear that he practised by observation, examination and prescription based on empirical knowledge of the medicines he used. It is a worthwhile exercise to quote his book here because, although circumstances have radically changed over the century since he wrote, his examples demonstrate that homoeopathy has a very definite and curative role to play in the treatment of patients with cancer. Let's take the first case in the book:

'Miss Jessie S-, 20, having had her left breast condemned at a well-known London Hospital, excited my sympathy and I had her brought to me, offering to treat her for nothing as she is but a poor orphan.

'She came on May 24th 1888 and informed me that two years previously a lump came in her left breast which lump persists in growing, and pains. In the left mamma there was a tumour in its outer lower fourth, about the size of a baby's fist. I have pointed out in my book "Tumours of the Breast" that, in my experience, mammary tumours are most commonly of ovarian origin. It was so here. The left ovary was hyperaesthesic and the menses had always been too frequent, at the time in question, every fortnight. Patient was a large salt eater. The mammae were rather unduly large. She had been recommended by the physicians and surgeons at the hospital to have very nourishing diet and to take as much milk as possible!!

'In three months the menses were normal: the tumour was gone and thus far has not returned. Thuja 30, Acid Nit. 30 and Sabina 30^{17} were used in infrequent dose and each given during one month by itself alone and in the order named.'

As this case appeared among others in a homoeopathic magazine in which there was an editorial comment, Burnett adds a postscript:

'P.S. – The "Hahnemannian Monthly" and the "Review" both observe that I was very fortunate in having patients who persevered with my treatment so long. That may be but as the earliest and most tedious cases paid me, for the most part nothing, no fees at all, I have not felt the "fortune" further than it justifies my motto – "Keep on pegging away."'

And peg away he did. Often his patients gave him a surprisingly long time to do his work though in some cases he was chided for being slow to effect a cure. The second case he relates is of a woman whose tumour resolved within three years. Her husband crossly pointed out that Burnett had told him that it would take two years. The good doctor confesses that:

'I lost my temper with the good squire, which I regret, for on reflection it is manifest that he did not understand, could not understand how the opinion of a homoeopath could possibly be as good as or better than that of Sir James (*the hospital surgeon*)...'

This case leads Burnett on to discuss the speed at which homoeopathy initiates healing in patients with cancer. He remembers the case of a woman with a tumour in the nose that had been successfully treated by him. So pleased was she that she recommended others to consult him. One woman, having asked how long the treatment for her ovarian tumour might be, was told by the cautious doctor that two years would be sufficient. The woman preferred to go through an operation and six weeks recuperation. Burnett observed that it took an even shorter term as she died shortly after the surgery. He further recollects the gentleman who refused his help on behalf of his wife suffering from a breast tumour. Two years was too long and the woman was sent to the surgeon who successfully operated on her.

'...nine months later she was again thoroughly cured of another tumour by a perfectly successful operation; a few months thereafter she was again successfully operated on for another tumour and, just as she was getting well – she died.'

The hint of acerbity is no doubt due to his frustration at knowing that he could have offered the patient a far better chance of success. Here is another case with brief commentaries to explain with what craft and elegance he set about his work.

'On November 14th 1884 a childless married lady of thirty years of age came to see me for a swelling in the left side of the abdomen that had been slowly growing about a year. Patient suffered most severely at the menstrual period and for many years from most severe and distressing leucorrhoea. She also suffers somewhat from haemorrhoids.

'In the recumbent position, with relaxed muscles, one feels in the left iliac region (*lower left abdomen*) a hard tender circumscribed mass of the size of an orange. It came gradually, subsequently to a fall she had about a year before. There are furfuraceous (*scurfy*) patches on the pubes and skin of the neck.

Remedy: Tincture of Bellis Perennis 3x.'

(This woman was not entirely well before her fall that resulted in the tumour as her pre-existing symptoms indicated. It was the fall that triggered the manifestation of cancer. *Bellis Perennis*, the common daisy, is a remedy that is indicated after injuries from blows or falls; it is also indicated when soft tissue becomes indurated [abnormally hardened], particularly that of the abdominal viscera. Further it is especially known to help relieve symptoms of the left side of the body.)

> 'Dec. 4th. – Did much good, at first particularly; decidedly better; the piles bleed; profuse menorrhagia (*excessive menstrual flow*); leucorrhoea sanguineous (*bloody vaginal discharge*) and severe. Tumour not perceptibly smaller.
> Remedy: Tincture of Thuja 30.'

(The 'much good' that the *Bellis* did, refers to the setting up of the discharges and the patient's increased sense of well-being. *Thuja* is noted for its influence over tumours of any description. It is rare indeed for *Thuja* to be absent from the list of remedies required by patients with cancer. It is also often used as an intercurrent remedy when other well-indicated medicines fail to do all their work. It therefore has the ability to help 'stuck' cases. This case was not stuck but Burnett used *Thuja* as he knew that the tumour itself, in spite of the patient's increased sense of well-being, was not showing signs of change. He would not have been concerned overly about the excessive bleeding from the piles or the period as the patient's body would have been using the blood as a discharge of waste material.)

> 'Jan. 6th 1885. – Very much better in her general feelings; only very little pain in left ovarian region; whites better; last period less excessive; the tumour is about the same size but very much less tender.
> Remedy: Repeat.'

(Sure that he was now causing this woman's body to create its own health, he continued *Thuja*. It is a foolhardy homoeopath who switches away from a remedial action that has had positive results just for the sake of speeding things up or to see if more can be achieved.)

> 'Feb. 5th. – Leucorrhoea worse; tumour much smaller; last period much less painful. Complains of a good deal of pain in the left eye and temple.

Remedy: Tincture of Bellis Perennis 1; 5 drops in water three times a day.'

(Burnett would have thought that the worsening of the leucorrhoea was a good sign as it was a discharge that was carrying toxic debris out of the body. He returned to the *Bellis* as he knew that this was the remedy that was indicated for the original trigger of the tumour. He would have seen that the *Thuja* had influenced the body to reduce the tumour. Doubtless he was ignoring the head pains when he prescribed the *Bellis* this time.)

'March 3rd. – Leucorrhoea better; tumour about half its original size; but still tender and when she hurries it drops. Last period less painful.
Remedy: Psorinum 30.'

(It was Burnett's habit to introduce intercurrent doses of nosodes when he wanted to keep the dynamic reaction to a remedy going. In this case he chose *Psorinum* as the patient probably showed more signs of a generally psoric constitution than a syphilitic, tubercular or sycotic one – and the scurfy patches of skin would support this. The effect of the remedy, however, was to highlight something far more sinister – a syphilitic 'layer'.)

'March 24th. – Some of her relatives have been paralysed; she gets nightmare; hands go dead; leucorrhoea worse; much dragging down.
Remedy: Syphilinum 200.'

(Sometimes the action of a remedy does nothing for the pathology itself but brings out a particular aspect of the general case that was hitherto unsuspected or ignored. Here Burnett realised that the nightmares, the family history of paralysis [though he doesn't specify further] and greater degree of discomfort at night-time all indicated that syphilism was behind the generation of cancer. He did not prescribe the *Syphilinum* to treat the tumour; he gave it to eliminate the miasmatic influence that would have been more powerful an energy than any other remedy could have dealt with. The report for the next visit speaks for itself.)

'May 22nd. – Says she feels well, so much good has she felt from the powders; tumour nearly gone, whites also. Is costive (*constipated*).
Remedy: Medorrhinum 30.'

(Burnett knew well that *Medorrhinum* complements *Syphilinum*, especially in cases of cancer. All the nosodes cover constipation as well as many other bowel symptoms and a sluggish bowel is not conducive to swift elimination of toxicity. He had used the *Psorinum* before and its result had not been shown up in any physiological way. He went for *Medorrhinum* which complements *Thuja*, *Bellis* and *Syphilinum*.)

'June 9th. – Tumour rather larger; whites nearly well.
    Remedy: Syphilinum 200.'

(Burnett returned to what had made the most dramatic difference to the tumour. He would have noted that the leucorrhoea was better when in fact it should still have been flowing. He would have wanted to see the tumour reduced in size before the discharge stopped. He may well have felt that he had given the *Medorrhinum* a little too soon or, more likely, that the potency had not been able to go deep enough into the system to effect a change.)

'June 20th. – Tumour much better; whites also.
    Remedy: Silica 6.' (*Probably one each day.*)

(The *Syphilinum* caused more of a swift response in the system this time; a reduction of the tumour in less than three weeks. Expecting the remedy still to be working, Burnett used *Silica* here because it too is complementary and also expulsive in its action. He wanted to make sure that there was no leucorrhoea left behind to cause more of the same trouble later.)

'July 4th. – Leucorrhoea again bad; piles bleeding.

July 16th. – The leucorrhoea is less bad; the left ovarian region is again very tender; pains in the eyes in the morning on waking.
    Remedy: Medorrhinum 100.'

(He waited on July 4th because he knew that the aggravation was to do with the *Silica* expelling the last of the leucorrhoea. He used the *Medorrhinum* [at a higher potency] again to complement the *Syphilinum* and because the ovarian region – especially the left – has a particular affinity for *Medorrhinum*.)

'August 22nd. – Pains in the eyes gone; left side much less tender.
  Remedy: Medorrhinum 200.'

(He simply repeats but in a higher potency – in order to reach deeper into the body's resources – what has worked most recently.)

'September 3rd. – No trace of the tumour can be found either by palpation or percussion. All she now complains about is that she so easily catches cold. She now dances and runs and bends herself at will without feeling the side at all.
  Remedy: Psorinum 100.'

(Catching cold easily is not much of a symptom to prescribe on. Nevertheless, Burnett knew that at the end of successful treatment of a chronic state it is very common to find the patient back in a psoric or tubercular mode; just where one should be. This is especially true of patients who have been in the carcinogenic state. To be in psora after cancer is indicative of an excellent prognosis – and 'catching cold easily' can very often be psoric in character. So it proved to be here for he discharged the patient as fit and well on October 27th. It had taken just under a year for this patient to restore her being to health. Burnett was assured of the full efficacy of his work as he saw the woman on several occasions after. She was still well in 1892.)

All his cases were demonstrable proof for Burnett that homoeopathy was of service in treating patients with cancer. Though he called his book *Curability of Tumours* he was really treating the whole person. He recognised that by regarding the diseased part as representing the sickness of the whole he could arrive at remedies which would cause the body to react in the direction of its own cure.[18] He never let the cancer obscure his view of the whole picture. He always relied on his acute powers of observation to let him know whether the vital energy of the patient or that of the disease was uppermost. Though Burnett and the other homoeopaths like him who had the confidence to treat such patients were working before the beginning of the twentieth century, nothing as far as these guidelines for prescribing is concerned has changed. Nor will it for the body's ability to heal itself, even of potentially terminal pathology, is immutable unless suppressed – or, even more controversially, the patient has a different agenda and more powerful reason for not getting better; strange to those of us who want to maintain our optimum health but nonetheless distressingly common.

But circumstances have changed and are such that the role of homoeopathy in the treatment of patients with cancer or other potentially terminal illnesses cannot, except in rare cases, be more than complementary. Even where homoeopathy could secure well-being for the patient it is unlikely he or she would choose to be treated exclusively with homoeopathic medicines. The overwhelming prestige of technology and the professionalism of its advocates are far too great for patients to resist being swayed by allopathic persuasion. Nor should homoeopaths complain at having to make compromises when their patients take the option of surgery, chemotherapy and radiotherapy as well as continuing to use remedies. They are, after all, exercising their right to choose.

What has also changed so radically since Burnett's day is the allopathic system. In his time surgery was radical. A tumour of the breast meant the removal of the breast. There were no sophisticated methods of control over drug prescribing. Today the cytotoxic drugs used are horrendously powerful, not to say lethal, though there is far more awareness of the awesome responsibility that goes with their use. The same goes for radiotherapy. The almost cavalier attitude of Burnett's contemporaries to the use of X-ray and radiation amounted to negligence and naivety. A century of experience has led to far greater respect for such an insidiously destructive tool. Furthermore, modern allopathy is much more aware of the need for psychotherapeutic support. The idea that psychosomatic causes might play a part in chronic diseases such as cancer used to be greeted with derision – far less so now. This vastly improved care when attended by the superb professionalism and technology has meant that patients can feel huge relief and tremendous support. Both of these can be prerequisite to getting better. The arguments that may rage over the philosophies of healing are so often silenced by a firm but gentle bedside manner – especially when the patient is riddled with angst.

But there is still more that has changed since Dr Burnett set about demonstrating the efficacy of homoeopathy in serious pathology cases. The patients were of a different constitutional make-up than we are today. Their intrinsic and basic constitutional health was far better than ours. They ate unpolluted food grown comparatively locally. They lived in houses that were not stitched up with electricity cables. They lived at a far slower pace and had fewer extravagant expectations of life. They were neither subjected to multiple vaccination programmes nor able to resort to repeated prescriptions of antibiotics and steroids for minor (or major) acute conditions. (Those who were too susceptible to severe acute conditions and unable to fight off infection died. It was more a case of survival of the fittest.) Nor had they been through two World Wars – events that had a devastatingly traumatic effect on humanity in general. Nor did they live in a world over which a pall of radioactivity and global warming hangs, as we do today.

If Burnett were alive today he would perhaps have adjusted to a subtly different mode of practice. The *principles* of his prescribing would all be the same; the natural laws of homoeopathy are unchanging. He would, though, have moulded his approach to take account of these changes that have undoubtedly had a detrimental effect on us all. Though he would have recognised all the positive advances that we have made he would not have ignored the fact that so many people eat appalling diets, live at a ridiculously hectic pace and place far too much importance on material things. He would have inveighed against the fact that we overdose on sugar, caffeine, alcohol and chemical additives; that we consume quantities of frozen and packaged foods wrapped in health damaging polythene and cellophane.

He would have been vituperative that we now inoculate our children against an ever increasing number of acute diseases thus permanently weakening their immune systems; that we take hormone drugs to control our rates of hormone output; that hallucinogenic drugs are more or less taken for granted; that we spend so long in cars driving at speed, building up stress that even the toughest constitutions would find hard to support; that our education system is geared to produce intellectual clones; that our political system has been lulling us into a false sense of security for decades while our individual freedom is whittled away; that we live with the violence of the world spewing out from the television into our sitting rooms to the point where we are inured to the traumatic effect it has on us.

Burnett had the skill and the patience to adapt his craft and would have been able to encompass the multiple layers of carcinogenic damage that we inflict on ourselves and which is inflicted on us. He would have been among the first to recognise that a patient with cancer would not achieve well-being without taking into consideration all those stress factors that contribute to the 'layers' of pathology. He would have practised medical archaeology on every patient. He would, though, have despaired that he would not have been given the time to treat patients without drug and surgical intervention. It is not that he would have failed to recognise cases that require some surgical assistance. He knew well that some patients are unreachable by homoeopathic remedies as their disease has gone too far, too fast. His problem would have been that which every homoeopath today faces – that allopathy is only superficially a medical system of choice.

For all the extraordinary care given by doctors and specialists, their philosophy remains the same – crude necessity to suppress symptoms, even ones that are not particularly threatening. So the apparent choice in cancer therapy is between either following the oncologist's advice which has been based on X-rays, blood tests, body scans and statistics ... or not. Those who do best are those who choose the necessary minimum of allopathic intervention and complement it with the alternative therapy of their choice. Yet patients who do question everything that they are offered are often made aware that they are risking death by not accepting the specialist's analysis and advice. This puts the specialist in an impossible position of false responsibility for no-one mentions that there is just as great a risk of death from the suppression of cancer. It is not observed that cancer is a state of being that informs the whole, not simply a disease of a part to be eradicated.

With the degeneration of our constitutions from all those factors identified above, we are obliged to accept that cancers are potentially faster growing and more destructive than they were a century ago. (The syphilitic element is far more widespread now.) So we do not, on the whole, have the leisure to treat tumours and other cancers in the way Burnett did.[19] If homoeopaths are consulted by a patient with cancer they are necessarily asked to treat the diseased part, the history of the condition including allopathic intervention, the miasmatic influences, the history of emotional traumas, the history of previous ailments and their suppression which possibly contributed to the existing condition and any present psychosomatic circumstances. The whole picture is not yet complete.

There would also be the dietary and nutritional aspect – cytotoxic drugs tend to wipe out a person's ability to assimilate nutrition from food. There is also the fact that radiotherapy, when it is used, tends to create or enhance the potential for metastasis as it cripples the body's protective auric energy – the electrodynamic field of energy that we all generate through the electrical activity of the nervous system.[20] As allopathic treatment of patients with cancer tends to change the constitutional health within such a short time span, the whole picture from the homoeopath's point of view is never stable. At least for Burnett, his patients only reported to him about the effects of *his* treatment; he did not have to follow a switchback of changes induced by other treatments. Yet, there is still every reason for homoeopaths to 'keep pegging away'. With their remedies they *can* stimulate whole bodies into creating the necessary changes for well-being despite the scorched earth policy of chemotherapy and radiotherapy.[21]

A case of cancer that never happened

Jemima, a woman in her late thirties, came for treatment. She had mastitis, she said, affecting her right breast; it was painful, sensitive to the slightest touch, red and hot. She had been to the doctor who had given her antibiotics but the prescription was having no effect. She had a very similar problem several years before when the youngest of her four children had been weaned. (She had to have three lots of antibiotics then before it would clear up.) She said that she also felt 'flu-like symptoms and that the glands under her arm were very sore and swollen. She felt a 'gathering' sensation in the right side of the breast where the pain was at its most severe. The diagnosis would, perhaps, have been better described as an abscess in the top right quarter of the breast.

The physical symptoms of this apparently acute condition were not difficult to identify as indicative of the remedy *Phytolacca*, a bushy plant that grows in America, Africa and China. It is a remedy that has a widespread reputation for its affinity with the breasts (especially the right) and the glandular system. What is more, the patient's mood fitted well with the psychological symptoms of the medicine: irritable and restless, fearful of the pain and that she had something seriously wrong with her, indifferent to her work – about which she was normally enthusiastic – and with a thoroughly negative attitude to everything. Jemima was given several doses of the 200th potency to take over the next 24 hours and asked to stop taking the antibiotics. The breast and glands returned to normality within a day, after a long sleep during which she sweated profusely. She rang to say that she did not need any further help.

Within a few days she rang to say she was suffering unbearable pains in one of her upper right molars. The dentist was insisting that she should go on antibiotics before he would treat her. This time her symptoms were different: she was extremely cold, very irritable and sensitive to noise, draught and "*anything that moves!*" She could find no comfort in anything at all except a hot drink. The diagnosis was clear – she had an abscess around the root of a molar. The remedy was also clear – *Hepar Sulphuricum*, one of the standbys in the treatment of dental abscesses. She was asked to take three doses of a high potency (1M). The result was complete relief within 24 hours though the abscess drained spectacularly. During the night her mouth filled with foul-tasting pus and blood that woke her. The drainage continued for some while though she complained of how revolting the process was.

Such a case seems to have no relevance in this chapter but you have not heard the rest of the facts. Before the breast abscess had flared up Jemima had asked for help over a traumatic situation that she had been struggling with for some two years – her husband, some five years her junior, had been having an affair with her best friend. Jemima had known about it from almost the beginning but had decided not to say anything. She had not known how to deal with the situation, not least because she had a demanding and stressful job working for social services that meant that she had little energy left when she returned home. She felt she was a loser either way. She had begun to lose her confidence and self-esteem. She was not doing her work well and she feared her team leader was breathing down her neck. When she got home she found she was ratty with the children and that she only wanted to crawl into bed and sleep. She felt confused about her moods: one moment she was irritable, then she was tearful, then frightened, bitter and angry by turns. She also felt that physically she was on the point of having a cold that would never quite come out. She felt as if 'flu was constantly lurking.

This quite common picture of long-held acute grief with an inability to find resolution plus a sense of loss of direction indicates that the cancer miasm is stirring. This is especially true when that feeling of lurking infection is there. Jemima was given several remedies for this condition and she felt her old enthusiasm resurfacing, her confidence returning and more balance to her emotions. She felt "*distanced*" from the relationship problem; she felt that she was in a vacuum so that she did not have to do anything about it. She expected it to resolve itself. But of course it didn't.

Two weeks before the breast abscess appeared she had been given *Carcinosin*. In homoeopathic terms, the abscess was an 'aggravation'. This was the result of her body parcelling up her general condition into one angry agony through physical symptoms. Because there was no vent for the breast abscess her body invented a route for the toxic waste to take. An abscess in the jaw is safer than one in glandular tissue. The thorough drainage that occurred from the base of the molar was a safe expression of all that had gone before.

All of which would signify nothing if it were not for the fact that Jemima began to come to terms with her emotional situation. She realised that she could not live in a vacuum; that she had to speak to her husband; that she needed to express her deep hurt that her best friend had cheated on her. However, she also realised that her creative energy and attention were too focused on her work and not on the home and children. She acknowledged that her husband had felt lonely – she tried not bring her work home and never spoke about the day's events. When she had spoken out she felt enormous relief. Husband and wife went to Relate, the counselling service for couples. They determined to try and resolve the turmoil that had been created by the incapacity of both to express their deepest emotional needs. Jemima continued well in spite of the very difficult times she went through.

Why is this a case of cancer that did not happen? Breast abscesses that involve the whole body are indicative of a systemic disease. Jemima's abscess was not simply of the breast but involved her lymphatic system and general energy as well as her psyche. If this abscess had been suppressed it is likely, as she was constitutionally quite strong, that it would have returned in the near future and then with increasing frequency. Without homoeopathic medicine she would have been obliged to use antibiotics. Eventually, the breast would have been unable to support the disease any more in the form of gathering pus with local fever. Her body would have 'hardened off' the abscess and its new name would have been carcinoma. This is not uncommon.

A case of cancer in which the patient was treated by two systems at once

Wendy was in her late forties when she came for help through the menopause. It had started early as she had fibroids with severe menstrual bleeding which had necessitated a hysterectomy. She had tried HRT but it had disagreed with her. She was worried about osteoporosis as she felt that she was at risk without taking any supplement to strengthen her bones. She was a slight person with fading orange hair. She wore an expression of wounded pride and puzzled anxiety. This may have been to do with the unhappiness in her marriage. Her husband was "*quite unable to understand me, I believe*". He was taciturn and morose and given to taking long leaves of absence without warning and with no explanation. Yet he could be extremely needy and helpless about practical matters. They had a son who was equally unused to explaining his actions. He had been involved with the police on several occasions. If she attempted to question him she would simply provoke a violent tirade of abuse and a week of silence.

Wendy was used to feeling very low in energy. She had suffered glandular fever on several occasions. These bouts had first begun when she was a teenager. (She was going through her exams at a time when her father returned home from living abroad. He had been another person of few words and black moods who consistently denigrated her so that she lost all sense of self-confidence.) She also had a history of swollen glands in and around her throat. They went up and down frequently and without warning or any specific infection being obvious.

"*I never feel well. I haven't felt well for years; not since I was a child probably. I always feel I'm on the brink of coming down with something. It doesn't matter what I do to help myself – diets, exercise, meditation, drinking more water – I can't feel really well.*" This state, when combined with a history of glandular fever, is very suggestive of the cancer miasm. Through her treatment over the next year or so, Wendy was given remedies that reflected this condition – including *Carcinosin*, which did give her a little more energy for a while though only after she came out with a thorough dose of 'flu. (A good sign!)

However, her home situation continued just as before. She found no solution to her relationship problems within the home. What she found was a lover. He was the most solicitous person she had met; a complete contrast to the dour, glowering male presences she was used to. The relationship made her ecstatically happy but extremely anxious in case she was found out. Within five months she had developed a breast lump and so went to the doctor. He told her that it was a cyst. She was sent to the hospital where it was drained. The biopsy suggested that something rather more radical should be done. Wendy went through an operation for the removal of the lump, the tissue around the lump and the lymph nodes in the armpit.

She was then referred to hospital for radiotherapy treatment. This lasted three weeks. After this she was put on the drug Tamoxifen "*for life*". They explained that it was a preventative and was obligatory. Throughout the whole procedure she was "*speechless with terror*". She had not been able to see anyone or speak to them. She had been afraid of her husband's reaction as he hated anything to do with illness. They never referred to her hospital appointments and he visited her in hospital only once, to bring her a fresh set of nightclothes. (Her son chose this time to move in with his girlfriend who lived in a caravan.)

During this "*whole ordeal*" she was given various remedies. She was given *Arnica* to help with the operation; *Opium* was needed to help her come round from the anaesthetic; remedies such as *Aconite* and *Oak* [22] for the psychological trauma. There had been remedies to discourage metastasis and to ensure that the lymph system was working as efficiently as possible. There were remedies for the burns from the radiotherapy and to remove the harmful radiation from the whole system. [23]

As a result of the supportive treatment Wendy was able to deal with the trauma of losing much of her breast. She had no swelling of the left arm due to the loss of her lymph glands. She found that her operation site and scar healed rapidly. She experienced none of the tiredness and listlessness commonly felt by those undergoing radiotherapy and none of the typical pains in her left arm after the treatment. Though terrified of being in hospital she realised that she actually had resources to deal with extraordinary situations that she did not know she had. "*I realise that I'm not such a mouse!*"

Her life changed radically. She decided that she wanted a divorce. She left home to live with her lover whom she married as soon as the divorce was made absolute. She stopped work and began coaching examinees from the local schools in French which she thoroughly enjoyed. She also decided that she was "*not having any truck with Tamoxifen as the wretched stuff brought back all those hot flushes*". Some five years later she continued well and with no sign of any return of glandular trouble.

The quality of life is more important

A very old gentleman was brought by his son for treatment to complement the surgery that had been performed to remove cancer of the stomach. At first it had been thought that Douglas had a stomach ulcer; doubtless, that is how the problem had first begun. He had been put on antibiotics but the condition deteriorated. The doctors found that the surgery was not going to prevent the disease as they discovered that it was too extensive, but there might be more chance that the cancer would be 'slowed down' by a short course of radiotherapy. Douglas explained that what troubled him most were the pains which were so much worse at night. He was not one to complain and he was anyway a man of few words. He clearly wished to present himself with dignity and he succeeded. It was evident he knew that he was terminally ill.

He wanted to go through with the radiation treatment and was happy to take the drugs for pain relief though he said that in the night they were ineffective. What he wanted from homoeopathy was something that would help him sleep and perhaps that would help him keep his food down – he would feel choked, distended and then nauseated; he would belch but feel no benefit. His son explained later that the oncologist had told him that his father possibly had no more than two months to live. He was anxious that Douglas should enjoy what life was left to him.

Ornithogalum, star of Bethlehem, is a plant with the characteristics that Douglas showed in his symptoms. He was given this remedy in the 6th potency and asked to take it up to six times per day. In addition he was given *Syphilinum* 30 to take at bedtime on two nights of each week. *Syphilinum* covers the pains of ulcerative cancer that are worse at night and it complements the *Ornithogalum*. Within a few days Douglas's son reported that his father was more comfortable. The vomiting had reduced and he had a slightly improved appetite. He still remained extremely tired but it was felt that this was due to the radiation treatment that had begun. He was given *Radium Bromide* 30 twice a day to help cope with this which it evidently did as he showed more sign of animation through the day and slept longer and more satisfactorily at night.

It was also reported that he was more cheerful since going on the remedies. He had confessed before to feeling extremely depressed and disinclined to move. This had been unheard of for him. He had even shown no interest in taking his much loved dog for a walk. Douglas was an outdoors man and he had never in his life been at a loose end before. Now he wanted to get back outside and take a turn round the garden. He wanted to hear about the grandchildren again. He looked forward to having a short gossip with his neighbour who came round once a day.

Then one evening he went to bed a little earlier than usual after a busy day with a visit from the grandchildren. In the morning it was found that Douglas had died quite peacefully in his sleep. He had not outlived the oncologist's expectations but the quality of his final weeks had been greatly enhanced.

Other aspects of the cancer miasm

It is comparatively acceptable these days to believe that cancer is often the result of emotional suppression. The 'stress factor' is no longer dismissed. Yet there are many people who develop cancer without being able to tell its origins; those with apparently healthy lives who are suddenly smitten out of the blue and for no discernible reason.

Even if we accept that there are some cancerous conditions that really are triggered by, say, radiation pollution – and there is absolutely no proof that this is not so – or heavy metal toxicity, there are still plenty of other cases that could not be laid at the door of outside influences or emotional suppression of the individual's life force.

In cases of apparently inexplicable origin we turn to other factors that point to the roots of this multifaceted condition. Heredity is one obvious place to start. It is not only a history of cancer in the family that should be suspect. Certainly, if it does morbidly decorate the family tree there will be a far greater likelihood of its appearance again even in the otherwise robustly healthy. This is going to be exaggerated in those whose forebears had the disease at a young age,[24] who were intrinsically unable to survive the early onset of the condition and yet were able to pass on their affected genes. But heredity is a very inexact gauge of who gets what and when.

Of a group of five siblings say, whose parents both had cancer and, perhaps, one or two of the grandparents also did, there is no certainty that all or any of them will develop the disease themselves. If only two were to develop cancer and the others remain healthy, there is every reason still to note that heredity played a part in creating the situation but no inherent explanation why it should be just those two who develop the disease – unless it were the two girls, for example, in the family that produced the cancer, leaving the boys without any hint of ill health. This is meat and drink to those who play the statistics game. What statistics never take into account is anything more than the *measurable* details – age, sex, weight, type of cancer, blood group and so on. Seldom is anything mentioned of the emotional background of the patient and never that of the parents. Yet this background is vital to a deeper understanding. There are patients who develop the symptoms of cancer as a way of expressing not just their own negative energies but that of their parents or of the family tree. It is as if the suppressed emotional history within the immediate forebears becomes a hereditary factor as much as facial features. *The energy of unresolved emotional trauma in a previous generation is passed on to the next generation for resolution.*

When this situation seems to arise it always does so in a manner that is illustrative of the patient's circumstances with which the patient was more or less content *before* the advent of the disease. In other words, the status quo before the advent of the cancer was just how the patient had arranged his or her life to fit most comfortably with their vision of how things should be. *This status quo almost always reflects the parental and familial influences impressed on the patient by his or her upbringing.* The disease unsettles this and makes the status quo seem like dutiful complacency; at least, it does if the patient rises to the creative challenge of getting better. For those who fight to maintain their prior circumstances, the disease becomes more threatening than the life changes that are being avoided.

This could be why a fifty-year-old menopausal woman with, to the outside world at least, a happy home and plenty of material comforts and only the suggestion of raised blood pressure developed cancer of the uterus. Her mother loathed her much loved father and *"hounded him to an early grave"* while the harridan herself *"succumbed to breast and liver cancer some ten bitter years later – she was a silly woman and I probably haven't forgiven her"*.

Perhaps we also have an explanation here for the young woman who was surrounded with half a dozen miserable spinster and bachelor relatives all with chronic terminal illnesses who demanded her caring attention constantly; which she all too willingly gave to the detriment of her energy and her marriage. This older generation, all victims of emotional straitjackets imposed by their parents and unable to climb out of their depression, lived and leached on their young relative who proceeded to produce ovarian cancer as her similarly gentle mother before had done.

We might see in the same light the man who developed stomach cancer in his sixties who had, till then, a marvellous life doing pretty much whatever he wanted to do but always with purpose and intent. He had a happy marriage and delightful children. Nevertheless, he had an irascible father who in turn had suffered, by all accounts, from his own rage-fuelled father.

The grandfather had died early of TB – which we know to be related miasmatically to cancer – and his father had died of lung cancer "*as he was an inveterate smoker of cheroots*". It was no surprise to hear that as a boy he had been frequently sick with anxiety because of fear of his enraged parent; "*but that was something I grew out of very quickly*", he said dismissively. (What was also relevant was that this gentle man's death – which was both peaceful and at home – caused his emotionally disturbed daughter to seek help – one of the things her father had long wished for her to do.)

There are cases of children who suffer potentially terminal cancers. They too produce disease from a cause. It is not 'unfair', though it feels so to the desperate parents. We can blame a malign fate but this is to miss the point. There are always roots in miasmatic history and there is always purpose in the cancerous end result even if we do not see what that is either at the time, in the future or ever. We might blame pollution, previous misdiagnosis or any other thing that could lighten the burden of grief. Ultimately though we have to look into the past, not just at the family history of sickness or the threads of miasmatic influences but also the pulsing body of emotional baggage that dominates the recent ancestors.

We might find the idea utterly repugnant but it can seem to be that many children come into this world with the express purpose of acting as a focus for the ills of their families. They produce sickness that draws people in and offers time for reconciliation or the release from the bondage of a loveless union. It offers time for consideration of values. It stops the mad clock of competitive activity and starts the slow ticking of understanding. Children with such serious disease can fill loved ones and those who have to tend them, with extraordinary humanity. At least, this is how it can be when those affected choose to witness the illness creatively in terms of their own lives. It is, though, not uncommon for parents of afflicted children to fail to get beyond the stage of feeling guilt and remorse that they were unable to do anything more to save them. Paradoxically, this is an emotional state familiar to dutiful children who, when young, were unable to help their parents to remain together. Feelings of helplessness and having no control are regular precursors to the cancer miasm stirring itself to manifest as pathology.

An apparently acute case can illustrate the controversial premise.

A mother phoned to say that her son had a very high fever. She had given *Belladonna* but it had not held. His temperature was 104°F and he had "*gone all floppy*". This mother was forever anxious. She was also racked with guilt as she blamed herself for the stillbirth of a daughter some seven years before. As well as the eldest son, who had been born before the tragedy, she had had two more children since. Her life was constantly in turmoil for she had no spare time. Her husband worked in the Middle East and was forever back and forth on flights at all hours. She had a soft-furnishing and interior design business that she ran from home.

Her little boy who had the fever had recently started at playgroup and seemed to love every minute of it even though he would howl until his mother was out of sight every morning. Then, the night before the fever began, there had been a power cut and the boy had woken suddenly and in great distress. His mother had known no peace since then, some three days now. The child's symptoms of fever were classically those for which *Belladonna* is best known yet it did nothing more than give half an hour's respite. High potencies were used to no avail. The only comfort the boy had was from a few moments breastfeeding – he was almost weaned but his mother was reluctant to finish completely. "*This is going to be my last child but I know I'm going to have to stop very soon.*"

The fever continued to rise and fall at certain times of day but never went below 101°F. The child had had fevers before when *Belladonna* had worked promptly. He had also had remedies to work on the tubercular miasm that was so prevalent in his family history and that can prevent the resolution of acute fevers. Something else was causing the block. He was given *Carcinosin* in a very high potency. The result was swift. The mother phoned to ask if it could be that her son had realised that it was time to give up the breast and if he could be expressing doubt, confusion, distress and insecurity. When told that children can produce fevers for such reasons it brought back a flood of suppressed emotion about her stillborn child. It seemed that only when the mother began to release her own emotions in waves of sobbing (and anger that her husband was so often away from home) did the child start to improve.

How long would this child have held the emotions that prompted the fever if he had not received the appropriate treatment? What would have happened if the fever had been suppressed by deliberate cooling of the body or antibiotics? Would the mother have been able to release her own emotional pain and so relieve the general emotional tension?

Summing up the cancer miasm

The cancer miasm is a multilayered weave of the threads of the other miasms. Yet it is a force in its own right and a force with a purpose. It is a state of being that is so profoundly disordered that it can manifest in disease of the building blocks of our life. It can be expressed spiritually or emotionally and cause psychological symptoms that should announce distress plainly. If no-one observes this it can go on to be expressed physically on the microcosmic level of cells which is where it causes us the most fear. We often do not notice until it is too late how the refined but perverted energies of the spirit and the emotions transmute into the characteristic physical pathology. We do not realise most of the time when a carcinogenic state of mind is most in need of help. This is not surprising when the active cancer miasm is the ultimate negative expression of suppression.

There are many triggers for the awakening of this miasm including pollutants of all descriptions from radioactivity to childhood vaccines, from physical accidents and shocks to lifelong grief. Some can bear the brunt of these far better than others and this is to do with the quality of their basic health, the very fabric of which they are made. Others, usually highly sensitive people with deeply tubercular family histories, struggle for years with building up a backlog of unresolved and suppressed illnesses that must at some point bring the body to find an ultimate resolution.

There are many signs from the almost indistinguishable to the glaringly obvious. Those who never have colds at all and those who have frequent bouts of 'flu; those with a repeated history of glandular fever and those who suffer the usual childhood illnesses badly in their adult years; those who have a history of infantile jaundice and/or hepatitis; those with a history of repeated suppression of venereal disease or allergic reactions; those who never leave home and never gain their own independence; those who become 'doormats', and without a word to say of spirit; those who find it impossible to come to terms with something long gone, all these have a tendency sooner or later to stir this ruthless energy into activity. 'Ruthless' because the body has an unwavering and unsentimental determination to seek resolution of all negative states be they mental, emotional, spiritual or physical.

Cancer is therefore a life lesson which demands that we stop what we are doing and pay attention to another inner voice from the one we have been listening to for too long. This other, quieter inner voice asks that we move in a different direction, an event that inevitably causes changes, whether we like it or not, in the lives of loved ones as well. Continued ignorance of the presence or stifling of 'the other voice' leads to a depressing prognosis. The more syphilitic or sycotic the patient is, the less likely he will be to hear it; the more tubercular or psoric, the better the chances of hearing the whole body's message.

What makes the cancer miasm different from the other miasms is that while their acute forms are quite specific, cancer pathology has no single entity involving a bug. (Though 'flu, in all its viral forms, is considered to be related to this miasm.[25]) In the microcosm of the other disease states there are reflected specific negative traits of the macrocosm of the whole body in distress. (The TB bacillus, the gonorrhoeal diplococcus and *Treponema pallidum* thus have characteristic behavioural 'signatures' that parallel and reflect the different psyches of their hosts.) In cancer, the microcosm has lost its programme altogether and the self is subsumed beneath years or generations of suppression. Cancer is a coming together of the strands of family history, multi-miasmatic heredity and layers of neglected and suppressed personal pathology and distress. Yet it is our way out of the thicket; the cancer miasm is as necessary for humanity as all the other miasms.

The treatment of this disturbing and disturbed state is ostensibly the easiest of all to initiate. We are only required to move forward in a positive direction – even if we keep making mistakes.[26] So for those who receive the benefit of advance warning either through their chosen form of treatment or from their own inner voice, there is little threat. For those who see change on the horizon and retreat from it with urgency there is only stagnation. What lies at the heart of that is fear. To deal with the fear of moving forward we need to be given emotional and spiritual tools – tools that our parents perhaps neglected or were unable to provide – which is why support is vital for everyone who attempts to regain his or her well-being. Yet so often the cancer miasm engenders a fatal state of denial.

"*I'll be fine.*"

Saying this and *knowing* it are two different things.

CHAPTER 26

MINOR MIASMS

AIDS

Homoeopathic thinkers speculate about the AIDS miasm. There is a homoeopathic remedy made from the blood of an AIDS patient that is used as a nosode. Even though we are beginning to learn that the human immuno-virus is anything but as straightforward as the spider mite, the spirochete, the diplococcus or mycobacterium that are representative of the other miasms, we should consider its claims as a physical metaphor for a deeper human condition; one in which the tendency might be described as the degradation and depreciation of the human spirit as the result of the loss of self-reliance and of choice in an increasingly materialistic world. Part of our modern world is the corruption of its natural resources for our own short-term gain; in AIDS we might be seeing a reflection of this macrocosm within the microcosm of the human body – in which all the fabulous intricacies of the self-healing mechanism break down.

AIDS is not a disease as such: it is a syndrome, the definition of which is a set of symptoms that occur together but that might not constitute the recognised 'package' of symptoms that could be labelled definitively as a specific disease. There are many different ways to express AIDS. What is more, it is clear that both syphilis and TB have an intimate relationship to AIDS as both are frequently suffered as part of the symptom complex.

Perhaps it is too early to speculate on just how deeply AIDS is a miasmatic influence on our lives in general. Nevertheless, while the nosode is in use and gradually building up a repertory of symptom states to which it is similar, it is incumbent on practitioners to keep an open mind on the significance of the broader miasmatic implications. Homoeopaths need to feel free to use their educated intuition to judge whether a patient is displaying the traits that would be similar to whatever underlying states might best be energetically represented by the *AIDS nosode*. *Carcinosin* had to undergo a period of trial. Even in the 1980s *Carcinosin* was something of a controversial remedy with many practitioners either avoiding its use or criticising those who did prescribe it for being too precipitate. Now, both miasm and remedy are indispensable in most homoeopaths' practices and the controversy is largely forgotten. So it may well prove with the *AIDS nosode*. As many see the syndrome itself to be an example of iatrogenic disease (sickness that has resulted from the misguided practice of physicians), it may well turn out that the miasm for which AIDS is representative is a lot to do with autoimmune disease generally – something which many already believe to be true. As autoimmune problems are increasingly rampant in our time, it would not be surprising if Nature were providing us with the means for self-healing what has so far eluded even today's most suppressive methods of treatment.

Diphtheria

Diphtheria is a very nasty disease that is mercifully no longer as prevalent in its acute form as it used to be. The last major epidemic occurred in the 1920s; it is well worth reading Dr Dorothy Shepherd's description of her experience in south London in her book *Homoeopathy in Epidemic Diseases*.

Diphtheria is a disease in which the mucous membranes of the throat are affected. It was most usual in the autumn – especially after deficient rainfall as Dr Shepherd tells us. It begins as a sore throat with headache and a feeling of general malaise. The membranes of the throat begin to swell and change to a deeper colour of red or even purple. The glands in the neck can become painful. The breath becomes foetid and the saliva thicker and stickier. A gelatinous pseudomembrane develops over the surface of the affected area. In severe cases the throat can seem to close up almost completely and make swallowing very difficult. In the worst cases the throat can bleed. There are many variations: green, brown or scarlet tongue; red, mottled or pale face; watery or dry eyes; passive or aggressive mood; desperate thirst or none at all. If complications set in then the heart and nervous system can be permanently affected.

Despite the fact that diphtheria has not made any serious attempt at resurfacing in Britain for so long, there is ample reason for suspecting that there is a memory of it that lurks in the gene pool of some patients.

A boy of fifteen developed a sore throat – again. He was prone to them and had a history going back to much earlier in his childhood of tonsillitis and fever. He had received homoeopathic treatment previously, each time his bad throat had begun – the remedies proved effective at relieving the symptoms. (This was in marked contrast to his previous experience of needing antibiotics for each acute episode.) On this occasion the symptoms were rather severe. He had considerable pain in the left side of his neck and the glands were swollen. He found it very difficult to turn his head to the left. He had a foul taste in his mouth, his tongue was furred and swollen, the tonsil area was dark red and his teeth were hypersensitive. This is the picture of *Mercurius Iodatus Ruber* (red iodide of mercury). He was given a 200 potency of this remedy but made no appreciable response.

As he was extremely thirsty and had a problem with deciding whether he was hot or cold, he was given *Mercurius Solubilis* 200. This made a little improvement but not much. As his condition worsened overnight he was then prescribed *Syphilinum* because of its affinity for and ability to enhance the action of *Mercury*. This, too, only made a slight difference. The lad was still clearly far from well and not making any substantial improvements. At this point, because of the thickness of the mucus, the threateningly swollen state of the throat and the lack of reaction to indicated remedies, he was given *Diphtherinum* 200. This remedy is made from diphtheritic material; it is a nosode. From the moment he took it he began to recover. Not only that, as he came out of the recuperation his general health began to show a marked improvement – as if he had thrown off some burden of malaise that had kept him from being a typical teenager bursting with energy and vitality.

It might be said that the *Diphtherinum* had removed an acute disease that had arisen from a compromised immune system that had once been pro-foundly affected by the DPT injection and struggled for years to express the iatrogenic toxicity. This case might not really be illustrative of an inherited disease pattern; of a miasm. Yet this is not an isolated case. *Diphtherinum* has often produced similar reactions in people of various ages suffering from severe tonsillitis that does not respond to the usual remedial agents and, what is more, in those who have never been inoculated against diphtheria. It has even been prescribed when there was no acute infection; the prescription being based on no more than a history of debilitating throat infections in a person who seemed not to be able to react satisfactorily to other well-indicated remedies that had been given for general constitutional reasons.

> In one case *Diphtherinum* had been given to a person who had never felt well since having her throat painted with calomel for quinsy, some 30 years before. Calomel is otherwise known as mercurius dulcis and is a less corrosive form of the liquid metal. She had recently presented a condition over several months that seemed to indicate that her system needed *Mercurius* as a homoeopathic dose yet this had not proved effective in any way. She was then given *Diphtherinum* on the assumption that a diphtheritic throat infection had been suppressed and waiting to express itself again ever since. The result of the prescription was that she developed a bad sore throat and a cold after which she felt *"better than I have for absolutely years – I can't remember when!"*
>
> Although diphtheria is hardly a widespread miasm in the sense that TB is, it would appear to be a condition that has left its mark on the system for future generations to have to deal with. This is true in those who come from families that have a history of inflammatory conditions of the throat, larynx and nasal passages and tonsils; it is reasonable to surmise from this evidence that the family tree bears its fair share of the tubercular inheritance.

Malaria, typhoid and cholera

There are other pandemic diseases that might be considered as representative of further miasmatic states: malaria, typhoid and cholera. These three have been scourges on humanity since time immemorial. Though we do not trouble ourselves about any of them in Britain today unless we are travelling abroad, all of them were at one time or another present in western Europe. It is only in the last 120 years or so that hygiene, drainage and common sense have meant comparative security from such sicknesses.

Malaria

> is different from the usual run of diseases in that it is spread by a mosquito which delivers the infection directly into the bloodstream from whence it migrates to the liver.

Typhoid

> is a contagious disease for which the body creates a fever with a rash, and that is spread by means of sewage, faeces and lack of hygiene.

Cholera

> is an infectious disease in which diarrhoea and dehydration can cause dangerous debility, and that is spread via unsanitary conditions or a tainted water supply.

Each one has its own distinct disease 'picture' though none seem to have as rich a tapestry as any of the six main miasms. Why they are worth considering as miasms is because the symptom pictures of each are sometimes mirrored by acute or chronic states in patients who are not actually suffering from them and yet, to all intents and purposes, do appear to be producing symptoms that in some way are 'like'.

While much more research is continuing in parts of the world where these diseases are part of the general practice of medicine, in Britain examples of patients suffering from malaria- or cholera- or typhoid-type conditions are comparatively rare. We would be hard pressed to think of examples of chronically ill patients who had conditions that would make us think at once of using the nosodes of any of these specific diseases – they do not much impinge on our medical consciousness except as historical data. Yet this should not dull our minds to the potential for using the nosodes of the specific diseases. We can also think laterally about conditions that occur in people who may never have travelled further than their local supermarket but are nevertheless expressing their sickness in a way that might be markedly similar to one or other of the diseases and who have never responded satisfactorily to the indicated remedies. Here is a curious example.

A man of sixty-two who had been receiving treatment over some time for arthritic hips and with no appreciable benefit, called to say that he had come down with some sort of bug. His symptoms were: overwhelming weakness and tiredness, intermittent chills with rigors (shivering) followed by sweats and fever; he ached all over; he was very thirsty for cold water; he was very trembly. On being asked what may have brought on this attack he replied that he had been fishing a lot recently and he felt that he had caught a chill while sitting by the marshy lake.

The picture of this set of symptoms belongs to *China Officinalis* (quinine) and he was given three doses of the 200 potency. Nothing happened. He was then given *Malaria* 30 based on the similarity of the two remedies in acute fevers. He became well within 24 hours. Not only that but his hips were, for a time, less stiff and less painful. *China* has a reputation for helping those who have suffered long and debilitating conditions especially where there is sensitivity and irritability – both of which he suffered through his rheumatic arthritis.[1] Other, similar cases of acute feverish symptoms that appeared to be very similar to what was once described in the medical textbooks and throughout literature as 'ague', have responded well to *Malaria* in homoeopathic potency.

Though writers in countries where malaria is rife have made use of this nosode in cases of chronic ill health with good effect, I have no personal experience worth more than hearsay. Having prescribed *Malaria* for those with chronic symptoms that have similarities to the disease and who have not responded to well-indicated remedies, it is disappointing not to have had more convincing proof of the lasting effects of the miasmatic tendency of a problem that beset the people of Britain for so many generations. To show how it is well worth trying to use *Malaria* here is another case.

Michael, a man in his sixties, robust, hard-working but with a history of arthritic problems following various accidents, came for treatment "*for my waterworks*". He suffered from slow urination, a slightly hypertrophied prostate and an agonising, sharp pain that occurred from time to time in the urethra. This symptom picture quickly responded to remedies. He was given *Colocynth*, *Thuja* and *Medorrhinum* at various intervals and these were followed and supported by *Rhus Toxicodendron* and *Sulphur* when he developed unbearably hot, burning feet with rheumatic pains through the legs.

He came to see and accept that in receiving treatment for the waterworks he had initiated the unravelling of a lot of old symptoms that he had always suffered from but that he had either ignored or had suppressed. Indeed, he became very interested in the whole process. Various of his symptoms had a habit of creeping back till they were unbearable: the aching in his legs, the hot feet, rheumatic pains in his arms and night sweats. Then suddenly his blood pressure rose. He went to the doctor and was given drugs which he felt disagreed with his system. Despite this unfortunate muddying of the picture it did emerge that many of his symptoms were similar to the descriptions of ague as it would have been recognised by Shakespeare and his contemporaries. There was intermittent fever, rigors, aches and pains in the limbs, night sweats and chills alternating with thirst. He also had indigestion with bloating, wind and acidity. He was given *China Off.* for these acute episodes which did ease the symptoms and helped him to recover enough to get back to work.

On the third occasion of this acute episode the symptoms were quite a bit more severe. When *China* failed to relieve as before, Michael took *Malaria* 30. The effect was remarkable in that all the symptoms completely disappeared within a few hours leaving him feeling considerably better. This might have been an important breakthrough except for one thing. Though he did not suffer any further acute attacks he did continue with the aches and pains at night, with the sweating and thirst as well as the acidity and other digestive symptoms. It was then noticed that he had a mouthful of amalgam fillings; his persistent symptoms had suggested that an oral examination might prove of interest. When Michael heard what significance mercury fillings might have in terms of his long-term treatment he straight away went to the dentist and arranged for the fillings to be replaced over a period of several months. As the dental treatment proved to be so effective in restoring much of Michael's well-being, energy and reduction of his blood pressure it is not possible to claim that *Malaria* did more than provide a swift answer to a difficult acute flare-up. However, the results of its use on this occasion are perhaps sufficiently satisfactory to continue keeping it in mind for cases that appear to mimic a condition that was once endemic to Britain.

Much the same might be written of cholera and typhoid. Both have quite well-defined basic symptom pictures which, with lateral thinking, might suggest their role in chronic pathology. Cholera is defined by cramps in the limbs, nausea, vomiting and then abdominal cramps that are followed quickly by profuse and severely dehydrating bouts of diarrhoea with the passing of quantities of mucus and blood. Little water is passed and there is a significant drop in blood pressure – all of which leaves the patient feeling exhausted and in a state of profound shock. Despite the fact that cholera is associated with the comma-shaped *Vibrio cholerae* and Crohn's disease has been tentatively associated with one of the tubercular mycobacteria, there are obvious similarities between the acute effects of the two conditions. The same is true of ulcerative colitis. In those cases where the similarities are inescapable and other, more obviously indicated remedies fail to act cura-tively, it might be justified to pursue the use of the *Cholera nosode*.

Typhoid is not so clear-cut. This is a disease that is associated with one of the salmonella bugs. By spreading through the blood and lymph and multiplying in the liver, spleen and bone marrow, the bacteria eventually colonises the whole system. All discharges from the body are infectious. There are four phases:

i)   a rise in temperature with a loss of appetite, insomnia, severe headache, general aching and constipation;

ii)   a rosy red rash which lasts for some three days, spreads over the chest and abdomen and is followed by diarrhoea, often with yellow stools; there is abdominal distension and signs of bronchitis set in;

iii) lethargy, weakness, tremor and blood in the stools set in;

iv)   recovery starts and proceeds slowly.

There are no chronic illnesses, either specific or not, that leap to mind with this description that might be similar enough to typhoid to think of using the nosode to clear a miasmatic tendency. However, many children do suffer from bouts of malaise followed by fever and a rosy rash over the torso with tummy ache and headache that is accompanied by constipation. Whether this is enough to consider using *Typhoidinum*, the remedy, will be food for thought for individual practitioners. To date, the most practical use of *Typhoidinum* is when patients suffer from the bad effects of the typhoid vaccine which induces a bewildering state of pain and feverishness that is like galloping 'flu.

Lots more time and experience is needed before anything more definite can be set down in the homoeopathic textbooks for others to use with confi-dence. Yet, as homoeopathy can do no harm except through a practitioner's neglect, educated experimentation is justified in the face of conditions that do not improve on indicated remedies.

CHAPTER 27

FROM MIASMS TO KARMA

There is no orthodox *scientific* proof that any of the foregoing information on the miasms is true. Hereditary disease is one consideration; geneticists are beginning to unravel the codes that determine whether a person might hand on cystic fibrosis, breast cancer or heart disease. Inheriting a state of being that is coloured by a universal 'disease theme' such as is exemplified by leprosy or syphilis is another matter. To assume that any particular 'disease theme' could be responsible for a wide range of identifiable specific diseases is adding inflammatory material to a smouldering fire.

Homoeopathy does not stop there. We risk having any serious debate doused with ridicule when we assert that each 'disease theme' is *purposefully* part of our inheritance and therefore ultimately necessary to our well-being. Nature has intended that over years and even generations, our whole bodies may creatively develop through processing the miasmatic threads in the fabric of our genes. The only way we have of measuring the truth behind this assumption in terms of health is the experience of clinical observation.

Every patient has a story that is unique. Yet every patient displays characteristics that are imbued with one miasmatic thread or another or, at times, several. Every patient is on a journey of exploration that includes the necessity for *purification* of all three of the integrated bodies: spiritual, emotional and physical. The gross, physical body, being the channel through which distress in the other two bodies becomes manifest, is our earthbound means of expressing what we least understand or are least willing to investigate about ourselves.

Ultimately, disease and health are inextricably linked into an essentially spiritual process – 'soul growth' as it might be called. The need for physical and emotional purification can only be, surely, because there is 'spiritual purpose'. Contemporary conventional medicine, giving itself no brief to find a cure for souls, ensures its permanent limitations by restricting its vision and tool kit to the realms of chemistry. When Church and Medicine divorced, monks and medics stopped speaking the same philosophical language. Ancient practitioners of shamanism would have been quite at a loss to understand how anyone interested in the bodily health of a fellow man could have abdicated responsibility for the welfare of that person's soul. Any prehistoric practitioner[1] would have appreciated what homoeopathy teaches us – the cleansing of the physical body as a vehicle for the balanced emotional body that supports the spirit's life purpose. It would never occur to him that there was any reason to separate these bodies for the purposes of treatment. To him it was enough that the patient had a story to tell which held the key to healing and that every positive change made as a result of asking for help was a step on a personal journey of discovery.

Homoeopathic remedies, even those made from disease material, being solely the characteristic energy of their material form are only aids to be used when indicated while on this journey. As pure energy they cannot, as drugs will do, impose anything on patients who take them; they cannot divert the course of a patient's progress away from natural physical elimination, emotional expression and increasing spiritual awareness though they can and do promote these things.[2]

Homoeopathy is not just the search for the 'right' remedy, the one that will eliminate a set of symptoms. It is also a rooting out of 'blocks to cure', influences that prevent the patient's own life force from dealing completely with the prevailing disease energy. These maintaining causes are often to do with the individual's lifestyle, catalogue of accidents and traumas or even such abstruse things as cellular memory of birth trauma. Such details belong firmly within the patient's own life experience.

There is also what is inherent in the gene pool which we avoid limiting to labelled diseases such as arthritis or osteoporosis or cancer.[3] We see genetic inheritance as a tapestry of miasmatic influences that, according to whichever one is uppermost at any given time, will *dictate the physical, emotional and mental expression of pathology* – bearing in mind that this expression is the body's method of signalling the need to redress an imbalance – and describe in the language of symptoms what remedies are indicated.

The miasms colour and shape our biographies; they give form and substance to our pathology. For those who seek to improve health in order to pursue their life's course creatively there will always come a time when one or other of the miasmatic dragons will awake. When it does, its manifestation will be apparent by its characteristic features. It is only necessary to recognise these in order to be able to treat the beast into submission to the creative spirit of the individual. The miasms in short, *afford the opportunity for the patient to grow. The negativity of pathology leads to the positive strengthening, through recognition and healing, of the creative force.* It is through their recognition that we know how to work towards a patient's recovery. It is one of the practitioner's chief skills, to act as pilot around the miasms; none of us present for treatment a simple case of psora or sycosis, tuberculism or syphilism. Though the nosodes may not form part of every prescription – indeed, may only be needed infrequently – all conditions bear the tidemark of one or other of the six. The pull of the current as the patient moves back towards health, should always be in the direction of psora even if the journey takes a circuitous route. If this does not occur then the patient will be one of those individuals who does not improve; will remain stuck in the whirlpool of negativity – but even this has its purpose in the grand scheme of things. For where this happens, nine times out of ten, there will be a relative or relatives affected by that patient's negativity – who will be witnessing the lack of progress and becoming increasingly frustrated by it, triggering their own desire for self-healing, away from such negativity – away, ultimately, from the syphilitic state. One person's refusal to choose the route back to health can act as a spur to another to take up the challenge.

Beyond the miasms and other maintaining causes there is another influence at work, one we shall approach with caution as it is hard to grasp – especially from the patient's point of view – and touches on the least apparently *medical* aspect of healing; spiritual philosophy. We refer to Karma, essentially a Buddhist concept and one that can easily be dismissed as a fashionable, exotic graft onto the stump of woolly western religious and alternative thinking. Before looking into Karma more deeply we should make sure we are on as firm a ground as possible by taking one more panoramic sweep of the miasms, not least as *they are an integral part of our karmic development.*

The karmic choices of the miasms

Psora

> obliges us to come to terms with our limitations; though not to feel their restrictions but their structure and support.

Sycosis

> obliges us to make the choice of whether to become subservient to another energy (either human, institutional or spiritual); to give away our life force to another's influence or keeping.

Tuberculism

> forces us to make the choice between exploration for its own sake and discovering that which is necessary to one's own existence.

Leprosy

> shows us the futility of isolation from the rest of humanity; that clustering in groups of similarly wounded souls only serves to perpetuate the reasons for being outcast.

Cancer

> offers us the ultimate choice of accepting change as a positive force or of living in a state of complete stasis induced by the fear of change as an inevitable negative influence.

There is no compromise in syphilism. It is ready to take control of a diseased body that refuses or is refused the light and flow of positive energy. Though it is the product of psora, it is ultimately the agent of destruction in the survival of the fittest. ('Destruction' is indicative of what happens to the physical body and its negative energies.) It can be subtly cruel or remarkably gentle; it can lead to long drawn-out illnesses marked by hideous deformity and continuous pain or it can be as mercifully quick as a sudden fatal heart attack. Syphilism offers us the starkest choice – the darkness or the enlightenment – the place to which all other miasms lead eventually if we do not heed their warning signals. Syphilism is a rite of passage: it is where we choose to progress purposefully in our own right whatever the difficulties and handicaps (thus drawing us back to the psoric state); or to pursue living under the destructive influence of other syphilitics, in the 'victim state', or by the systematic manipulation of people and circumstances for one's own ends till the effort involved extinguishes one's present life force. Working through and beyond one's miasmatic influence is part of Karma.

Karma

It is through our collective Karma that the world is in the state it is. We are as much part of the Earth's whole as a single cell would be of a person's body – with all the information about that whole body that it carries. As the saying goes 'As above, so below'.

Karma is probably many things and yet only one thing: one of those infuriating paradoxes of oriental origin. As it is an eastern philosophy why should we in the West need to know about it or be aware of it? We have seemingly done well enough without it up until the second half of the twentieth century. What does Karma have to do with medicine – or with healing, at least? It seems, too, that having been adopted by many in the alternative medicine culture, the word 'Karma' has subtly shifted in definition so that it now carries broader meaning than it did before. It is sensible to define the main aspects of Karma that are relevant to this book.

The original concept

In Buddhist teaching the law of Karma states that for every action or event that happens, another, caused by the first, will occur and that this second happening will be either pleasant or unpleasant, positive or negative relative to the first event. A positive event (termed 'skilful') is seen as one that was not initiated or produced from any

   i)   'craving' (personal desire for gain or gratification),
   ii) resistance (the prevention of a natural occurrence from fear, anger, malice), or
   iii) delusion (misapprehension of the real and natural state of things from faulty judgement due to mistaken preconceptions).

A negative event (termed 'unskilful') is one that is the result of any of these. Implicit in this is that every negative action is the responsibility of the one who initiated or committed it.

This might appear to be no more than common sense until we apply it to that which precedes action, i.e. *thought*. It is considered that thought is a form of energy that can be directed. Just as creative thought can become physically manifest when a cook bakes a cake or an author writes a book, so can a negative thought become hurtful to another (or to oneself) when given form either as words, deeds or resistance. Any sense of gratification at another's lack of success, discomfiture or pain is seen to be negative or bad Karma. Buddhist philosophy takes this to its logical conclusion by saying that only in those who are utterly selfless and who truly are aware of the 'oneness' of everything is unalloyed Karma possible. This leaves the rest of us in a hole. We struggle daily; patient and practitioner alike.

> Two Buddhist priests, a monk and his acolyte, came to a fast-flowing stream where they found a young woman weeping. She was unable to cross the stream because the ferry boat had been swept away. The older monk at once offered to give the woman a piggyback; he forded the stream and set her down safely on the other side. She went off in one direction and the monks in another. After two miles the acolyte could not contain himself any longer, being full of turmoil and doubt about what had happened.
> *"Tell me, how could you have allowed yourself to carry that woman over the stream when you know so well that it is forbidden to us to converse with women, let alone touch them?"* The older man said, *"I put the woman down as soon as we had crossed the river. You are still carrying her."*

The younger man's thoughts – which implied criticism of his master – obsessed him to the point where he was unbalanced in his view. His anxiety prevented him from seeing either his master's charity or that his critical viewpoint showed that he could not allow the rules that governed his life to be flexible.

We often let anxiety and inflexibility colour our opinions and from this come so many personal misunderstandings that lead to disappointments, criticism, offence and anger; then on into sadness. If these are allowed to fester they become the seeds of fixed ideas and depressive tendencies. It is not necessary to be Buddhist to believe just how potentially harmful this is to relationships, family or friends. So familiar with the processes of negative thought patterns are we that television holds up a mirror for us in soap operas in which people tear themselves to shreds because of repeatedly mistaking sentiments and situations and basing negative judgements on them.

Yet, Karma is more. All past negative or unskilful Karma continues to exist until expiated and forgiven – forgiveness is a cardinal skilful event. So for any of us who harbour regret about things that were said and done causing hurt to others or ourselves, we await the moment of forgiving. We need to be released from an unskilful event that has impinged sufficiently on another or on ourselves to cause emotional damage. Such damage is always recorded on the emotional body much as a mechanical trauma is on the physical body. Similarly, we also need resolution for those events that we have misinterpreted and acted upon negatively thus hurting ourselves.

This all may seem rather petty until one realises just how often little hurts occur and how big resentments can build up as time runs away from what first inspired them. We have an amazing capacity to bury hurt; it is often viewed as antisocial not to – our lives would be impossible if we left bleeding chunks of emotional meat where all could see them. Burying them, though, is not only insufficient to deal with bad Karma; it is conducive to further negative Karma and damaging to the general whole body health. Negative Karma is as foreign to a balanced body as any chemical toxin. The body can store toxins – and often has to – but it is not built to be a permanent receptacle for them. If buried negative Karma is harboured for too long, the body will convert it into chronic physical pathology. This is classed – sometimes rather witheringly – as psychosomatic disease. As the psyche *is* involved in all chronic pathology it is essential to see the importance of Karma being resolved.

Stephen was a retired solicitor, a few years older than his wife. She was also a solicitor but now worked for various charities. Stephen suffered from migraines and had a peptic ulcer. Lillian, full of energy and drive, never suffered from anything. They had two children living, a third had died in her teens from multiple burns sustained in a car accident. Stephen pottered. He loved gardening and golf; he saw himself as a collector of antiquarian books "*in a very small way*". Lillian was seldom at home as she sat on various committees and organised events. She also sat on the local parish church council. She was generally acknowledged to be popular, efficient, enthusiastic and dynamic. People were at a loss to know where she found the energy to do all the things that she did. Stephen, too, was very sociable and much liked by his local community though they probably saw him more as a support for his wife.

Stephen's migraines had begun some two years after the death of their daughter. His ulcer had begun to cause him trouble intermittently some three or four years later. He was very open and matter-of-fact about his condition and his circumstances. He appeared, above all, to want to get better. In describing his migraines it was clear that the symptom picture was best matched by *Sanguinaria*.[4] The ulcer caused acute symptoms that were matched by *Lycopodium*.[5] The general constitutional picture was also similar to *Lycopodium* in that Stephen was cautious until sure of his ground, preferred to keep space between him and his fellow man despite his outward and genuine friendliness; he admitted to a vague sense of apprehension when faced with anything that demanded any self-confidence. Despite this, there was also an underlying sense of unresolved grief about him. He said very little that suggested that he was emotionally wounded but it was clear from 'body language' and choice of words that his daughter's death lay unresolved in his heart.

Stephen came for treatment for many months yet however well chosen the remedies might have been he made little general progress. The *Sanguinaria* did nothing for his headaches at all. *Lycopodium* gave him more energy and relief from his digestive symptoms but was unable to heal the ulcer which, whenever he was stressed, caused him acute pain. Remedies chosen for their reputation for dealing with grief at the deepest levels made no appreciable difference. He spoke neither more nor less about his past than before. When he was stressed the migraines came on every few days. When he was able to stay quietly at home, pottering, then they left him in peace for a while longer. He continued to take prescription drugs for the relief of the pain because nothing else helped him.

What was the stress factor? Lillian was forever asking him to accompany her to all the functions that she organised; to "*put on a good show*" when she invited important guests for dinner. Stephen felt obliged to be Lillian's support and shadow. As many of the events involved meeting medical people, both doctors and journalists, he felt out of place as his natural inclination was to pursue an alternative route – not simply medical but in other aspects as well: diet, the environment and politics. His wife resented his views and she made it clear to him that his condition, she thought, was much too serious to be handled by charlatans and quacks. He needed proper medical attention or he would be "*really ill*".

Stephen loved his wife and found it painful that she dismissed his ideas so readily. He was confused by her attitude and, while he felt that he understood *"where she was coming from"*, he thought that she should be able to let him find his own way. Yet he could see that his interest in alternative therapy in some way reflected negatively, at least in his wife's mind, on what she was involved with.

He did go (privately) to see the consultant that she recommended. He started to take the medication that was prescribed and when he felt so much worse he stopped taking it. He then felt guilty because he did not tell his wife. He went to see a counsellor but gave that up as he felt that the therapist *"harped on about Mary's death all the time"* and he saw no point in *"raking over old ground"*. He went to a reflexologist and found that very beneficial: he felt calm and less stressed than he had done for ages. The treatment also afforded him at least ten days without a migraine. He also had all his amalgam fillings removed; he had both amalgams and gold in his mouth and he periodically showed signs of mercury poisoning that did always respond to homoeopathic remedies. After the removal he, at first, felt no difference but within four months he felt that he was *"less toxic"*. Stephen understood the concept of elimination of both biochemical and emotional waste and he did everything that he could to initiate the process – to no avail with the headaches and the ulcer. Despite the comfort he found in all the alternative paths he took, nothing shifted these two physical symptom generators.

He began to be so affected that he was forced to cancel all engagements. Lillian became increasingly concerned especially when she learnt that he had stopped seeing the specialist and was not on the medication. She suggested that he should see the local GP to find out if he thought that Stephen was depressed. The GP did think so and recommended a psychiatrist. Stephen obliged once again and was put on Prozac. Within three weeks he felt so anxious and dizzy and had so little appetite that he stopped taking the antidepressant. Shortly after this he discovered that if he went for a reflexology session and then followed it with a visit to the cranial osteopath while intermittently taking *Oak*, the remedy, he could function much better and stave off the migraines for considerably longer. Here was a change that he felt confident about.

Within a few weeks Lillian developed breast cancer. She was given a biopsy and a mastectomy followed by radiotherapy for several weeks. When she came home she was completely changed. She was in permanent pain and depression. She needed Stephen's help for everything and he waited on her hand and foot. Though he became exhausted the migraines stayed away for the most part. He asked her if she would see a homoeopath and she said she would as she had nothing to lose. However, so bad did Lillian's depression become that the GP referred her to a psychiatrist who gave her several sessions of counselling and put her on an antidepressant. Within a month she was feeling better. She was more cheerful and showed some of her old energy by ringing up various contacts to find out what had been happening. As soon as she started to improve Stephen began to have migraines again. He came for treatment with the osteopath and said that he was going to try the orthodox approach again because "*nothing else seems to have worked*". He said that Lillian was relieved when he agreed to see another specialist.

So where is the Karma in this case? Lillian and Stephen shared a grief. While he pottered, she drove herself and others to a point where there was no space to feel pain. She poured all her efforts into charitable works. To do this well she felt the need of her husband's support. He gave this support but at the expense of what he most loved doing. Though he willingly gave his time and energy he was hurt that his wife did not appreciate that he had another philosophical point of view that was not particularly sympathetic to the world in which she moved. His undoubted love for Lillian and his loyalty to her had become the maintaining causes of his physical symptoms; symptoms that had most likely been initiated by the death of their daughter – an event about which they had rarely spoken. For Stephen to have said clearly that he no longer wanted to accompany her to social functions, no longer wanted to take any orthodox medicine, would have been a betrayal (in his view) he could not commit.

Lillian was unable to see that her expectations of Stephen were part of the maintaining cause for his physical pain. Nor could she see that her lifestyle was partly a compensation for the loss of their daughter. The subtle understanding between them that only Stephen was partly aware of and that was entirely subliminal in Lillian, was that if she stopped working she would have to face the sickening consequences of long-buried grief. Breast cancer is not uncommonly the result of a mother's grieving process. It was no coincidence that Stephen's considerable but temporary improvement was followed by Lillian's illness. It would be a mistake to blame Lillian for their situation. They were two people who were attempting to work out an intractable dilemma in the ways they knew best. Both of them were capable of making other choices than the ones they made.

The only successful resolution we see is the one in which both will face what they have so efficiently buried without expecting the other to bend their existence to support any compensatory activity that masks the route to resolution. If we become partisan it is because we recognise their hurt from our own and empathise more with one than the other. Practitioners also run the risk of unskilful Karma when they prescribe from bias. But practitioners can never prescribe *on* Karma; they can only prescribe on the effects – the resultant symptom picture and the miasmatic inheritance that supports it.

In Stephen's case while he was willing to try alternative means to travel through his pathology and could see the esoteric value of it, Lillian was not and the greater pull belonged to her. Lillian was not so much cured of cancer as given a temporary reprieve. She found a way of returning to the state she was in before her illness. Yet, if she were to remain in 'stuck Karma' then her body would either return to the metastasised cancer or it would invent another way of demonstrating its distress at having to support unresolved issues.

Herein lies a further definition of Karma, broader than skilful or unskilful thought forms with their consequences. Karma is the journey to resolution; the process of acceptance of history, forgiveness of self and others and the steady movement forward into purposefulness. It is a journey where negative Karma is released and it is one that only the patient can make.

Unfortunately, many choose not to make it. All homoeopaths have cases which tell of patients who simply do not respond on any deep level to treatment. While it is always possible to put this down to the practitioner's inability to see what needed to be done, it should also be remembered that many people do not want their deepest levels of feelings and spirituality disturbed. They have so securely battened down the hatches that their emotions have 'calcified', so to speak. Quite often they are completely unaware that they have buried anything, so efficiently have they done the job.

Inheritance of Karma

There is another aspect of Karma which is borne out of the general philosophy. This is inherited Karma. What happens when someone who has lived a life full of negative Karma dies? Do they take it all with them? Is Karma resolved by death? What happens to those people left living who have been negatively affected by the deceased? Is their Karma resolved by the passing or are they condemned to put up with unresolved hurt, buried or otherwise? The hurt carried still is as much negative Karma as was the initial inspiration for it. It is simply that the infliction of hurt is aggressive or yang while the feeling of pain is submissive or yin.[6] Delia's case can illustrate the subtle workings of Karma from both sides of this question.

Delia was born in the late 1940s to a ferocious virago, frequently gripped by hormonal hysteria, and a thoroughly cowed older and enfeebled father who was dominated by his wife. Delia was an only child and bore the brunt of her mother's violence. She was beaten and verbally abused for much of her childhood. She was also raped at the age of six by a distant relative; an incident that she admitted she only remembered through having a dream (when she was forty) which she felt *"explained so much that I had not understood"*.

Delia came with a complicated and convoluted symptom picture. Chiefly, she was permanently tired. *"I feel that it is a mental, physical, emotional and spiritual tiredness and I think that it goes back many years."* She felt sleepy all the time and had no energy even to cook for herself. She was confused and indecisive and tended to cry quietly a great deal. She became anxious about many things, usually little day-to-day things. Her sleep was disturbed by bad dreams. She also felt as if she were not quite within herself; as if she were at a distance from herself. She could see with her eyes but her body was elsewhere. Her work as a secretary was increasingly difficult as she became muddled and inefficient. Her self-confidence was *"around my ankles at the moment"*.

It was quite difficult to hear everything that Delia said as she was so quietly spoken. Tears were not far away as she spoke of her life and the tedious work she did.

"I know that I'm not really suited to my work. I feel that I should really be doing something else. I find that the office is uncongenial but I've always found myself in places where I don't fit in. I didn't fit in at home, I s'pose. I was always afraid in childhood. My mother was always so cross. I realise, looking back, that she had a difficult time with her cycle. She had bad mood swings and they were always worse around the full moon. And my cycle was always regularly at the full moon. I stopped mentioning things like that because people thought I was odd but actually I've never found anything like that peculiar. I was always able to see things. I was always aware of 'energies', I s'pose you'd call them. I

escaped into another space and that allowed me to get on with things – one side of me learnt what to expect from my mother and the other was where I went to get away as I knew she couldn't reach me there. I think my father understood.

"*Then my mother had a stroke when she was fifty-one shortly after she had a hysterectomy. She must have had a tendency to high blood pressure. When she was angry you could see the veins on her temples stand out. That was rather frightening; I always thought that they would burst. When the storm passed she would often be rather dizzy and have to sit quietly. She was very overweight too. She had another stroke at fifty-nine and that left her very weak and then not long after she had a heart attack and died. It sounds terrible but it was a relief to me. My father had died about five years before and I dreaded having to look after her especially if she was incapacitated.*

"*The strange thing is that I don't feel that she has left me. I still feel her around – not all the time but quite often. She's become a bit like a ball and chain. It's not frightening any more but it is a burden. It's as if she is the one that is frightened – it's taken me some time to see that but that is how it feels.*"

Delia was given *Ayahuasca* 1M (as a single dose) and *Thuja* (in a liquid form to be taken as a drop each day). The former because it re-establishes, on an esoteric, energetic level, family links – at least, that is how it seems as those who take it while in circumstances of strain between family members (especially mothers and children) find that they are able to resolve their potentially negative pathological emotions. The latter because this remedy helps to reintegrate the two halves of a divided psyche. The result of this prescription was extraordinary. Within a few weeks Delia phoned to say that she had developed a severe sore throat after a week of intense emotional upheaval during which she wept copiously. So bad was her throat that she found it difficult to swallow and felt that she would suffocate. There was terrible pain especially on the left side and her glands were swollen, her breath was rank and what she could see of her tongue was dark red veering on maroon.

Delia also felt irritable, even angry. She wanted to hide away from any contact; she felt as if she would be very sharp with anyone if they were to talk to her. This was a feeling that was completely foreign to her. (On the phone her manner seemed grim and brittle and it was obviously hard for her to answer the questions as she seemed somewhat confused.) She also complained of feeling hot – even though she had no temperature – and "*muzzy headed*". Her last comment was that her mother had a history of regular sore throats very similar to this.

The remedy that covered this acute condition was *Lachesis*. She had to wait until the next day before it arrived in the post but she later reported that the effect of the remedy was almost instantaneous. The pain disappeared within an hour, the tonsils began to reduce in size, she no longer felt afraid of suffocating, she was able to drink and swallow and the neck glands disappeared from view. Within 48 hours she felt the episode was completely over. She also felt that she was no longer so mentally tired. She found that she was contemplating doing things that she had not considered for a long while: making a patchwork quilt, getting out her knitting machine and going for long walks. She felt her brain was clearer; her thinking processes were no longer clouded.

"And there is something else: while I had the throat I talked to my mother about the symptoms; I knew that she must have felt like this herself. I told her about the dreadful choking feeling. I asked her to take that away. Then the remedy came. It's so odd, I just don't feel my mother is anywhere around me anymore. It's extraordinary; it's as if a huge load – and all that ugly crossness with it – it's been taken off my back – I'm not carrying it round with me anymore. It's a new experience for me. I feel that I'm not someone's little girl anymore. It's quite scary but exciting at the same time."

Why this is significant is that Delia's mother, rocked as she must have been by her hormonal problems, had she been a patient of homoeopathy, would have needed *Lachesis* as a remedy for her long-term chronic state. Delia's description of her mother was a classic example of the remedy: mood swings, unpredictable, unstable temperament, furious, impatient, cruel, spiteful, jealous and full of suspicion. It may well have been that she would have needed *Lachesis* to deal with her chronic recurrent tonsillitis as well. Furthermore, *Lachesis* is often required to deal with conditions that precede strokes or that are consequent on high blood pressure. It is a medicine famed for its ability to influence hormonal imbalances. Delia had never at any time in her history shown any sign of pathology or temperament that would have needed *Lachesis* yet here she was relating her experience with this inimitable medicinal energy. It was as if she had to reproduce her mother's symptom pattern in order to be free of her mother's influence.[7] By shedding her mother's pall she was able to start her life afresh.

Even more intriguing was that soon after the acute sore throat episode, Delia came to her next appointment feeling extremely shy, retiring and vulnerable. She felt that she could not do her work effectively because her self-confidence was so low. The rest of the mental/emotional picture she described indicated the remedy *Baryta Carbonicum*, that is often prescribed for those who are entering second childhood or who suffer from stunted growth; it is a remedy that is so often needed for anyone who suffers from retarded development of any description.

779

The result of this prescription was no less remarkable as she returned after three months to say that she had decided to hand in her notice, to put her house on the market and move to Wales where she wanted to take up painting, a hobby that she had always had but never allowed anyone to know about. She had an old school friend in mid-Wales who ran a craft workshop and who would be happy to help launch her. With the mother-layer lifted, it was as if she were able to go back to her suppressed childhood and deal with the stunted development of her very capable mind. *"I've no idea how it'll work out but I feel I must try. This is what it must feel like for a teenager to leave home for the first time."*

Where is the Karma in this? If one is comfortable with the concept of souls passing from this life into the next and that some souls might, at the point of death, not be able to complete the passage fully due to intense fear or anger, then it is not too much of a leap of imagination to see that someone living still and close to the deceased might unwittingly take responsibility for the reluctant deceased, stuck in a state of irresolution.

The fact that Delia emerged from treatment as if she had been through a metamorphosis suggests certain things. One is that there are many such people who have unique but similar stories to tell; there are countless people who have close relatives who died 'unsatisfactory' or 'uncompleted' deaths and who feel that the deceased have not left them and are in some way a continued burden even though they no longer have a physical body. Such a situation reflects on people's health in a way that can be read in terms of symptoms, both chronic and acute. These symptoms are also susceptible to treatment with natural healing methods. A further thought is that the resolution of Karma may be one of the most imperative of all maintaining causes – unless Delia had shed her mother's influence in the way that she did, she would never have made the developmental, purposeful progress that resulted.

Delia's story must stand as representative for many similar cases; it is only unique as far as the personalities are concerned. It is not unusual for people to show all the symptoms of needing to deal with family Karma. Like Delia, the patient might be repressed, mild-mannered and have the sense that they have never 'found' themselves. Yet this same person may have been a survivor of extraordinary events, displaying a toughness of constitution that does not quite fit with the picture of vulnerability. The patient can appear to be the very image of a victim yet they have a persistence and tenacity that are remarkable and seemingly maintained against the odds. Their patience and humility can seem either biblical or dog-dumb, leaving us to wonder why on earth they could not have seen for themselves the suppression of their life force from abuse, humiliation and degradation.

There are others who may not appear to be 'victim' types at all; they may even be aggressive. They have lives in which patterns of behaviour suggest that they cannot undo those attitudes imposed by inadequate parentst, attitudes that force them into relationships in which the abuse, humiliation and grief match that of a previous generation. What these people share is a sense of responsibility. At first, they seem to feel responsible for their failures, for their inadequacies – for that is what they were taught. They more often than not feel responsible for any troubles that exist between their parents or they assume a protective role for their siblings – sometimes both. Then they become responsible for their own lame relationships and for their parents' old age or for the boss or institution they work for. Duty is strong and enough to silence the inevitable resentment. Most importantly, they are responsible for hiding the pains of their own childhood from the next generation. Never, they vow, will the trouble brought on them by their own damaged parent or parents filter through to a third generation – but it does in some way or another; often because they have married people who, damaged themselves, have been attracted to yet more similar damage (*like finds like!*)

Appalling negative events in childhood usually stop with adulthood but the pattern of inflicted pain continues and the patient finds ways of repeating the pattern, *not necessarily to continue being a victim but to reproduce conditions and feelings similar to the original circumstances, in order to find a solution.* For these patterns to be resolved there has to be a resolution not only of the patient but also those others who inculcated it. This is why so many patients who live through such tragic childhoods of physical and sexual abuse and who go on to suffer persistently from humiliation and abuse do not become released entirely from their burden. Though they may go through long periods of therapy and counselling, though they may change their lifestyles radically to reflect a growing confidence and vitality, though they may seem to embrace changes to their central purpose, they are never entirely free unless there is atonement for the Karma.

We may see a patient who might be unrecognisably different from the person who first acknowledged the pain and grief but who is now suffering physically from heart and circulation problems or from cancer. We might see someone who, having managed to survive a grievous childhood and having suffered a repressed youth, finds a voice to vent their anger and goes on to take charge of their lives but is now dangerously manipulative of others. It is as if the patient has found within (and beneath their suppressed self) a new sense of personal power and a confidence in wielding it that gives them such an attractive force that delving further into forgiveness and understanding would threaten to undo it; it is hard indeed to relinquish the very power that would, had it been theirs in childhood, have been the means of avoiding all that pain.

In all these people there is movement towards healing, towards the lifting of suffering but there is no resolution of the negative energy that was *'first cause'* of the troubles. That first cause can originate from generations back. The patient alone can resolve the results of these first causes as he or she is the one attempting to heal the negative energy patterns set up so long before and so effectively buried in history and deep within the core of the emotional body and probably in the spiritual body as well.[8]

Just as we have pain-killing chemicals in the physical body to deal with extreme physical trauma, so we have the ability to kill emotional pain by consigning memories to the furthest recesses of the mind. Unfortunately (or fortunately, if we are going to attempt any self-healing), the *physical* body is still able to register the memories that we would rather keep buried in the psyche. If we do not seek healing for them then the physical body must remind us by producing relevant or even symbolic symptomatology[9]; some-times by taking us to the brink of threatening or terminal pathology. The body is simply extraordinary and extraordinarily simple in its ability to create symptom metaphors.

To know the truth of this it is only necessary to hear the stories of those who recover fully from cancer; they all become aware of the importance of past, unresolved issues that involve forebears. Women fully restored to health from breast cancer often have had to dredge up memories of their mothers and resolve in their hearts issues with them that were long since buried. And if not with their mothers then with some other relationship in which frustrated nurturing was a powerful element. Others who have come through uterine cancer have had to heal themselves through understanding and forgiving perverse fathers, uncles or older cousins, perhaps, who made them feel so mortally self-disgusted; then, after them, the string of men with whom they may have had relationships in an attempt to reproduce the original circumstances of their pain. Or they have perhaps had to deal with the agony of having had an abortion – or even that they were themselves threatened with abortion by mothers who could not initially bear the thought of pregnancy.

Smokers, so long addicted as a way of suppressing heart-hurt sustained in infancy or childhood, who develop cancer of the lung but recover, at some point will have faced their terrible sadness by conjuring up the memories of those who imposed their 'unskilful' thoughts, strictures and obligations on them and understanding what it was that drove that previous generation to act as it did. The first step a patient makes to freeing the soul of its negative Karma is to acknowledge the unresolved past that is perpetuated by negative spirit-energy influencing those to whom it is attached.

It must be remembered that the medicines are prescribed only on a patient's symptom picture and not on the practitioner's judgement of the state of the patient's soul and karmic journey. It is not possible for anyone to prescribe symptomatically or therapeutically on Karma; only on what characteristic energy pattern is described by a patient's words and from the objective observation of his general physical symptoms. The events of a patient's karmic journey become clear only once the patient returns having experienced the particular, peculiar and personal effects that the last prescription has had. It is as if the remedies are keys to unlock doors; no more than that. It remains with the patient alone as to which doors are opened or whether they are opened at all. The fact that we might be able to take such journeys to the interior of the mind and soul is extraordinary enough. That there are natural healing agents to assist us to make them is miraculous.

Irrational medicine

Can rational minds really contemplate any of this? What would any of it have to do with ordinary men, women and children who visit their GPs' surgery or who walk down hospital corridors to visit sick relatives or who lie in a clinic bed waiting for a hip replacement or to have an appendix removed? The speed of disease and the intensity of the effort to combat it with the sophisticated technology now at the disposal of medical science precludes the idea that any esoteric consideration needs to be taken into account. A doctor does not need to know that a man dying of congestive heart failure has led a life of suppressed emotions as the result of a repressive father. He has no time to ask what would happen to the man's spirit if he could not re-vive the failing body. He could not be aware of family dynamics beyond the obvious worry and grief of those relatives in the corridor waiting for news. The urgency of a hospital ward is no place to consider occult medicine. Nor is the local surgery. It is not possible to notice the emerging signs of a per-son's spirit-quest within the short time a GP is able to offer. Even if it were possible, the doctor could not prescribe conventionally on what he ob-served. Drugs are meant to cover symptoms not to uncover truths.

Karma cannot be studied as if it were a science. It can be scrutinised only at the level of witnessed experience; this is no better than hearsay. It is, from the practitioner's point of view, medicine with hindsight. It took me many, many months to be able to write about this area of healing purely because Karma is so arcane and so far out of reach of anything remotely to do with most people's experience of improving their health. I found it hard to be-lieve that more than a few people who were seriously interested in alternative therapy would go so far as to accept the premise that Karma is as important to our well-being as any of the other, more obvious, maintaining causes. Though years of practice have offered me the opportunity of meet-ing many patients who do explore their karmic histories (mostly unwittingly) and thus allow their life purpose to flow fully, there are many more who make the choice, after initial treatment for particular problems, not to go further. While many understand – and are even fascinated by – the multiplicity of different maintaining causes that might prevent them from returning to balanced health and are quite prepared to go along with advice and even referrals to other and complementary alternative therapies, when it comes to delving into the effects upon themselves of their own and others' Karma they withdraw and the self-healing stops.

> The very determined Polish woman in her late seventies who came to the college clinic when I was a student. She was Jewish and, judging by her very lined face, seemed to have had a difficult life. She complained of rheumatism of the knees. She said that she had taken *Rhus Toxicodendron* for the problem. At first it had worked but now it was ineffective. She said that she needed another remedy but she issued an injunction that we should do no more than treat her knees.
>
> Her case was considered collectively by the class and after much discussion the remedy chosen for her was *Thuja*. This remedy has similar symptoms to *Rhus Tox.* in the treatment of rheumatism and is often chosen when *Rhus Tox.* appears to fail. When the patient returned she was furious. She was bitterly disappointed and had only returned to complain. She appeared anxious, resentful and haggard. She had dark circles under her eyes and her facial expression, when she relaxed from her tirade, was drawn with grief. As she stalked out it was apparent that her walk was brisk and steadier than on her first visit. For some years I was nervous of using *Thuja* because of this – absurdly ascribing the cause of the woman's distress to the remedy. I felt that we had prescribed wrongly; that it had been our fault that the woman had experienced aggravation. In my mind I invested *Thuja* with the power to impose on a patient something that was disadvantageous or even harmful. I did not see that the woman had invested her lame knee with the physical pain of her grief.

We cannot tell how long it was before what I took to be her emotional aggravation settled down. The case does suggest, though, that she knew, on some subliminal level perhaps, that homoeopathy was capable of initiating her self-healing in a way that might disturb her psyche and possibly memories of wartime horror. Our only other option that day would have been to say that there was no other remedy that we could suggest beyond *Rhus Tox.* But that would leave us with the idea that all prescriptions (especially of *Thuja*) might risk a patient's carefully self-preserved balance – even if that balance is a false one, achieved at the cost of physical pathology and the lack of a final resolution of long-held grief. Practitioners can only speculate as to what any prescription will do and then go by what they observe; they can only be witnesses. Speculation may well be based on individual experience of years of practice and on the collective experience of over two centuries of homoeopathy but, in the final analysis, every patient is still about to embark on a unique experience with every 'constitutional' prescription that is taken and this precludes any absolute certainty as to the outcome. Healing thus mirrors life itself.

This lack of foreknowledge of a remedy's effects is less important in terms of biochemistry than it would be for a doctor prescribing drugs because the physical body is only going to react to energy medicines in ways that are within the bounds of its capabilities. The results may sometimes be initially uncomfortable but the eventual outcome is always going to be positively eliminative. (And any reaction that threw up symptoms would be susceptible to complementary supporting remedies.) It is the body that reacts to a stimulus; not the remedy that creates any organic changes. It is well to remember this when considering the lack of certainty about reactions to remedies in the emotional body. Though we cannot know precisely the how, when, why, where and what, it will still be the psyche that produces the reactions and not the remedy.

We can be sure that the soul's journey through the self-healing process, only obvious to us through hindsight, is absolutely out of the practitioner's hands because the only evidence on which remedies can be prescribed is the information supplied by the physical, mental and emotional bodies – the soul has no symptomatic voice on its own level. Some would argue with this and say that the colours of the body's aura change when the soul is sick. However, it is still comparatively rare to find a practitioner who can genuinely see and read the coloured energy that flows in, through and around a living body. Even those homoeopaths who do will always check the physical and emotional symptoms for confirmation of their extrasensory perceptions as they know that whatever distress there is in the soul will always be registered in the more earthbound levels of the body.

We can summarise Karma as far as homoeopathy is concerned in the following way:

  i)   It is a sequence of historical events (either in thought or action) from the past of the patient that leaves its mark and requires resolution in the form of acceptance or forgiveness. It is unfinished business that lies buried in the psyche and that, left unattended, will eventually create emotional disturbance and then physical pathology.

ii)   The events (usually both in thought and action) that began in previous generations have created a pattern of behaviour and thinking in the present generation so that the patient is able to find a resolution to that pattern by working through symptomatic conditions that mirror the original disturbance.

iii)   It is a maintaining cause that does not preclude the beneficial effects of remedies in acute conditions or in many lesser chronic ones but does preclude complete resolution of the deepest chronic pathology if the patient is reluctant to face and answer questions posed by his life circumstances.

iv)   It is not treatable through any system of medicine though many alternative therapies are able to facilitate the resolution of Karma when the current symptoms of mind, emotions and body are considered as a whole.

v)   It is resolved gradually not least by working through the miasmatic inheritance which we all have and with which it is inextricably linked.

vi)   It is only witnessed through hindsight and is always accompanied in its resolution by forward, developmental movement in the patient's life purpose.

Every prescription potentially creates a window of karmic opportunity. Yet, in practice, what usually occurs is that a patient gradually improves until a point when one particular prescription seems to afford the opportunity for a far greater leap of self-healing than before. It is as if the series of remedies given over several months or even years has a cumulative effect and, when the patient is ready, a major breakthrough happens and a balanced sense of true purpose comes through. At this moment the homoeopath's work comes to fruition; the patient has made creative use of the treatment by taking full responsibility for his or her health, by accepting the inevitability of change and understanding the need to let the negative past rest.

This last state is perhaps the most difficult. Whatever bad thing happens when we are at our most vulnerable, when we are most needy, when we should be able to expect to have absolute trust and faith in those who care for us, becomes indelibly imprinted on the psyche. We take it to heart. Yet this is to fail to see the karmic significance of such events; how we can find resolution by reproducing their effects and finding the answer to them from within. Homoeopathic remedies, by stripping away the accretions of old chronic and miasmatic patterns, allow more and more awareness of karmic patterns to be brought to the surface which, when they are understood from within, can be seen to be either habitual out of fear, anger or grief (i in the list above) or to be nature's insistence that negative history must be resolved (ii above).

One final case will serve to illustrate these points.

Megan was eight years old when she was brought for treatment. She was very bright and not in the least shy. She was having problems at school as so many of her friends were being unkind to her. Her best friend now ignored her and had teamed up with a girl new to the school. Megan was devastated by this, her mother explained. She no longer wanted to go to school and had "*abdominal migraines*", pains in the gut, each morning except for Saturdays and Sundays. She had wet the bed on several occasions. She had become tearful and overdependent on her mother, a single parent since her father had left the home for another woman.

Megan was given *Pulsatilla* in the 50M potency, a potency that is regarded as extremely high but that is useful in cases where there is a possible risk of trauma becoming a deeply established pattern. The result was that Megan had no further 'accidents' at night and stopped being so clingy. What emerged though, was a different picture but one which the mother said had been there, underneath, since her husband had left. She was often pessimistic and disgruntled. When like this she could be spiteful and hurtful, even lashing out at her much younger brother. She was haughty and contemptuous in a way that a teenager might become. She refused to play games suggested by anyone other than herself. She skimped the household chores that she knew were hers – she left her bed unmade, she did not put her plates in the dishwasher. She spent a long time preening in front of the mirror; she refused to wear the clothes that her mother put out for her. (Her mother laconically commented that this reminded her of Megan's father's new girlfriend.) A further symptom was that Megan always tried to listen in on phone calls; she would rush for the phone to answer it or, if too late, she would surreptitiously pick up the extension to listen in. So marked was her suspiciousness that her mother felt that she was being watched by her own daughter.

Megan was given the snake venom, *Lachesis*. Her mother reported within four weeks that the remedy seemed to have settled the atmosphere. Where before it had been heavy with gloom and a sense of "*almost menace*", it was now much lighter. Megan was more biddable, less imperious. She no longer smacked her brother and she had returned to making her bed and tidying her room. Nonetheless, she was still sad and inclined to pessimism. She complained of headaches which seemed to coincide with periods of worry; by odd things that she said she appeared anxious for the family's safety. She was tense and nervy and tired much of the time.

This is not a symptom picture that many parents would take a great deal of notice of – not because they would not care but because it seems nebulous and insufficient for an appointment with the GP. It is a picture that is common and one that has many variations and it is often neglected as being a 'phase'. 'She'll grow out of it, I shouldn't worry if I were you.'

Yet one never grows out of it; it is, like a fallen building, overgrown in time by other things. Layer upon layer of superseding events bury it until it is forgotten deep in the memory's archives. In itself this one passage of time might be insignificant in comparison with more dreadful events that might happen. Yet, in an eight-year-old mind such feelings of anxiety, anticipation and sadness are not insignificant at all.

Megan was given the remedy made from *Amethyst*. This remedy covers symptoms of anxiety and tension that stem from a state of mind that sees everything in a negative light. People who need it tend to expect the worst to happen. They become introspective and pessimistic. They wonder what will become of themselves; they have no positive sense of a secure future. The ancient Greeks considered the stone to impart great courage in battle; it is a remedy that encourages those who falter from lack of confidence in the face of emotional challenges.

Megan was violently sick on the night of taking the remedy, though strangely she brought up very little of her evening meal; it was mostly mucus and bile. By the next morning she was manifestly better. Within a week or two she was back with her friends in the school; she felt included in their circle. What was more significant was that she now told her mother about all that went on when she went off to visit her father – how she felt so confused and angry with him and his new girlfriend; that he spent more time on her rather than his daughter; that he was forever criticising everybody, especially 'Mum'. Yet she related it all from the perspective of someone who had come to a decision not to let it disturb what was most important in her life: home, friends, school, family outings, sleep.

The situation had been loaded with what could have become a severe karmic burden. Megan might have buried her confusion, anger and grief and then gone on to experience years of intolerance between her separated parents. She would have learnt to judge them both from the perspective of an eternal eight year old but laden with other baggage – gathered successively from the classroom and the playground, from early and later boyfriends, from the social cocktail of university, from the competition of the workplace. By thirty her entrenched beliefs would only have allowed her a warped image of her mother and father. So many people, when eventually they come to resolve their relationships with parents, realise that the reality of history is so different from what they had believed. The parents are exactly the same as they ever were but the one-time child's understanding offers such a different view of them. For Megan, this time at least, there was no need to form a set, negative pattern of attitudes coloured by sadness and anger. She managed to find a view of the situation that let her understand enough to realise that she did not have to be part of her parents' feud even if it made her feel sad. She achieved a sense of objectivity that enabled her to express her feelings openly to her mother. She was able to *"let go"*.

Pulsatilla, Lachesis and *Amethyst* are not 'karmic' remedies any more or less than any others. They were prescribed simply on the symptom pictures available at the moment. It was Megan's own innate common sense that was able to come through while allowing her also to experience all the natural feelings of any child learning to live in such circumstances. She was able to feel the pain of separation without apportioning blame or seeking retribution. Megan was sparing herself a long history of 'unskilful' thoughts towards others that would lead to yet more pain both for them and herself.

It is in the light of these illustrative cases that Karma should be seen as a profoundly important maintaining cause. Yet, paradoxically, it is one – it is the only one – for which we are not permitted by nature to 'medicate'. It is only for us to observe in hindsight as the patient's own achievement. Yet, when it is there to be seen it affords the greatest satisfaction to the prescriber. It is then that we know that the job has been well done.

CHAPTER 28

A POSTLUDE TO THE MIASMS

In the introduction to these chapters on inherited disease patterns it was said that the separating out of the miasms was arbitrary for the purpose of understanding. From the individual descriptions it is possible to see just how different they all are and yet how closely related to the original psora. Though psora may seem to be far less dark, brooding, manipulative or lethal than syphilism; less divorced from reality and certainly less addictive than sycosis; less dissatisfied with life and less determined to embrace constant change for its own sake than tuberculism; less isolated than leprosy; less lost to the state of purposelessness and suppression than cancer, it nevertheless is the soil from which the roots of all the others grow. From the chapter on cancer you will have seen how this miasm is eventually arrived at through the neglect or suppression of any or all the others. You will also have seen how tuberculism grows out of not only psora but either syphilism or sycosis as well.

From psora all the others 'inherit' something of the core theme of being susceptible to playing *host*;

> – firstly to the idea of being fundamentally inadequate (psora),
> – secondly to the 'worm' of both self-seeking manipulation and ultimately self-destruction (syphilis),
> – thirdly to the sense of separation from both self and the real world (sycosis),
> – fourthly to the sense of dissatisfaction and distraction and the urgent quest to find the solution outside oneself (tuberculism),
> – fifthly to the sense of isolation and the inevitability of fate (leprosy) and
> – finally to the fundamental sense of lost purpose (cancer).

The trunks of these miasmatic trees are not even really separate once they achieve their maturity; once they are sufficiently influential to cause the manifestation of their characteristic pathology. They are interdependent, one with the others. We saw with smallpox, the disease used to be manifest in different ways: in one it was mild and appeared not much more than a serious dose of chickenpox (psoric); in another it might have been characterised by pus-filled pocks (sycotic); in yet another it was terrifyingly fatal and characterised by internal haemorrhaging from confluent lesions in the lungs (syphilitic). We saw that tuberculosis can be either syphilitic (rapidly destructive of the tissues of vital organs) or sycotic (where the patient is full of mucus and pus) – in much the same way that asthma can differ. Eczema can be either dry, scaly and itchy (psoric), inclined to fester with staphylococcal infection (sycotic) or have a tendency to suppurate and bleed and be accompanied by distress at night as well as depression (syphilitic/ tubercular) – and indeed can shift back and forth between. Yet not everything can be so neatly compartmentalised as all this might imply.

Suppose we take the case of a child who suffers from intolerance to milk. The common symptoms would be a history of ear infections with the production of thick pus and wax from one or both ears (glue ear); a history of throat infections with swollen tonsils and neck glands; the constant production of mucus from the nose with a post-nasal drip that might well cause stomach aches and occasional bouts of nausea and vomiting of frothy, mucous matter. There would be an inevitable history of antibiotics to suppress the many fevers that the patient would have created in an effort to throw off the toxic effects of cow's milk. Quite commonly – and without any apparent connection to the milk and dairy intolerance – there is also a history of tantrums between acute bouts of pain and fever. It is increasingly obvious that many such children also suffer from some form of learning difficulty; anything from dyslexia, dyspraxia and dyscalculia to chronic inability to concentrate on a set task.

The simple solution is to remove dairy produce from the patient's diet altogether. What this will almost certainly do is to remove all the acute symptoms. It should also improve the patient's ability to concentrate – though not necessarily as much as one would like. What it does *not* do is to deal with the susceptibility to being affected by dairy produce – which is chiefly peculiar to tuberculism. If we look at the symptom picture of the patient while he was still taking the dairy products then we can see that underlying the condition is actually a mixture of tuberculism and sycosis. There is the thick, green or yellow pus and mucus (features of both miasms); there is the tendency to swollen glands with high fever (mostly tubercular in children though it is common to both miasms). There is, rather more controversially, the vaccination factor (sycotic) which often triggers the whole problem off – usually around the age of three to nine months; shortly after the DPT inoculation.

The tendency to tantrums may initially seem to be the deciding factor to determine from which miasm any continuing problem stems: if the child has bouts of fury which are triggered by frustration, tiredness and admonishment then he is in the tubercular miasm; if he has rages that suddenly erupt for no apparent cause, are totally unreasonable and are impossible to placate until exhaustion sets in then he is in the sycotic miasm. It is very common for children (particularly) to display symptoms of first the tubercular and then the sycotic state.[1] What happens in practice, however, as constitutional treatment unfolds the case, is that remedies are needed to deal with first one miasm and then another.

In childhood conditions where a miasmatic tendency acts as a maintaining cause and thus blocks further treatment, the miasmatic influence is taken as the focus of the prescription. It is frequently observed that this 'sets the ball rolling' and reveals more work to be done that may in turn bring up another miasm to be so dealt with. This is no less true in adults. It is often the case that a particular condition – say, rheumatoid arthritis or gout, for example, which are chiefly sycotic – progresses well until a subtle shift in the symptom picture betrays the evidence of another miasm. This is not to say that the treatment causes additional problems; it is to say that miasmatic and constitutional treatment with remedies will not necessarily stop with the removal of the patient's initial, presenting symptom picture if there are other underlying features of potential disease.

Once started on the course of self-healing initiated by the first remedies, the body is not likely to stop demanding further treatment for the remaining subliminal negative energies still left in play. A patient, unhampered by any avoidance tactics as the result of an emotional agenda, has every reason to

persevere even when symptoms, seemingly unrelated to the presenting illness, arise. Unless a remedy is being taken frequently and consistently
(which might suggest any new symptoms being an inadvertent proving),
such new symptoms would be highly likely to be evidence of an underlying
tendency coming to the surface for attention – they would in fact be 'old
symptoms' returning.

Let's take gout as our example. A patient with gout is a psoric, usually
well into sycosis. There is swelling, redness – due to excesses (sycosis) – and
the formation of uric acid crystals in the spaces between the small joints (a
psoric solution to a toxic problem).[2] *Sulphur* is a common remedy in gout
and is identified by swelling of the big toe with redness and burning of the
foot, especially at night; it is also frequently the remedy of choice when the
acute attack is caused by overindulgence in red wine. *Sulphur* often works
well here but equally often fails to stop the next attack. *Medorrhinum* is
commonly prescribed to support the action of *Sulphur*. But then the patient
may return to complain of a developing chronic pain in the knee of the
other leg; it is achy but not swollen, causes the patient to feel restless and to
want to move it about and to feel that the whole limb is weak. There might
be other more fleeting pains as well, in the ankle and thigh. This might be
viewed as further evidence of the gout, on the move, so to speak. As the new
symptoms are covered by other sycotic remedies such as *Thuja* and *Rhus
Tox.* it may take several attempts to tell us to look deeper into the system
than these common remedies.

We may well have to look into the psyche: the patient has generally
begun to feel restive and intolerant of his immediate surroundings; perhaps
he has even decided to move house or he has thoughts of changing his job
or he is desperate to have a holiday and go off to the Bahamas. This is actually the moment when the patient is expressing the tubercular aspect of the
arthritis that has been provoked by the gout treatment. It is *Tuberculinum*
that will cause the Vital Force to ease the new symptoms that had initially
looked so much part of the chronic gout picture but were, in fact, something from another level that had surfaced as a result of treating the true
gout layer.

What happens in so many chronic cases is that patients begin to unravel
their *whole* miasmatic inheritance and they do so as if they were peeling off

the layers of an onion. If we follow patients who have been through many years of treatment then it is possible to see the cyclical patterns they go through; they travel, so to speak, through one miasmatic territory after another, doing each one in turn, layer by layer. The body, restless in its search for optimum health, takes every opportunity to dig deep into its history. Each prescription is equivalent to the next layer of soil stripped from the surface of an archaeological site. *Each prescription is a chance for the body to remember how it should function.*

As so many of the patterns that have been laid down in the course of a person's life and those of previous generations are so multilayered and intricately woven, it would be well nigh impossible for any of us to eliminate all the influences of a miasm with just one prescription. The amount of work necessary on each of the miasms that we hold is too much for us to be able to produce curative eliminative reactions in one go; so we do things more gradually, more safely, bit by bit. Each return to a miasmatic state is characterised by the same elements as before but each turn is less dramatic, less severe.

Sometimes a return will make its appearance through a different part of the body; if so, that part would be less significant in terms of vital function. For example, someone with a history of kidney infections characterised by excruciating pains, bleeding and general lassitude and 'flu-like symptoms might well initially have needed *Syphilinum* to support remedies such as *Nitric Acid* and *Terebinth* (oil of turpentine). Once the threat of further dangerous infections is past, the patient may well reveal a tendency to sycotic infection – which underlay the now quietened syphilitic acute episodes. The symptoms might include aching and tenderness in the testicle (often the left), thick and turbid urine, a tendency to a forked stream of urine and a marked loss of energy in the daytime. This is a typical picture of someone requiring *Medorrhinum* and *Thuja*. There might, perhaps at the same time next year, be a further need for a very similar series of prescriptions but, on this occasion, for redness and swelling of the foreskin with first a few painful spots on the glans (*Syphilinum/Nitric Acid*) and, later, itching (*Medorrhinum*). The body is simply continuing to manifest a bit more of the syphilitic and sycotic states but in a way that is safer and further from vital organs – and doing it cyclically and, quite often, seasonally.

It is not uncommon, either, for relatively well patients who come for relief from symptoms to do with poor energy and difficult emotions, at some point to start to produce physical symptoms that require quite different strategies of prescription. What had been treatment at the level of the psyche becomes treatment at the level of the physical body. The whole will have been processing negative energy towards being physically expressed so that the very cells of the body are included in the healing. This is to recognise that patients need to do more than gnash their teeth or weep and wail; if the physical body is not part of the process of eliminating chronic patterns of negative energy then there is no permanent healing. The microcosm of the body's cells must reflect the macrocosm of the psyche.

Mapping the miasms

By knowing the characteristics and personalities of the individual miasms and understanding how each one grows out of the same rootstock, it is possible to use them as a route map and guide to prescribing appropriately. We can follow a patient's progress as he or she gradually self-heals their way through the different miasmatic territories. For those who are willing and who seek transformation through their self-healing, gradually unravelling the miasmatic threads is absolutely fundamental. None of us, at least in the western world, are free of the miasms.

We know that all the great remedies have different miasmatic aspects to them. *Sulphur* can be:

   i)   fat and jolly (sycotic);
   ii)   unkempt, lean and hungry (psoric);
  iii)   restless, asthmatic and hot in bed – in both meanings of the phrase (tubercular);
   iv)   emaciated, fragile, alcoholic (syphilitic);
   v)   hot-bodied yet emaciated and plagued by either constipation or diarrhoea (cancer).

Calcium Carbonate can be:

   i)   fair, chubby and flabby (psoric);

ii)   thin, pale, blue-eyed and with frequently swollen glands and
      throat infections (tubercular);

iii) dropsical, chilly and costive with a tendency to overheat in bed
      or with exertion (sycotic);

iv)   emaciated with suppurating glands, ulceration and fistulae and
      easily floored by deathly lethargy (syphilitic);

v)   troubled with athlete's foot and fungal infections
      (leprotic/tubercular).

The list is endless. We also have the nosodes which can be seen both as remedies in their own right, with unique *Materia Medica* pictures, and as remedies to support other indicated medicines that have miasmatic affinities but that are, on their own, insufficient to deal with the whole condition because of the underlying miasmatic impediment.

Every student of homoeopathy must study the miasms as a musician perfects his technique and studies the mechanics of his instrument with the theory and history of music. Without this basic grounding there is no possibility of practising the science of homoeopathy as a profession. Yet each student must arrive at his or her own unique understanding of the miasms from the standpoint of his or her own life experience. Only when this is achieved can students truly practise the art of homoeopathy. Applying knowledge from medical books is 'healing by numbers'. There must come a time when the practitioner closes the books and hears only what the patient has to say.

NOTES

Preface

1 Allopathy: 1842 (German *allopathie*; Hahnemann). "The curing of a diseased action by the inducing of another of a different kind, yet not necessarily diseased." 'Opposite of Homoeopathy', *Oxford English Dictionary*, by which is meant that the practitioner, seeing that the patient is suffering a particular condition, seeks to suppress that state by introducing a drug (a chemical) that will be stronger than the cause of the symptoms with the result that the cause would no longer be able to sustain those symptoms. Today the word 'allopathy' carries the less precise meaning of 'conventional' medicine.

2 This is not to say that homoeopaths would ignore the vital role of testing and surgical equipment.

3 Except where I quote from scientific sources to make a point.

PART I

Chapter 1

1 Many remedies are well known for what are called time aggravations. *Lycopodium's* aggravation of symptoms between 4 and 8 p.m. is an example. Other remedies cover symptoms that are exacerbated at different times of day: *Belladonna* and *Apis* deal with fevers that are worse around 3 p.m.; an asthma attack that comes on at midnight usually calls for *Aconite* etc.

Chapter 2

1 That the inherent faculty for self-healing is 'intelligent' is denied or disputed from the beginning of homoeopathic literature; it is viewed much as a sailor would regard a gyroscope – only responsive to the loss of balance and a shift of direction. Certainly, the intelligence is not evident in primarily physical conditions. By reading further you may find that it becomes easier to believe in the possibility of something akin to intelligence motivating that self-healing as you become acquainted with cases where the mind, emotions and spirit are far more in evidence. Whether the intelligence is inherently part of the 'faculty' or is in some arcane way what drives it, must remain a subtle point for debate beyond the scope of this book.

2 *Arnica* is not only a remedy for acute bruising; it is also a remedy that is indicated in chronic cases of rheumatism in one whose temperament has become morose and who is physically restless because his pains make it impossible for him to find a comfortable position to settle in.

Chapter 5

1 Bleak though the idea seems, epidemic acute diseases often assume the role of culling in times of disaster. The net result is that it is the fittest who most often survive.

Chapter 6

1 In 1845 Hering wrote the Preface to the American edition of Hahnemann's *The Chronic Disease* in which he stated the four principles of the Law of Cure.

2 An 'intercurrent' remedy is one that is given to support or promote the action of another that would otherwise not be able to complete its action. This is common when a patient arrives at a point in their treatment when there is a block to cure: this is often a hereditary disposition.

Part II

Chapter 7

1 Remedies that support indicated remedies are either remedies that are used to strengthen weakened organs while otherwise indicated remedies do their work, or they are nosodes that are given to ensure that any hereditary or historical block to cure cannot interrupt the effectiveness of the chosen main remedy.
2 See Part III on the miasms.
3 There are times, as mentioned before in the first part of the book, when allopathic medicines and homoeopathic remedies must work alongside each other. This is most common in long-term chronic pathology. For example, antibiotics can be lifesavers in cases of cystic fibrosis where the menace of powerfully entrenched bacteria – often of more than one type – is stronger than the effect of remedies. However, there are also occasions when people resort to drugs to get over a temporary flare-up of an acute episode – say, impetigo in an eczema patient. This is not good practice and is often unnecessary as remedies are quite capable of dealing with such problems but the damage from the suppression is usually relatively negligible.
4 The way to minimise aggravations is to select the dosage of the appropriate remedy accurately and to know when to support it with complementary remedies.
5 The remedy that solved this problem of the stuck sphenoid was made from sycamore seed, a remedy that has an affinity with this particular cranial structure. However, the chance of its success was greatly enhanced by the fact that an osteopath was involved in the treatment as well.
6 *Carcinosin* is a remedy that is very hard to pin down to a single characteristic portrait unlike the other remedies mentioned in this section. This remedy is discussed more broadly in Part III. Suffice it to say that it is a remedy that is often called for when patients suffer from an overwhelming sense of fear that they will develop cancer – especially when this is accompanied by a confused mix of symptoms that seem to call for various other identifiable remedies.

Chapter 8

1 Several practitioners in Boulder, Colorado, which is just a short distance from Rocky Flats where the USA government held much of its plutonium stocks, report that patients do better if their treatment is first begun with a dose of *Plutonium* 30c or 200c.
2 X-ray has its own distinct homoeopathic picture which first emerged from a proving undertaken in 1897 by Dr Bernhardt Fincke and published in 1910 by Dr H.C. Allen. The symptoms of the woman in the case cited here did not match those of the remedy, thus suggesting evidence that X-ray was curative only because it was homoeopathic to the return of the disease after exposure to the mild doses of radiation from the scan.
3 Something that is worthy of further research is that people with a natural inclination to be vegetarians seem to have less trouble with coffee and it may not be so much of a cause for homoeopathic concern.
4 One should avoid toothpaste that contains fluoride. The statistical research that proves that it is effective in oral or dental hygiene is both suspect and flawed. Fluoride is a poison which primarily affects the glandular system. The tonsils, the first line of internal defence of the body and in close proximity to the mouth, are the most immediately vulnerable organs.

Chapter 11

1 Isopathy in cases of drug toxicity seems not to be thoroughly successful as often as one might wish, because the energy created by the poisoning effect of the drug on the patient's system is not always precisely matched by, and is not necessarily truly similar to, the

energy of the homoeopathically prepared drug remedy. The poisoning effects of every drug may have some or many aspects in common from one patient to another, but in effect each individual patient is going to respond in his or her own individual way to any particular drug. A drug such as lithium has so many and varied side effects – from gastrointestinal upset to coma, from fine tremor to hypothyroidism – that it would be quite impossible for a patient to produce all of them. Lithium as a homoeopathically prepared remedy would not necessarily cover all the symptoms that it creates as a material substance.

Chapter 12

1 Wild yam is known to homoeopaths as *Dioscorea*. This remedy is well known as a healer of terrible colic.
2 This aspect is looked at in greater depth in Part III, The Miasms.
3 The majority of the population is blood group O.
4 Chorea is involuntary jerking movements – a condition of the nervous system. Chloasma is discoloration of the skin due to liver dysfunction.
5 It is very often surgical intervention to remove cancerous breast tissue that sparks off metastasis, the spread of disease from one site to another.
6 'Some Effects of Oral Contraceptives on Carbohydrate Metabolism' – Prof. V. Wynn: *Lancet*, Oct. 1966.
7 The Walnut Creek Contraceptive Drug Study: Centre for Population Research Monograph NIH Bethesda 1981. (S. Ramcharan et al.). 'Oral Contraceptives, Smoking, Migraine and Food Allergy', *Lancet*, Sept. 1978. One of the statistics showed the following: that of 81 women who had recently died of vascular disease 6 per cent had never smoked or used the Pill; 10 per cent had smoked; 19 per cent had used the Pill; 65 per cent had both smoked and used the Pill. Interestingly enough this was used as proof that it was quite safe to take the Pill as long as you did not smoke as well. Once again logic seemed to elude the researchers who ignored the fact that the figures also demonstrated that it was 9 per cent more dangerous to take the Pill than it was to smoke.
8 'Adenocarcinoma of the Vagina, Association of Maternal Stilbestrol Therapy with Tumour Appearance in Young Women', A.L. Herbst et al. *New England Journal of Medicine*, 1971.
9 DES is still used today even though it carries warnings about its considerable toxicity. Ironically it is used in the treatment of breast cancer in menopausal women and occasionally in prostate cancer in men. Its list of side effects all bear out the discoveries made in 1971.

Chapter 13

1 I am thoroughly indebted to the contributors to a paper put out on the Internet called 'The Amalgam Issue' edited under the auspices of DAMS Inc. and the Consumers for Dental Choice, a project of the National Institute for Science, Law and Public Policy, 1424 16th Street, NW suite 105 Washington DC 20036. It can be found at www.amalgam.org
2 Some vaccine producing companies are now, belatedly, producing mercury-free vaccines following protests from concerned parents and pressure groups.
3 See *Trace Element Imbalances in Isolated Subcellular Fractions of Alzheimer's Disease Brains* (D. Wenstrup, W.D. Ehmann, and W.R. Markesbery) Brain Research, 533 125–131 Elsevier Science Publishers (1990) as quoted in The Dental Amalgam Issue DAMS Inc. Also see *Mercury Vapour Inhalation Binding of GTP to Tubulin in Rat Brain: Similarity to a Molecular Lesion in Human Alzheimer Brain* (Pendergrass, Haley Boyd, Murray, Winfield and Lorscheider) quoted in the same publication.
4 The study quoted in the DAMS Inc publication cited above is *Heavy Metals and Infertility* (Gerhard, Monga, Waldbrenner and Runnebaum. 1998)
5 *Marked Elevation of Myocardial Trace Elements in Idiopathic Dilated Cardiomyopathy Compared with Secondary Cardiac Dysfunction* (Frustaci, Magnavita, Chimenti, Caldarulo, Sabbioni, Pietra, Cellini and Maseri: Dept. of Cardiology, Catholic University, Rome) as quoted in The Dental Amalgam Issue by DAMS Inc.
6 T-lymphocytes are cells that identify foreign microbial bodies and 'label' them so that killer cells can be sent to despatch the intruders. Tests carried out in the USA strongly

suggest that mercury kills off these vital cells. (See the *WDDTY Dental Handbook* published by What Doctors Don't Tell You.)

7 See *What Doctors Don't Tell You: Dental Handbook* which includes a brief but comprehensive article by Dr Hal Huggins on the findings of Weston Price, an American dentist determined to prove the fallacy of several long-held beliefs about dentistry.

Chapter 14

1 Ibid.

Chapter 15

1 Usually by overenthusiastic alternative-minded medical journalists.

2 One only has to think of the cow which, by eating quantities of grass, can produce 8–10 pints of milk per day that is rich in calcium. She could not possibly donate such excessive amounts of calcium from her own bones on a long-term daily basis without succumbing to rickets. The answer is that her system is programmed to synthesise it, just in far larger quantities than a biochemist would expect from a grass-eater.

3 Osteoporosis is a disease that is usually post-menopausal and characterised by bone becoming brittle and porous. It is considered to be associated with heredity. It most commonly affects the lower back and causes the spine to curve.

4 It is interesting to note that the metal cadmium sulphate, in its homoeopathic potency, is a very efficient remedy at encouraging the elimination of side effects of cytotoxic drugs from patients who are going through or have been through chemotherapy for cancer.

5 Liver is not to everyone's taste not least because modern farming methods of pumping cattle full of antibiotics and hormones cause the meat to be so unpalatable – morally and gastronomically. The best way to deal with this is to soak the liver (or kidneys) in milk for 6-8 hours before cooking. The milk draws out all the toxic waste still in the liver and leaves it tender and nutritious.

6 See What Doctors Don't Tell You *Guide To Your Heart*.

7 There are no diets that should ever be regarded as specific any more than there are specific remedies for particular pathologies. Every individual must be assessed on their individual needs. The Hay diet of food-combining might suit some people but for others it can create intestinal havoc. Weight Watchers has been going for years basing its system on the simple premise that counting calories and cutting out what is excessive and potentially bad for you is best, but it does not work for everyone. There are not a few patients who discover to their surprise that a diet with a heavily increased intake of animal protein and a reduction of vegetable consumption causes a significant weight loss. It seems that there are no set rules for diets and dieting. However, the idea that one's dietary requirement is dictated by one's blood type does deserve great attention. Most recently promulgated in the books *Eat Right for your Type* and *Live Right for your Type* by Dr Peter D'Adamo (Putnams/Michael Joseph) this theory, based on the human evolution of blood types, has a great deal to recommend it. It has the merit of being very simple and not being based on restrictions of quantity. (The best diet for blood group O is nothing less than what has been dubbed the Atkins diet.)

Chapter 16

1 *A Shot in the Dark* by Harris Coulter (1985) Harcourt Brace Jovanovich, New York, is a salutary exercise in chronicling the haste of medical science. Also *Vaccination: The Medical Assault on the Immune System* by Viera Scheibner – ISBN 0646 15124 X. It is to this exhaustive study of hundreds of scientific journals and articles both for and against vaccination and on the history of inoculation that I am indebted for much of the evidence used in this chapter.

2 It might be noted that *Thymus gland*, prepared as a homoeopathic remedy, has no full orthodox proving as yet. It is used here as a support remedy to more constitutional prescribing.

3 A sobering article by Viera Scheibner published in *Nexus* magazine (Vol. 5 #5 – Aug '98) [www.nexusmagazine.com] homes in on the co-incidence of DPT vaccination and 'shaken baby syndrome'. As the article points out, it is remarkable how many parents or

minders, who are subject to investigation on a charge of maltreating their children or charges, do not realise that the babies may have been reacting to the DPT jab.

4 Essential reading is *Everything There is to Know about Vaccination,* Joanna Karpasea-Jones, (1999) VAN UK, PO Box 6261, Derby, DE1 9QN. Website: www.vaccine-info.com.

5 An illuminating exercise is to search the Internet for web sites about 'vaccine damage': just these two words will bring up more than 200,000 possible sites. A large number of them refer to litigation and compensation sought for damage and death. So widespread is the need for legal expertise that there are law firms that specialise in this one aspect of medical justice.

6 Reported in *The Daily Telegraph,* 28 September 2004.

7 What Doctors Don't Tell You – www.wddty.co.uk

8 The term 'celiac disease' originally was applied to the potentially fatal inability of an infant's gut to deal with gluten that is in wheat products; the symptoms were no less than the effects of poisoning. Today, the term has come to be used to describe intolerance to wheat generally, even in those with comparatively mild symptoms.

9 *Silica* is another remedy for vaccinosis and was chosen in this case for its close affinity with *Pulsatilla* and its reputation for working on glands and ears. It has a centrifugal effect on the body which starts to eliminate any foreign matter from tonsils and ears, particularly in children. It is usual for children who need *Pulsatilla* to need *Silica* as a support remedy whether or not they are vaccine damaged.

10 Hahnemann did not, of course, know anything about the physics and chemistry of heredity. It was his clinical observation based on his many cases that led him to postulate that we inherit disease patterns, best described as susceptibilities. His work is not negated by our contemporary knowledge but complemented. We need only to read his work in the light of the as yet incomplete information we have respecting DNA and genetics in general to realise how very far advanced he was in his thinking.

Chapter 18

1 *Ant. Tart.* is a remedy that is most often used in the acute state. It is particularly known for its effects on the lungs when there is a great build-up of mucus that threatens to congest the airways. The patient is obliged to sit up to cough and there is a tremendous amount of rattling of phlegm. It has been known to pull patients back from the brink of an emergency situation.

Chapter 19

1 See the section on the Pill above. This case also illustrates that *Folliculinum* is a remedy that can be prescribed for other reasons than a history of having taken oral contraceptives.

2 The general rule is that remedies are entirely harmless in any circumstance but it is also true that there are occasions, as has been illustrated in Part I, when a patient with severe physical pathology might respond too rapidly to eliminative remedies and thus be in danger of becoming too depleted too quickly.

3 *Proteus* is a bowel nosode; that is a remedy made from the natural bacterial bowel flora that is found in the gut. It has been found in excess in those who have suffered the difficulties and ignominy of becoming exiles or immigrants.

Part III

Introduction

1 The personalities that populate the fairy stories of the brothers Grimm, of E.T.A. Hoffmann and of Hans Christian Andersen are equally redolent of miasmatic characteristic behaviour, being motivated by love, faith, hope, grief, despair, villainy and violence. No less are the tales of Beatrix Potter and J.K. Rowling. The tales of these authors all share the same purpose: to identify the motivational energy that drives people to be what they are and to do what they do.

Chapter 20

1 John Henry Clarke (1853-1931), author of the *Dictionary of Practical Materia Medica*, Homoeopathic Publishing, 1900 and *The Prescriber*, Keene and Ashwell, 1885 (revised 1925) was a prolific author whose works are still in constant use today.

2 This may have been due to the suppression or neglect of the frequent bouts of erysipelas that he suffered.

3 When these two great constitutional remedies are influenced by any of the other miasms then we find it necessary to qualify the basic, fundamental, psoric descriptions. For example, a *Calcium* person who is essentially tubercular may still be chilly, costive, anxious and methodical but he will also be restless, easily dissatisfied, irritable, oversensitive to his environment and given to disease of glandular tissue, the chest and skin. It is also far more likely that diseases will appear quickly with stress and leave deeper impressions on the body's memory. When the characteristic restlessness of the tubercular miasm affects a *Sulphur* person then the result is to create an inveterate traveller; someone who must go in search of interest and excitement and who finds it hard to stick to a career or put down roots.

4 See *Portraits of Homoeopathic Medicines*, Catherine Coulter, North Atlantic Books, 1988.

Chapter 21

1 It is increasingly common for children to produce shingles.

2 In the following chapter, on sycosis, it will be seen that the lesions of chickenpox and shingles can also be sycotic as well as syphilitic.

3 Psoric chickenpox can transform into sycosis (i.e. the gonorrhoea miasm) if the symptoms are manifest with that miasm's typical characteristics – inflammation and heavily infected pus.

4 It is noteworthy that antibiotics are only useful in eradicating *Treponema* when the spirochetes are initially active. Once they cross the 'blood-brain barrier' – the point where the circulating blood enters the part of the brain that contains no red cells but only cerebrospinal fluid – they are quite beyond the reach of most antibiotics.

5 The late twentieth-century history of the HIV virus, in any of its numbered forms, illustrates this point. Before it became common knowledge in the 1980s that HIV was 'responsible' for creating the AIDS epidemic, HIV was simply a relatively harmless virus that no scientist bothered much about. Viruses are opportunists though, and with the increasingly frail immune systems of those groups of patients most at risk, HIV graduated to become something far more sinister. It is no accident that those groups – homosexuals, drug users and poverty-stricken Third World communities – are also the ones most in need of frequent suppressive treatment. It is among them that syphilis and gonorrhoea are most rife and this created a high demand for antibiotics. Nor is it an accident that AIDS in its many guises can look so like syphilis.

6 It ought to be said that some commentators deny that Schumann's final illness was tertiary syphilis as the medical evidence is too sparse. In spite of a suspicious scar on his foreskin that he had had since youth and all the circumstantial evidence, any preferred diagnosis is obstinately elusive though schizophrenia and 'primary psychiatric illness' have been put forward – both of which, incidentally, are often regarded as syphilitic in homoeopathy.

7 As we shall see in the chapter on sycosis, there is a difference between syphilitic and sycotic suicide; one seeks to leave a trail of trauma and devastation while the other almost seeks to minimise the event while creating out of it a *cri de coeur* ; they often make several botched attempts, seeking easy options and leaving notes of sorrow and apology.

8 There is often a strong desire among syphilitic suicides to leave behind them a scene of tragedy that is their powerful and indelible mark of punishment or vengeance. Sometimes it is specifically aimed at one person – in Anna's case, she is determined that her lover shall pay for his callousness – and in other cases at the world in general.

9 It is intriguing that Emma swallows arsenic, the very poison that would, in homoeopathic potency, have done Flaubert himself some good. He was a perfectionist to the point of fastidiousness about his work; so much so that it might have been responsible for the only very small body of work that he produced.

10 Remember William Gladstone: he suffered from erysipelas on and off for years. This disease is psoric/syphilitic and, though he always got through the acute episodes, eventually his body gave up on producing it and he developed the far more threatening cancer of the face that eventually killed him.

11 It remains a moot point whether or not antibiotics would have made a significant difference to either of these composers – or any other great artist denied this form of suppressive treatment by history. As antibiotics weaken the immune system and as most gifted creators – at least those who do not remain in psora – tend greatly to exceed their energy limitations through pursuit of ideas, it is more than likely that there would have been little difference in the outcome of their lives as far as their art was concerned. The suppression of their state would more than likely have led to their deaths from some other terminal condition such as cancer. (A sweeping statement perhaps, except that most of the great syphilitic composers – Mozart and Smetana included – left a satisfyingly complete body of work despite the unfinished pieces remaining on their desks at their deaths. Their work, created with extraordinary intensity, described their individual life journeys.)

12 It is extremely unlikely that herbal preparations alone would be able to effect a cure of syphilis today, not because the plants used do not have the efficacy they once had nor because early observers were not strictly scientific enough and reported inaccurately about 'cures' that never really happened. The problem is that over the last hundred years we have become such a complex of miasms that plants would not be able on their own and in their material form to unravel the tangle of disease taints on which the acute form of syphilis would become engrafted.

13 Clarke was a homoeopath but his knowledge of herbalism was profound. He was not constrained by any limitations and happily used herbal tinctures where he felt they were needed.

14 *Corydalis* has not had a full proving in any of its potencies. Any prescription of it must therefore have been made based on the information gained from reports of cases 'cured'.

15 Fortunately for posterity, mercury was not used on either Schubert or Schumann. Paganini, the famous virtuoso violinist, was not so lucky. Though tubercular/syphilitic by nature, he may not have suffered syphilis at all but he was given mercury to swallow by various practitioners for a chronic throat condition. The result was that he never got better and spent years becoming more and more gaunt, wracked by disease of the lungs and bowels and increasingly hypochondriacal. He died a ruined recluse. He is, perhaps, a prime example of a patient expressing the syphilitic miasm and 'choosing' a peculiarly apt method (the use of mercury) to determine the declining course of his health – as if he had a death wish. (He was one of the very first performing celebrities, much swooned over by ladies in withdrawing rooms; he was reputed to be in league with the Devil because of his prodigious virtuosity – a nineteenth-century Jimi Hendrix!)

16 Some of these 'mind' symptoms may seem rather extreme when everyday prescribing has mostly to do with mainly physical conditions. Yet it is actually common enough to see degrees of these psychic states very commonly in those suffering from acute infections. Feverish children brewing tonsillitis can easily appear restless, agitated and frightened. An adult hatching a tooth abscess can readily produce mood swings, irascibility and anguish with pain that can induce a feeling of becoming demented.

17 *Mercurius* is a remedy for heartburn and other acid problems of the gut such as ulceration. In intractable cases it is often worth considering the patient's amalgam fillings as contributing to the problem.

18 Other remedies that have a reputation for positively affecting MS symptoms include *Causticum*, *Phosphorus*, *Nux Vomica* and *Lathyrus* (chickpea).

19 It is far more usual than not for a homoeopath to find it impossible to select his or her own remedies except in the most obvious acute situations.

20 Leucorrhoea, sometimes called 'the whites' (inappropriately as it can also be yellow, green, pink, brown, grey or khaki), is a vaginal discharge.

21 The recognition of the syphilis gene might be unlikely for some time to come. Who would claim to have discovered and labelled a kink on a gene as syphilis, an acute disease, after

all? What is required here is the toleration of the idea that acute diseases such as syphilis, gonorrhoea and tuberculosis might be hereditarily transmissible and might contribute to the susceptibility to so many of the ills that we suffer and that are read off the gene printout as other named conditions – while at the same time accepting that emotions and psyche share the responsibility for manifesting disease.

22 See Chapter 16, note 8.

23 She had *Pulsatilla* 30s and 1M because, apart from the phlegm (which *Pulsatilla* matches well), she was susceptible to heat and stuffiness (which made her feel faint), drank very little in the way of fluids and was dependent on her husband and friends for company which she felt was so important – all of which are keynotes of *Pulsatilla*. She also had *Tuberculinum* 200 because her grandfather had had TB in the 1920s (see the chapter on TB).

24 For this picture she was given *Sepia* 200 which is a well-known remedy for women who are worn out and 'sag' – the back aches, the abdomen hangs heavy, the pelvic floor feels incompetent to support the internal organs any more. Though she responded quite well to this initially, the improvement did not last. The prescription was only superficial.

25 Tonic spasms are those which are continuous and with no relaxation; clonic spasms are those in which there is repeated spasm and relaxation.

26 Strangely, sexual relations were not abandoned; thrush was a frequent problem to be treated in both and was reported as being the result of intercourse. Each saw the other to blame though neither actually said so.

Chapter 22

1 It should be noted that warts are not exclusively sycotic. Warts do appear in psora and syphilis as well. They also crop up in the TB and cancer miasms though the appearance and behaviour of the warts and of their owner is what guides the practitioner to recognise which miasm is showing and to the appropriate prescription for their removal. Psoric warts tend to be slow growing, dry and painless; syphilitic ones tend to crack, bleed, have a blackened surface and be sharply painful.

2 Interestingly, the virus associated with molluscum contagiosum is comparatively large and very similar in appearance to the smallpox virus. It is like two bulbous ends with a narrow waist between; this gives it something in common with the diplococcus which is associated with gonorrhoea.

3 It is also worth mentioning in this context that Edward Jenner began his pioneering work with vaccination in 1798, a year *after* the war with the colonists.

4 Sycosis has its very humorous moments too such as the delicious comedy of hundreds of flower-power hippies attempting to raise the Pentagon off the ground with the collective power of thought.

5 It could be justly said that the practitioner was at fault in this case, in asking about the suppressed gonorrhoea when it was quite obvious that the acute disease had been present in either the boy's parents or, possibly, in the grandparents. It was unnecessary to highlight the gonorrhoea for successful treatment to have taken place.

6 Indulging in gossiping is a very common if non-pathological symptom of sycosis.

7 The equally sycotically driven prince was so repelled by his spouse that he locked her out of their joint coronation.

8 Jalap or jalapa is a form of convolvulus, *Ipomoea purga*.

9 The psoric either views party politics with distaste and a jaundiced eye or would want to contribute on a local level.

10 It is worth quoting from Dr Clarke's *Dictionary* here: 'A school of 200 children was 'internally variolated' with *Variolinum* CMM (the homoeopathic dose) on the evening of Feb. 18th and the morning of Feb. 19th Of the two school mistresses one was not at all affected; the other was two days in bed ill. On the 21st many of the children were ill; by the 23rd all except 40 were, the symptoms being the usual preliminary symptoms of Smallpox and later Swan [*the homoeopath*] found pustules on many. After the varioloid [*i.e. the proving of the remedy*] had passed off but before the children had recovered their vitality, 23 were vaccinated [*materially*] without Swan's knowledge. All but one 'took' and had

terrible ulcers on the arms and had to be remedied by *Vaccininum* CMM.' (i.e. Swan had to use the homoeopathic *Vaccininum* as the direct antidote to the material vaccine.)

11 An oft-quoted case is that of the woman who went to hospital for treatment with her legs wrapped up in brown paper and string. She did this, she explained, because she felt that her legs were so fragile that they would shatter.

12 Quoted from Dr Clarke's *Dictionary*. These are from cases cured by *Thuja*.

13 For a fuller appraisal of the miasmatic tendencies behind learning difficulties, see Chapter 23 on tuberculosis. It is often confusing to realise that *Thuja* can be both a sycotic and a tubercular remedy and that either miasm might call for *Thuja*'s services – sometimes in the same case.

14 The tubercular miasm is also to be reckoned with in eczema and asthma but it is itself a product, as we shall see in the next section, of the other three miasms.

15 Verrucae or plantar warts, being a type of wart, are essentially sycotic though they have echoes within the other miasms. They are often useful indicators of how well a patient is discharging on a miasmatic level. As such they should be strictly left alone unless painful or infected. Contrary to popular belief, verrucae are not contagious. They are expressions from within the body of miasmatic inheritance.

16 *Thuja* covers this curious symptom – the sensation in the abdomen of a foetus moving around.

Chapter 23

1 It should be taken into account that in the nineteenth century the distinction between acute and chronic disease was not so clearly defined; it is harder to ascribe causation to emotional and spiritual conditions when considering acute and epidemic diseases. Even these days, over a century later, it is assumed that stress is restricted to causing only chronic and, often, indeterminate conditions such as irritable bowel syndrome or ME.

2 See the reference to the poet, Keats' death on p. 606

3 See *Béchamp or Pasteur*, by Ethel Douglas Hume for a devastating reappraisal of Pasteur's work on anthrax.

4 Pasteur 'attenuated' his vaccines by cultivating the bacteria in isolation in a series of cultures. Into each culture he put a drop of the preceding culture so that the last of the series was then able still to provoke the disease symptoms but only so weakly that the host's immune system would deal with the resulting infection. Though this procedure has direct parallels with the homoeopathic preparation of medicines, the essential difference is that there is no succussion in Pasteur's method; what is more, there is still disease material in the vaccine.

5 In her book Miss Hume is careful to give the dates of submission to the Academy of Science by the two men thus showing that Béchamp's work preceded that of Pasteur. It is also clear from the *Comptes Rendus* that Pasteur originally concluded that the generation of fermentation was spontaneous, an idea that he later became famous for scorning.

6 Today microzymas only appear in the dictionary; the word used now is microsome though the phrase *chromatin granules* has also been used. Interestingly, Béchamp is credited in the *Oxford English Dictionary* with the word *zymase* (1875).

7 Enzymes, also named after the Greek word for fermentation or leavening, are complex organic substances that cause transformation of material in plants and animals and are associated with digestion. Through their action, bacteria are formed that break down foods so that they can be absorbed and assimilated into the body. This is very much akin to what Béchamp and Estor observed in microzymal activity. Where they went further was to show how microzymas influence the chemistry of a living being to produce bacteria that are pathogenic as well as others that are beneficial.

8 *Comptes Rendus de l'Académie des Sciences* 66, p. 421 (1868). The operative word in the statement being 'spontaneously'.

9 *La Théorie du Microzyma*, p.116. (Béchamp)

10 *Pasteur Exposed*, Ethel Douglas Hume. (Bookreal, Australia, 1989)

11 Quoted in *Pasteur Exposed*, Ethel Douglas Hume.

12 TB only occurs in humans or in animals that are intimately connected or negatively associated with them.

13 Clean, crisp, mountain air is what tubercular people crave and it was frequently prescribed as part of the cure – hence the famous Swiss sanatoria.

14 There is only one *Psorinum* and only one *Syphilinum* but there is now a second *Medorrhinum* (*Med. Americana*, made from the gonorrhoeal pus from an American patient) and there are several different remedies made from cancerous material.

15 Isopathy is the treatment of a condition by the agent of its cause. Snake venom might be administered to one bitten by the same snake for example; bee-sting venom might be given to heal bee stings. This is similar to 'like cures like' but very much more limited in its scope. It nevertheless has a relatively solid tradition. Koch's idea was to use a preparation of the TB bacillus (in fact a glycerine extract) to combat the disease.

16 It also has some value to chicken fanciers and farmers. A dose of *Tuberculinum Aviare* is very helpful in improving the constitution of the birds, notorious as they are for poor recovery once sickened. (One dose of the 200th potency in the communal drinking water every three to four months is highly recommended though you may like to consult a practitioner first.)

17 Wallowing in nostalgia is usually peculiar to sycosis.

18 There are some forms of insanity that some people would ascribe to possession.

19 *Stramonium* and *Belladonna* belong to the same plant family - the *Solanceæ* (the nightshade family). It is common for one to follow the other or to be mistaken for it.

20 *Tuberculinum* is by no means the only remedy that is prescribed for those who have experienced sexual abuse and the consequent emotional trauma. Even those who have received expert counselling after such an ordeal find that homoeopathic remedies still bring up the unresolved trauma for final resolution. It is a condition for which there is no substitute but to consult a qualified practitioner and it often behoves those in this situation to seek help from both disciplines.

21 In the earlier chapter on sycosis, a case of learning difficulties was related that responded to *Thuja* and *Medorrhinum*. It should be remembered how similar *Tuberculinum* and *Medorrhinum* can appear to be and that *Thuja* is as tubercular a remedy as it is sycotic. It is often the subtle nuances that differentiate for us which remedy or which miasm is indicated. Indeed, it is not uncommon for *Tuberculinum* to be indicated in a case that has just responded to *Medorrhinum* and vice versa. Just why this should be will appear in the following pages.

22 *Lycopodium* is a well-known remedy of service to those who suffer from low blood sugar – hypoglycaemia. It is also very common for it to be indicated after a dose of *Anacardium* has been prescribed; the two remedies are closely related in terms of their energy.

23 For further reading on the homoeopathic aspect of treating children with learning and behavioural difficulties then go to *Ritilin-Free Kids* by Judith Reichenberg-Ullman and Robert Ullman, Prima Publishing, Rocklin, CA (1996).

24 It is not surprising that the younger the patient, the more likely it is the difficulties will gradually diminish while under treatment. This is because there has been less time for the child to form alternative methods of using brain pathways in order to cope with tasks that usual brain pathways would make simple. Older children and young adults with learning difficulties will have formed their own compensatory ways of dealing with the demands on brain function and the consequence of this can be that it is harder for the remedies to effect major change.

25 This susceptibility to colds, coughs, ear infections and glandular swellings that is so typical of *Silica* is also redolent of those who suffer vaccine damage. No surprise then to find that *Silica* is one of the main remedies that are useful in dealing with vaccine damage in children.

26 In describing eczema as tubercular/*Calc. Carb.* what is meant is that the miasm so influences the pathology that *Tuberculinum* is very highly likely to be needed to complement the indicated *Calc. Carb.* to effect a lasting healing. Similarly so with psoric/*Calc. Carb.* eczema or sycotic/ *Nat. Sulph.* asthma or, say, syphilitic/*Aurum* heart disease.

Chapter 24

1 It is likely that there were a few remaining institutions dedicated to lepers more recently than this.

2 When the tubercular fire of creativity is turned onto religion then the result is often highly persuasive to those who might be seeking spiritual support.

3 It is Dr Vakil's proving of the leprosy nosode that provides us with the bulk of the psychological picture of the miasm. We, in northern Europe, need to learn how to apply what appears in the general proving among Indian patients to patients of our very different culture. A small example: the leprotic patients in the proving expressed a strong dislike for the colour black and would not wear black clothing but preferred white – bearing in mind that the subjects would be poor and unlikely to be able to afford expensive textiles. In the West it is likely that this aversion to black would not be so strongly expressed but that the patient might wear white and pastel shades exclusively. The modern trend for pastel colours suits leprotic people as they tend to encourage anonymity. Similarly, European patients are not likely to express their aversion to begging; it is far more of an everyday occurrence in India. This aspect, as far as western patients are concerned, needs to be seen more as a reluctance to ask for and receive financial or moral support. There is in all cases a definite aversion to being pitied.

4 This should not surprise us as it is well known that there are also quite a number of drugs in orthodox medicine that are used for more than one type of condition.

5 One might cite the example of a film star who, confused by fame and money, suddenly retires from the showbiz world and retreats to become involved with an obscure religious order and immerses himself in charitable work.

6 The cases are quoted in the *Proceedings of the 1991 Professional Case Conference* published by the International Foundation for Homoeopathy in which *Leprosinum* was first presented to American homoeopaths.

7 It is worth noting that *Tuberculinum* (close relative to *Bacillinum*) is a listed remedy for leprosy.

Chapter 25

1 For those interested in astrology, it might be noted that one of the governing principles of Cancer is 'I seek myself through what I feel'. Another is the protection and nourishment of one's roots, i.e. home. The disease is so frequently about these very issues. Though it may be fanciful to some, perhaps others would not find it remarkable that Cancer 'rules' the breasts, so commonly the primary site of this disease. The breasts also represent 'nurture' and the mother-child link; cancer is often about unresolved relationships.

2 Normal is 98.4°F.

3 These were typical remedies used from the 1940s. *Carcinosin* began to be widely used in the 1980s though it was, at first, controversial among homoeopaths: despite the fact that Dr Foubister of the London Homoeopathic Hospital had done so much to introduce it as a major remedy *Carcinosin* has not replaced *Thuja* or *Silica*; it complements them.

4 ME should be differentiated from chronic fatigue syndrome. CFS is usually found to be the result of misalignment of the musculoskeletal system. ME is the result of a profoundly inadequate immune system. CFS patients also have a different outlook on life: they really want to throw off their ill health. ME patients, despite frequent calls for treatment, often relapse due to being unwilling to relinquish their dependency on the help of others. (The acronym thus becomes rather apposite even though the full title is virtually meaningless.)

5 Most of these symptoms are also to be found among other remedies. However, when there is a collection of these miscellaneous signals in the one body at one time, then *Carcinosin* is very possibly the indicated similar remedy.

6 Catherine's father may have loved his daughter in his own fashion but this did not deter him from ignoring her piteous and perfectly justified pleas for assistance in favour of diplomacy.

7 Extracts of letters to Queen Victoria from her daughter as quoted in *An Uncommon Woman* by Hannah Pakula, Weidenfeld and Nicholson, 1995. (First published in the USA by Simon & Schuster Inc.)

8 Vicky's one stroke of revenge was that she managed to have her correspondence smuggled out of Germany before her son was able to stop it. The letters were eventually edited and published in the 1920s as a refutation to a twisted and self-congratulatory memoir written by the ageing but unrepentant Wilhelm.

9 Catherine's final, deathbed letter to Henry was an example to us all of a desire for peace and understanding between them. Her plea for God's pardon of him and her own forgiveness may have been hard won but it was genuine – and might have caused Henry a little moment of conscience had he ever read it.

10 This description of Grainger's health does not take account of the possibility that he himself might have suffered from venereal disease. It is highly unlikely that he contracted syphilis because the nature of his final illness developed slowly over a number of years whereas truly syphilitic cancers tend to be very fast and very malignant in their nature. He might have suffered from gonorrhoea at some time and had it suppressed. This is a condition that can eventually raise the susceptibility to prostate cancer.

11 We agonise when we watch film tragedies in which somebody fails to ask someone else a vital question. This only reflects our fear, guilt, shame or another emotion that we cannot for some reason allow to be seen – a form of suppression. The drama in our own hearts has been touched.

12 Cancer cells are graded in terms of their differentiation. The more differentiated, the less malignant is the dynamic of the cell. Stage 1 carcinoma of the breast indicates well differentiated cells in an unfixed tumour – i.e. one that can be thoroughly examined all round and is not fixed to the chest wall. The prognosis of this is comparatively good.

13 *Arsenicum* has a very considerable reputation among homoeopaths for relieving the symptoms that come up in those suffering with cancer. It is often called for as not only does it cover the burning pains and nausea but also the anxiety and restlessness especially in those whose symptoms are worse at night.

14 It is perhaps worth noting that the remedy *Nitric Acid*, as a major part of its characteristic mental picture, covers the inability to forgive even those hurts of very long standing.

15 This should not imply that the doctor does not care about the rest of the patient. Oncologists are fully aware of the potential damage to their patients' welfare from the extraordinarily dangerous drugs that they use.

16 'Empiricism: the use of empirical methods in any art or science i.e. based on or guided by the results of observation and experiment only.' (*Oxford English Dictionary*) This is as opposed to the application of the science or art by adherence to strict rational theories based on logic. All results of inspirational ideas are essentially empirical. Unfortunately they become rational (fixed by means of immutable logic) when they are used as the basis of theoretical laws. Once this happens practitioners wish to abide by the law rather than what they observe; so variation in nature is ignored.

17 All three remedies have acknowledged influence over the female organs. *Thuja* is particularly well documented as being of use in treating patients with cancer. *Sabina*, from the juniper tree, is a very close relative of *Thuja*. *Nitric Acid* is often indicated in such cases when the characteristic needle and shooting pains, sometimes felt in tissue or bone close to tumours, are present.

18 This approach to healing a threatening pathology is in contrast to the 'classical' approach which would still consider the symptoms of the beleaguered psyche as paramount (i.e. despite the symptoms manifest by the affected organ or part, the symptoms of the whole person would be prescribed on). Burnett saw that the diseased part should actually be the focus because the *energy of the disease* in that part is stronger than that of the whole. By taking the 'personality' of the symptom picture of the stricken part, the body is then able to restore the integrity of that part and reintegrate it with the whole. The corollary of this is that once the diseased organ or part is restored to its full integrity, the next step to maintaining health is to prescribe on the whole constitution.

19 It should be noted that Burnett was not alone in successfully treating patients who had cancer. There were others before and after. Burnett has been chosen for my purpose here because he was the best writer on this subject (not least as he avoided all embellishment) and he had such a clear spirit of practical humanity towards his patients.

20 For those who are able to 'see auras', radiation appears to strip away the layers of colour they are normally able to see, leaving holes in the aura.

21 Some homeopaths refuse to treat patients undergoing chemo- and radiotherapy on the grounds that the allopathic treatment would antidote their remedies. The remedies might well be partially compromised (depending on the intensity of the allopathy) but they still are quite capable of benefiting patients while not undermining the intended chemical effects of the allopathic prescription. There is no excuse for not trying, for not offering the body an alternative, *complementary* and simultaneous healing potential to help reduce the discomfort of pernicious side effects and even the risk of metastasis of the cancer.

22 Both *Aconite* and *Oak* are important for situations when the patient is in abject terror. *Aconite* is used for stark fear; *Oak* is indicated when patients have to face an ongoing ordeal where judgements are being made either with or about them and they have to keep a level head.

23 These include *Radium Bromide*, *Radium Iodatum* and *Sol*. *Calendula* (common pot marigold) was also used for the healing of the surface skin. *Urtica Urens* (stinging nettle) was used to relieve the appalling itching that surfaced (curatively) after the use of the other remedies.

24 The older the age at which a forebear produces cancer, the less significant a feature it is when looking into the family history of a patient. The younger the relative was, the weaker their constitution was and therefore the more susceptible the constitution that is handed down.

25 Surely it was no accident of nature that the First World War was succeeded by the most devastating epidemic of 'flu ever suffered that despatched more people than had died in the previous five years of fighting.

26 In sycotic patients one of the difficulties can be that they believe their forward step is in the direction of opening themselves up to spiritual awareness. Though this is important for all of us, the sycotic goes into it with such enthusiasm that they fail to see how 'ungrounded' they have become. So often the effect is that they abdicate the responsibility for the cure of the condition to 'the higher self'; this is a long way from psora.

Chapter 26

1 Though the *Malaria* 30 undoubtedly did this man good generally he was unable to sustain the improvement. Within a short time his arthritic condition went back to its usual state though this has to be weighed against the fact that his wife, already chronically ill physically, became so confused and abusive with the onset of Alzheimer's that she had to be *"put away"*. Shortly after she died and he had a double hip replacement.

Chapter 27

1 It is not good enough to dismiss ancient shamanism as belonging to unsophisticated cultures in which the short life expectancy was a measure of the fundamental ignorance of their medical knowledge. Many ancient cultures were civilised enough to have very profound knowledge of herbal medicine – the application of which would have been homoeopathic – primitive surgical techniques and even early forms of acupuncture.

2 Despite the assertion that homoeopathy is one of the safest techniques of medical therapeutics it should be added here that there are some remedies that are commonly used that, when given too frequently in high potency or, particularly, in a series of descending potencies, can inadvertently set up in very sensitive patients a state of proving which can destabilise the course of treatment. The remedy most likely to cause this problem is *Lachesis*. This is one of the reasons why practitioners are so thoroughly taught to recognise sensitive patients.

3 Remember Florence Nightingale's dictum: 'Diseases are adjectives, not noun substantives.'

4 *Sanguinaria Canadensis* (bloodroot) covers the symptoms of right-sided headache which starts in the back of the neck or head and travels up and over the head to the right forehead and settles over the eye. The arteries of the temple become visibly distended and blood rushes to the head creating a feeling of bursting and congestion. The pain is accompanied by throbbing in the head and chilliness of the body. There is nausea and vomiting as well.

5 The ulcer pains of *Lycopodium* are gnawing. This is accompanied by abdominal bloating and flatus, hiccoughing and hunger pangs.

6 The conflict in Northern Ireland has shown the stark contrast between those who can forgive and even pray for those who inflict pain and those others who seek revenge and retribution thus perpetuating negative Karma.

7 It is worth noting that *Lachesis* has yet another aspect to it; some of those who require it develop symptoms of what might be called a supernatural order. They are able to predict events accurately before they happen; they may have prophetic visions or they suffer delusions that they are under superhuman control. Though such patients might well be considered to be under delusions in strictly conventional medical terms, it is startling just how accurate and perceptive they can be in reality. As time and space are mentally disordered for them it is reasonable to see their condition as sickness but the energy of the state they are in seems to allow for a genuine channel of extrasensory perception. It is not uncommon for patients who have to deal with the Karma of past relatives (in the manner suggested by Delia's case), to need remedies that cover delusions or otherwise psychically disturbed conditions – remedies that they would never normally have needed for their own personal healing purposes.

8 *Staphysagria* is the most commonly used remedy to heal those who have suffered from humiliation and grief after physical violence and sexual abuse. It is noticeable how often the remedy, when being taught to students or discussed, elicits passionate, heated responses. It is also worth adding that with experience of prescribing this remedy, it is noticeable that though patients may feel initially better, they do not ever let go of the deepest well of their pain. *Staphysagria* is often ultimately a disappointment for it cannot always help people to find the resolution that they need. The remedy that does help such patients to find resolution is made from the flower of the white chestnut tree.

9 Relevant symptoms such as Delia's *Lachesis* sore throat and symbolic symptoms such as Lillian's breast cancer.

Chapter 28

1 It is also frequent enough to mention that children go from the tubercular miasm to the syphilitic; if tantrums are being treated (or are central to the case), syphilitic rages are characterised by manipulation and emotional calculation. Where tubercular and sycotic fury is 'hot', syphilitic wrath is 'cold'.

2 Psora has the tendency to harden waste excreta by crystallisation and calcification.

INDEX